Pediatric Nursing

Pediatric Nursing

Third Edition

Parul Datta MSc (N) (Delhi University)
Senior Sister Tutor
School of Nursing
Shambhunath Pandit Hospital
Kolkata, West Bengal, India

Presently, Senior Sister Tutor
Department of Neonatology
Institute of Postgraduate Medical Education and Research (IPGMER) and
Seth Sukhlal Karnani Memorial (SSKM) Hospital
Kolkata, West Bengal, India

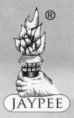

JAYPEE

JAYPEE BROTHERS MEDICAL PUBLISHERS (P) LTD

New Delhi • London • Philadelphia • Panama

Jaypee Brothers Medical Publishers (P) Ltd.

Headquarters
Jaypee Brothers Medical Publishers (P) Ltd.
4838/24, Ansari Road, Daryaganj
New Delhi 110 002, India
Phone: +91-11-43574357
Fax: +91-11-43574314
Email: jaypee@jaypeebrothers.com

Overseas Offices

J.P. Medical Ltd.
83, Victoria Street, London
SW1H 0HW (UK)
Phone: +44-2031708910
Fax: +02-03-0086180
Email: info@jpmedpub.com

Jaypee-Highlights Medical Publishers Inc.
City of Knowledge, Bld. 237, Clayton
Panama City, Panama
Phone: +1 507-301-0496
Fax: +1 507-301-0499
Email: cservice@jphmedical.com

Jaypee Medical Inc.
The Bourse
111, South Independence Mall East
Suite 835, Philadelphia, PA 19106, USA
Phone: +1 267-519-9789
Email: jpmed.us@gmail.com

Jaypee Brothers Medical Publishers (P) Ltd.
17/1-B, Babar Road, Block-B, Shaymali
Mohammadpur, Dhaka-1207
Bangladesh
Mobile: +08801912003485
Email: jaypeedhaka@gmail.com

Jaypee Brothers Medical Publishers (P) Ltd.
Bhotahity, Kathmandu, Nepal
Phone: +977-9741283608
Email: kathmandu@jaypeebrothers.com

Website: www.jaypeebrothers.com
Website: www.jaypeedigital.com

© 2014, Jaypee Brothers Medical Publishers

Inquiries for bulk sales may be solicited at: jaypee@jaypeebrothers.com

Pediatric Nursing

First Edition: 2007
Second Edition: 2009
Reprint: 2010

Third Edition: **2014**

ISBN: 978-93-5152-148-8

Printed at Replika Press Pvt. Ltd.

Preface to the Third Edition

It gives me immense pleasure to present the third edition of *Pediatric Nursing*. This textbook was first published in 2007 and second edition was done in 2009 with reprint in subsequent years. I like to express my sincere gratitude to all the readers for their exceptional and remarkable acceptance of the textbook.

As per opinion of some readers and reviewers, the textbook provides a concise overview of child health nursing, as it is designed to make learning easier by including more practical, relevant and important aspects but avoiding huge details of information. The textbook is very useful for all nursing students of diploma and undergraduate courses, because the content of the textbook includes different aspects of common childhood conditions in illness and wellness which are seen in the community and facility levels. Both general nursing and midwifery (GNM) and BSc Nursing students can refer the textbook to clarify basic concepts of child health nursing.

The third edition of the textbook is enriched with latest statistical data related to Child Health and Neonatal Resuscitation Protocol, 2010. This edition also has some additions of important topics on neonatal problems and child welfare.

I hope the textbook will serve as a useful guide for explanation of fundamental ideas of child health care towards significant contributions by the nursing professionals working for the children in hospitals and community, especially in low resource settings. Suggestions and comments will be gladly accepted to modify the textbook more useful in next edition.

At the end, I like to convey very special thanks to all members of M/s Jaypee Brothers Medical Publishers (P) Ltd of both Delhi and Kolkata office for their excellent expertise in publication.

Parul Datta

Preface to the Third Edition

Preface to the First Edition

"With the birth of every child, man may calculate that God is still hopeful about the World He created" (Wordsworth). But healthy survival of the children is threatened in every moment. Child health problems are shocking and alarming throughout the world, especially in the developing countries. Expert and empathetic approach is essential to minimize these problems and to reduce the inexcusable causes of childhood morbidity, mortality and disability.

A pediatric nurse is the key person in child care team. It is expected that a pediatric nurse should have competence and good judgment based on specialized up-to-date knowledge, skill and positive attitude. A clinical nurse should be enriched to understand the problems of the children and to help them whenever needed. So the pediatric nurse needs special preparation in child health to contribute towards healthy child, the future productive and creative individual.

Being a teacher of General Nursing and Midwifery (GNM) Curriculum for 15 years, I felt the need for a textbook on Pediatric Nursing for GNM students. When I received the proposal, I had decided to accept this work in spite of my hardwork schedule.

This book is fully in accordance with the new GNM syllabus as recommended by the Indian Nursing Council (INC). Keeping in mind the level of the students, I have tried to use simple language and clarify the complicated aspects concisely with rational, as relevant for the need of the students.

It seems that the book will be helpful to the nurses working in the clinical areas and community to review their knowledge and practice in different aspects of child care. I think interest and practice with up-to-date knowledge will contribute to develop confidence in them.

Most references used in the preparation of this title are from the books and journals, written by the eminent Indian authors. Foreign books, WHO newsletters, journals and periodicals are also reviewed for preparation of the contents. I have tried with best effort to prepare and enrich the book considering the level of the students and placement of the course according to the INC Syllabus. Unintentional mistakes are regretted and will be rectified.

Suggestions for further enrichment of the book will be gladly accepted. Constructive criticism and comments are always welcomed. I hope my efforts will be useful to the nursing students and nursing personnel working for the children.

Parul Datta

Preface to the First Edition

Acknowledgments

It gives me immense pleasure to acknowledge all renowned authors and publishers of various medical and nursing books, journals, manuals and periodicals, which I have used as guidelines for preparation and updating the content of the *Pediatric Nursing*.

I would like to extend my special thanks to all members of M/s Jaypee Brothers Medical Publishers (P) Ltd, New Delhi, India, for their intense effort for publication and promotion of the textbook. I am really grateful to all members of Kolkata branch of Jaypee Brothers Medical Publishers (P) Ltd for constant encouragement towards completion of third edition of the book.

Special acknowledgments are made with my heartfelt thanks to all reviewers, students and readers of this textbook for exceptional acceptance of this textbook. My sincere gratitude is due to all my seniors, colleagues, friends and well-wishers for their cooperation.

I wish to express my indebtedness to my parents, teachers and family members for continuous support for preparation of third edition of this textbook.

Contents

1. Introduction to Child Health   1

*Concept of Child Health 1; Trends in Child Health Care 3; Child Health Problems 5;
Disease Patterns in Children 6; Statistics Related to Child Health 6; Child Health Care in India 9;
Rights of the Child 9; Universal Children's Day 10; National Policy for Children 11; Children Act 11*

2. Introduction to Pediatric Nursing   13

*Concept of Pediatric Nursing 13; Goals of Pediatric Nursing 13; Qualities of Pediatric Nurse 13;
Role of the Pediatric Nurse 14; Functions of Pediatric Nurse 14; Trends in Pediatric Nursing 15;
Emerging Challenges in Pediatric Nursing 16; Nursing Process Related to Pediatric Nursing 16*

3. Preventive Pediatrics   22

*Concept of Preventive Pediatrics 22; Family Health 23; Maternal and Child Health 23; Reproductive and
Child Health 23; Baby Friendly Hospital Initiative 24; Integrated Child Development Services 25; National
Rural Health Mission 26; Under-five's Clinic 27; School Health Service 29; Integrated Management of
Neonatal and Childhood Illness 31; Child Labor 31; Street Children 32; Gender Bias 32; Female Feticide 33;
Child Abuse and Neglect (CAN) 34; National Health Programs for Children in India 34; Nursing
Responsibilities in Preventive Pediatrics 35*

4. Immunization   36

*Vaccine Preventable Diseases 36; Immunizing Agents 36; National Immunization Schedule 37;
Immunization of Children 38; Cold Chain 43; Nursing Responsibilities for Child Immunization 44*

5. Nutrition in Children   46

*Nutritional Requirements in Children 46; Breastfeeding 50; Complementary Feeding or Weaning 56;
Artificial Feeding 57; Feeding Problems 58; Balanced Diet for Children 59; Assessment of Nutritional Status 60;
Nutritional Counseling and Guidance 61; National Nutritional Policy 62; National Programs on Nutrition 63*

6. Newborn Infant   64

*Healthy Newborn Infant 64; Common Health Problems of the Newborn Baby 73; High Risk Neonates 102;
Kangaroo Mother Care 107; Grades of Neonatal Care 112; Transport of Sick Neonates 112*

7. Growth, Development and the Healthy Child   113

*Growth and Development 113; Needs of the Healthy Child 127; Health Promotion of Children and
Guidance to Parent for Child Care 134*

8. **Sick Child**   137

*Setting of Pediatric Illness Care Delivery 137; Hospitalization of Sick Child 138; Child's Reaction to
Hospitalization and Prolonged Illness 138; Effects of Hospitalization on the Family of the Child 139;
Role of Nurse to help to Cope with Stress of Illness and Hospitalization of Children 140; Nursing
Interventions and Adaptations in Nursing Care of Sick Child 141*

9. **Common Health Problems during Childhood**   162

*Fever 162; Excessive Cry 163; Vomiting 164; Diarrhea 165; Constipation 165; Abdominal Pain 166;
Abdominal Distension 166; Allergies 167; Poisoning 168; Bites and Stings 170; Foreign Bodies 172;
Multiple Injury 173; Failure to Thrive 173; Developmental Disorders 174*

10. **Behavioral Disorders in Children**   177

*Behavioral Problems of Infancy 178; Behavioral Problems of Childhood 179; Behavioral Problems of
Adolescence 182; Nursing Responsibilities in Behavioral Disorders of Children 184*

11. **Congenital Anomalies**   185

*Concepts of Congenital Anomalies 185; Etiology of Congenital Anomalies 186; Diagnostic Approaches 187;
Common Congenital Anomalies 188; Prevention of Congenital Anomalies 191; Genetic Counseling 192;
Nursing Responsibilities Towards Congenital Anomalies 192*

12. **Nutritional Deficiency Disorders**   194

*Ecology of Malnutrition 194; Assessment of Nutritional Problems 195; Protein-energy Malnutrition 195;
Vitamins and their Deficiency Disorders 200; Minerals and their Deficiency Disorders 205; Community
Nutrition Programs 207*

13. **Fluids, Electrolytes and Acid-base Disturbances**   208

*Body Fluids 208; Electrolyte Composition of Body Fluids 209; Acid-base Balance 209;
Fluid Imbalance 210; Electrolyte Imbalance 211; Acid-base Imbalance 213; Clinical
Conditions Requiring Fluid Therapy 215; Monitoring of Fluid and Electrolyte Imbalance 215*

14. **Common Communicable Diseases in Children**   217

Common Viral Infections 217; Common Bacterial Infections 232; Common Parasitosis in Children 245

15. **Respiratory Diseases**   259

*Acute Respiratory Infections 259; Bronchiectasis 262; Emphysema 264; Atelectasis 265;
Pleural Effusion 265; Empyema 266; Pneumothorax 267; Lung Abscess 267;
Bronchial Asthma 267; Drowning and Near-drowning 271; Cystic Fibrosis 272*

16. **Diseases of Gastrointestinal System and Liver**   273

*Diarrheal Diseases 274; Dysentery 278; Malabsorption Syndrome 279; Ulcerative Colitis 280; Hypertropic
Pyloric Stenosis 281; Esophageal Atresia with Tracheoesophageal Fistula 282; Gastroesophageal Reflux*

Disease 284; Intestinal Obstruction 285; Acute Abdomen 287; Appendicitis 288; Hirschsprung's Disease 289; Anorectal Malformations 291; Umbilical Malformations 293; Hernia 294; Rectal Prolapse 296; Pancreatitis 296; Jaundice (Icterus) 296; Hepatomegaly 297; Extrahepatic Biliary Atresia (EHBA) 298; Liver Abscess 298; Indian Childhood Cirrhosis 299

17. **Heart Diseases in Children**   301

Fetal Circulation 301; Congenital Heart Disease 303; Congestive Cardiac Failure 310; Acute Rheumatic Fever 311; Rheumatic Heart Disease 313; Infective Endocarditis 315; Cardiomyopathy in Children 316

18. **Childhood Blood Dyscrasias**   318

Anemia 318; Iron Deficiency Anemia 320; Megaloblastic Anemia 322; Hereditary Spherocytosis (Congenital Hemolytic Anemia, Familial Acholuric Jaundice) 323; Sickle Cell Anemia 323; Aplastic Anemia 323; Thalassemia (Cooley's Anemia, Mediterranean Anemia) 324; Hemophilia 327; Leukemia 329; Bleeding Disorders/Purpura 332; Disseminated Intravascular Coagulation 334; Immunodeficiency 335

19. **Disorders of Kidney and Urinary Tract**   337

Congenital Abnormalities of the Kidney and Urinary Tract 337; Wilms' Tumor (Nephroblastoma) 340; Nursing Management of the Child with Urologic Surgery 341; Acute Glomerulonephritis 342; Chronic Glomerulonephritis 343; Urinary Tract Infections 344; Nephrotic Syndrome 344; Acute Renal Failure 346; Chronic Renal Failure 349; Care of the Child who Undergoes Dialysis 350

20. **Burns and Skin Diseases**   352

Burns in Children 352; Common Skin Diseases in Children 358, Scabies 358, Superficial Fungal Infections 358, Candidiasis 358, Dermatophytosis 359, Superficial Bacterial Infections (Pyoderma) 359, Psoriasis 360, Acne 360, Atopic Dermatitis 360

21. **Diseases of Central Nervous System**   362

Child in Coma 362; Meningitis 365; Encephalitis and Encephalopathies 368; Guillain-Barré Syndrome (Infective Polyneuritis) 369; Convulsive Disorders 370; Cerebral Palsy 374; Mental Retardation 376; Down's Syndrome (Mongolism) 378; Neural Tube Defects (Myelodysplasia, Dysraphism) 379; Hydrocephalus 381; Intracranial Space Occupying Lesions 385; Brain Tumors 385; Head Injury (Craniocerebral Trauma) 386

22. **Endocrine Disorders in Children**   390

Short Stature 390; Disorders of Pituitary Glands 391; Diabetes Insipidus 392; Disorders of Thyroid Glands 393; Disorders of Parathyroid Glands 395; Disorders of Adrenal Glands 396; Congenital Adrenal Hyperplasia 396; Ambiguous Genitalia 397; Undescended Testes (Cryptorchidism) 397; Precocious Puberty 399; Delayed Sexual Development (Delayed Puberty) 399; Menstrual Abnormalities 400; Obesity 401; Diabetes Mellitus 402

23. **Eye, ENT and Orodental Problems in Children**   406

Diseases of the Eye 406; Ear Problems in Children 411; Disorders of the Nose 415; Disorders of Throat 416; Dental Problems 419; Problems of Oral Cavity 420; Cleft Lip and Cleft Palate 420

24. **Musculoskeletal Disorders in Children**   **423**

    Disorders of Muscles 423; Disorders of Bones 425; Diseases of Joints 434

25. **Handicapped Children and Child Welfare**   **437**

    Handicapped Children 437; Welfare of Children 440

Appendices   **447**

    Appendix I: Basic Care of the Baby at Birth Plea of a Baby at Birth 447

    Appendix II: Children Learn what they Live 448

    Appendix III: Prelude 449; His Name is 'Today' 449

    Appendix IV: Height and Weight of Indian Boys and Girls from 1 to 18 years 450

    Appendix V: Normal Blood Pressure Values at Various Ages 451

    Appendix VI: Calculation of Approximate Surface Area from Weight in Children with Normal Physique 452

    Appendix VII: Mean Urine Output at Different Ages 452

    Appendix VIII: Normal Biochemical Values 453

    Appendix IX: Acid-base Status (Arterial) 454

    Appendix X: Normal Hematological Values 455

    Appendix XI: Cerebrospinal Fluid Constituents 456

    Appendix XII: Modified Glasgow Coma Scoring System 457

    Appendix XIII: Oxygen Therapy and Delivery Devices 458

    Appendix XIV: Basic Life Support (BLS) Maneuvers of Cardiopulmonary Resuscitation (CPR) 459

    Appendix XV: Optimal Timing of Surgical Correction 460

    Appendix XVI: Neutral Thermal Environmental Temperatures 462

    Appendix XVII: Neonatal Resuscitation Program Guideline-2005 463

    Appendix XVIIA: Newborn Resuscitation Algorithm: 2010 (AAP) 464

    Appendix XVIIB: Neonatal Resuscitation Program™: Reference Chart 465

    Appendix XVIII: Identifying Intrauterine Growth Retardation in a Newborn 467

    Appendix XIXA: Gestational Age Assessment (Ballard) 468

    Appendix XIXB: Maturational Assessment of Gestational Age (New Ballard Score) 469

    Appendix XX: Routine Examination of Newborn Infants 470

    Appendix XXI: Transient Abnormalities in the First Few Days of Life 471

    Appendix XXII: Overview of Common Neonatal Medical Problems 472

    Appendix XXIII: Fetal-infant Growth Chart for Preterm Infants 473

Appendix XXIV: IMNCI Case Management Process 474

Appendix XXV: Emergency Triage Assessment and Treatment (ETAT) 475

Appendix XXVI: Neonatal Drug Chart 477

Appendix XXVII: Pediatrics Drug Dosages/Regimens 478; Management of Pediatric Tuberculosis under the Revised National Tuberculosis Control Program (RNTCP) 479

Appendix XXVIII: Safe Disposal of Hospital Waste 481

Appendix XXIX: IMNCI Protocol 482

Suggested Readings   *491*

Index   *493*

PLATE 1

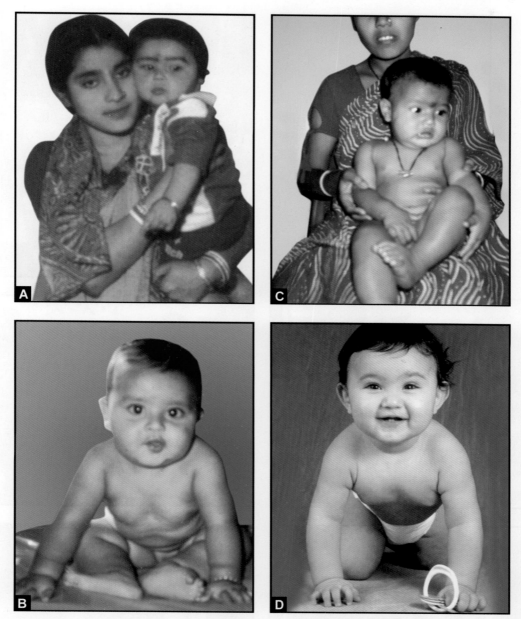

Figs 1.1A to D: Healthy mother and healthy children: (A) Healthy mother and child of a rich family; (B) Healthy infant of 6 months age;
(C) Healthy mother and healthy child of a poor family; (D) Healthy infant of 9 months age

PLATE 2

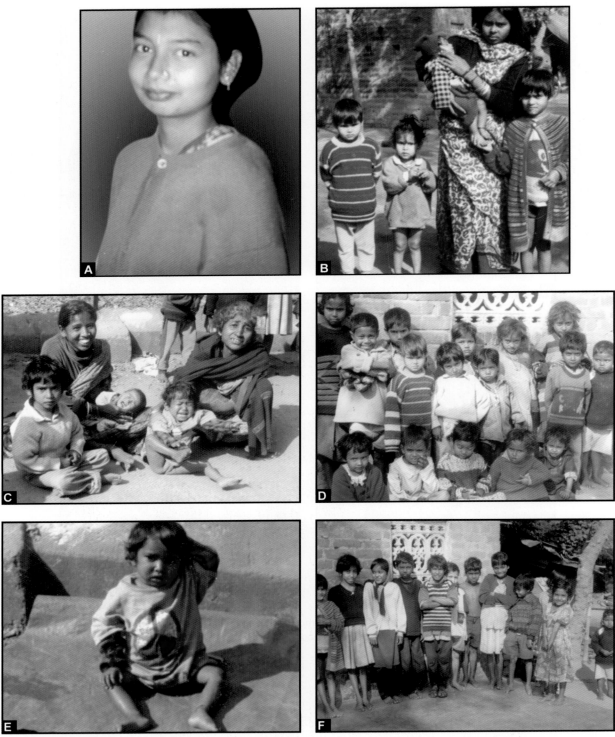

Figs 1.2A to F: Children in need for support services: (A) Teenage mother (second gravida); (B) Young mother with four daughters waiting to have a son; (C) Smiling lady in presence of several problems; (D) Malnourished children of urban slum; (E) Malnourished child of 2 years; (F) Children in need

PLATE 3

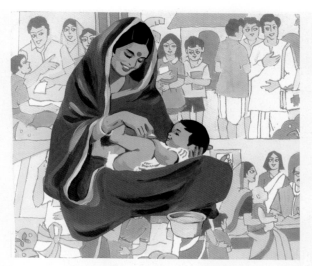

Fig. 3.2: Preventive pediatrics

Care in illness

Adequate nutrition

Immunization

Fig. 3.3: Symbol for under-fives clinic

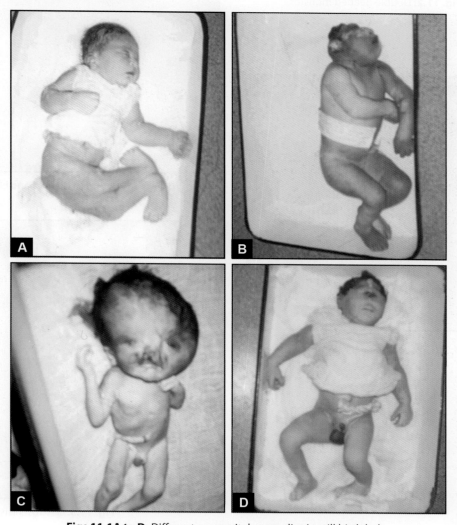

Figs 11.1A to D: Different congenital anomalies in still birth baby

PLATE 4

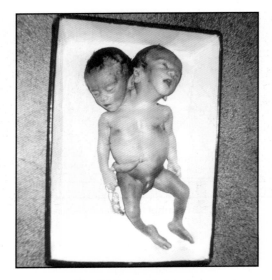

Fig. 11.2: Double headed monster

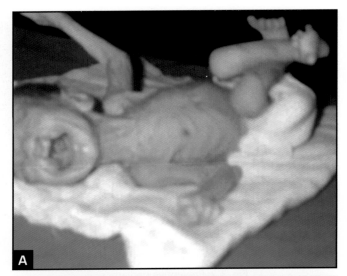

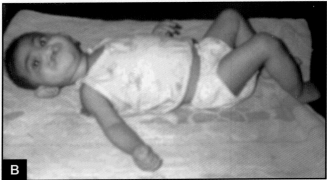

Figs 11.4A and B: Cleft lip and cleft palate

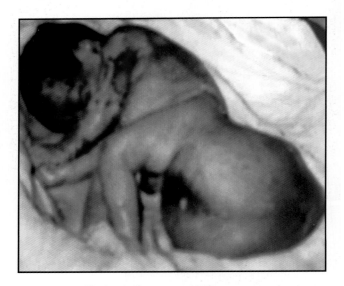

Fig. 11.3: Sacrococcygeal teratoma

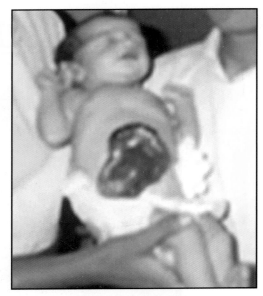

Fig. 11.5: Gastroschisis

PLATE 5

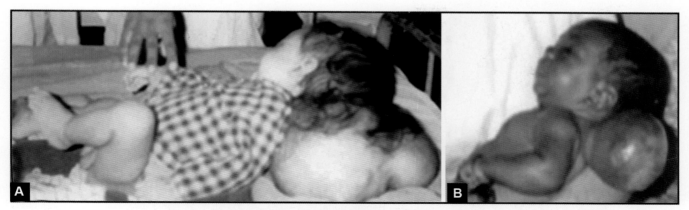

Figs 11.6A and B: Meningoencephalocele

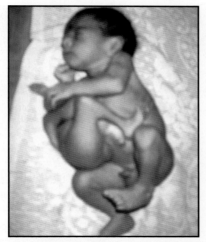

Fig. 11.7: Conjoined twin, one twin baby is without head

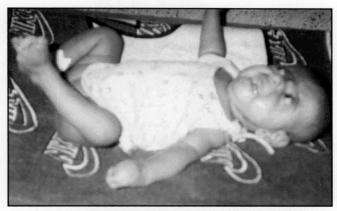

Fig. 11.8: Multiple congenital anomalies

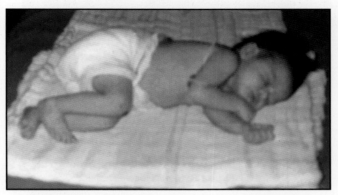

Fig. 11.9: A neonate with congenital obstructive jaundice

PLATE 6

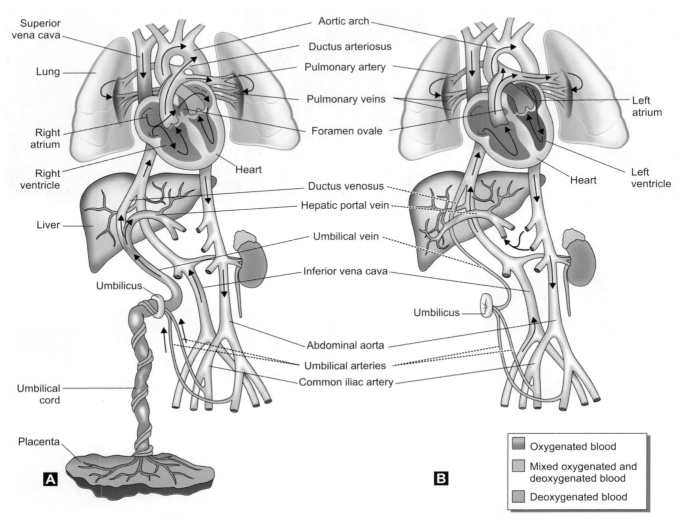

Labels on left (A):
Superior vena cava
Lung
Right atrium
Right ventricle
Liver
Umbilicus
Umbilical cord
Placenta

Center labels:
Aortic arch
Ductus arteriosus
Pulmonary artery
Pulmonary veins
Foramen ovale
Heart
Ductus venosus
Hepatic portal vein
Umbilical vein
Inferior vena cava
Umbilicus
Abdominal aorta
Umbilical arteries
Common iliac artery

Right labels (B):
Left atrium
Left ventricle
Heart
Umbilicus

Legend:
Oxygenated blood
Mixed oxygenated and deoxygenated blood
Deoxygenated blood

Figs 17.1A and B: (A) Fetal circulation before birth; (B) Changes to the fetal circulation at birth
(*Source:* Ross and Wilson. Anatomy and physiology by Churchill Livingstone: Elsevier)

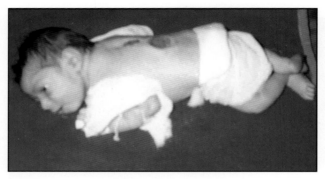

Fig. 21.3: Meningocele

PLATE 7

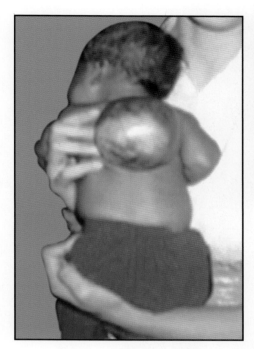

Fig. 21.4: Myelomeningocele

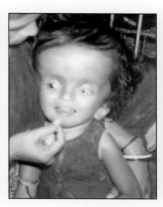 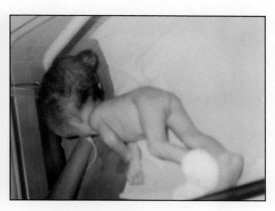

Figs 21.5A and B: Hydrocephalus

Introduction to Child Health

1

- Concept of Child Health
- Trends in Child Health Care
- Child Health Problems
- Disease Patterns in Children
- Statistics Related to Child Health

- Child Health Care in India
- Rights of the Child
- Universal Children's Day
- National Policy for Children
- Children Act

CONCEPT OF CHILD HEALTH

The term 'pediatrics' is derived from the Greek words, 'Pedia' means child, 'iatrike' means treatment and 'ics' means branch of science. Thus, pediatrics means the science of child care and scientific treatment of childhood diseases. Pediatrics is synonymous with child health.

Pediatrics can be defined as the branch of medical science that deals with the care of children from conception to adolescence in health and illness. It is concerned with preventive, promotive, curative and rehabilitative care of children.

Children are major consumers of health care. In India, about 35 percent of total population are children below 15 years of age. They are not only large in number but also vulnerable to various health problems and considered as special risk group. Majority of the childhood sickness and death are preventable by simple low-cost measures. Disease patterns and management of childhood illness are different than that of adult. Children always need special care to survive and thrive. Good health of these precious members of the society should be ensured as prime importance in all countries. As said by Karl Meninger "What is done to children, they will do to the society." Children are the wealth of tomorrow.

A child is unique individual, he or she is not a miniature adult, not a little man or woman. The childhood period is vital because of socialization process by the transmission of attitude, customs, and behavior through the influence of the family and community. Family's cultural and religious belief, educational level and ways of living influence the promotion and maintenance of child health. Children are vulnerable to disease, death and disability owing to their age, sex, place of living, socioeconomic status and a host of other variables. They need appropriate care for survival and healthy development.

The triad problems, poverty, population explosion and environmental stress are great threat towards child health in developing countries. Better nutrition, education (especially of girls) and family planning are essential aspects to improve child health. Healthy well nourished children develop better mentally and benefit more from education. Better education associated with more health knowledge, better health practices and more use of health services.

Factors Affecting Child Health

The important factors affecting the health of children are mainly maternal health, family health, socioeconomic situation, environment, social support and available health care facilities.

Maternal health is a major determinant of child health. The healthy mother brings forth a healthy baby with better chance of survival (Figs 1.1A to D). Child health is adversely

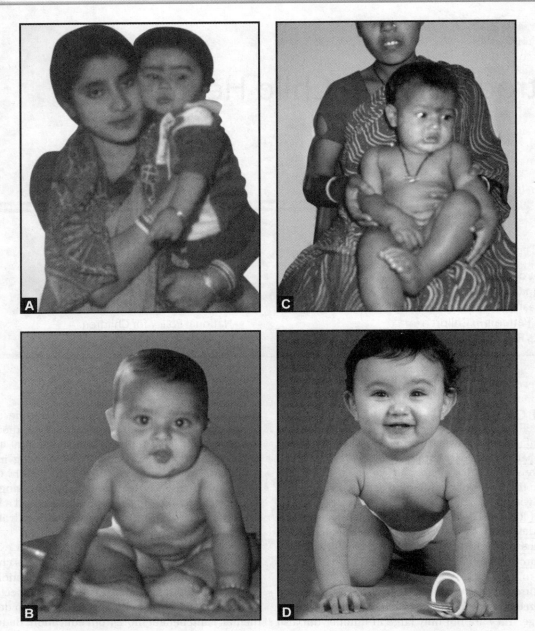

Figs 1.1A to D: Healthy mother and healthy children: (A) Healthy mother and child of a rich family; (B) Healthy infant of 6 months age; (C) Healthy mother and healthy child of a poor family; (D) Healthy infant of 9 months age *(For color version, see Plate 1)*

affected, if the mother is malnourished or diseased. Mother's age, parity, prepregnant health, antenatal care and lack of spacing between two children affect the health of the child.

Child health is greatly depending upon family health. It depends upon family's physical and social environment which includes the lifestyle, culture, customs, taboos, rituals, religious practices, traditional habits, child bearing and child rearing practices, like son-complex, neglect to female child, etc. Family size, family relationship and family stability also influence the child health. For example, number of episodes of childhood diarrhea increases with the size of the family and prevalence of malnutrition increases with more than four children in a family. So, fewer children would mean better nutrition, better health care, less morbidity and lower infant mortality.

The socioeconomic condition of the family is a very important factor in child health. The physical and intellectual development of children varies with the socioeconomic status of the family. Parent's education, profession, income, housing, urban or rural living, industrial life, etc, are significant factors which influence on child health. Poverty, ignorance, superstition, illiteracy especially mother's illiteracy and sickness pass from one generation to the next. The differences in health status between rich and poor can be observed in all age groups but particularly striking among children.

Environment plays a very great role as determinants of infant and childhood morbidity and mortality. Insanitary and hostile environment are responsible for various illnesses like infections, infestations, accidents, etc. Home and family hygiene, local epidemiological conditions, insufficient supply of safe water, inadequate disposal of human excreta and other waste, an abundance of insects and other disease carriers are the continuous threat to child health. Healthy environmental stimulation as interpersonal relationship is an essential factor for child's development. Congenial family relationship, healthy interaction with neighbors, teachers, schoolmates and playmates, exposure to mass media like radio, television, magazines are significant requirements for psychological and intellectual development of children.

Social support measures from the community and organized health care systems are indispensable for improvement and maintenance of health status of children (Figs 1.2A to F).

TRENDS IN CHILD HEALTH CARE

Historically, the concept of pediatrics was limited to the curative aspects of diseases peculiar to the children. Hippocrates (460-370 BC) made many significant observations on disease found in children and devoted a great part of his treatize to children. Galen of Rome (1200–1300 AD) wrote on the care of infants and children. Rhazes of Arab (850–923 AD) devoted much of his treatize to the subject of childhood illness. The first printed book on Pediatrics was in Italian (1472) by Bagallarder's *"Little Book on disease in Children"*. The first English book on children's disease was *"Book of Children"* written by Thomas Phaer (1545 AD).

The world's first Pediatricians were two Indians, Kashyapa and Jeevaka, of sixth century BC. Their pioneering works on child care and childhood disease are as relevant today as many of the modern concepts of child health. Sushruta, also wrote many aspects of child rearing and Charka wrote about care and management of newborn.

Child health care has changed dramatically in recent years due to advances in medical knowledge and understanding of emotional response of children. Advancement of understanding of different aspect of human development influences the changing concept of health. Health exists when an individual meets minimum physical, physiological, intellectual, psychological and social aspects to function appropriately for their age and sex level. Illness is the situations when individual experiences a disturbance in any of these areas that prevents functioning at appropriate level. Thus, attention is directed to psychosocial as well as physiological characteristics of health and illness.

Modern concept of child health emphasizes on continuous care of 'Whole child'. According to UNICEF, assistance for meeting the needs of children should no longer be restricted to only one aspect like nutrition, but it should be broad based and geared to their long-term personal development ensuring holistic health care of children.

At present, in child health care more emphasis given on preventive approach rather than curative care only. Primary health care concept with team approach and multidisciplinary collaboration are adopted for child care. The challenge of this time is to study child health in relation to community, to social values and social policy. Increased public awareness, consumerism and family participation in child care are newer trends. Family health, a new concept is accepted for the care of children in their families and families in society. Need based, problem oriented, risk approach care is practiced for better child health.

In developed countries child health care extended up to adolescent, whereas in developing countries and in India, child care is extended up to 10 to 12 years of age. Recently special emphasis is given on adolescent health through RCH package services in our country. Special attention is given on the children at-risk like, orphans, destitute, disastrous, pavement dwellers, slum dwellers, child labors and handicapped children. Movement against gender bias, female fetocide, child abuse and neglect and maltreatment are in highlight at present.

Interest of the political leaders and understanding the importance of child health, constitution of national health policy for children and implementation of various health programs for improvement of child health are great achievements for children. Population control and family welfare approach, improvement of educational status specially women education and women empowerment, involvement of government and nongovernment organizations, political commitment and special budgetary allocation for child health activities, international guidance by WHO, UNICEF and other child welfare organizations for improvement of child health are promising aspects towards survival, health and well-being of children.

Growth of subspecialities for the superspecialized care of children is recent trend. The subareas are neonatology, perinatology, pediatric surgery, pediatric cardiology, pediatric neurology, pediatric hematology, pediatric nephrology, preventive pediatrics, child psychology, child psychiatry, pediatric intensive care unit, neonatal intensive care unit, etc.

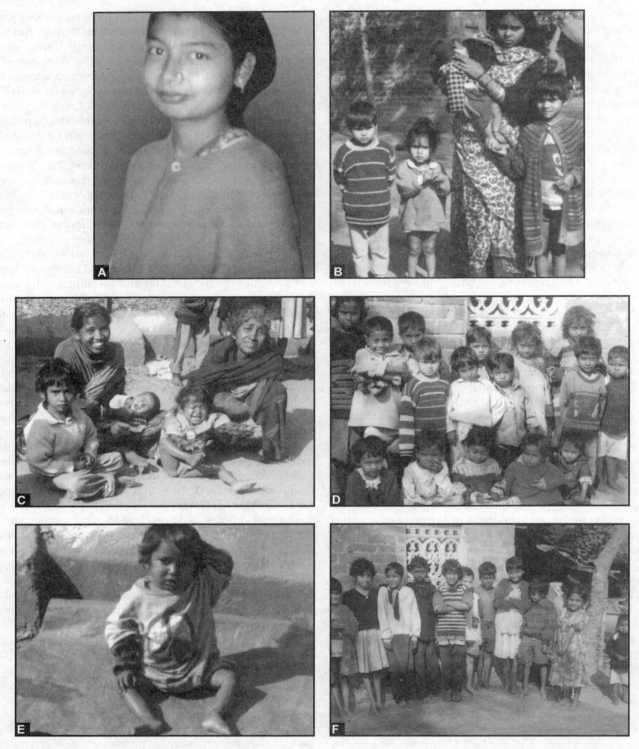

Figs 1.2A to F: Children in need for support services: (A) Teenage mother (second gravida); (B) Young mother with four daughters waiting to have a son; (C) Smiling lady in presence of several problems; (D) Malnourished children of urban slum; (E) Malnourished child of 2 years; (F) Children in need *(For color version, see Plate 2)*

Medical science is advancing in every moment. So child health will also progress by various movements towards the aims to improve the survival and well-being of all children, as per WHO theme of the year 2005, "Healthy mothers and healthy children."

CHILD HEALTH PROBLEMS

In the developing country like India, the child health care givers are facing a large numbers of problems. The major health problems include low birth weight, malnutrition, infections and infestations, accidents and poisoning, behavioral problems, etc. (Figs 1.3A to E).

1. **Low birth weight (LBW):** It is the single most important determinant of the chances of survival, and healthy development of children. In countries, where the incidence of LBW infants is less, their preterm birth is the major cause. But where the proportion is high (e.g. in India), the majority of cases are related to fetal growth retardation, i.e. IUGR (Intrauterine growth retardation). WHO estimated that globally about 17 percent of all live births are LBW babies. In India, it is about 26 percent of all live births, in which more than half of these are born at term. Government of India wished to control this problem and decrease the incidence to 10 percent by the year 2000 but not achieved till now.

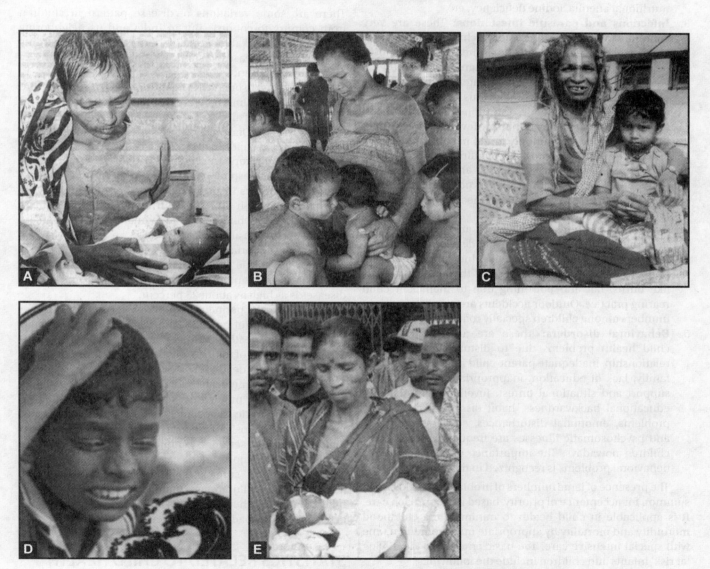

Figs 1.3A to E: Child health problems: (A) Poor maternal health; (B) Children in refugee camp; (C) Street child; (D) Child in disaster; (E) Neonatal death

2. **Malnutrition:** It is the most widespread condition affecting health of children. Inavailability and scarcity of suitable food, lack of money for purchasing food, traditional beliefs and taboos about child's diet and insufficient balanced diet are resulting in malnutrition. It is the underlying and associated cause of childhood illness and death among the under-five age group. It makes the child susceptible to infection, slower recovery from illness and higher mortality. Malnutrition in infancy and childhood leads to growth retardation. Undernourished children do not grow to their full potential of physical and mental abilities. The most frequent nutritional deficiency states are protein-energy malnutrition, vitamin— 'A' deficiency, nutritional anemia, iodine deficiency, etc.

3. **Infections and parasitic infestations:** These are very common in children. The leading childhood infections are diarrhea, respiratory infections, measles, tuberculosis, pertussis, poliomyelitis, neonatal tetanus and diphtheria. HIV/AIDS is the emerging life-threatening infection and children are innocent victims of this condition. Beside these infections, systemic infections like meningitis, encephalitis, hepatitis, typhoid fever, urinary tract infections are also commonly found in children. Malaria and intestinal parasitosis including round worm, hookworm, tapeworm, giardiasis and amebiasis are frequently seen in children due to poor environmental sanitation, inadequate hygienic measures, unhygienic food and unsafe water.

4. **Accidents and poisoning:** These are relatively more important child health problems in developed countries. But in developing countries like India, accidents are frequent among children especially the home accidents like burns, fall and poisoning due to inefficient child rearing practice. Outdoor accidents are also increasing in numbers among children specially road traffic accidents.

5. **Behavioral disorders:** These are another increasing child health problems due to disturbances in family relationship, inadequate parent-child interaction, broken family, lack of education, inappropriate socioeconomic support and situational unrest. Juvenile delinquencies, educational backwardness, habit disorders, personality problems, emotional disturbances, sexual promiscuity and psychosomatic illnesses are frequently observed in children nowadays. The importance of special care for behavioral problems is recognized in most countries.

The presence of large numbers of problems in child health summon for acceptance of priority-based risk approach care. It is applicable in child health to minimize the childhood morbidity and mortality by appropriate management in time with special intensive care. The basic criteria for identifying 'at risk' infants and children include the followings:

- Birth weight less than 2.5 kg
- Twin births
- Birth order 5 or more

- Spacing of children less than 2 years
- No breastfeeding or insufficient breastfeeding along with artificial feeding
- Failure to gain weight during three successive months
- Weight below 70 percent of the reference standard
- History of death of two or more siblings before the age of 24 months
- Death of either or both parents
- Children with PEM and severe acute infections like diarrhea, measles, pertussis, etc.

DISEASE PATTERNS IN CHILDREN

There are some variations of disease pattern in children from country-to-country. But in India and its neighboring countries, a remarkable similar pattern is observed regarding frequency of diseases responsible for hospitalizations of infants and children.

It is observed in our health institutions that up to one-third of total pediatric admissions are due to diarrheal diseases and up to 17 percent of all deaths in indoor pediatric patients are diarrhea related. Diarrheal diseases are major public health problem among children under the age of 5 years.

Acute respiratory infections (ARI) are another major cause of death. Hospital records show that up to 13 percent of inpatient deaths in pediatric wards are due to ARI. The proportion of death due to ARI in the community is much higher as many children die at home. About 14 percent hospital admission are due to ARI.

Another important cause of pediatric admissions in hospitals is vaccine preventable diseases, that is approximately 15.5 percent. Death due to vaccine preventable diseases is as high as about 25 percent.

Neonatal and perinatal conditions are responsible for about 4.6 percent of hospital admission and approximately 13 percent of all deaths. Other various conditions are responsible for one-third of total hospital admission in children and also for childhood death.

The common medical conditions found in the pediatric units are mainly meningitis, encephalitis, typhoid fever, hepatitis, nephrotic syndrome, acute glomerulonephritis, malaria, tuberculosis, kala-azar, thalassemia, etc. Gross malnutrition and serious systemic infections are found in combination in majority of the cases.

The common surgical conditions requiring hospital admissions in children are mainly related to congenital malformations. Other conditions are intestinal obstructions, acute abdomen, road traffic accidents, burns, fractures, etc.

STATISTICS RELATED TO CHILD HEALTH

Vital statistics are considered as indicators of health. Important vital statistics are birth rate and death rate. Child health status is assessed through measurement of mortality and morbidity. Morbidity data collected in specific survey can serve as indicators of comprehensive and specific health aspect. But morbidity data are scarce and poorly standardized. Measurement of growth and development is also an important indicator of child health status. Attention has been paid, recently, for systemic collection, interpretation and dissemination of data on growth and development.

In many countries, mortality rates are still the only sources of information about child health. The frequently used mortality indicators of child health care are perinatal, neonatal, postneonatal, infant and under 5 mortality rates.

Perinatal Mortality Rate

World Health Organization (WHO) expert committee on prevention of perinatal mortality and morbidity recommended a precise formula of perinatal mortality rate, i.e. "Late fetal and early neonatal deaths weighing over 1000 gm at birth expressed as a ratio per 1000 live births weighing over 1000 gm at birth." It is calculated as:

$$\text{Perinatal mortality rate} = \frac{\text{Late fetal and early neonatal deaths weighing over 1000 g at birth}}{\text{Total live birth weighing over 1000 g at birth}} \times 1000$$

Perinatal mortality rate has assumed greater significance as a yardstick of obstetrics and pediatrics care before and around the time of birth. It gives a good indication of the extent of pregnancy wastage as well as quality and quantity of health care available to the mothers and children.

Perinatal mortality is a problem of serious dimensions in all countries. It now accounts for about 90 percent of all fetal and infant mortality in the developed countries. In India, the perinatal mortality rate was reported about 32 per 1000 total live births with about 35 for rural and 22 for the urban areas (2010) as per SRS estimates. The national goal was to achieve a perinatal mortality rate between 30 and 35 by the year 2000 AD.

A number of social and biological factors are known to be associated with perinatal mortality. The risk factors are low socioeconomic status, high or low maternal age, high parity, short stature mother, bad obstetrical history, maternal malnutrition and severe anemia, multiple pregnancy, etc.

The causes of perinatal mortality are mainly antenatal, intranatal or postnatal asphyxia, LBW babies, congenital anomalies, birth injury and perinatal infections.

Reduction and prevention of perinatal mortality can only be possible with better maternal and child health services.

Neonatal Mortality Rate

Neonatal deaths are deaths occurring during the neonatal period, i.e. from birth to 28 completed days of life. It is calculated as:

$$\text{Neonatal mortality rate} = \frac{\text{Number of deaths of children under 28 days of age in a year}}{\text{Total live birth in the same year}} \times 1000$$

Neonatal mortality is most difficult part of infant mortality to change. In India, it was about 33 per 1000 live births (2010). About 70 percent of all infant deaths occur within neonatal period and approximately 80 percent of neonates die during the first week of birth and first 24 hours is the greatest risk time.

Neonatal mortality is greater in boys throughout the world due to more fragility of boys than girls. The common causes of neonatal mortality include LBW, perinatal asphyxia, birth injury, difficult labor, congenital anomalies, hemolytic diseases of newborn, conditions of placenta and cord, diarrheal diseases, ARI and tetanus. Neonatal deaths can be reduced by adequate antenatal and intranatal care including essential neonatal care at all levels by preventing and managing the causes.

Postneonatal Mortality Rate

Postneonatal mortality rate is defined as the ratio of the postneonatal death in a given year to the total number of live births in the same year, usually expressed as a rate per 1000. It is calculated as:

$$\text{Postneonatal mortality rate} = \frac{\text{Number of deaths of children between 28 days and one year of age in a given year}}{\text{Total live birth in the same year}} \times 1000$$

Postneonatal mortality is dominated by exogenous factors, i.e. environmental and social factors. The main causes of death during postneonatal period are diarrhea and ARI. Malnutrition is the additional factor, which predisposes various infections. In developed countries, it is mainly caused by congenital anomalies. Postneonatal deaths increase with birth order and the girl children die more frequently than boys due to neglected care to the female children in terms of nutrition and health care.

In India, postneonatal mortality rate is estimated to be 20 in rural areas, 16 in urban areas and 19 per 1000 live births combined in rural and urban areas (2007).

Infant Mortality Rate

Infant mortality rate (IMR) is defined as "the ratio of infant deaths registered in a given year to the total number of live births registered in the same year, usually expressed as a rate per 1000 live births". It is calculated by the formula:

$$\text{Infant mortality rate} = \frac{\text{Number of deaths of children less than one year of age in a year}}{\text{Number of live births in the same year}} \times 1000$$

Infant mortality rate is universally regarded as a most important sensitive indicator of the health status of community. It is considered as an indicator of level of living of people and effectiveness of MCH services.

There are wide variations between countries or regions in the level of infant mortality. The world average of IMR for 2004 has been estimated at about 54 per 1000 live births. The worst rates were in Afghanistan (121.63) and the lowest IMR of less than 3 per 1000 live births in Japan, Sweden Hongkong, Singapore and Monaco.

India is still among high IMR countries, though it has come down to 44 per 1000 live births in 2011. There is statewise variation with highest in MP—59, and UP and Orissa—57 and Kerala as low as 12 per 1000 live births. National target is set to bring down the IMR to less than 28 per 1000 live births within the year 2015.

The principal causes of IMR in India are LBW, ARI, diarrheal diseases, congenital malformations, and infections, especially umbilical sepsis. There are several factors which interact to cause infant mortality. Biological and socio-economical factors influence more on the infant death. There is no single specific health program or a single set of action that can reduce IMR. As the etiology of IMR is multifactorial, so it requires multipronged approaches. Certain important measures to reduce IMR include lowest birth rate, highest literacy rate, specially female literacy and improvement of primary health care. Other preventive measures include prenatal nutrition, prevention of infections including six-killer diseases, exclusive breastfeeding, growth monitoring, family planning, environmental sanitation, simple hygienic measures and socioeconomic development.

Under-Five Mortality Rate (Child Mortality Rate)

United Nations International Children's Emergency Fund (UNICEF) defines the under-5 mortality rate as the "annual number of deaths of children aged under 5 years, expressed as a rate per 1000 live births". The rate is computed by the formula:

$$\text{Under-5 mortality rate} = \frac{\text{Number of deaths of children less than 5 years of age in given year}}{\text{Number of live births in the same year}} \times 1000$$

Child mortality rate measures the probability of dying in between birth and exactly 5 years of age. The UNICEF considered this rate as the best single indicator of social development and well-being rather than GNP per capita. It reflects nutritional status, income, health care and level of basic education of the population.

The global average for under-5 mortality rate in 2008 was 65 per 1000 live births. In developed countries the rate was 7

per 1000 live births and in least developed countries, it was 158 per 1000 live births in 2002.

In India, child mortality rate in 2010 was 59 per 1000 live births. It is about 34 percent of all deaths. It was 242 per 1000 live births in 1960 and has declined significantly during the past years due to decline in infant mortality. This reduction is largely related to drop in deaths due to vaccine preventable diseases as well as drop in deaths from ARI and diarrhea.

The major causes of child mortality among children under 5 years in developing countries are acute respiratory infections, neonatal and perinatal threats, diarrhea, malaria, pertussis, neonatal tetanus, tuberculosis, measles, mal-nutrion, accidents and HIV related diseases.

The basic measure of infant and child survival is the reduction of under-five mortality. The difference in the survival rates of children in developed and developing countries is a grim pointer to the third world's need for preventive services. The child survival can be best achieved by breastfeeding, adequate nutrition, clean water supply, immunization coverage, oral rehydration therapy and birth spacing.

On the occasion of World Health Day, 2005, WHO reported that one child in twelve does not reach his/her fifth birthday. Each year 10.6 million children under the age of five years die from a handful of preventable and treatable conditions. Nearly all these deaths occur in low and middle income countries. WHO, celebrated World Health Day on 7th April, 2005, with the theme "Healthy mothers and healthy children" and the slogan "Make every mother and child count", to make the health of women and children a higher priority and to improve survival, health and well-being of these precious group.

Selected Statistics Related to Child Health in India

A.	Distribution of population below 15 years of age	–	32.1 percent of total population (2007)
B.	Crude birth rate	–	22.1 per 1000 midyear population (2010)
C.	Crude death rate	–	7.2 per 1000 midyear population (2010)
D.	Mortality indicators:		
	a. Infant mortality rate	–	44 per 1000 live births (2011)
	b. Under-5 mortality rate	–	59 per 1000 live births (2010)
	c. Neonatal mortality rate	–	33 per 1000 live births (2010)
	d. Postneonatal mortality rate	–	19 per 1000 live births (2007)

e. Early neonatal mortality – 25 per 1000 live births
rate (2010)
E. Prevalence of LBW babies – 28 percent of all
live births (2003–2008)
F. Services coverage:
  a. Infants fully immunized – 43.5% (2008)
    i. BCG vaccination – 87% (do)
    ii. DPT and OPV – 66% (do)
     vaccination
    iii. Measles vaccination – 70% (do)
  b. Pregnant women- – 83.4% (do)
    Tetanus toxoid
  c. Antenatal care – 75% (do)
  d. Institutional delivery – 47% (2007–2008)
G. Total fertility rate – 2.6 (2009)
H. Urban and rural population – 31.16 : 68.84 (2011)
ratio
I. Literacy rates – 74.04% (2011)

CHILD HEALTH CARE IN INDIA

Children are the most important age group in all societies. Health status and health behavior of later life are laid down at this stage. Child health care should include specific biological and psychological needs that must be met to ensure the survival and healthy development of the child, the future adult.

Childhood period can be customarily divided for purpose of effective care into the different age-groups, i.e. infancy, preschool, school age, and adolescence.

Children under the age of 5 years are grouped with the mothers considering as vulnerable and risk group comprising about 32 percent of total population in India.

The mother and child health (MCH) services is the method of delivering health care to these special groups. The MCH services contain the preventive, promotive, curative and social aspects of obstetrics, pediatrics, family welfare, nutrition, child development and health education. The ultimate objective of MCH services is life-long health. The specific objectives for the services include reduction of morbidity and mortality rates for mother and children and promotion of reproductive health along with child health. Promotion of physical and psychological development of the child within the family can be possible by family participation in the comprehensive care of children through the MCH services.

The components of MCH services include six subareas, i.e. maternal health, family planning, child health, school health, care of handicapped children and care of children in special setting such as day care centers.

The MCH services, at present, are provided through reproductive and child health (RCH) program. The RCH program incorporates the components related to child survival and safe motherhood (CSSM), family planning and prevention of RTIs/STDs and AIDS. The services are provided in client-oriented, target-free, demand driven, high quality, participatory and decentralized approaches on the basis of needs of community.

Other than RCH program, various health programs are initiated by the Government of India to improve the survival of children. Nongovernment organizations and child welfare organizations also contributing towards better child health. Other child health services include integrated child development services (ICDS) scheme, under-5 clinics, school-health services, postpartum services through PP units, baby-friendly hospital initiative, child guidance clinic, etc.

Child health services are delivered through *anganwadi* centers (ICDS-center) at village level, subcenter clinics, PHC clinics, outreach services by home visit and camps and in hospital as indoors and outdoors. The child care is planned in various health institutions by the health workers in integrated and risk approach. Primary health care is now recognized as a way of making essential health care available to all, including children, by the multipurpose health workers, professional health workers, voluntary workers and field workers, like community health guides, traditional birth attendants, *anganwadi* workers, etc. The services are available both in urban and rural areas through different infrastructures. The specific low cost simple measures are organized for the child health care through various approaches for saving life of millions of children on priority basis.

RIGHTS OF THE CHILD

The united nations adopted the "Declaration of the Rights of the Child", on 20th November, 1959, to meet the special needs of the child. India was a signatory to this declaration to give the child pride of place and to make the people aware of the rights and needs of children and duties towards them.

The *ten basic rights* of the child are:
1. Right to develop in an atmosphere of affection and security and protection against all forms of neglect, cruelty, exploitation and traffic.
2. Right to enjoy the benefits of social security, including nutrition, housing and medical care.
3. Right to a name and nationality.
4. Right to free education.
5. Right to full opportunity for play and recreation.
6. Right to special treatment, education and appropriate care, if handicapped.
7. Right to be among the first to receive protection and relief in times of disaster.
8. Right to learn to be a useful member of society and to develop in a healthy and normal manner and in conditions of freedom and dignity.

9. Right to be brought up in a spirit of understanding, tolerance, friendship among people, peace and universal brotherhood.
10. Right to enjoy these rights, regardless of race, color, sex, religion, national or social origin.

A nongovernmental organization (NGO), Defence for Children International, Geneva; has been in operation since 1979, the International Year of the Child, to ensure ongoing, systemic international action, especially directed towards promoting and protecting the Right of the Child.

UNIVERSAL CHILDREN'S DAY

November, 14th is observed as universal children's day. It was started by the International Union for Child Welfare and the UNICEF. In 1954, the UN General Assembly passed a formal resolution establishing universal children's day and assigned to UNICEF the responsibility to promote the celebration of this annual day.

The World Summit for children (1990) agreed on a series of specific goals for improving the lives of children including measurable progress against malnutrition, preventable diseases and illiteracy. The vital vulnerable years of childhood should be given priority on society's concerns and capacities. A child has only one chance to develop normally and demands protection and commitment that never be superseded by any other priorities.

The realization that children have special needs and hence the special rights has given birth to an international law in the shape of convention on the 'Rights of the child'. The provisions of the convention were confirmed in 1990 by the World Summit for Children.

The convention defines children as people below the age 18 years whose best interests must be taken into account in all situations. It protects children's right to survive and develop to their full potential with highest attainable standard of health care.

The social goals that have been accepted by almost all nations following the 1990 World Summit for Children were:

Overall Goals (1990–2000)

A one-third reduction in under-five death rates (or to 70 per 1000 live births, whichever is less):
- A halving of maternal mortality rates.
- A halving of severe and moderate malnutrition among the world's under-fives.
- Safe water and sanitation for all families.
- Basic education for all children and completion of primary education by at least 80 percent.
- A halving of adult illiteracy rate and achievement of equal educational opportunity for males and females.

- Acceptance in all countries of the convention on the rights of child including improved protection for children in especially difficult circumstances.

Protection for Girls and Women

- Family planning information and services to be made available to all couples to prevent unwanted pregnancies and birth which are 'too many and too close' and to women who are 'too young or too old'.
- All women should have access to antenatal care, a trained attendant during child birth and referral facilities for high-risk pregnancies and obstetrical emergencies.
- Universal recognition of special health care and nutritional needs of females during early childhood, adolescence, pregnancy and lactation.

Nutrition

- A reduction in the incidence of low birth weight (below 2.5 kg) to less than 10 percent.
- A one-third reduction in iron deficiency anemia among women.
- Elimination of vitamin 'A' deficiency and iodine deficiency disorders.
- Information to all families about the importance of supporting women in exclusive breastfeeding for first four to six months of a child's life.
- Growth monitoring and promotion need to be institutionalized in all countries.
- Information to increase awareness about household food security in all families.

Child Health

- Eradication of poliomyelitis
- Elimination of neonatal tetanus and 90 percent reduction in measles cases and 95 percent reduction in measles deaths.
- Achievement and maintenance of at least 90 percent immunization coverage to infants and universal tetanus immunization for women in the child bearing years.
- A halving of child deaths caused by diarrheal diseases and 25 percent reduction if its incidence.
- A one-third reduction of child deaths caused by acute respiratory infections.
- Elimination of Guinea worm disease.

Education

- Expansion of primary school education and improvement of essential knowledge and life-skills of all families by mobilization of present day's vastly increased communication capacity.

NATIONAL POLICY FOR CHILDREN

The Government of India adopted a National Policy for children in August 1974, keeping in view the United Nations Declaration of the Rights of the child and the constitutional provisions.

The policy declares "it shall be the policy of the state to provide adequate services to children, both before and after birth and through the period of growth, to ensure their full physical, mental and social development. The state shall progressively increase the scope of such services so that, within a reasonable time, all children in the country enjoy optimum conditions for their balanced growth."

According to the declaration, the development of children has been considered as integral part of national development. The policy recognizes children as the "nation's supremely important asset" and declares that the nation is responsible for their "nurture and solicitude". It also emphasizes the priorities of children's program and special focus on child health, child nutrition and welfare of the handicapped and destitute children.

A number of programs were introduced by the Govt. of India, after the declaration of national policy for children. The important programs are ICDS scheme, programs of supplementary feeding, nutrition education, production of nutritious food, welfare of handicapped children, national children's fund, CSSM programs, etc.

The principles of India's National Policy for Children are as follows:

1. A comprehensive health program for all children and provision of nutrition services for children.
2. Provision of health care, nutrition and nutrition education for expectant and nursing mothers.
3. Free and compulsory education up to the age of 14 years, informal education for preschoolers and efforts to reduce wastage and stagnation in schools.
4. Out of school education for those not having access to formal education.
5. Promotion of games, recreation and extracurricular activities in schools and community centers.
6. Special programs for children from weaker sections.
7. Facilities for education, training and rehabilitation for children in distress.
8. Protection against neglect, cruelty and exploitation.
9. Banning of employment in hazardous occupations and in heavy work for children.
10. Special treatment, education, rehabilitation and care of physically handicapped, emotionally disturbed or mentally retarded children.
11. Priority for the protection and relief of children in times of national distress and calamity.
12. Special programs to encourage talented and gifted children, particularly from the weaker sections.
13. The paramount consideration in all relevant laws is the "interests of children."
14. Strengthening family ties to enable children to grow within the family, neighborhood and community environment.

CHILDREN ACT

The children Act, 1960 (amended in 1977) in India, provides for the care maintenance, welfare, training, education and rehabilitation of the delinquent child. It covers the neglected, destitute, socially handicapped, uncontrollable, victimised and delinquent children. In Article 39(f), the constitution of India provides that "the state shall in particular direct its policy towards securing that childhood and youth are protected against moral and material abandonment."

The Juvenile Justice Act, 1986, provides a comprehensive scheme for care, protection, treatment, development and rehabilitation of delinquent juveniles. The new Act has come into force from 2nd October 1987, after rectification of the inadequacies of the Children Act (1960). This Act was amended again in 2000 and 2006.

Juvenile Justice Act 2000

Juvenile Justice (Care and Protection of Children) Act 2000, now amendment Act 2006 is an Act to consolidate and amend the law relating to juveniles in conflict with law and children in need of care and protection. The Act defines a juvenile/child as a person who has not completed the age of 18 years. It has two chapters—one for juveniles in conflict with law and other for children in need of care and protection. It also contains an exclusive chapter concerning rehabilitation and social reintegration of children. This Act promotes proper care, protection and treatment by catering to the developmental needs of children and by adopting a child friendly approach in the best interest of children and for their ultimate rehabilitation.

The needs of children and our duties towards them are enshrined in our constitution. The relevant articles are as follows:
a. Article 24 prohibits employment of children below the age of 14 years in factories.
b. Article 39 prevents abuse of children of tender age.
c. Article 45 provides the free and compulsory education for all children until they complete the age of 14 years.

Other important Acts for child welfare are: "The Child Labor (Prohibition and Regulation) Act, 1986", "The Child

Marriage Restraint Act 1978" "The Hindu Adoptions and Maintenance Act, 1956", "Infant Milk Substitute, Feeding Bottles and Infant Foods (Regulation of Production, Supply and Distribution) Act 1992 and Prenatal Diagnostic Techinique (Regulation and Prevention of Misuse) act 1994.

Special attention has been given to the welfare of children in the five-year plans by the Government of India. Various schemes and programs have been introduced and implemented to achieve the goals of child health services.

Healthy children are future healthy citizens of the countries. So every attempts should be made towards better tomorrow for better survival of this precious group and to help them to grow into healthy adult. Promotion of child health should receive priority attention in all levels as new challenge of the 21st century. WHO, in 2005, emphasizes on healthy mothers and children. The aims and objectives of World Health Day, 2005, is to create momentum that compel national governments, international community, civil society and individuals to take action to ensure the health and wellbeing of mothers and children. These can be achieved by raising awareness, increasing understanding about the existing solutions and generating movement to stimulate collective responsibility and action to improve the survival, health and well-being of all mothers and children.

Introduction to Pediatric Nursing

2

- Concept of Pediatric Nursing
- Goals of Pediatric Nursing
- Qualities of Pediatric Nurse
- Role of the Pediatric Nurse
- Functions of Pediatric Nurse
- Trends in Pediatric Nursing
- Emerging Challenges in Pediatric Nursing
- Nursing Process Related to Pediatric Nursing

CONCEPT OF PEDIATRIC NURSING

Health of the children has been considered as the vital importance to all societies because children are the basic resource for the future of humankind. Nursing care of children is concerned for both the health of the children and for the illnesses that affect their growth and development. The increasing complexity of medical and nursing science has created a need for special area of child care, i.e. Pediatric nursing.

Pediatric nursing is the specialized area of nursing practice concerning the care of children during wellness and illness. It includes preventive, promotive, curative and rehabilitative care of children. It emphasizes on all round development of body mind and spirit of the growing individual. Thus, pediatric nursing involves in giving assistance, care and support to the growing and developing children to achieve their individual potential for functioning with fullest capacity.

Pediatric nursing practice is concerned with:
- Well-being of the children towards optimal functioning.
- Integration of developmental needs of children into nursing care with holistic approach.
- Integration of scientific principles and theory related to child health into nursing practice.
- Delivering care to the family-child unit.
- Interdisciplinary team approach to plan and provide child care in comprehensive manner.
- Focusing on the ethical, moral and legal problems regarding child care.

GOALS OF PEDIATRIC NURSING

- To provide skillful, intelligent, need based comprehensive care to the children in health and sickness.
- To interpret the basic needs of the children to their parents and family members and to guide them in child care.
- To promote growth and development of children towards optimum state of health for functioning at the peak of their capacity in future.
- To prevent disease and alleviate suffering in children.

QUALITIES OF PEDIATRIC NURSE

A pediatric nurse should have all desirable and preferable qualities of a professional nurse. More than those a professional nurse should possess the following qualities to be a pediatric nurse:
- She should be a loving person and have liking for the children.
- She should have patience, pleasant appearance and ability to understand the child's behavior.
- She should be able to maintain good interpersonal relationship and to provide safety and security to the children.
- She should be friendly, honest, gentle, diligent and humorous.
- She should have good observation, judgement and communication ability-based on scientific knowledge and experience.

- She should be well-informed, skillful, responsible, truthful and trustworthy.

ROLE OF THE PEDIATRIC NURSE

The ever expanding demands of medical and nursing practice, emerging challenges in different aspects of child care, consumer demands and improved technology have necessitated the highly specialized roles of pediatric nurse.

The role of the pediatric nurse is both caring and curing. Caring is a continuous process in both wellness and illness. It refers as helping, guiding and counseling. Curing refers to the act of diagnosis and management, usually during illness. Pediatric nurse have the responsibilities of providing nursing care in hospital, home, clinic, school and community where children and their parents have health and counseling needs.

The role of the pediatric nurse may vary from one health institution to others, but the basic responsibilities remain the same. It may vary depending upon the educational preparation of the pediatric nurse and exposure to the specialized training. The characteristics social behavior of the pediatric nurse as role model for the child care can be summarized as follows:

1. **Primary caregiver:** Pediatric nurse should provide preventive, promotive, curative and rehabilitative care in all levels of health services, as therapeutic agent. She/he acts as case finder and compassionate skilled caregiver as needed by the today's society. In hospital, care of the sick children, i.e. comfort, feeding, bathing, safety, etc. are the basic responsibilities of the pediatric nurse. Health assessment, immunization, primary health care and referral are basic responsibilities at the community level as quality care provider.

2. **Health educator:** Important role of the pediatric nurse is to deliver planned and incidental health teaching and information to the parents, significant others and children to create awareness about healthy lifestyle and maintenance of health. Change in health behavior and attitude and to develop healthful practice regarding child care should be initiated by the pediatric nurse as change agent, teacher and health educator.

3. **Nurse-counselor:** Problem solving approach and necessary guidance in health hazards of children to minimize or to solve the problem and to help the parents and family members for independent decision-making in different situations are essential role of the pediatric nurse in the present health care delivery system.

4. **Social worker:** Pediatric nurse can do case work especially for children and try to alleviate social problems related to child health. She/he can participate in available social services or refer the child and family for necessary social support from the child welfare agencies.

5. **Team coordinator and collaborator:** Pediatric nurse should work together and in combination with other health team members towards better child health care. She/he should act as liaison among the members and maintain good interpersonal relationship. The nurse interprets the objectives of health care to the family and co-ordinates nursing services with other services necessary for the child. Co-operations and good communication among team members should be promoted by the nurse.

6. **Manager:** The pediatric nurse is the manager of pediatric care units in hospital, clinics and community. She/he should organize the care orderly for successful outcome with better prognosis and good health.

7. **Child care advocate:** Child or family advocacy is basic aspect to comprehensive family centered care. As an advocate, the pediatric nurse can assist the child to obtain best care possible from the particular units. Advocacy can range from consulting dietary department for special foods to arrange team meeting to discuss plan of care.

8. **Recreationist:** This supportive role of pediatric nurse is important for the child to adjust to the crisis imposed by illness or hospitalization. She/he can organize play facilities for recreation and diversion for child's emotional outlet.

9. **Nurse consultant:** The pediatric nurse can act as consultant to guide the parents and family members for maintenance and promotion of health and prevention of childhood illness. The nurse can promote self-care within the family and prepare self-care agent for the children who are unable to take care of their own health. The nurse can help the older children to become responsible for their own lives. The nurse assesses the children's ability to do self-care activities and assist them in developing the ways of self-care and self responsibility.

10. **Researcher:** Nursing research is an integral part of professional nursing. Pediatric nurse should participate or perform research projects related to child health. Clinical and applied research provide the basis for changes in nursing practice and improvements in the health care of children.

Beside the above roles, pediatric nurses have to respond to the social need with expanded roles. The independent role of pediatric nurse reflect the expansion of the role as pediatric nurse practitioner, pediatric clinical nurse specialist, etc. New roles and responsibility can be added to the pediatric nurse in changing situations of child care in future.

FUNCTIONS OF PEDIATRIC NURSE

The dynamic nature of nursing profession has had an impact on trends in pediatric nursing care and functions of pediatric nurse. Nursing care of children is directed towards understanding of nature and nurture of children and environmental influence on their development. The core activity of pediatric nursing practice is developing a therapeutic relationship with parents and children and then applying the nursing process.

The use of nursing process for both independent and dependent nursing functions provides significant assistant in planning and implementing care. Based on assessment, the nurse determine the nursing diagnosis and make planning for necessary care on priority basis. Interventions and evaluation of care help to implement nursing action with necessary modification. Nursing process can be used both in hospital and community during illness or in maintenance of health.

Implementation of physical care to the children through provision of rest, comfort, hygienic measures, dietary arrangement, administration of medications and other therapies, maintenance of safe and supportive environment, performance of diagnostic procedures and caring in special management schedule are essential functions of pediatric nurse for hospitalized children.

An important function of pediatric nurse is the psychological care that helps children and parent to adapt in illness and hospitalization. Emotional support to child and family, encouragement of children and parental participation in child care, preparation of children and parents for procedures and surgery, allowing child to express feelings about illness and hospitalization, promotion of therapeutic relationship, strengthening coping mechanism and monitoring emotional reactions of child, parents and family members during illness and hospitalization are the delicate functions of pediatric nurse.

The vital function of pediatric nurse is to contribute to increase knowledge and understanding of parents and family members about child health. Information to be provided about illness, hospital procedures, treatment plan, discharge plan and possible outcome of the illness. Health counseling about different aspects like prevention of diseases, promotion of healthful practices, child rearing and family welfare are also important. Information about community resources, health care facilities, referral services, available social and economical support should be provided by the pediatric nurse for necessary child care.

Pediatric nurse should function as a member of the health team and acts in co-operation and co-ordination towards better child care. Clinical rounds, case study, case discussion, etc. are essential aspects of team approach to the solution of child's problems.

Thus, the functions of pediatric nurse are directed towards the welfare of children and their family, promotion of growth and development towards highest possible state of health of children, prevention of diseases and injuries, meeting health needs and rehabilitating children in the family and community.

TRENDS IN PEDIATRIC NURSING

Remarkable changes have occurred in the field of pediatric nursing in recent years due to changing needs of society, medical and technological advances, political interests and changing trends within the nursing profession. Other influencing factors are consumers demands, increased public awareness and greater understanding of child health problems along with psychological aspects of illness and hospitalization.

Modern approach of child health care emphasizes on preventive care rather than curative care. Most childhood diseases are preventable and nurses play pivotal role in preventive health services, e.g. immunization, nutrition demonstration, health education, etc. So nurses are considered as key person in child care.

Growth of specialization within the field of pediatric medicine has had an impact on nursing care of children. There is need for specialized well trained pediatric nurses with continuous reorientation about the advancement of technical aspect of child care. Nurses are assuming an increasing share of the services to children in health and illness and working significantly towards the promotion of child health. Pediatric nurses are performing specialized care in neonatal intensive care unit, pediatric intensive care unit and in any special care system of child care.

Because of growth and maturation of the nursing profession, nurse may become an independent practitioner who can fulfill an autonomous position as a member of an interdisciplinary health team. Pediatric nursing is the area where independent practices are mostly accepted, especially in the community services for improvement in the child care. The large number of child population with various health problems required more numbers of health care providers along with specially trained nurses. So special importance are given in basic nursing curriculum to prepare the nurses with specialized knowledge and skill on child health.

Acceptance of family centered care of children impart more responsibility on pediatric nursing and pediatric nurse. The nurses are working in liaison with the health team and family to prepare mutually developed plan of care and to minimize psychological trauma in relation to holistic approach of child care.

Pediatric nursing practices are influenced by the research findings of nursing sciences and other health disciplines. Psychological approach of child care; acceptance of beneficial traditional practices, newer diagnostic and treatment modalities are the different aspects which have impact on pediatric nursing towards modernization.

Consideration of ethical, moral and legal dilemmas in child care create problems and nurses may need to decide to perform nursing activities based on professional and personal judgement. Ethical decision-making, legal safeguards and quality assurance are the recent trends in nursing practice in all fields including pediatric nursing.

EMERGING CHALLENGES IN PEDIATRIC NURSING

In the changing trends and changing attitude towards care of children, the pediatric nurse has to face various challenges on the following aspects.

Emergence of medical speciality and superspeciality of pediatric care need specialized education and training of pediatric nurse. Nurses required to be up-to-date in the field of specialized care to be at per with their coworker and team members especially medical counterpart in intensive care, neonatology and in any special care system.

Increasing numbers of HIV infected innocent children create problems in pediatric care and nursing practices which need for specialized approach.

Increasing numbers of psychological problems among children due to unhealthy competition, comparison, single parent and family disruption call for special attention of pediatric nurse in child care.

Ethical decision-making in ethical dilemmas about issues like refusal of treatment (discontinuing life support system, with-holding or withdrawing nutrition and fluids), euthanasia, prolongation of life, prenatal genetic screening, abortion, *in vitro* fertilization, allocation of scarce medical resources and rights of children in health care research, etc. are the new challenges in pediatric nursing.

Moral dilemmas for pediatric nurses arise from power conflicts about treatments in which the nurse may need to decide whether to continue to co-operate with the health team and follow the physician's directions or not to follow them.

Legal issues related to Consumer Protection Act, malpractice and negligence are great challenges in all areas of nursing practice and also in child care.

Poverty and illiteracy are two big obstacles need to overcome to improve child health. Nurse must be confident and engaged to advocate for the child's protection in these situations in hospital and community.

Childhood illness leads to frustrating and stressful situations, nurses also need to adjust and cope with those situations and develop tolerance of own feelings.

Emphasis on 'quality care' and increased complexity of medical and nursing practices, required for highly specialized, expert and competent practitioners, with special preparation for superspecialty areas. It calls for better education in pediatric nursing for specialized knowledge and skill of motivated pediatric nurse for better contribution as health team members towards improvement of child health.

NURSING PROCESS RELATED TO PEDIATRIC NURSING

Nursing process is the core and essence of nursing. It is central to all areas of nursing practice. It is an organized and systematic method of giving individualized nursing care that focuses upon identifying and treating unique responses of individuals or groups to actual or potential alterations in health. It is holistic in focus considering both present problems and the effects of the problems. It follows a logical sequence towards the objectives by problem solving approach through quality nursing care.

Definition

The nursing process is an orderly, systematic manner of determining the clients' (patients') problems, making plans to solve them, initiating the plans or assigning others to implement it and evaluating the extent to which the plan was effective in resolving problems identified. It should be planned, client-centered, problem-oriented, goal-directed, dynamic and continuous phenomenon.

The term 'client' is used to denote any recipient of care and may refer to a child, a mother, a father, another family member or the family.

Purposes

The purposes of use of nursing process in child health are the followings:
- It assists to deliver optimum, need-based nursing care to the children effectively and intelligently.
- It guides nurses to take deliberate steps to identify clients problems to set realistic goals and to intervene individualized care.
- It encourages for identification and utilization of client's strength.
- It enhances communication and interpersonal relationship with clients and team members.
- It provides continuity of care by reducing omissions and duplications of actions.

Steps in the Nursing Process

The nursing process has been described by many authors as having five basic steps: assessment, diagnosis (nursing diagnosis), planning, implementation (intervention) and evaluation. The acronym used for these steps is "ADPIE". Another acronym used to denote the steps is 'SOAPIE', i.e. subjective data, objective data, assessment, planning, implementation and evaluation (Figs 2.1 and 2.2).

Assessment

Assessment includes gathering of subjective and objective data. It is done by collection of data through history taking, physical assessment, review of investigations reports and record analysis. It comprises comparison of data with the normal value and analysis of the data gathered to ascertain

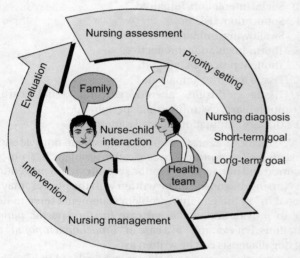

Fig. 2.1: Nursing process

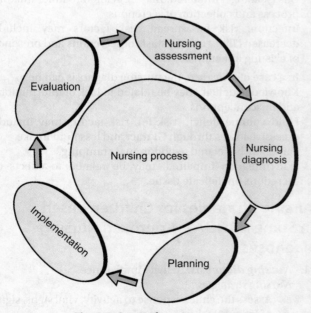

Fig. 2.2: Steps of nursing process

the clients condition and identify problems. Analysis of data helps to establish nursing diagnosis and to formulate short-term and long-term goals. Types of data include, subjective data, i.e. facts expressed by the patients or relatives which are not observable and measurable. Objective data are the facts observable and measurable by health personnel.

Nursing Diagnosis

Nursing diagnosis are judgments and conclusions made by the nurse after analyzing the data base. It indicates actual or potential problem or unmet need of the client/patient. It differs from medical diagnosis. Medical diagnosis refers to disease, whereas nursing diagnosis refers to difficulty experienced by the patient due to disease process. Nursing diagnoses are made in all areas of health care, i.e. health promotion, health maintenance and health restoration. It is written in the form of patient problem statements, also known as 'PES' format, (problem, etiology, signs/symptoms). The phrase "may be related to" in the patient's problem statements serve to help one to provide individualized care for the specific patient situations.

Planning

Planning includes establishing goals, setting priorities, determining resources, stating nursing strategies and assigning care. It is a written document with intervention strategies and outcome of nursing actions as nursing care plan, which should be available for all members of the nursing team. Client's participation in planning of care is an important aspect in terms of effectiveness.

Implementation

It is putting the plan into action to achieve the goals. It includes performance, assistance or assignment of nursing actions and completion of plan of care. This phase involves decision-making, observation and communication among client, nurse and other team members. It requires up-to-date and correct knowledge with skill and competency to perform the activities. Implementation is concluded when the nurse's action are completed and client's reactions and results have been documented on the permanent record. Parents' involvement in the care of children is essential for total care in holistic approach.

Evaluation

Evaluation helps to measure the extent of achievement of goals and effectiveness of interventions. Attention should be given to the client's response in the planned nursing action. During this step, the nurse also will be able to identify omissions from the assessment, planning and implementation phases of the process. A decision can be made to continue, modify or terminate all or part of the nursing care plan.

The nursing process provides an organized nursing assistance to the child and the family towards better outcome.

List of Approved Nursing Diagnoses

North American Nursing Diagnosis Association (NANDA) approved a list of nursing diagnoses through the 12th conference, 1996. Some of them are given below in alphabetical order:

1. Activity intolerance.
2. Activity intolerance, risk for.
3. Adjustment, impaired.
4. Airway clearance, ineffective.
5. Anxiety.
6. Aspiration, risk for.
7. Body temperature, altered, risk for.
8. Bowel incontinence.
9. Breastfeeding, ineffective.
10. Breathing pattern, ineffective.
11. Cardiac output decreased.
12. Communication, impaired, verbal.
13. Comfort, altered, pain.
14. Confusion.
15. Constipation.
16. Coping, ineffective, individual.
17. Coping, ineffective, family.
18. Diarrhea.
19. Diversional activity, deficit.
20. Family process, altered.
21. Fatigue.
22. Fear.
23. Fluid volume, deficit, risk for.
24. Fluid volume, excess, risk for.
25. Fluid volume deficit.
26. Gas exchange, impaired.
27. Growth and development, altered.
28. Hopelessness.
29. Hyperthermia.
30. Hypothermia.
31. Infant feeding pattern, ineffective.
32. Infection, risk for.
33. Injury, risk for.
34. Knowledge deficit.
35. Memory, impaired.
36. Mobility, impaired, physical.
37. Noncompliance.
38. Nutrition, altered, less than body requirements.
39. Nutrition, altered, risk for, more than body requirements.
40. Oral mucous membrane, altered.
41. Pain, acute.
42. Pain, chronic.
43. Parenting, altered.
44. Parental role conflict.
45. Poisoning, risk for.
46. Post-trauma response.
47. Protection, altered.
48. *Self-care deficit:* Feeding, bathing/hygiene, dressing, toileting.
49. *Sensory alteration:* Visual, auditory, tactile, etc.
50. Skin integrity, impaired.
51. Skin integrity, impaired risk for.
52. Sleep pattern disturbance.
53. Social interaction, impaired.
54. Suffocation, risk for.
55. Swallowing, impaired.
56. Thermoregulation, ineffective.
57. Thought processes, altered.
58. Tissue integrity, impaired.
59. Tissue perfusion, altered, cerebral, renal, cardio-pulmonary, gastrointestinal, peripheral.
60. Urinary elimination, altered patterns of.

A "risk for" diagnosis is a potential problem not evidenced by signs and symptoms, because the problem has not yet occurred and nursing interventions are directed at prevention.

Nursing diagnosis can be written with the phrase "may be related to" in the patients' problem statements serve to help one to provide individualized care for the specific patient situations. For example, in a case of "*Bronchopneumonia*" the nursing diagnosis can be written as:

a. Airway clearance, ineffective may be related to bronchial inflammation and edema.
b. Gas exchange, impaired, may be related to inflammatory process and collection of secretions.
c. Infection, risk for spread, risk factors may include decreased ciliary action, stasis of secretions and presence of existing infections.

In a case of '*diarrhea*', the nursing diagnosis can be:

a. Knowledge deficit, may be related to lack of informations and misconceptions.
b. Fluid volume deficit, risk for, risk factors may include excessive losses through GI tract and less fluid intake.
c. Pain, may be related to abdominal cramping.
d. Skin integrity, impaired, may be related to effects of excretions on delicate tissue.

Nursing Strategies for Children Based on Some NANDA—Approved Nursing Diagnoses

1. ***Nursing diagnosis:*** Activity intolerance.
   Nursing strategies:
   a. Assess the child response to activity, vital signs, signs of fatigue, lack of interest in play, etc.

b. Provide uninterrupted sleep/rest, tender loving care and diversional activities.

c. Change the position every 1 to 2 hours in the day and 2 to 4 hours at night.

d. Administer medications as prescribed.

e. Teach the parent/child to plan activities to conserve energy.

2. *Nursing diagnosis:* Airway clearance, ineffective.
   Nursing strategies:
   a. Assess child's respiratory status, vital signs and orientation according to normal level for age group.
   b. Position with head elevated, if condition permitted and suction to remove secretion as needed.
   c. Encourage coughing to remove secretions or by postural drainage.
   d. Teach the parent/child about importance of coughing and clear airway.

3. *Nursing diagnosis:* Adjustment impaired.
   Nursing strategies:
   a. Assess child's problem solving abilities.
   b. Allow the child to verbalize fear and anxieties and utilize therapeutic play to assist child to express feelings of anger.
   c. Encourage child to participate in decision-making and planning for care, diet, activities, etc. and involve the child in problem solving process.
   d. Provide contact with family members and peers.

4. *Nursing diagnosis:* Anxiety.
   Nursing strategies:
   a. Assess the child's behavioral pattern at home and during illness and hospitalization.
   b. Encourage to express feelings and concerns about illness and hospitalization.
   c. Provide age-appropriate toys and physical contact for the child. Allow to play out or draw pictures that describe concerns.
   d. Provide opportunity for parent to express concerns.
   e. Encourage child/parent to write or ask questions and to discuss with health team members.

5. *Nursing diagnosis:* Aspiration risk for.
   Nursing strategies:
   a. Assess respiration pattern, risk for entry of oro-pharyngeal or GI secretions, level of consciousness, swallowing ability, cough and gag reflex, feeding behavior, neurological status, presence of endotracheal tube, etc.
   b. Position the child with slightly head elevated or head turned to one side or in lateral position or prone position.
   c. Monitor the child's condition continuously with close supervision.
   d. Do suctioning to remove the secretions, whenever necessary.

6. *Nursing diagnosis:* Body temperature, altered, risk for.
   Nursing strategies:
   a. *Assess child's physiological status:* Skin temperature, vital signs and environment for heat or cold.
   b. Provide stable environmental temperature and adequate clothing.
   c. Administer extra fluids to the child having temperature elevation.
   d. Teach the parent to monitor child's temperature and provide a constant environmental temperature.

7. *Nursing diagnosis:* Breast feeding ineffective.
   Nursing strategies:
   a. Assess infants sucking, swallowing and rooting reflex and features of illness.
   b. Assess mother's breast and nipple for presence of any problems.
   c. Look for any pain and anxiety in mother.
   d. Ask the mother about urine output of the infant.
   e. Weigh the baby to identify the gain and loss of weight.
   f. Explain and reassure the mother to make her confident.
   g. Demonstrate breast feeding technique to the mother.
   h. Assist for latching and appropriate positioning of the baby with mother.
   i. Ensure about sufficient water and food intake of mother.
   j. Do back massage of the mother to make her relax.
   k. Manage the mother's problem like, retracted nipple, sore nipple and engorged breast as per recommended guidelines.

8. *Nursing diagnosis:* Breathing pattern, ineffective.
   Nursing strategies:
   a. Assess respiratory status, lung sounds, vital signs, skin color, activity level, etc.
   b. Position the child with elevated head or side lying to improve the use of respiratory muscles.
   c. Provide tender loving care and support to decrease anxiety which can cause breathing difficulty.
   d. Encourage to use breathing exercises through play activities.
   e. Administer prescribed medications.
   f. Teach child and parents to use positioning and breathing exercises to improve respiratory status.

9. *Nursing diagnosis:* Cardiac output, altered, decreased.
   Nursing strategies:
   a. *Assess cardiac function:* Vital signs, skin color and activity level according to age.
   b. Provide a quiet supportive environment and simple explanation for all aspects of care.
   c. Position the child for maximum respiratory function.
   d. Administer prescribed medications.

e. Provide tender loving care, support and play to decrease anxiety.

f. Provide support to family members by listening, teaching and facilitating access to health team.

g. Teach the child and parents to improve cardiac output by rest, relief of stress, monitoring and use of medications.

10. ***Nursing diagnosis:*** Comfort, altered, pain.
Nursing strategies:
a. Assess child for pain, vital signs, changes in behaviors, change in activities of daily living, change in sleep, lack of interest in play, etc.
b. Provide supportive care by rest, change of position, tender loving care and favorite play.
c. Administer medications on a routine basis or on request to provide continuous comfort level.
d. Encourage the child to express emotions.
e. Explore the use of nonpharmacologic pain control measures.
f. Explain and inform child and family members about the course of the disease and plan of treatment.

11. ***Nursing diagnosis:*** Constipation.
Nursing strategies:
a. Assess bowel sounds, bowel patterns and frequency of bowel movement.
b. Encourage more fluid intake, and roughage or bulk food in diet unless contraindicated.
c. Provide opportunities for increased activity level if possible.
d. If nursing strategies are not effective, administer laxatives or enema as per medical advice.
e. Explain the need of fluids, bulk foods and exercise to prevent constipation, to the child/parents.
f. Discuss the need for regular bowel habit.

12. ***Nursing diagnosis:*** Diarrhea.
Nursing strategies:
a. Assess frequency and nature of diarrheal bowel movement, bowel sounds, bowel patterns and degree of dehydration.
b. Monitor fluid and electrolyte status, intake and output.
c. Assess vital signs and child's body weight.
d. Provide fluids oral or IV fluid therapy and foods, as appropriate.
e. Clean rectal area immediately after loose stools, keep the area dry and apply ointment whenever needed.
f. Practice hand washing and medical asepsis in providing care to prevent cross infection.
g. Provide tender loving care and medications if prescribed.
h. Teach the family members/parent about specific care of the child with diarrhea.

13. ***Nursing diagnosis:*** Fluid volume deficit.
Nursing strategies:
a. Assess for signs and symptoms of fluid volume deficit and its specific cause.
b. Monitor fluid intake according to the prescription for oral intake or, parenteral fluid administration.
c. Monitor accurate intake and output and keep accurate records and monitor laboratory values.
d. Provide frequent mouth care and application of emollient to lips.
e. Provide skin care and apply emollients to dry skin areas and use no soap.
f. Change position frequently to prevent pressure sore.
g. Involve parents and teach the care specific to fluid intake, mouth care and skin care.

14. ***Nursing diagnosis:*** Growth and development altered.
Nursing strategies:
a. Assess the child's physical growth parameters, ability to perform self-care skills and developmental milestones based on age norms.
b. Provide stimulation using appropriate developmental level of activities.
c. Develop a plan to assist the child to acquire identified skills and physical growth.
d. Assist parents to determine goals, realistic for their child, and refer for appropriate treatment.

15. ***Nursing diagnosis:*** Infection, risk for.
Nursing strategies:
a. Assess child for changes in vital signs and laboratory findings, physical changes, behavioral changes, signs of infection and response to treatment.
b. Use universal precautions for prevention of infections.
c. Administer medications as prescribed.
d. Use nursing measures to provide comfort for child by rest, fluid intake, cool environment and application of heat as required.

16. ***Nursing diagnosis:*** Knowledge deficit.
Nursing strategies:
a. Assess child and family for level of knowledge, specific to health problem or concern.
b. Develop teaching plan about present health problem for the child and family.
c. Provide opportunity for child and family to ask question, to discuss about problem and to observe demonstration of care.

17. ***Nursing diagnosis:*** Mobility, impaired, physical.
Nursing strategies:
a. Assess child's physical activity, movements of limbs, vital signs, pain and other associated signs and symptoms.
b. Assist child to change position, and ambulate.
c. Perform passive and/or active range-of-motion exercises to increase mobility.

d. Provide safe environment for mobility and prevention of injury.

e. Encourage the child to perform self-care, as able.

f. Teach the parent about the importance of allowing the child to perform the activities, as per capability.

18. **Nursing diagnosis:** Nutrition altered less than body requirements.

Nursing strategies:

a. Assess the child for nutritional intake, nausea, vomiting, inability to eat, appetite, etc.

b. Take daily weight of the child and compare with previous weight record chart.

c. Provide balanced diet based on child's nutritional and caloric needs.

d. Encourage the child to increase intake of food and fluids.

e. Offer favorite foods and encourage the family to bring favorite foods from home.

f. Serve food in pleasant environment and attractively.

g. Teach the child and parent about the importance of eating well-balanced diet to support nutritional needs.

h. Teach about the sources of nutrition from available food items.

19. **Nursing diagnosis:** Self-care deficit, feeding, bathing/hygiene, dressing, toileting.

Nursing strategies:

a. Assess child's ability to provide self-care based on growth and development and physical abilities.

b. Encourage the child to perform self-care whatever able to do to boost self-esteem feeding, bathing, dressing and toileting.

c. Provide basic care that the child is not able to complete for self.

d. Discuss with parents the need to foster independence in self-care in their child with self-care deficit.

20. **Nursing diagnosis:** Skin integrity, impaired.

Nursing strategies:

a. Assess the child's skin for redness, edema, blisters, abrasions or open lesions. Assess the skin condition every 2 to 4 hours.

b. Change the child's position hourly during day and 2 hourly during night.

c. Expose the skin to the air to avoid moist and to prevent bacterial growth.

d. Give back care and massage the child's skin to stimulate circulation.

e. Bathe the child on a routine basis to remove secretions and stimulate circulation.

f. Involve family member during care of the child.

21. **Nursing diagnosis:** Trauma, risk for.

Nursing strategies:

a. Assess the child's environment for potential dangers in which falls, burns and other injuries can occur.

b. Teach parents the dangers of a child climbing out of cribs, falling down stairs, playing with matches or sharp toys, etc.

c. Discuss selection of appropriate toys and play materials according to developmental level.

d. Teach children the safety measures for home, school and hospital, to be practiced.

e. Instruct the parent to keep an eye on the child and to anticipate the risk of injury.

22. **Nursing diagnosis:** Tissue integrity, impaired.

Nursing strategies:

a. *Assess the child's tissue intactness:* Mucous membranes, skin, subcutaneous tissue, cornea, etc.

b. Keep the skin dry and clean.

c. Provide soft, bland diet when mucous membranes are impaired.

d. Apply a patch on the eye when cornea is impaired.

e. Stimulate circulation by nursing measures like turning, massaging and maintaining hygiene.

f. Provide a safe environment by removing harmful irritants, chemicals, secretions and medications.

g. Teach parent about the assessment and immediate care of impaired tissue integrity.

23. **Nursing diagnosis:** Tissue perfusion, altered, cerebral, cardiopulmonary, renal, gastrointestinal, peripheral.

Nursing strategies:

a. Assess the child for alteration in skin temperature, color, vital signs, mental status, output, fluid retention, nausea, vomiting, diarrhea, etc.

b. Provide physical support for the child by warmth, rest, fluids, medications, food, orientation, etc.

c. Teach child/parent/family members to adapt self-care in altered condition and encourage to discuss feelings.

24. **Nursing diagnosis:** Urinary elimination, altered patterns of.

Nursing strategies:

a. Assess child for urinary output, volume, color, pain, frequency, incontinence, etc.

b. Maintain accurate output for child, according to age.

c. Encourage increased intake of fluids, unless contraindicated and restricted.

d. Use comfort measures to decrease pain, burning sensation, etc. by fluid, warm baths and other nursing measures.

e. Teach child/family members about bladder training, safety measures to prevent trauma and specific medical instructions.

f. Refer child for evaluation of cause.

Preventive Pediatrics

3

- Concept of Preventive Pediatrics
- Family Health
- Maternal and Child Health
- Reproductive and Child Health
- Baby Friendly Hospital Initiative
- Integrated Child Development Services
- National Rural Health Mission
- Under-Five's Clinic
- School Health Service

- Integrated Management of Neonatal and Childhood Illness
- Child Labor
- Street Children
- Gender Bias
- Female Feticide
- Child Abuse and Neglect
- National Health Programs for Children in India
- Nursing Responsibilities in Preventive Pediatrics

CONCEPT OF PREVENTIVE PEDIATRICS

Child health depends upon preventive care. Majority of the child health problems are preventable. Preventive pediatrics is a specialized area of child health comprises efforts to avert rather than cure disease and disabilities.

Preventive pediatrics has been defined as "The prevention of disease and promotion of physical, mental and social wellbeing of children with the aim of attaining a positive health". Pediatrics is largely preventive in its objectives.

Preventive pediatrics been broadly divided into antenatal preventive pediatrics and postnatal preventive pediatrics.

Antenatal preventive pediatrics includes care of the pregnant mothers with adequate nutrition, prevention of communicable diseases, preparation of the mother for delivery, breastfeeding and mothercraft training, etc. Pre-pregnant health status of the mother also influences the child health. Promotion of health of girl child and nonpregnant state should be emphasized as the future mother, who is soil and seed of future generation.

Postnatal preventive pediatrics includes promotion of breastfeeding, introduction of complementary feeding in

appropriate age, immunization, prevention of accidents, tender loving care with emotional security, growth monitoring, periodic medical supervision and health check-up, psychological assessment, etc.

Another new concept of child health care is social pediatrics. The challenge of the time is to study child health in relation to community to social values and to social policy.

Social pediatrics has been defined as "The application of the principles of social medicine to pediatrics to obtain a more complete understanding of the problems of children in order to prevent and treat disease and promote their adequate growth and development, through an organized health structure". It is concerned with the delivery of comprehensive and continuous child health care services and to bring these services within the reach of the total community. It also covers the various social welfare measures—local, national and international—aimed to meet the health needs of a child.

To ensure adequate physical, mental and social growth of the child, total health needs should be provided as:
- Healthy and happy parents
- Balanced and nutritious diet
- Clean, healthful house and living environments

- Developmental needs like play, recreation, love and affection, safety and security, recognition and companionship as emotional food
- Educational provisions and opportunities.

For the comprehensive services to the mothers and children, primary health care strategy is adopted by the health care delivery system. Government of India accepted a national policy for children in 1974 and implemented various health programs for preventive and social services along with curative care for the millions of children.

FAMILY HEALTH

Child health depends upon the family's physical, social, economical and environmental conditions, which include family size, family income, standard of living, parents' education, culture, customs, traditional habits, child bearing and child rearing practices, family relationship, family stability, etc.

Family health means the overall health of the individual family members. It is influenced by the inter-relationship and interdependence of the physical and mental health status of the individual members of the family. It is determined by the effective functioning of the family as biological and cultural unit.

Aims of family health services:
- Reduction of maternal, infant and child mortality and morbidity rates
- Improvement of family planning practices and to ensure planned parenthood
- Improvement of nutritional status of all family members
- Increasing health awareness through health education in all preventive, promotive, curative and rehabilitative aspects of health care.

Sub-areas of family health:
- Maternal and child health service including immunization
- Family welfare services
- Nutritional services
- Health education.

Factors influencing family health:
- Environmental factors—housing, sanitation, drinking water supply, pollution, etc.
- Economical factors—income and expenditure in the family
- Educational factors—parents education especially mother's education and level of literacy of other family members
- Social factors—culture, customs, food habit, health habit, family size, fertility rate, etc.

The success of family health program can be achieved by the continuous preventive and promotive health care through primary health care services at the door step of the family and involving the family to assume responsibility of the health and welfare of its members. Family health program should be supported by adequate referral system for better community health.

MATERNAL AND CHILD HEALTH

Maternal and child health (MCH) refers to the promotive, preventive, curative and rehabilitative health care for mothers and children.

The components of maternal and child health include the sub-areas of maternal health, child health, family planning, school health, handicapped children, adolescence and health aspects of care of children in special care setting, e.g. day care centers.

The specific objectives of MCH care are:
- Reduction in maternal, perinatal, infant and child mortality and morbidity.
- Promotion of reproductive health, e.g. postponing unwanted arrival of child, adequate spacing between two children and containment of population explosion
- Promotion of physical and psychological development of the child and adolescent within the family.

The important health problems affecting the mother and the child are mainly malnutrition, infections and hazards associated with uncontrolled reproduction or fertility. MCH services in India are now delivered as a 'package' services against these problems to promote continuity of care and to reduce number of visits by mother, for herself and for the child.

The MCH care package services include, antenatal care, intranatal care, perinatal care, postnatal care, nutrition advice, immunization, primary health care and rational family planning.

The MCH services should always be flexible and based on local needs and resources of the community it serves. It is organized in integrated and risk approach and delivered as priority element of primary health care. MCH services highlight the concept of mother and child as one unit because the child health is closely related to maternal health and a healthy mother only can bring a healthy child.

REPRODUCTIVE AND CHILD HEALTH

The reproductive and child health (RCH) program was formally launched by Government of India in October 1997 as per recommendations of International Conference on Population Development at Cairo, in 1994. The RCH program covers the components of child survival and safe motherhood

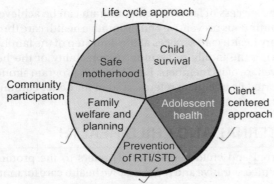

Fig. 3.1: Component of RCH program

(CSSM) program and family welfare program with addition of two new interventions, i.e. prevention and management of RTIs/STDs and adolescent health (Fig. 3.1).

The RCH services are planned and implemented on the basis of the needs of the community with client-centered approach. Other management strategies of this services are target-free, demand-driven, decentralized, participatory, bottom-up planning with life cycle approach. This program is implemented in the community level, subcenter level, primary health center level and FRU/district hospital level.

The RCH program is not just a new package of services. The program lays emphasis on quality of services and satisfaction of the consumers. The package of services offered by RCH program are as follows:

For the Children
(Child Survival Components)

- Essential newborn care
- Exclusive breastfeeding for 6 months, semisolids to be started after six months of age
- Immunization against six-killer diseases
- Appropriate management of diarrhea and ORT
- Appropriate management of ARI
- Vitamin 'A' prophylaxis
- Treatment of childhood anemia.

For the Mothers
(Safe Motherhood Components)

- Early registration of all antenatal mothers
- Minimum three antenatal check-up
- Immunization against tetanus
- Prevention and treatment of anemia
- Early identification of maternal complications and referral
- Deliveries by trained personnel
- Promotion of institutional deliveries
- Management of obstetrical emergencies

- Minimum three postnatal check-up.
- Birth spacing.

For the Eligible Couples

- Promotion of contraception to prevent unwanted pregnancies
- Safe services for MTP.

Other New Services

- Prevention and management of RTIs and STDs
- Adolescent health and counseling on family life and reproductive health.

Life cycle approach has been adopted in the RCH package services. A healthy pregnancy ensures a healthy child. A healthy child grows up into healthy adolescent. Good health during adolescent years leads to healthy reproductive years and the cycle continues into next generation.

RCH-Phase II began from 1st April, 2005. The focus of the program is to reduce maternal and child morbidity, and mortality with emphasis on rural health care.

Major strategies under 2nd phase of RCH program include: (1) Essential obstetric care (2) Emergency obstetric care and (3) Strengthening of referral system. New initiatives under RCH-II are training of MBBS doctor, setting up of blood storage centers and *Janani Suraksha Yojana* (JSY) with NRHM along with ASHA (Accredited Social Health Activist). Child health components emphasis on IMNCI, F-IMNCI, home based newborn care, facility based newborn care (FBNC), nutrition rehabilitation center, RCH camps RCH-out reach scheme, *Navjat Shishu Suraksha Karyakram*, etc.

BABY FRIENDLY HOSPITAL INITIATIVE

Baby Friendly Hospital Initiative (BFHI) was launched in 1992 in India, as a part of 'Innocenti declaration' on breastfeeding. The historic Innocenti Declaration on the promotion, protection and support of breastfeeding was produced and adapted by participants at the WHO/UNICEF policy makers' meeting on breastfeeding in the 1990s, held at the Spedale degli Innocenti, Florence, Italy, on July 30 to August 1st, 1990. The global initiative was cosponsored by the USAID and SIDA.

The baby friendly hospital campaign was launched by the WHO/UNICEF, in mid 1991 in Ankara to boost the breastfeeding practices and to counter the trends of bottle feeding.

The goals of the declaration included a call to the various governments in the word to act and create an environment for exclusive breastfeeding from birth of the baby till she/he is 6 months old and to continue breastfeeding with adequate complementary foods for up to two years.

Baby friendly hospitals are required to adopt breastfeeding policy and to follow the 'Ten steps of successful breastfeeding' as recommended by code of practice of WHO/UNICEF.

1. Have a written breastfeeding policy, that is routinely communicated to all health care staff.
2. Train all health care staff in skills necessary to implement this policy.
3. Inform all pregnant women about the benefits and management of breastfeeding.
4. Help mothers to initiate breastfeeding within half an hour of birth.
5. Show mothers how to breast-fed and how to maintain lactation even if they should be separated from their infants.
6. Give newborn infants no food or drink other than breast milk, unless medically indicated.
7. Practice rooming-in. Allow mothers and infants to remain together 24 hours a day.
8. Encourage breastfeeding on demand.
9. Give no artificial teats or pacifiers (also called dummies or soothers) to breastfeeding infants.
10. Foster the establishment of breastfeeding support groups and refer mothers to them on discharge from the hospital or clinic.

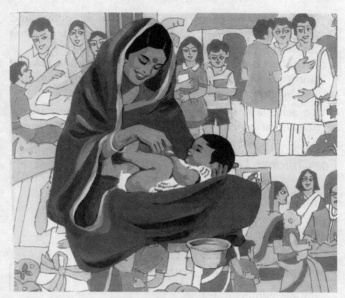

Fig. 3.2: Preventive pediatrics *(For color version, see Plate 3)*

Indian hospitals are till in early stages of joining this movement. The National BFHI task force was formed in 1992, towards the efforts to improve the breastfeeding practices. The task force comprising of Government of India, UNICEF, WHO and professional organizations (TNAI, BPNI, NNF, IMA, FOGSI, IAP, CMAI, CHAI, IBFAN, ACASH) is working for evaluation of breastfeeding practices in the hospitals and appropriate certification as 'Baby Friendly Hospital'. The certificate needs re-recognition on every two years to ensure the standard and quality for successful breastfeeding.

Besides promotion of breastfeeding, baby friendly hospital initiative in India also proposes to provide:
• Improved antenatal care
• Mother friendly delivery services
• Standardized institutional support of immunization
• Diarrhea management
• Promotion of healthy growth and good nutrition
• Widespread availability and adoption of family planning.

Government of India has made significant efforts to promote and protect breastfeeding by enacting a law 'The Infant Milk Substitutes, Feeding Bottles and Infant Food Act, 1992'. The act prohibits advertizing of infant milk substitutes (IMS) and feeding bottles to public, free sampling, hospital promotion and gifts of samples of IMS to health workers. Violation of the act can lead to fine or imprisonment.

INTEGRATED CHILD DEVELOPMENT SERVICES

At present, the most important scheme in the field of child welfare is the Integrated Child Development Services (ICDS) scheme. In pursuance of the national policy for children, Government of India, started ICDS program in 1975, under the Ministry of Social and Women's Welfare.

The ICDS program was initiated for the welfare of the children and development of human resources. It is designed for both preventive and development effort through a integrated package services. The beneficiaries of the program are children up to 6 years, adolescent girls (11-18 years), pregnant women, nursing mothers and women of 15 to 45 years.

ICDS scheme is working at village level in rural areas and also in urban and tribal areas. In 1975, number of ICDS projects was only 33, which was started on experimental basis. At present, the ICDS projects are functioning in 5422 blocks all over the country. The *Kishori Shakti Yojna*, Adolescent girls scheme is sanctioned in 2000 ICDS blocks as special interventions for the benefits of 3.51 lakhs adolescent girls in the age group of 11 to 18 years. NGOs are also involved in running *anganwadi* centers in 67 ICDS projects. World Bank assisted ICDS projects are also working in some states (Fig. 3.2).

Objectives

The objectives of the ICDS scheme are:
• To improve the nutritional and health status of children in the age group of 0 to 6 years.
• To lay the foundations for proper psychological, physical and social development of the child.
• To reduce mortality, morbidity, malnutrition and school drop out.

- To achieve an effective co-ordination of policy and implementation among the various departments working for the promotion of child development.
- To enhance the capability of the mother and to provide nutritional needs of the child through proper nutrition and health education.

To achieve the above objectives the following package services are provided to different categories of beneficiaries.

For Children Less than 3 Years

- Supplementary nutrition
- Immunization
- Health check-up
- Referral services.

For Children in Age Group 3 to 6 Years

- Supplementary nutrition
- Immunization
- Health check-up
- Referral services
- Nonformal preschool education.

For Adolescent Girls 11 to 18 Years

- Supplementary nutrition
- Nutrition and health education.

For Pregnant Women

- Health check-up
- Immunization against tetanus
- Supplementary nutrition
- Nutrition and health education.

For Nursing Mothers

- Health check-up
- Supplementary nutrition
- Nutrition and health education.

Other Women of 15 to 45 Years Age Group

Nutrition and health education.

Delivery of Services

The services are delivered by the *Anganwadi* worker (AWW) at the ICDS center for about 1000 population. She is assisted by a local women, who is usually uneducated and unskilled person. AWW has 4 months training in fundamentals of child development, nutrition, immunization, personal hygiene, environmental sanitation, antenatal care, breastfeeding, care and treatment of common day to day illness, identification and management of at-risk children, preschool education, functional literacy and record keeping.

The activities of AWW are supervised a supervisor or *mukhyasevika*, who is a graduate and having special training for two months. Each supervisor is responsible for 20 to 25 AWWs. The Child Development Project Officer (CDPO), is the incharge of ICDS projects, supervises the activities of four *mukhyasevika* or supervisor.

The administrative unit of an ICDS project is the 'community development block' in rural areas, the tribal development block in tribal areas and a group of slums in urban areas.

ICDS scheme is an important aspect of child welfare to improve the health, nutrition and education status of the underprivileged children and mothers. It is much more than a health program.

The impact of program on the lives of children is evident in several important indicators, i.e. increased birth weight, reduced incidence of malnutrition, increased immunization coverage and a reduction in infant and child mortality rate in areas covered by the ICDS.

NATIONAL RURAL HEALTH MISSION

National Rural Health Mission (NRHM) was launched by the Government of India on April 2005 for the period of 7 years (2005–2012). The mission seeks to improve rural health care delivery system on nutrition, sanitation, hygiene and safe drinking water by making necessary changes in basic health care delivery system. It also brings the Indian system of medicine (AYUSH) to the main stream of health care.

The main aim of NRHM is to provide accessible, affordable, accountable, effective and reliable primary health care and bridging the gap in rural health care through creation of a cader of Accredited Social Health Activist (ASHA).

Strengthening of subcenters, PHCs and CHCs are important plan under NRHM. District becomes the core unit of planning, budgeting and implementation of programs. According to NRHM plan all vertical health and family welfare programs at district level should be merged into one common 'District Health Mission' and at state level into 'State Health Mission'. There should be provision of mobile medical unit and public private partnership (PPP model) under this program.

Goals to be achieved by NRHM were formulated clearly. Role and responsibilities of ASHA, *Anganwadi*, and ANMs were well defined under this program. Monitoring and evaluation of activities is planned and done based on process indicators and outcome indicators of the mission.

UNDER-FIVE'S CLINIC

The concept of under-five's clinic is derived from the Well Baby clinic of the west, for comprehensive health care of children below five years of age. This clinic provides preventive services along with health supervision, treatment, nutritional surveillance and health education. The services are economical within available resources for a large numbers of young children.

Under-five age groups are vulnerable and special risk group constituting a major portion of total population with high death rate. The important causes of morbidity and mortality of this group are mainly, ARI, diarrhea, neonatal and perinatal diseases, infections and accidents. These conditions are mostly preventable with adequate health care. This age group also needs regular monitoring for growth and development. For these reasons, the under-five age group children are provided with special health care through this clinic services.

The services provided by the clinic are set out in the symbol, which has been proposed for under-fives clinics in India (Fig. 3.3).

The apex of the large triangle represents care in illness, the left triangle represents adequate nutrition, the right triangle represents immunization and the central red triangle represents family planning. The line bordering the big triangle represents health teaching to the mother.

Care in Illness

The care of illness for children provided in the under-5 clinics includes the followings:
1. Diagnosis and treatment of:
   a. Acute illness, e.g. oral rehydration therapy.
   b. Chronic illness including physical, mental, congenital and acquired abnormalities.
   c. Disorders of growth and development.
2. X-ray and laboratory services.
3. Referral services.

Care and treatment of sick children are rendered by the trained health worker on the basis of the felt need of the mothers. Research studies have shown that 70 to 90 percent of the care of sick children can be managed but the trained nurses with effective training and responsibility for managing the child health care service.

Adequate Nutrition

Adequate nutrition is vital for growth and development of children. The health worker should ensure about adequate breastfeeding, weaning and balanced diet of the under-5 children. Almost all nutritional disorders like PEM, anemia, rickets, nutritional blindness occur in this age group.

Attempts to be made to identify early onset of growth failure and malnutrition. One of the basic activities of the under-fives clinic is growth monitoring. It is done by weighing the child periodically at monthly intervals during the first year, every 2 months during the second year and every 3 months thereafter up to the age of 5 to 6 years. The child's weight is plotted on 'Road to Health Card' as 'growth curve' which helps to detect early onset of growth failure (Figs 3.4 and 3.5).

Health check-ups are done every 3 to 6 months by physical examination of the child and appropriate laboratory tests. The 'child health card' is maintained which assist to identify 'at risk' children who can be enlisted for special care and referral for better treatment.

Food supplementation or on-site feeding are often an integral part of intervention strategies.

The ICDS projects has taken up the supplementary feeding of children below 6 years of age. Nutrition education to the mothers is an important aspect of the clinic.

Immunization

Immunization of six killer diseases, viz. tuberculosis, diphtheria, pertussis, tetanus, poliomyelitis and measles, are administered as per national immunization schedule recommendation. The health worker should motivate and promote the immunization acceptance to prevent morbidity, mortality and disability hazards by these six killer diseases.

Family Planning

The family planning program is successfully conducted through these clinics. The mothers attending the clinic receive counseling with different aspects of family planning practices, which is a significant concern for the health and well-being of the child.

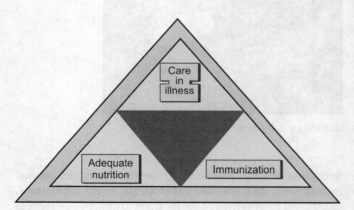

Fig. 3.3: Symbol for under-fives clinic *(For color version, see Plate 3)*

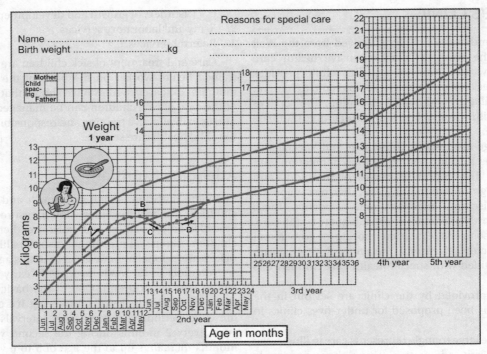

Fig. 3.4: Growth chart

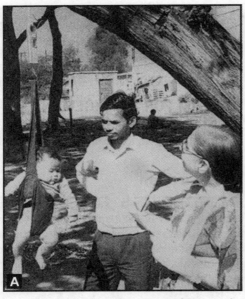

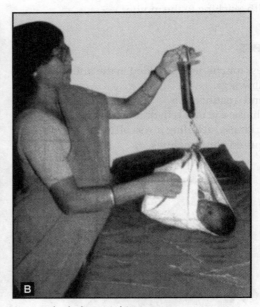

Figs 3.5A and B: Growth assessment by baby weighing

Health Education

Health education to the mother is an essential and compulsory activity of the under-fives clinic. The mothers should receive the information on various aspects of child care and child rearing practices. Preventive measures against malnutrition, ARI, diarrhea tuberculosis, worm infestations, etc. should be informed to the mothers to improve awareness about the disease and its prevention.

The under-fives clinic is usually located in village or a slum or a labor colony. It is managed by trained health worker. She also visits home to educate the mothers and to make sure that children are brought to the clinic for regular check-up. She maintains child registers and records related to child care given and health check-up done. She distributes supplementary food, vitamin 'A' oil and iron-folic acid tablets and keep accounts of expenditure. She arranges health exhibitions, well-baby competitions and mother craft training program. Thus, 'under- fives' clinics provide a low-cost comprehensive care through preventive promotive, curative and rehabilitative health care services to the under-five children.

SCHOOL HEALTH SERVICE

School health service is an important economical and powerful health care delivery to improve community health especially of future generations. It is comprehensive care of the health and well-being of children throughout the school years.

The school health committee was constituted by the Government of India in 1960 to assess the standards of health and nutrition of school children and to suggest recommendations to improve them. As per recommendation of the committee, the school health program was initiated in 1962 but minimum services are provided to the school children due to shortage of resources and insufficient facilities.

School-going age is relatively safe from health point of view. Health problems of school children may vary with local health problems, cultural practices, socioeconomic status and available resources. The common health problems, which require special emphasis, include malnutrition (PEM, nutritional anemia, vitamin 'A' deficiency), infectious diseases, intestinal parasitosis, skin diseases, dental caries and diseases of eye and ear. Presently, reproductive tract infections or sexually transmitted infections are requiring special attention in relation to adolescent health.

Objectives

The objectives of school health service are as follows:
1. The promotion of positive health.
2. The prevention of disease.
3. Early diagnosis, treatment and follow-up of defects.
4. Increasing health awareness in children about good and bad health.
5. The provision of healthful environment.

Aspects of School Health Service

The school health service may vary according to local priorities. Some important aspects of a school health service are as follows:

- Health appraisal of school children and school personnel.
- Remedial measures and follow-up.
- Prevention of communicable diseases.
- Healthful school environment.
- Nutritional services.
- First aid and emergency care.
- Mental health.
- Dental health.
- Eye health.
- Health education.
- Education of handicapped children.
- Maintenance and use of school health records.

Health Appraisal

Health appraisal should be done for the students by periodic medical examination and daily morning inspection by the class teacher. Health appraisal of teachers and other personnel is also necessary.

Medical examination to be done for each and every child at the time of school entry and thereafter every 4 years or less. Basic investigations like urine, stool and blood tests should also be done. Recording of weight and height should be done quarterly and vision testing annually. Daily morning inspection helps to detect any deviation from normal health status or changes in child's appearance or behavior that suggest illness or improper growth and development. A teacher should be trained about the common health problems of children during basic training and later in-service training courses.

Remedial Measures and Follow-up

Appropriate treatment and follow-up should be arranged after medical check-up. Special clinics should be conducted for school children at primary health centers in the rural areas and in dispensaries or in one of the selected schools in the urban areas. Special attention should be paid to dental, eye and ENT problems. There should be provision for referral along with further investigations and treatment of the specific problem.

Prevention of Communicable Diseases

Immunization program should be planned for the prevention of common communicable diseases like tetanus, typhoid, hepatitis 'B', etc. Record of all immunizations should be maintained and this record should accompany the school leaving certificate.

Healthful School Environment

A healthful school environment with good sanitation is essential requirement for the best emotional, social and personal health of the students.

The school should be located centrally with approaching roads but at a far distance from busy markets, cinema house, factories, etc. The school campus should be fenced and free from dampness or any other hazards. The land must be high and properly drained. Playground should be made available for the students.

The school structure should be single storied for nursery and secondary schools and multistoried for higher schools. Walls should be heat resistant. Verandas should be attached to class room. No class room should accommodate more than 40 students. Doors and windows should be broad and should be placed for cross ventilation.

Furniture of the class room should be appropriate for the age of the students. Class room inside wall should be painted white and periodically white washed should be arranged. Class rooms must be well lighted. There should be provision of safe and potable water supply, preferably continuous and distributed from taps. Provision for separate room for mid day meal or tiffins should be made. Separate toilet facilities must be made for boys and girls, with one urinal for 60 students and one latrine for 100 students.

Nutritional Services

Diet for the school children should receive first attention for the maintenance of optimum health. Nutritional disorders are widely prevalent among school children. To prevent malnutrition and improve the health of school children, it is now accepted procedure to provide a good nourishing meal to school children. Mid-day school meal can be brought form home or provided by the school on a 'no profit no loss' basis. UNICEF assisted applied nutrition program or specific nutrients supplementation may also available to the school children.

First Aid and Emergency Care

First aid and emergency care should be provided by the teachers in such situations like accidents, fainting, vomiting, diarrhea, convulsions, injuries, etc. Teacher should have adequate training regarding first aid and emergency measures.

Mental Health

The school is an important place for development of child's behavior and promotion of mental health. The school teacher has positive and preventive role to help the children to attain mental health and to develop into mature responsible and well-adjusted individual. In the school hours, there should be provision for relaxation between periods of intense work. There should have no unhealthy comparision or discrimination in religion, caste, social status, etc. Provision

of vocational and psychological counseling are a great need for the school children. Juvenile delinquency, maladjustment, drug addiction are becoming problems among school students and need early preventive interventions.

Dental Problems

Dental caries and periodontal disease are two common dental problems among school children. There should be provision for dental examination once in a year to detect problems. Guidance for maintenance of dental hygiene and improvement of dental appearance should be emphasized during dental checkup. Improvement of dental health is a part of school health program.

Eye Health

Early detection of eye problems in school children is essential to prevent further complications. Refractive errors, squint, Vitamin 'A' deficiency conditions (like night blindness, xerosis, etc.) and eye infections should be detected early and referred for necessary treatment.

Health Education

The health education is the most important aspect of school health program to bring about the desirable changes in knowledge, attitude and practices related to health.

The essential areas of health education to the school children are related to different aspects of personal hygiene, environmental health and family health including human reproduction and sexual hygiene.

Community health nurse has great responsibility in health education programs at schools. Teachers are the key persons in the presentation of the materials to the children but they should get help from school health nurse and other health team members.

Education of Handicapped Children

The school health service must have facilities for assisting handicapped children and their families to achieve maximum potential to become as independent as possible and to become productive and self-supporting member of society. This requires the co-operation of health workers with social welfare and educational agencies.

School Health Records

Maintenance of school health records is an useful function to have cumulative information on the health aspects of school children to provide continuing health supervision. It helps to evaluate school health programs and provides useful link between home, school and community.

The maintenance of health of school children is the responsibility of parents, teachers, health care providers and the community. In India, school health service is administered jointly by the Dept of Health and the Dept of Education. According to School Health Committee (1961), school health program should be continuous and self-supporting by the formation of school health committees at the village level, block level, district level, state level and national level.

As an integral part of general health service, the primary health center is responsible to deliver school health service. Primary health nurse (PHN), health supervisor and health workers are key persons to conduct school health program with the necessary guidance of medical officer. Periodic visit, health checkup, immunization, health education, nutritional education, referral and health recording are important functions of them.

INTEGRATED MANAGEMENT OF NEONATAL AND CHILDHOOD ILLNESS

WHO and UNICEF have developed new strategy for management of common childhood illnesses, in an integrated manner, which are responsible for main causes of morbidity and mortality among children. The overall objective of this strategy is to reduce under-five morbidity and mortality in the developing countries by improved performance of health workers.

Three remarkable components of this strategy are: (a) improvement of case management skills of health care providers, (b) provision of essential drug supplies and (c) optimization of family and community practices in relation to child health, mainly care-seeking behavior. This Integrated Management of Childhood Illnes (IMNCI) approach emphasized on both preventive and curative health services including vaccinations, breastfeeding, complementary feeding, micronutrient and vitamin 'A' supplementation, counseling on health problems and case management of ARI, diarrhea, worm infestations, malnutrition, measles, malaria, etc. It also includes home based and community-based interventions for improvement of nutritional status and appropriate care-seeking behavior with treatment compliance. Health care providers practice the case management skills through provisions of locally adapted guidelines and training activities to promote their use.

The Indian version of IMCI has been renamed as Integrated Management of Neonatal and Childhood Illness (IMNCI) as it includes the first 7 days of age in the program. It is the central pillar of child health interventions under RCH-II strategy. The case management process is presented on two different sets of charts:

1. For children aged 2 months to five years
2. For infant up to 2 months of age.

Presently emphasis is placed on F-IMNCI strategy. F-IMNCI is the integration of facility based care package with IMNCI package for the improvement of quality of management of newborn and childhood illness at the community level as well as the facility level especially in low resource setting.

CHILD LABOR

Child labor may be defined as employment of children in gainful occupations even at the expense of their physical, emotional and social wellbeing. Child labors have consequences on their growth and development and health status resulting various health hazards.

A large number of growing children of poor socio-economic group are employed in various occupation as child labor. These children work outside their own family and earn for livelihood. They work with physical strength or patience without any skill or training.

Numbers of child labor are increasing. India has the largest numbers of child labors in the world, among them 90 percent are from rural areas. Every third house has a working child and every fourth child is employed.

These children are working both in unorganized sectors or in organized sectors. In *unorganized* sectors, the child labors are found as domestic servants, as helpers in shops, *dhabas* and restaurants, as vendors, as agriculture worker, as shoeshine boys, rag pickers, etc. In *organized* sectors, only a small proportion of working children are found. Actually, child labors are mostly seen in *semiorganized* sectors, i.e. carpet weaving, *sari* embroidery, precious stone polishing, *bidi* making, bangle manufacturing, leather industry, match and fire works factory, balloon factory, building construction, petrol pumps, automobile workshops and garages.

The factors responsible for this problem are mainly poverty, lack of education, unemployment, exploitation by selfish and lazy parents, bad company, beggar-gang, school dropout, maladjustment in the family, broken family, death of parents, child of unmarried pregnancy, etc.

There are numbers of health hazards resulting in the working children, which include hygienic problems, drug addiction, smoking, STDs, accidents and injuries, malnutrition, juvenile delinquency and even prostitution. High morbidity is related to respiratory infections, tuberculosis, diarrheal diseases, parasitic infestations, scabies and pyodermas. Working conditions are mainly harmful to the health of child labor, than the hazards of work.

Child labor is a social problem and needs special attention from all levels to eliminate the basic causes behind it. It is now difficult to abolish child labor in the present situation of our country, but these children can be protected from health hazards, abuse and exploitation. Working conditions for these children can be improved and regulated. Regular health check up and early detection of health problems with necessary treatment should be arranged for them.

Indian constitution emphasized on protection against exploitation in childhood. The Child Labor *Protection and Regulation* Act, 1986, provides guidelines about the restriction related to child labor. The Supreme court of India, in 1996, directed all state government and union territories to take concrete steps to abolish child labor and instructed for setting up of child labor rehabilitation welfare fund. Elimination of child labor can only be possible with combined effort of parent, community, government, nongovernment and voluntary agencies. Creation of awareness about the evil is the prime responsiblity to prevent and abolish it.

STREET CHILDREN

A large number of homeless children are seen as pavement dwellers in urban and semiurban areas. They live and work on the streets usually without family or with family. The numbers of these children are increasing day by day. These children are vulnerable to various health problems and psychosocial problems.

The contributing factors responsible for this social problem are poverty, rapid urbanization, rural to urban or cross country mobility, broken family, loss of parents, natural or manmade disasters, accidents, child abuse and neglect and population explosion.

The street children are at high risk of different health problems like malnutrition, diarrhea, ARI, skin diseases, tuberculosis, STDs, HIV/AIDS, intestinal parasitosis, etc. They are also prone to psychosocial problems like juvenile delinquency, sexual abuse and exploitation, drug addiction, prostitution and criminal activities.

These children need support from government and NGOs to overcome their problems and to grow as an healthy individual. Free educational facilities, provision of health and welfare services, housing facilities, job opportunities, promotion of adoption, and rehabilitation services will be useful to reduce the problem to some extent. These children need guidance and counseling facilities towards self-support and problem-solving.

The government and nongovernment agencies are working for the prevention of various problems and to promote the living standards of the street children. Child Relief and You (CRY), an Indian organization, was set up by Rippon Kapoor, in 1979, for helping these deprived children of streets and slums with food, shelter and education. The networks of CRY centers are working in major cities in India. *The City Level Program of Action (CLPOA)* was established in 1994, in Kolkata, by the initiative of government and NGOs for the welfare of street and working children. They have undertaken, a number of services for these underprivileged children in the areas of health, education, recreation, nutrition, vocational training, counseling and protection in response to rights of the child.

GENDER BIAS

Gender bias or discrimination against females is more prominent in India and in developing countries. The cultural pattern of 'Son-complex' of Indian family leads to discrimination against female child and creates gender gap between male and female children. Furthermore, the social system like dowry, fear of sexual molestation or exploitation of girl child influence and insist the gender bias and early marriage of female child mainly in rural areas among poor and illiterate groups.

Discrimination against girl child starts before birth as female feticide and afterwards found as female infanticide and inappropriate rearing of girl child. In spite of legal opposition on abortion of female fetus, following identification of sex by diagnostic tests (amniocentesis and ultrasonography), the people from all socioeconomic groups are practicing this evil. After birth, female infants are reared up carelessly with inadequate nutrition, education, love and affection, as a result, those female children suffered from malnutrition, ill health and other health problems. Physical and sexual abuse are also more evident in female child. Girl child of poor family are more exploited as child labor mainly in household activities and also force into commercial sex workers.

For the promotion of status of girl child, UNICEF mentioned and emphasized on the long-lasting effects of the unfolding of potentialities of female child and empowerment of women. The SAARC declared the year 1990, as 'The Year of Girl Child' and the decade 1991-2000 AD, as the 'Decade of the Girl Child' with the view of generating awareness to improve the status of female child and to reduce the gender gap.

Government of India and various NGOs also planned several programs towards disappearance of gender bias and promotion of health of female child with equal opportunities as male child (Figs 3.6A to F). Care of female child should be emphasized considering them as the seed and soil of future generations.

Ten recommended practical action plan by the National conference on status of girl child, held at Mumbai are:
1. No discrimination on the basis of sex and equal opportunities for girls as boys with stress on welfare of girl children.
2. Strict implementation of total ban of female feticide in all states and union territories.
3. Emphasis on creation of awareness on care of girl child, e.g. education, health care, legal status, etc. through local and mass media programs.
4. Improvement of nutritional status of girl child by mid-day meal program, special nutritional supplementation program, vitamin 'D' supplementation program, etc.

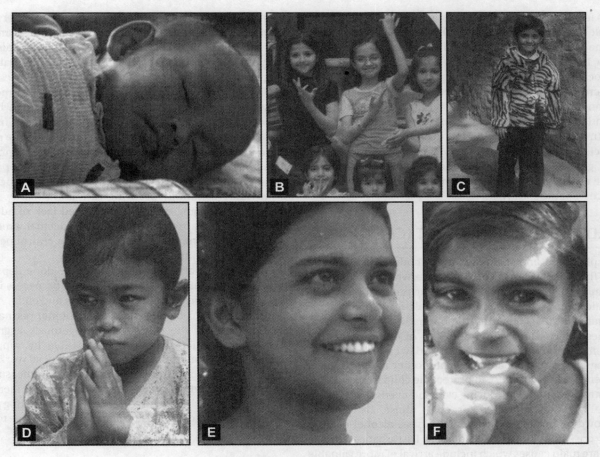

Figs 3.6A to F: Healthy girl children

5. Free education of all girls up to secondary school level in all the states of India. Education of girls should be the priority and should be planned according to the needs and requirements of the particular community.
6. Compulsory immunization to all female children. Record of complete immunization should be an essential requirement along with birth certificate during school admission which will help to increase the immunization status of the children.
7. Stress on health status and problems of female child during home visits by the community health nurse to avoid negligence on care of female child by the family.
8. Revision, simplification and implementation of child labor act and laws pertaining to exploitation of children especially girls in regards to sexual exploitation.
9. Motivation for adoption of female child especially handicapped one needs to be stressed. Mass adoption should be promoted by voluntary organization.
10. Job opportunities for handicapped and socially deprived girls should be arranged by government and nongovernment agencies.

With the implementation of these practical action plan, status of the girl child can be improved to reduce the incidence of gender bias.

FEMALE FETICIDE

Female feticide is a challenging social problem related to gender bias especially in India. It is an important issue of discrimination against the girl child which begins even before birth. Ultrasonography and amniocentesis facilities during pregnancy help to detect the sex of the unborn fetus. These diagnostic interventions are actually performed in pregnancy to assess the fetal wellbeing and to detect the presence of congenital anomalies in the fetus. But presently these diagnostic procedures indirectly promote the practice of prenatal sex determination and termination of pregnancy with female fetus by abortion. This practice is observed in all socioeconomic groups, as an affinity to male child or son-complex. It is also influenced by dowry system and fear of sexual victimization of girl child. Outcome of this practice results in reduction of number of females to male, i.e. female to male ratio in the society (940:1000 in 2010 in India). In some state of our country, number of females is less than 800 for 1000 males. Ultimately this problem may disturb the total social structure and cultural harmony.

There is legal ban on sex determination tests during pregnancy. Prenatal diagnostic technique (Regulation and prevention of misuse) Act 1994 came into force from January 1996. In spite of legislation till this evil practice is present in our society and allowing more gender gap. Public awareness about gender discrimination and prevention of female feticide are the most significant approach to reduce this evil practice from the society.

CHILD ABUSE AND NEGLECT (CAN)

The exploitation and maltreatment of children are age old event. The broader concept of child abuse, which also includes battering, is of recent origin by the caring professions.

Child abuse includes physical violence (75%), sexual molestations (20%), mental and emotional (5%) maltreatment with negligence, deprivation and lack of opportunity. The children are abused at home, school, day care centers and working places by the care takers and other adults. Neglect is evident as chronic failure to protect the child from physical danger and to provide the loving care and needs.

The factors responsible for child abuse are poverty, overcrowding in the family, mental illness, alcohol or drug abuse, crisis situations and violence. Disturbances in the family are main causes which include arrival of more valuable child, unwanted pregnancy, single parent, immature parent, angry frustrated parent and parents who were abused in their childhood. The children, who are abused, mostly due to negative behavior, temper tantrum, bed wetting, habitual crying, mental subnormality and who are working as child labor.

The consequences of child abuse are physical injury, malnutrition, lack of hygienic care, growth failure or non-organic failure to thrive due to lack of emotional stimulation and foods, behavioral problems, mental retardation, rape, sexual injury and even death.

Child abuse may be found in the form of 'battered baby syndrome'. It is a clinical condition in young children especially below 3 years of age, who have received non-accidental injury wholly inexcusable violence or injury, on one or more occasions, including minimal as well as severe fatal trauma, by the hand of an adult, in a position of trust generally a parent, guardian or foster parent. In addition to physical injury there may be deprivation of nutrition, routine care, love and affection. Battered baby syndrome has been found in all social groups with risk of mental and neurological complications. It results from excessive anger or an attempt to teach discipline to the children by parents or other adults. It can represent as burns, bruises, belt or stick marks, multiple trauma or fracture, failure to thrive, cerebral palsy and emotional deprivation. These children need hospitalization and psychotherapy for both parents and child.

The term 'maternal deprivation' is used for emotional abuse and neglect to denote circumstances during which an infant is deprived of the opportunity of forming an initial tie with a mother figure. It also implies deprivation of the mother figure after a meaningful tie has been formed. Deprivation of mothering may also occur without physical separation whenever the mother is emotionally or physically incapable of providing continuity of loving care and security for the child. The damaging effects of prolonged lack of adequate mothering are inappropriate motor, intellectual, emotional and social development, as the infancy is a critical period of psychosocial and intellectual maturation.

Management of child abuse should be done depending upon type of injury. Hospitalization may be necessary and psychotherapy may be needed for parents and child. Abused child may need to be kept away from home, permanently or temporarily, if the parents are dangerously aggressive. Prevention of child abuse can be possible by supportive home visits by community health nurse or social worker and increasing legal help against child abuse. Other measures for prevention of child abuse are mothercraft training, increasing awareness about child rearing practices and educating people about acceptance of children at sufficient mature age to be an adequate parents.

NATIONAL HEALTH PROGRAMS FOR CHILDREN IN INDIA

Various national health programs are currently in operation for the improvement of child health and prevention of childhood diseases. The brief lists of these programs are:

- Reproductive and Child Health Program
- Universal Immunization Program
- Intensified Pulse Polio Immunization Campaign and Pulse Polio Immunization Program
- Integrated Child Development Services Scheme
- School Health Program
- Integrated Management of Neonatal and Childhood Illnes (IMNCI)
- Nutritional program, e.g.
  - Mid-day Meal Program
  - Special Nutrition Program
  - Nutritional Blindness Prevention Program.

Beside these, there are other several national health programs which directly and indirectly promote child health along with other members of the community.

Those programs include:
- National Tuberculosis Control Program
- National Leprosy Eradication Program
- National Antimalaria Program
- Kala-azar Control Program
- National AIDS Control Program
- National STD Control Program
- National Surveillance Program for Communicable Diseases
- National Iodine Deficiency Disorders Control Program
- National Mental Health Program
- National Cancer Control Program
- National Diabetes Control Program
- National Water Supply and Sanitation Program
- Diarrheal Disease Control Program
- Minimum Need Program
- National Vector Borne Disease Control Program
- National Rural Health Mission
- Millennium Development Goals.

NURSING RESPONSIBILITIES IN PREVENTIVE PEDIATRICS

Pediatric nurse has a unique opportunity to work with parents and children in the family and community to provide good environment and adequate facilities to promote health and prevent childhood illness to attain their fullest potentials. Preventive care is better render by nurses by health assessment, health education, health counseling, anticipatory guidance, direct nursing care and referral.

Nursing responsibilities in preventive care of children begins with promotion of care of girl child and continues in prenatal, neonatal and childhood period till adolescence. Nurse should follow steps of nursing process, i.e. assessment, nursing diagnosis, planning, implementation and evaluation while providing care to children to attain, maintain and restore health.

The nursing responsibilities in preventive pediatrics can be summarized as follows:
- Creating awareness about the care of girl child and promotion of health of girls, the future mothers.
- Appropriate care of antenatal mothers to have healthy children and provision of mothercraft training.
- Adequate intranatal care to reduce perinatal hazards and neonatal problems.
- Promoting breastfeeding practices and providing essential care during neonatal period.
- Preventing vaccine-preventable diseases by improving immunization coverage following appropriate techniques.
- Nutrition education about weaning, balanced diet, feeding practices, food hygiene, prevention of malnutrition, etc.
- Health education and counseling on personal hygiene, hand washing practices, environmental sanitation, safe water, prevention of accidents, promotion of mental health and reproductive health, prevention of communicable diseases, and family planning.
- Promoting community hygiene by use of latrines, burning or burying household refuses, keeping the sources and supply of water safe and clean.
- Prompt and adequate care of sick and injured child in comprehensive approach.
- Promoting self-care abilities of children and parents in preventive measures.
- Health supervision at regular interval for early interventions of childhood illnesses.
- Participating in the implementation of health programs and promoting the preventive activities for improvement of child health.
- Promoting beneficial traditional child rearing practices for prevention of childhood illnesses.
- Involving family and improving community participation in promotion of child health and prevention of childhood diseases.
- Participating and contributing in the planning of child health programs.

Immunization 4

- Vaccine Preventable Diseases
- Immunizing Agents
- National Immunization Schedule
- Immunization of Children
- Cold Chain
- Nursing Responsibilities for Child Immunization

INTRODUCTION

Immunization is a process of protecting an individual from a disease through introduction of live, or killed or attenuated organisms in the individual system. It is one of the 'best buys' in community health and one of the most cost-effective health interventions. Immunization against vaccine-preventable diseases is essential to reduce the child mortality, morbidity and handicapped conditions. It is mass means of protecting the largest number of people from various diseases. It gives resistance to an infectious diseases by producing or augmenting the immunity. Artificially acquired immunity is developed by the immunization.

Immunity is the security against a particular disease and nonsusceptibility to the invasive or pathogenic effects of foreign microorganisms or to the toxic effect of antigenic substances. Acquired immunity can be active or passive.

Active immunity is produced by stimulating immunological defence mechanism through administration of antigen usually prior to natural exposure to infection. Active immunizing agents are known as vaccines.

Passive immunity is produced temporarily by supplying preformed exogenous animal or human antibody to suppress the disease, given soon after or prior to exposure of an infection. It is readymade antibodies. Passive immunity agents are antisera and immunoglobulins.

VACCINE PREVENTABLE DISEASES

Some infectious diseases can be prevented by vaccines. The diseases against which vaccines are currently available:
a. *Six-killer vaccine preventable diseases,* i.e. Poliomyelitis, Tuberculosis, Diphtheria, Pertussis, Tetanus and Measles.
b. *Other vaccine preventable diseases* include Hepatitis 'B', Mumps, Rubella, Hemophilus influenzae type B (Hib) infections, Typhoid, Meningococcal meningitis, Japanese encephalitis, Influenza, Pneumococcal pneumonia, Chickenpox, Rotavirus diarrhea, Yellow fever, Cholera, Malaria, Hepatitis 'A', Plague and Rabies.

IMMUNIZING AGENTS

The immunizing agents may be classified as vaccines, immunoglobulins and antisera.

Vaccines

Vaccines are immunobiological substances which produce specific protection against a given disease. It stimulates active production of protective antibody and other immune mechanisms. Vaccines are prepared from live attenuated organisms, or inactivated or killed organisms, extracted cellular fractions, toxoids or combination of these. More recent preparations are sub-unit vaccines and recombinant vaccines.

The ideal vaccines should induce permanent immunity, be free of toxic substances, have minimal side effects, not produce disease to the recipient and be easy to administer.

The following immunizing agents are currently used:

Live Attenuated Vaccines

- Bacterial—BCG, Typhoid (oral), Plague.
- Viral—Oral polio, Measles, Mumps, Rubella, Yellow fever, Influenza.
- Rickettsial—Epi. typhus.

Killed or Inactivated Vaccines

- Bacterial—Pertussis, Typhoid, Cholera, Plague, CS meningitis.
- Viral—Rabies, Hepatitis 'B', Influenza, Salk polio, Japanese encephalitis.

Toxoids	— Bacterial-Diphtheria and Tetanus.
Cellular fractions	— Meningococcal and pneumococcal vaccines.
Combinations	— DPT (Diphtheria, Pertussis, Tetanus)
	— MMR (Mumps, Measles, Rubella)
	— DT (Diphtheria, Tetanus)
	— Hib-Hep. B (*H. influenzae* 'B', Hepatitis 'B')

Immunoglobulins

The human immunoglobulin (Ig) system is composed of 5 major classes (IgG, IgM, IgA, IgD and IgE) and subclasses within them. The various classes and subclasses of Igs represent different functional groups that are required to meet different types of antigenic challenges. All antibodies are immunoglobulins, but it is still an open question whether all immunoglobulins are antibodies. The WHO recommends that the term "gamma globulin" should not be used as a synonym for "immunoglobulin".

Two types of immunoglobulin preparations are available for passive immunization. These are normal human immunoglobulin and specific (hyperimmune) human immunoglobulin. They are used in the prophylaxis of viral and bacterial infections and in replacement of antibodies in immunodeficient patients. The available human immunoglobulins are:

- Normal Human Ig—Hepatitis 'A', Measles, Rabies, Tetanus and Mumps.
- Specific Human Ig—Hepatitis 'B', Varicella and Diphtheria.

Antisera or Antitoxins

The term 'antisera' is applied to the materials prepared in animals. Originally passive immunity was achieved by the administration of antisera or antitoxins prepared from nonhuman sources like horses. Human Ig preparations exist only for a small number of diseases. Administration of antisera may have adverse effects like serum sickness and anaphylactic shock due to abnormal sensitivity of the recipient. The current trend is to use the immunoglobulins whenever possible. The important antisera which are still used for passive immunization are:

- Bacterial—Diphtheria, Tetanus, Gas gangrene, Botulism.
- Viral—Rabies.

NATIONAL IMMUNIZATION SCHEDULE

Immunization schedule should be planned according to the needs of the community. It should be relevant with existing community health problems. It must be effective, feasible and acceptable by the community. Every country has its own immunization schedule.

The WHO, launched global immunization program in 1974, known as Expanded Program on Immunization (EPI) to protect all children of the world against six killer diseases. In India, EPI was launched in January 1978.

The EPI is now renamed as Universal Child Immunization, as per declaration sponsored by UNICEF. In India, it is called as Universal Immunization Program (UIP) and was launched in 1985, November, for the universal coverage of immunization to the eligible population.

The Global Alliance for Vaccines and Immunization (GAVI) is worldwide coalition of organization, established in 1999, to reduce disparities in life-saving vaccine access and increase global immunization coverage. GAVI is collaborative mission of Govt., NGOs, UNICEF, WHO and World Bank. The GAVI and Vaccine Fund also adopted the objective of new introduction but under used vaccines in the developing countries, where the diseases like hepatitis-B and *H. influenzae* 'B' (Hib) are highly prevalent.

National Immunization Schedule as recommended by Government of India for uniform implementation throughout the country was formulated. It is shown in Table 4.1. The schedule contents the age at which the vaccines are best given and the number of doses recommended for each vaccine. The schedule also covers immunization of women during pregnancy against tetanus.

Note:
i. Interval between 2 doses should not be less than one month.
ii. Minor cough, colds and mild fever or diarrhea are not a contraindication to vaccination.
iii. In some states hepatitis 'B' vaccine is given as routine immunization.
iv. At 9 months of age, vitamin 'A' oil should be given orally with recommended dose and then to be continued at six months interval upto 5 years of age.

Table 4.1 National immunization schedule

Beneficiaries	Age	Vaccine	Dose	Route	Amount
Infants	At birth (for institutional deliveries)	BCG	Single	Intradermal	0.05 mL
		OPV	Zero dose	Oral	2 drops
		Hepatitis-B-0	Birth dose	Intramuscular	0.5 mL
	At 6 weeks	BCG (if not given at birth)	Single	Intradermal	0.1 mL
		DPT-1	1st	Intramuscular	0.5 mL
		OPV-1	1st	Oral	2 drops
		Hepatitis B-1	1st	Intramuscular	0.5 mL
	At 10 weeks	DPT-2	2nd	Intramuscular	0.5 mL
		OPV-2	2nd	Oral	2 drops
		Hepatitis B-2	2nd	Intramuscular	0.5 mL
	At 14 weeks	DPT-3	3rd	Intramuscular	0.5 mL
		OPV-3	3rd	Oral	2 drops
		Hepatitis B-3	3rd	Intramuscular	0.5 mL
	At 9 months	Measles	Single	Subcutaneous	0.5 mL
Children	At 16–24 months	DPT	Booster	Intramuscular	0.5 mL
		OPV	Booster	Oral	2 drops
	At 5–6 years	DT	Single Intramuscular 0.5 mL (*Note:* Second dose of DT should be given after 4 weeks, if not vaccinated previously with DPT)		
	At 10–16 years	TT	Single Intramuscular 0.5 mL (*Note:* Second dose of TT should be given if not vaccinated previously)		
Pregnant women	Early in pregnancy	TT-1	1st	Intramuscular	0.5 mL
	One month after	TT-2	2nd	Intramuscular	0.5 mL

v. Measles "Booster dose" is now recommended in children at the age of 16 to 24 months.

vi. Interruption of the schedule with a delay between doses not interfere with the final immunity achieved. There is no basis for the mistaken belief, that if a second or third dose in an immunization is delayed, the immunization schedule must be started all over again. So, if the child missed a dose, the whole schedule need not be repeated again.

IMMUNIZATION OF CHILDREN

BCG Vaccination

Bacillus Calmette-Guérin (BCG) vaccine is live attenuated bacterial vaccine produced from "Dannish-1331" strain of tubercle bacilli. It produces active immunity to protect the child from tuberculosis. The aim of BCG vaccination is to induce benign artificial primary infection which will stimulate an acquired resistance to possible subsequent infection with virulent tubercle bacilli and thus reduce the morbidity and mortality from primary tuberculosis among risk group.

The presently available and used BCG vaccine is heat stable and in freeze dried form. It should be kept away from direct light and stored in a cool environment below 10°C (2–8°C). Normal saline is recommended as a diluent for reconstituting the vaccine. The reconstituted vaccine may be used up within 3 hours and then the left over vaccine should be discarded.

The BCG vaccine is administered at birth in institutional deliveries or as soon as possible after birth, or at 6 weeks, if not given at birth. The standard site is the middle of deltoid muscle over the left upper arm, i.e. just above the insertion of the deltoid muscle. If it is injected too high, too forward or too backward, the adjacent lymph nodes may become involved and tender. The vaccine is given using a special tuberculin syringe in intradermal route. The dose is 0.05 mL in neonates and 0.1 mL in infants. A satisfactory injection should produce a wheel of 5 mm in diameter. The vaccine must not be contaminated with an antiseptic or detergent. If alcohol is used to swab the skin, it must be allowed to evaporate before the vaccine is injected.

Following BCG vaccination, a papule appears in 2 to 3 weeks at the site of correct intradermal injection of a potent vaccine. In 4 to 5 weeks, the papule grows in size and then subsides or breaks into a shallow ulcer. It may be open or covered with a crust. The ulcer heals in 8 to 12 weeks leaving a small scar.

Complications following this vaccination are uncommon or may be mild. Deep ulceration, local abscess formation, enlargement of axillary lymph glands, osteomyelitis, keloid formation over the injection site may develop.

BCG immunization is contraindicated if the child is suffering from generalized eczema, infective dermatosis, hypogammaglobulinemia, immunodeficiency conditions and HIV infected children with symptoms of AIDS related complex (ARC) or AIDS. All asymptomatic HIV infected children should receive the BCG vaccine.

The duration of protection is about 15 to 20 years. BCG vaccination is a fundamental component of National Tuberculosis Program and plays a valuable role in preventing severe form of childhood tuberculosis.

Polio Vaccination

Oral polio vaccine (OPV) was first described by Sabin in 1957. It contains live attenuated polio virus of three strains (types-1, 2 and 3). It is administered as trivalent (TOPV) vaccine. The recently available OPV is heat stabilized and can be kept without losing potency at 4°C for a year and for a month at room temperature. The nonstabilized vaccine should be stored at –20°C in a deep freeze. The OPV is cheaper, easy to administer, protects the individual child from poliomyelitis and prevents spread of wild pathogenic poliovirus in the community. It induces both humoral and intestinal immunity. The OPV is very safe vaccine without any adverse effects. Rare cases of vaccine associated paralytic polio may occur (one case per million vaccinated child). Vaccine potency can be effectively monitors using vaccine vial monitiors (VVM).

OPV is administered with 'zero' dose at birth in institutional deliveries and then 3 doses at one month interval from 6 weeks of age (6 weeks, 10 weeks and 14 weeks). OPV can be given with DPT and BCG at the same time and same day. The dose is two drops or as stated on the label of the vial and given orally. It is very important to complete primary course of OPV within 6 months. Because most polio cases occurs between 6 months and 3 years. One booster dose is recommended at 16 to 24 months of age.

The contraindications for the administration of OPV include, acute infectious disease, fever, diarrhea, dysentry, leukemias, malignancy and corticosteroids therapy.

After vaccination, breastfeeding can be given, if the child is hungry, but hot drinks, hot milk or hot water should be withheld for 1/2 hour. The OPV should be administered in cool room in the clinic rather than hot, humid and crowded room and the OPV vial should be kept on ice pack.

The problems with OPV are instability of the vaccine at high ambient temperature and frequent vaccine failure even with fully potent vaccines. Failure of 3 dose regimen has been reported and indicates a serious problem. In order to overcome this problem 5 doses of OPV is recommended by Indian Academy of pediatrics in clinic-based programs and 3 doses in community campaigns.

Inactivated (killed) polio vaccine developed by Salk administered in IM or SC route is expensive and produce short lived immunity which is not recommended in National Immunization Schedule.

Govt. of India, conducted Pulse Polio Immunization (PPI) campaigns towards the goal of eradication of poliomyelitis. The first round of PPI consisting two immunization days was started in 1995 targeting all children under 3 years of age irrespective of immunization status. Later on, as recommended by WHO, it was decided to increase the age from under 3 years to under 5 years. In PPIs extra doses of OPV is administered to all children below 5 years of age on fixed date in whole country. The term 'pulse' has been used to describe the sudden simultaneous mass administration of OPV on a single day. The OPV is given regardless to previous immunization during low transmission season of polio, i.e. November to February. Children should receive all their schedule doses of OPV and PPI doses. There is no minimum interval between PPI doses and scheduled OPV doses.

In India, NIDs (National Immunization Days) for PPI have become the largest public health campaigns ever conducted in a single country. The 1st day of NIDs/SNIDs (sub-NIDs) were booth based while on 2nd and 3rd days house to house search was made for missed children to vaccinate them to accomplish 100 percent immunization of eligible children. 'Mopping up' activities are usually the last stage of polio eradication. The strategy of mopping up involves door to door immunization in high-risk areas where wild poliovirus is known or suspected to be still circulating. All strategies for polio eradication in India are now implementing to achieve the goal in near soon.

DPT Vaccination

The DPT is a combined vaccine administered for the protection against three diseases, i.e. diphtheria, pertussis and tetanus. DPT vaccine is composed of diphtheria toxoid, tetanus toxoid and killed *B. pertussis* bacilli. The potency of diphtheria toxoid is enhanced by the pertussis component of DPT vaccine.

There are two types of DPT vaccine, i.e. plain and adsorbed. Adsorption is usually carried out on a mineral carrier like aluminum phosphate or hydroxide. Adsorption increases the immunological effectiveness of the vaccine. The WHO recommends that only adjuvant DPT vaccine to be utilized in immunization programs. The plain DPT vaccine can be used as a booster.

The DPT/DT vaccines should be stored between 4°C and 8°C temperature and should not be frozen. The vaccines will lose potency if kept at room temperature over a longer period of time.

For primary immunization, DPT vaccine is administered in 3 doses at 4 weeks interval at 6 weeks, 10 weeks and 14 weeks of age. Each dose is 0.5 mL and should be given deep intramuscularly as all vaccines contain mineral carriers or adjuvant. The site of injection for children below one year of age should be lateral aspect of thigh (vastus lateralis muscle). In older children, it may be given in upper and outer quadrant of the gluteal muscle.

The DPT vaccine may be given concurrently with OPV. BCG can be given on the same time along with DPT, but the site for the injection should be different.

The booster dose of DPT vaccine is given at 16 to 24 months of age followed by another booster dose of DT (Diphtheria, Tetanus) vaccine at the age of 5 to 6 years, without pertussis component.

The DPT vaccination usually not recommended after 6 years of age. So children above the age of 5 years, who received the primary course of DPT vaccine earlier, should receive only DT as booster at 5 to 6 years and those who have not received DPT, need only two dose of DT vaccines at 4 weeks interval.

Following DPT vaccination mild reactions are common. In 2 to 6 percent vaccines, mild fever (about 39°C) may develop and in 5 to 10 percent cases have swelling, or induration and pain occur for 48 hours. The most severe complications following DPT vaccination are neurological problems like encephalitis, encephalopathy, prolonged convulsions, infantile spasms and Reye's syndrome. These problems are thought to be due to the pertussis component of the vaccine.

The DPT vaccination is contraindicated in progressive neurological problems and with severe reactions of first dose DPT (i.e. shock like state, temperature above 40°C, persistent crying episodes, and convulsions). Subsequent immunization with DT only is recommended without pertussis component. Local reaction at the site of injection and mild fever do not prevent the administration of DPT. Minor ailments like cough, cold and mild fever are not contraindications of this vaccination, but seriously ill hospitalized children with these symptoms should not be immunized with DPT.

For immunizing children over 12 years of age and adults, the preparation of choice is DT, which is an adult type diphtheria-tetanus vaccine with 2 doses at an interval of 4 to 6 weeks followed by a booster, 6 to 12 months after the second dose.

Measles Vaccination

Measles vaccine is live attenuated and tissue culture vaccine, available as freeze dried product. It is safe and effective. Heat stable measles vaccine and its diluting fluid should be stored at 2 to 8°C temperature to maintain their potency.

The measles vaccine is administered at the age of 9 months, before this age maternal antibody protects the infants. Single dose of vaccine is given with 0.5 mL amount in subcutaneous route. The freeze dried vaccine should be reconstituted with diluting fluid and must be kept on ice and to be used within one hour. Left over vaccine must be discarded and never used after 4 hours of opening the vial. Previously no booster dose was recommended as the immunity usually appears for long duration. But presently, booster dose of measles vaccine is recommended at the age of 16–24 months.

After the measles vaccination, reactions may develop as fever and rash on 5 to 10 days after immunization and induces a mild measles illness but in reduced frequency and severity. This may found in 15 to 20 percent of vaccines. The fever may persist for 1 to 2 days and the rash for 1 to 3 days. Severe reactions may develop following this vaccination if the recommended temperature is not maintained; and necessary precautions are not followed. Toxic shock syndrome (TSS) may develop with contaminated vaccine or if the same vial is used for more than one session on the same day or next day. The features of TSS are severe watery diarrhea, vomiting and high fever which usually develop within few hours of measles vaccination. This condition may cause death within 48 hours and case fatality rates are high.

Measles vaccine is contraindicated in infants below 6 months of age, acute illness, convulsions, allergy, active tuberculosis, malnutrition, immunodeficiency states, malignancy and immunosuppressive therapy (steroids, antimetabolites, etc.).

Measles vaccine can be combined and effectively administered with other live attenuated vaccines such as mumps and rubella. MMR vaccine can be given at the age of 15 months, 3 months following primary measles vaccination. MMR vaccine is not included in National Immunization Schedule.

Hepatitis 'B' Vaccination

Hepatitis 'B' vaccination is now included in the immunization schedule, in some states of India, as routine vaccine. But due to economical constraints, it is not included as seventh vaccine, in the National Immunization Schedule.

Hepatitis 'B' vaccines are available in two forms: (a) plasma derived vaccine and (b) RDNA yeast derived vaccine.

Plasma derived vaccine is based on the surface antigen (HBs Ag) which is harvested and purified from plasma of human carriers of hepatitis 'B' virus. It is formalin inactivated subunit viral vaccine. Each 1 mL dose of the vaccine contains

20 mcg of hepatitis surface antigen formulated in an alum adjuvant. The vaccine is safe, effective and cheapest.

The hepatitis 'B' vaccine is given intramuscularly with the 3 doses in general at 0, 1 and 6 months or 4 doses at 0, 1, 2 and 12 months in highly endemic area. The dose of the vaccine is 0.5 mL for the child below 10 years and 1 mL above 10 years at the same time interval. Antibody response attained after 3 doses. Immunity levels provide protection for about 3 to 5 years. Booster doses may be administered after 3 to 5 years.

Hepatitis 'B' vaccine is given for pre-exposure and post-exposure prophylaxis. Examples of postexposure prophylaxis are protection of neonates born to carrier mothers and individuals accidentally exposed parenterally to HBV infection through transfusion, cuts, injuries and needle sticks.

High risk children for HBV infections should be immunized with hepatitis 'B' vaccine, e.g. repeated and multiple blood transfusion, (in case of thalassemia, hemophilia), hemodialysis, IV (intravenous) drug users, sexual contact with carriers of HBV, etc.

RDNA or recombinant DNA yeast derived vaccine is an alternate vaccine against hepatitis 'B'. It is a genetically engineered vaccine, safe, effective as the plasma derived vaccine and is more cost-effective. It can be given to the new born and children with one-half of adult dose. Protection appears to be excellent even up to 9 years and booster reimmunization is not routinely recommended.

Typhoid Vaccination

Immunization against typhoid does not give 100 percent protection, but it reduces the incidence and severity of infections. It can be given at any age after one year. Typhoid vaccine is not now included in National Immunization Schedule. It is recommended to the risk group (school-children, hospital staff), travellers, residents of endemic areas and mela or yatra attendance.

The available injectable typhoid vaccines are: (a) monovalent antityphoid vaccine, (b) bivalent antityphoid vaccine and (c) TAB vaccine.

Monovalent vaccine is prepared from killed *S. typhi*, as phenol-preserved vaccine and AKD (acetone killed and dried) antityphoid vaccine. Bivalent vaccine contains *S. typhi* and *S. paratyphi* 'A'. The traditional TAB vaccine contained *S. typhi, S. paratyphi* 'A' and *S. paratyphi* 'B'. The WHO recommended that the TAB vaccine should be discontinued.

Primary immunization with antityphoid vaccine should consist of 2 doses to subcutaneous injections, each dose of 0.5 mL, at 4 to 6 weeks interval. The children between 1 and 10 years required smaller dose with 0.25 mL. Immunity develops in 10 to 21 days after inoculation and gives protection for about 3 years. So booster dose is needed in every 3 years. This vaccines should be stored at 2 to 4°C temperature and should not be frozen.

Following typhoid vaccination, local reactions occur as pain, swelling and tenderness at injection site. General symptoms like malaise, headache and fever may occur and usually subside within 36 hours.

Recently *oral typhoid vaccines* (Typhoral) are available as safe and highly immunogenic. It is developed from live attenuated strains of *S. typhi. S. typhi*, Ty 21a is developed by swiss scientists and 541 Ty, by US scientists.

The Ty 21a vaccine is used in more than 50 countries including India. It is recommended for the children above 6 years of age and adults. One capsule of Typhoral is given on alternate days, 1, 3 and 5, irrespective of age, one hour before meal with cold milk or water. It gives protection for 3 years and required booster doses (same 3 doses) once every three years. The vaccine should be protected from light and stored at 2 to 8°C. This vaccine should not be given in immunodeficiency states, immunosuppressive therapy, acute febrile illness, acute intestinal infections and with antimalarial therapy.

Other Available Vaccines

Rabies Vaccines

Rabies or hydrophobia is a fatal disease and transmitted through bite of the infected animal. Incubation period of the disease is long, so postexposure prophylaxis is possible. There are three types of rabies vaccines available for vaccination, i.e.
1. Cell-culture vaccines
   - Human diploid cell (HDC) vaccines.
   - Purified chick embryo cell (PCEC) vaccines.
2. Duck embryo vaccines (DEV)
3. Older conventional, nervous tissue vaccines (NTV) derived from sheep brain or from suckling mouse brain.

The HDC and PCEC vaccines are effective and safe, but they are costly. These vaccines are recommended as subcutaneous or intramuscular injections on 0, 3, 7, 14 and 30 days for 5 doses and a booster dose on 90 days. These cell culture rabies vaccines can also be given for pre-exposure prophylaxis. DEV is not available in India.

The old NTV is cheaper but having high risk of neuroparalytic reactions. This old antirabies vaccine is administered in a dose of 1 or 2 mL for 14 days over abdominal wall or as prescribed depending upon the severity of bite exposure.

Haemophilus Influenzae Vaccines

H. influenzae type 'B' (Hib) is an important cause of meningitis and pheumonia among children below five years of age. At present several Hib vaccines are available which are safe and effective. The WHO recommends inclusion of Hib vaccine in routine infant immunization programs.

At least four conjugated polysaccharide Hib vaccines are available. Any one of these can be used. Hib vaccine is also available in combination with DPT as 'DPT-Hib' and with DPT and hepatitis 'B' as 'DPT-HB-Hib'.

Routinely, Hib vaccine can be given at the age of 2 months and second dose after 8 weeks along with DPT vaccine. A booster dose is recommended at 12 to 18 months of age. The dose is 1.5 mL and given in intramuscular route with no known adverse reactions or absolute contraindications except hypersensitivity to the vaccine.

When Hib immunization has not been started by the 7 months of age, only 2 doses are given and only one dose is given to unimmunized children of aged 15 months or more. For the children more than 5 years of age this vaccine is indicated in immune disorder or after splenectomy.

Combined DPT-HB Vaccines

The combined DPT and hepatitis 'B' vaccines are now available to protect from four disease. It is cost-effective, reduced numbers of visit for immunization and has better coverage. It can be given as primary immunization during first 6 months of age with three doses (0.5 mL each dose), intramuscularly at 4 to 6 weeks interval.

Combined DPT-HB-Hib Vaccines

The combined DPT-HB-Hib vaccines protect from five infections in one vaccination. It can be given as 3 dose primary course at 2–4–6 months or 1.5–3–5 months of age.

Hepatitis 'A' Vaccines

Several inactivated and live attenuated vaccines against hepatitis 'A' have been developed. The dose, age and time of the vaccination vary from one manufacturer to other. No vaccine is licensed for children below one year of age. A combined vaccine of inactivated hepatitis 'A' and recombinant hepatitis 'B' vaccine has been licensed.

Varicella Vaccines

Varicella vaccine is live attenuated vaccine for the protection against chickenpox. It is safe, well-tolerated but expensive. It is recommended as single dose with 0.5 mL subcutaneously for all age group. Another type of varicella vaccine can be administered as single dose for the children one year to 12 years and above 13 years as two doses at 6 to 10 weeks interval. If the vaccine is administered within 3 days of exposure to a case of chickenpox, it provides 80 to 90 percent protection.

Influenza Vaccines

Influenza vaccine is prepared from killed virus for protection against influenza type 'A' and type 'B' infections. It can be administered subcutaneously with 0.2 mL of an oily emulsion preparation or 1.0 mL of saline preparation as single dose. It should not be given during acute febrile illness. The vaccine is recommended for children older than 6 months. Previously unimmunized children should receive 2 doses at 4 weeks interval. Live attenuated vaccines and other newer vaccines for influenza are under trial.

Rotavirus Vaccine

Rotavirus is most common cause of severe diarrhea in infants. Now a tetravalent rhesus rota viral vaccine (RRV-TV) is available for protection of children below 2 years of age. It is recommended as oral vaccine of 3 doses at an interval of 4 weeks for the infants 6 to 26 weeks of age. No serious adverse effects have been observed.

Cholera Vaccine

Cholera vaccine is whole cell killed vaccine, available for parenteral administration having poor protectivety (approximately 50%), which lasts for only 3 to 6 months. The available cholera vaccine is administered by subcutaneous injection with two doses at 4 to 6 weeks interval. The dose is 0.2 mL for children below 2 years and 0.3 mL above two years. This vaccination may cause reactions like local pain, erythema, edema and abscess. Research for developing an improved and more potent oral cholera vaccine is in progress.

Mumps Vaccine

Mumps vaccine is a live-attenuated viral vaccine and gives long immunity with protective value of 75 to 90 percent. It is usually available, combined with measles and rubella vaccines as MMR, a trivalent vaccine. Mumps or MMR vaccine may be given after 12 to 15 months of age in subcutaneous route. Mumps vaccine is safe and effective.

Rubella Vaccine

Rubella vaccine is also a live attenuated viral vaccine protects against the occurrence of congenital rubella syndrome in offspring. The vaccine is administered to girls between one year of age and puberty. It can also be given to susceptible women of child bearing age provided they are not already pregnant and conception is unlikely in the subsequent 2 months. The dose is 0.5 mL subcutaneously, as single administration. The recommended minimum age is 12 to 15 months, only after maternal antibodies have disappeared.

The adverse reactions after rubella vaccine are transient skin rash, lymphadenopathy and arthralgia, which are usually self-limiting. The vaccine is contraindicated in pregnancy and immunosuppression.

The combined MMR vaccine (Mumps, Measles, Rubella) is now gaining popularity for economical advantage as well as for convenience.

Pneumococcal Vaccine

Currently available polyvalent pneumococcal vaccine can protect children from infections caused by *Streptococcus pneumoniae* resulting pneumonia, meningitis, otitis media, bacteremia, etc. The protection efficacy is about 60 percent. The vaccines are not immunogenic in children below 2 years of age. It is indicated in children above 2 years of age and having nephrotic syndrome, chronic renal failure, immunosuppressive conditions, malignancy, HIV infection, splenectomy, etc. The vaccine is given intramuscular or subcutaneously with 0.5 mL amount. Revaccination is recommended for children less than 10 years of age and are at high risk of severe pneumococcal infection. It is given after 3 to 5 years of primary immunization. The adverse reactions may found as anaphylaxis, local painful swelling, fever, GB syndrome, etc.

Meningococcal Vaccine

A quadrivalent vaccine is available of *Neisseria meningitidis* from subgroups A, C, Y and W135. Routine vaccination against meningococcal disease is not recommended. It is indicated during epidemics for all contacts and for high risk children with asplenia and complement deficiencies. During an outbreak of this infection, close contact cases must be protected with chemoprophylaxis also.

The vaccine is administered deep subcutaneously in single dose of 0.5 mL, in children older than two years of age. Second dose is needed after one year if the first dose is given between 2 and 4 years of age. When first dose is given after 4 years of age, than next dose should be administered only after another 5 years. The vaccine may have some adverse reactions like local tenderness, edema and fever.

Japanese Encephalitis Vaccines

Japanese encephalitis (JE) is an important viral disease causing fatal condition in children. Vaccination against JE is significant preventive measure as the specific drugs are not available for treatment.

At present three types of JE vaccines are available, i.e. mouse brain derived and inactivated viral vaccine, cell-culture derived inactivated vaccine and live attenuated vaccine.

The mouse brain derived JE vaccine is available internationally and stable at 4°C for at least one year. The vaccine is administered in 2 doses subcutaneously, with 0.5 mL amount to the children of 1 to 3 years age and with 1.0 mL for above 3 years age, at interval of 1 to 2 weeks. The 3rd dose can be given after 6 months and booster

dose every 3 to 4 years. Protective efficacy is about 90 to 95 percent. It is indicated in epidemics and endemics of JE and contraindicated in high fever, diabetes mellitus, liver and heart disease and immunodeficiency states. Live attenuated and cell culture vaccines are used in China.

COLD CHAIN

The 'cold chain' is a system of storage, transport and distribution of vaccines in the state of efficacy and potency at recommended temperature from the manufacturer to the actual recipient of the vaccine. The failure of cold chain system may lead to ineffective protection against the vaccine preventable diseases. Maintenance of cold chain is the corner stone for the success of immunization program.

All vaccines must be stored, transported and distributed at the recommended temperature by the manufacturer in the literature accompanying the vaccine, otherwise they may become denatured and totally *ineffective* with loss of potency. For successful cold chain system, three elements are essential, i.e. cold chain equipment, transportation system and motivation and training of the workers for maintenance of cold chain link.

Among all vaccines, polio is the most heat sensitive, requiring storage at –20°C. Polio and measles vaccines must be stored in the freezer compartment. DPT, DT, TT, BCG, Typhoid and diluents of vaccines must be stored in the cold part and never allowed to freeze. Vaccines must be protected from sunlight and contact of antiseptic. At the health centers, most vaccines, except polio, can be stored at 4 to 8°C for 5 weeks. Multidose opened vial, which is not used fully must be discarded, within one hour, if no preservative is present. It should be discarded within 3 hours or at the end of a session when preservative is used. Necessary instruction for the particular vaccine must be followed regarding maintenance of required temperature. Instruction for maintenance of vaccine vial monitor (VVM) especially for oral polio vaccine should be followed strictly.

Cold Chain Equipment

The cold chain equipments consist the following:

Walk in Cold Rooms

In the regional level, vaccines are stored for 4 to 5 districts in the walk in cold rooms (WIC), at recommended temperature upto 3 months.

Deep Freezers

Deep freezer is a top opening cold chain equipment and available as 300 liters or 140 liters capacity. Big deep freezer

(300 ltr) is supplied to all districts and the WIC locations along with ice lined refrigerators (ILR). Deep freezers are used for making ice packs and for storing polio and measles vaccines. A pair of deep freezer and ILR is connected to a common voltage stabilizer. Small deep freezers (140 liter) along with ILR are supplied to PHCs, urban family planning centers and postpartum centers.

Ice Lined Refrigerators

Ice lined refrigerators (ILR) is top opening refrigerator. Two types of ILR are available, one with ice tubes (electrolux) and other with ice packs (vest frost) as the ice lining. The bottom of the ILR is the coldest part. DPT, DT, TT and diluents should not be kept directly on the floor of the ILR as they can freeze and get denatured. These vaccines should be kept in the basket provided within the ILR. Temperature of the ILR should be recorded twice a day with the dial thermometer which should be kept inside the ILR, even if there is an in built thermometer. Defrosting should be done at regular interval with alternative arrangement of storing the vaccines. During electric supply failure or equipment failure, vaccines should be transferred to cold boxes and then to alternate storage.

Deep freezer and ILR should be kept in cool room, away from direct sunlight and at least 10 cm away from the wall. They will be kept in levelled and to be fixed through voltage stabilizer. The vaccines should be kept inside the ILR neatly with space in between for air circulation. The ILR should be kept locked and open only when necessary. Do not keep any object on the deep freezer or ILR. Never store any other drugs, drinking water, foods or date expired vaccines or more than one month requirements at PHC level and do not open these equipment unless required.

Cold Boxes

Cold boxes are available at all peripheral health centers. They are used for transporting vaccines and also for storing vaccines during failure of electric supply. Fully frozen ice packs are placed at the bottom and sides of the cold box before placing the vaccines in it. The vaccines should be first packed in cartons or polythene bags, then to be kept inside the cold box. DPT, DT, TT vaccines and diluents should not be kept in direct contact with the frozen ice packs.

Vaccine Carriers

Vaccine carriers are used to carry 16 to 20 vials of vaccines to out-reach sites to the subcenters, village, vaccination clinic or camp. Four fully frozen ice packs are placed for lining the sides of the carriers. DPT, DT, TT and diluents should not be placed in direct contact of frozen ice packs. The carrier must be closed tightly.

Day Carriers

Day carriers are used for nearby areas and only for few hours period with two fully frozen ice packs. It is used to carry small quantities of vaccines, i.e. 6 to 8 vials only.

Ice Packs

Ice packs are used for cold boxes and vaccine carriers. It is prepared in the deep freezer. Ice pack contains water, filled upto the level marked on the side. No salt is added to it. Leak ice pack should not be used.

At present, household refrigerator and flask are not recommended as cold chain equipment. Cold chain failure is commonly observed at subcenter and village level. So vaccines are not stored at subcenters and supplied for the day of use only. Nurses, especially the community health nurses have to play major role in maintaining cold chain to protect the potency of vaccines. Successful implementation of immunization program depends upon maintenance of vaccine potency at the delivery end of actual vaccination site.

NURSING RESPONSIBILITIES FOR CHILD IMMUNIZATION

Nursing personnel are mostly responsible for administration of immunization and its related activities. In collaboration with other health team members, the nursing personnel should shoulder the responsibility to organize the immunization sessions and to ensure the achievement of universal immunization. Administration of vaccines are the main assignment but other related activities are also vital for success of immunization program. The nursing responsibilities at various levels can be summarized as follows:

- Motivation of general people about the importance of immunization and its benefits.
- Estimation of beneficiaries of the area and identification of nonparticipants and dropouts of immunization.
- Assessment of problems and reasons for nonacceptance of immunization and intervening to solve the problems.
- Information, health education and communication about the immunization session, time, place, available vaccines and other health facilities related to immunization.
- Organization of immunization clinics at different health institutions, immunization camps, out-reach and home-based services.
- Arrangement and maintenance of required amount of vaccines and other necessary equipment and materials for the particular immunization center or clinic.
- Maintenance of cold chain system at immunization center or during transportation of vaccines to home or clinics with necessary precautions to preserve the efficacy and potency of the vaccines. Care of cold chain equipment and maintenance of recommended temperature for vaccines

are crucial aspects of the success of immunization program.

- Administration of vaccines are important responsibilities of the nurses at all levels of health care. Nurse should follow the basic nursing skills of aseptic techniques and check the vaccine vials or ampules. Reconstitution of vaccines should be done according to particular instructions with specific diluents. Selection of proper site, positioning of the child, maintenance of six-rights and steps of medication should be followed. Instruction of the vaccine manufacturer or physicians' directions or standing orders should be noticed and kept in mind during vaccination.
- Observation of possible reactions after vaccination and providing necessary instructions, about the care of the child following immunization, to the parent and family members.
- Information about the next date of visit to complete the immunization as per schedule and dangers of default.
- Maintenance of immunization card with required information and next date of visit.
- Maintenance of clinic records, registers, stocks, number of attendance for vaccination, vaccine used, etc.
- Reporting about immunization coverage and problems of the particular area.
- Participating in research activities and new approaches related to immunization program.
- Updating own knowledge and developing skill regarding advancement of immunization practices and changing attitudes.

Nutrition in Children

5

- Nutritional Requirements in Children
- Breastfeeding
- Complementary Feeding or Weaning
- Artificial Feeding
- Feeding Problems

- Balanced Diet for Children
- Assessment of Nutritional Status
- Nutritional Counseling and Guidance
- National Nutritional Policy
- National Programs on Nutrition

INTRODUCTION

Balanced and sufficient nutritional intake is most essential for children to promote optimal growth and development, to protect and maintain health, to prevent nutritional deficiency conditions and various illness and to reserve for starvation and dietary stress.

The word nutrition is derived from the word 'nutricus' which means to suckle at the breast. Nutrition is defined as combination of dynamic process by which the consumed food is utilized for nourishment and structural and functional efficiency of every cell of the body. It is the science of food and its relationship to health.

The term food refers to anything which nourishes the body. It includes solids, semisolids and liquids which can be consumed and which help to sustain the body and keep it healthy. Food and nutrition are different and having different meaning. Food is defined as what one feeds on and is a composite mixture of many nutrient substances ranging from a fraction of a gram in some cases to hundred of grams in others. Food stuff is defined as anything which can be used for food.

Foods can be classified by chemical composition as proteins, fats, carbohydrates, vitamins and minerals. They can be of animal origin or vegetable origin. On the basis of nutritive value, foods are broadly classified as cereals and millets, pulses, nuts and oilseeds, vegetables, fruits, milk and milk products, animal or flesh foods, fats and oils, sugar and jaggery, condiments and spices and miscellaneous foods. The functions of foods are mainly, bodybuilding, energy-giving and protection by maintenance and regulation of tissue functions.

Nutrients are organic and inorganic complexes contained in food. Each nutrient has specific functions in the body. Most natural foods contain more than one nutrient. There are about 50 different nutrients which are normally supplied through the foods we eat. Nutrients can be grouped as macronutrients and micronutrients. Macronutrients are proteins, fats, carbohydrates, which form main bulk of food and micronutrients are vitamins and minerals, which are required in small amounts.

NUTRITIONAL REQUIREMENTS IN CHILDREN

Nutritional requirements may vary from one individual to others and depends upon metabolic and genetic difference. No single food meets all the essential requirements for children except mother's milk, which provides all nutritional substances to the infant till 6 months of age. Afterwards healthy dietary habits depends upon cultural and social influence and contribute to personal and social enjoyment. So, to fulfil the nutritional requirements, child's diet should be planned by the parents and family members with different types of food items to provide balanced and nutritious diet. The child's diet should contain sufficient amount of fluids, calories, proteins, fats, carbohydrates, vitamins, minerals and salts to meet their daily nutritional needs. Food items should be digestible, palatable, attractive, choiceable and easily available. Nutritional requirements should be maintained with margin of safety and with right balance. A deficit or excess in nutrients could be harmful and should be avoided. The 'recommended daily intake' of nutrients with sufficient amounts to be provided to maintain needs of the body and good health.

Water

Water is most important for maintenance of life. It constitutes about 70 percent of body weight in children. The total water content of the body is comparatively higher in infants than in adults. Water is required for digestion, metabolism, renal excretion, temperature regulation, transportation of cellular substances, maintenance of fluid volume and growth of children.

The daily requirements of water is fulfilled by fluid intake, food and oxidation processes in the body. Water is absorbed throughout the intestinal tract. The balance of water depends on the protein and electrolyte intake, solute load, metabolic and respiratory rates and body temperature. Evaporation from the lungs and skin accounts for 40 to 50 percent water loss and 3 to 10 percent by fecal loss. The kidneys maintain the water and electrolyte balance by varying amount and concentration of urine. Excess loss of water can cause dehydration whereas an excess intake can result in water intoxication. Loss of water or dehydration is an important cause of death in children even than starvation. Water intoxication may found as edema, circulatory failure, abdominal distress or convulsions.

Daily requirements of water in different age group are given in Table 5.1.

Calories

The energy value of foods is measured in terms of 'large' calorie or kilocalorie. The production of energy varies during the oxidation of different foods. Children required more calories per kg of body weight than adults. Calorie requirements gradually decrease from infancy to adulthood. The average energy expenditure is 50 percent in basal metabolism 12 percent in growth, 25 percent for physical activity, 8 percent in fecal loss and 5 percent for specific dynamic action.

The calorie requirements of children depend upon body size and surface area, rate of growth, level of physical activity, food habits and climate. In a balanced diet, 50 percent of

Table 5.1 Daily requirements of water and calories

Age range	Water requirements (mL/kg)	Calorie requirements (cal/kg)
First 3 days	80–100	120
3–10 days	125–150	120
15 days to 3 months	140–160	120
3–12 months	150	105–115 (110)
1–3 years	125	100
4–6 years	100	90
7–9 years	75	80
10–12 years	50	70
13–15 years	50	60
16–19 years	50	50
Adult	50	40

calories is provided by carbohydrates, 15 percent by proteins and 35 percent by fat. Deficiency of calorie intake leads to loss of weight, growth failure and protein-energy malnutrition. An excess intake of calorie results in increased weight gain and obesity.

Daily requirements of calories in different age of children are given in Table 5.1.

Proteins

Proteins are essential for synthesis of body tissues in growth, and during maintenance and repair. They help in the formation of digestive juices, hormones, plasma proteins, enzymes, hemoglobin and immunoglobulins. They are needed for maintenance of osmotic pressure and acid base equilibrium. Proteins also act as source of energy, when the calorie intake is inadequate. Excess proteins, which are not used for building tissues or providing energy, converted by the liver into fat and stored in body tissues.

Proteins are made up of simpler substances called amino acids. There are 24 amino acids to be needed by the human body, of which '9' are called, essential amino acids, because the body cannot synthesize them in amounts of their need and therefore must be supplied in the diet. Both essential and nonessential amino acids are required for synthesis of tissue proteins.

Proteins are obtained from two main dietary sources, i.e. animal origin and vegetable origin. Proteins of animal sources are biologically complete protein with all essential amino acids and more easily digestible. Proteins of vegetable sources are incomplete and lack of one or more amino acids. The combination of vegetable proteins may provide all the essential amino acids. This is the reason that vegetarian diet

Table 5.2 Recommended protein allowances

Group	Age	Protein allowance g/kg/day	g/day
Infants	0–3 months	2.3 (milk protein)	-
	3–6 months	1.8 (milk protein)	-
	6–9 months	1.65 (mixed protein)	-
	9–12 months	1.5 (mixed protein)	-
Children	1–3 years	1.83	22.0
	4–6 years	1.52	30.0
	7–9 years	1.48	41.0
Adolescents	Males		
	10–12 years	1.46	54.0
	13–15 years	1.40	70.0
	16–18 years	1.31	78.0
	Females		
	10–12 years	1.45	57.0
	13–15 years	1.33	65.0
	16–18 years	1.21	63.0

should have mixing of 3 to 4 types of pulses or combination of wheat and legumes.

Protein requirements depends upon the age, sex, physical and physiological factors. It is maximum in neonates and early infancy but gradually decreases as age increases. Extra amount of protein should be provided during illness to compensate the destruction or degeneration of body tissue, e.g. in blood loss, surgery, etc. Deficiency of protein intake result in growth failure and protein-energy malnutrition.

The recommended daily protein allowance according to the ICMR is given in Table 5.2.

Carbohydrates

Carbohydrates are main source of energy and supply bulk in the diet. They contribute taste and texture of foods. They are essential for digestion and absorption of other foods.

Adequate carbohydrate intake in diet allow the use of protein for tissue synthesis, otherwise protein is also used for energy production and fat is metabolized with production of ketone bodies. Excess carbohydrates are stored in the liver and muscle. Carbohydrates play an important part in infant nutrition as they spare proteins to be fully utilized for growth and various repair processes.

Carbohydrates are consumed as monosaccharides (glucose, fructose, galactose), disaccharides (lactose, sucrose, maltose, isomaltose) and polysaccharides (starch, dextrin, glycogen, gum, fibers, cellulose). All carbohydrates are ultimately oxidized and converts to glucose. Glucose is used as fuel by brain and muscle or converted to glycogen and stored in liver and muscle. Excess carbohydrates are converted to fat.

The source of carbohydrate of infant's diet is in the form of lactose found in both human and cow's milk that should be provided up to 6 months. Afterwards cereals, legumes, fruits, tubers, pulses and vegetables are the main sources.

Lack of adequate carbohydrate intake may produce symptoms of starvation, undernutrition, constipation, fatigue, loss of body protein, ketosis, depression and carbohydrate malnutrition.

Excess carbohydrate in diet may lead to obesity, ischemic heart disease, cataract and dental caries in case of concentrated sugar intake.

Fats

Fat supplies 40 to 50 percent energy needed for infant. It provides protection and support for organs and insulation of the body as adipose tissue. It acts as carriers of fat soluble vitamins and components of cells and tissue. Fats and oils are concentrated sources of energy and make the foods palatable.

Fats are solid at 20°C and oils are liquid at that temperature. Fats and oils are termed as lipids. Lipids are classified as simple, compound and derived.

Simple lipids are monoglycerides, diglycerides and triglycerides, which are combination of glycerol and fatty acids. Compound lipids are combination of simple lipids with nonlipid substance such as glycolipids, phospholipids and lipoproteins. Derived lipids are produced during breakdown of simple and compound lipids, i.e. cholesterol and steroid hormones.

Fats are available from both animal and vegetable sources. About 98 percent of neutral fats are triglycerides and other two percent include free fatty acids, monoglycerides, diglycerides, cholesterol and phospholipids. Fatty acids are divided into saturated and unsaturated fatty acids, which are further divided in monounsaturated and polyunsaturated fatty acids.

Polyunsaturated fatty acids are mostly available in vegetable oils and the saturated fatty acids available in the animal oils. Exceptionally, fish oils contain poly- and monounsaturated fatty acids whereas coconut and palm oils have extremely high percentage of saturated fatty acids.

Essential fatty acids are those that cannot be synthesized in the human body and should be derived only from food. The most essential fatty acid is linoleic acid, which is abundantly available in vegetable oils. It helps in maintenance of good health.

Saturated fat should not be more than 10 percent of total fat intake. Cholesterol intake should be limited though it is essential for good health and synthesized in the body. It is found only is animal foods.

More fat intake in diet may results in indigestion as it remains longer in the stomach. Excess fat intake leads to excess accumulation of adipose tissue, obesity, NIDDM, cancer, artherosclerosis and hypertension.

Deficiency of all essential fatty acids may result in growth retardation, phrenoderma and skin disorders, susceptibility to infections, neurological and visual problems and decreased myocardial contractility.

The ICMR has recommended a daily fat intake of 25 g/day in young children and 22 g/day in older children. Total fat intake should provide not more than 20 to 30 percent of daily energy intake and at least 50 percent of fat intake should consist of vegetable oils rich in essential fatty acids.

Vitamins

Vitamins are organic substances and essential micronutrients for maintenance of normal health. They are available in many foods in small amounts. Since the body is generally unable to synthesize them sufficiently, they must be provided through diet. Balanced diet supplies all the vitamins needed for a healthy individual.

Vitamins act as cofactor in many enzyme systems and essential for energy production, hemopoiesis, reproduction, neurological functions, hydroxylation and synthesis of fats, amino acids, nucleic acids and nucleoprotein. They enable the body to use other nutrients and help in maintenance and protection of good health.

Vitamins are classified into two groups, i.e. fat soluble and water soluble vitamins. Fat solubles vitamins are vitamin A, vitamin D, vitamin E and vitamin K. They are stored in body fat and needed only in minimal amount in daily diet. Excess intake of these may produce toxic effects. The water soluble vitamins are vitamin B and vitamin C. They are not stored in the body and required in adequate amount in daily diet to prevent deficiency conditions. Water soluble vitamins are easily destroyed during food processing, preparation and storage. Each vitamin has a specific function to perform and deficiency of any particular vitamin may result in specific deficiency disease.

The vitamin requirements of the individual child may vary with the activity, age, body weight and the amount of calories consumed and the amount of carbohydrates in the diet. They may vary in certain physiological and pathological conditions.

Many factors are responsible for the vitamin deficiency conditions. They include poor dietary intake, faulty absorption, increased loss in chronic diarrhea, greater demand during fever, infections and metabolic diseases and poor utilization in chronic liver diseases.

Vitamin requirements is more in preterm babies. Infants get adequate vitamins from mother during lactation. Dietary intake of vitamins may be low or marginal during infancy and childhood. The minimum intake for the maintenance of health in respect of many of the vitamins has been determined. The daily requirement of some vitamins are given in Table 5.3.

Minerals

Minerals are inorganic elements, required by human body for growth, repair and regulations of vital body functions. They acts as catalysts in biochemical reactions. More than 50 minerals are found in the human body, all of which must be derived from foods. A well-balanced diet supplies a sufficient quantities of minerals.

Minerals are required for maintenance of osmotic pressure, supply of necessary electrolytes for the actions of muscles and nerves and for hemopoiesis.

Table 5.3 Recommended dietary allowance of vitamins

Age group	Vitamin 'A' Retinol	Corotene	Vitamin B$_1$	Vitamin B$_2$	Nicotinic acid	Pyridoxin	Vitamin 'C'	Folic acid	Vitamin B$_{12}$	Vitamin D
Birth to 6 months	350 mg	1200 mg	55 mcg/kg	65 mcg/kg	710 mcg/kg	0.1 mg	25 mg	25 mg	0.2 mcg	200 IU
6–12 months	350 mg	1200 mg	50 mcg/kg	60 mcg/kg	650 mcg/kg	0.4 mg	25 mg	25 mg	0.2 mcg	200 IU
1–3 years	400 mg	1600 mg	0.6 mg	0.7 mg	8 mg	0.9 mg	40 mg	30 mg	0.2–1 mg	200 IU
4–6 years	400 mg	1600 mg	0.9 mg	1 mg	11 mg	0.9 mg	40 mg	40 mg	0.2–1 mg	200 IU
7–9 years	600 mg	2400 mg	1 mg	1.2 mg	13 mg	1.6 mg	40 mg	60 mg	0.2–1 mg	200 IU
10–12 years	600 mg	2400 mg	1.1 mg	1.3 mg	15 mg	1.6 mg	40 mg	70 mg	0.2–1 mg	200 IU
13–15 years	600 mg	2400 mg	1.2 mg	1.5 mg	16 mg	2 mg	40 mg	100 mg	0.2–1 mg	200 IU
16–18 years	600 mg	2400 mg	1.3 mg	1.6 mg	17 mg	2 mg	40 mg	100 mg	0.2–1 mg	200 IU

Minerals are classified as macrominerals when the daily requirement is 100 mg or more and as microminerals when less than 100 mg is required daily.

Macrominerals are calcium, phosphorus, sodium, potassium and magnesium. Microminerals or trace elements required by the body in quantities of less than few mg per day and include iron, iodine, fluorine, zinc, copper, cobalt, chromium, manganese, molybdenum, selenium, nickel, silicon, etc. There are some trace elements or contaminants found in the human body, whose functions are not known. These include lead, mercury, barium, boron and aluminum.

Only a few mineral elements are associated with clearly recognizable clinical conditions. They are mainly calcium, phosphorus, sodium, iron, iodine and fluorine. Trace elements deficiencies are uncommon. Minerals deficiencies are less among vegetarians than nonvegetarians. Adequate amount of protein in daily diet prevents minerals deficiencies.

The recommended intake of important minerals as dietary allowance given in Table 5.4.

The adequate knowledge, attitude and practice of application of nutritional requirement must be the basis of infant feeding. The health and nutritional status of an infant and subsequent growth and development through childhood depend upon successful feeding practices. The socioeconomic status and education of the mother and family members have been known to influence child's feeding behavior. Nutritional counseling is the important responsibility of the nurse to promote the nutritional status of the children and to prevent nutritional deficiency diseases.

BREASTFEEDING

Breastfeeding is the best natural feeding and breast milk is best milk. The basic food of infant is mother's milk. Breastfeeding is the most effective way to provide a baby with a caring environment and complete food. It meets the nutritional as well as emotional and psychological needs of the infant. But recently there is tendency to replace the natural means of infant feeding and introduction of breast milk substitutes. So breastfeeding deserves encouragement from all concerned in the welfare of children.

UNICEF stated that every year over one million infants die and millions of others are impaired, because they are not adequately breastfed. Every day between 3000 to 4000 infants die from diarrhea and acute respiratory infections because the ability to feed them adequately has been taken away from their mothers. Thousands more succumb to other illnesses and malnutrition. Breastfeeding is now an endangered practice around the world, in both rich and poor countries. There is unanimous agreement on the need for, and the route to, global support for breastfeeding through various approaches and programs. Baby Friendly Hospital Initiative is one of the important interventions towards that goal.

Advantages of Breastfeeding

Breastfeeding is safest, cheapest and best protective food for infants. Superiority of human milk is due to its superior nutritive and protective value. It is perfect food for infants and provides total nutrient requirements for the first six months of life. When combined with appropriate weaning foods, it is an invaluable source of nourishment until past the second birth day. It prevents malnutrition and allow the child to develop fully.

The advantages of breastfeeding are as follows:

Nutritive Value

- Breast milk contains all the nutrients in the right proportion which are needed for optimum growth and development of the baby up to 6 months.
- It is essential for brain growth of the infant because it has high percentage of lactose and galactose which are important components of galactocerebroside.
- It facilitates absorption of calcium which helps in bony growth.
- It contains amino acids like taurine and cysteine which are important as neurotransmitters.
- Breast milk fats are polyunsaturated fatty acids which are necessary for the myelination of the nervous system.

Table 5.4 Daily requirements of minerals

Mineral	Age-group	Requirement
• Iron	• Infant	• 1 mg/kg
	• 1–3 years	• 12 mg
	• 4–6 years	• 18 mg
	• 7–9 years	• 26 mg
	• 10–12 years	• Boys—34 mg
		• Girls—19 mg
	• 13–15 years	• Boys—41 mg
		• Girls—28 mg
	• 16–18 years	• Boys—50 mg
		• Girls—30 mg
• Calcium	• Infant	• 500 mg
	• 1–9 years	• 400 mg
	• 10–15 years	• 600 mg
	• 16–18 years	• 500 mg
• Iodine	–	0.2 mg
• Sodium	–	2 mEq/kg
• Potassium	–	1.5 mEq/kg
• Zinc	–	0.3 mg/kg
• Copper	–	0.05–1 mg/kg
• Fluorine	–	0.5–1 mg

- It has vitamins, minerals, electrolytes and water in the right proportion for the infant which are necessary for the maturation of the intestinal tract.
- It provides 66 calories per 100 mL and contains 1.2 g protein, 3.8 g fat, 7 g lactose and vitamin 'A' 170 to 670 IU, vitamin 'C' 2 to 6 mg, vitamin 'D' 2.2 IU, calcium 35 mg, phosphorus 15 mg in 100 mL. The total amount of milk secretion per day is about 600 to 700 mL, which is sufficient for the baby. Its composition is ideal for an infant.
- It provides specific nutrition for preterm baby in preterm delivery.

Digestibility

Breast milk is easily digestable. The protein of breast milk are mostly lactoalbumin and lactoglobulin which form a soft curds that is easy to digest. The enzyme lipase in the breast milk helps in the digestion of fats and provides free fatty acids.

Protective Value

Breast milk contains IgA, IgM, macrophages, lymphocytes, bifidus factors, unsaturated lactoferrin, lysozyme, complement and interferon. Thus breastfed body less likely to develop infections especially gastrointestinal and respiratory tract infections, e.g. diarrhea and ARI.

It also provides protection against malaria and various viral and bacterial infections like skin infections, septicemia, etc.

Breastfeeding protects the infant from allergy and bronchial asthma. It also protects against neonatal hypocalcemia, tetany, necrotizing enterocolitis, deficiencies of vitamin E and zinc, neonatal convulsions and sudden infant death syndrome.

Exclusive breastfeeding baby has less chance of developing malnutrition, hypertension, diabetes mellitus, coronary artery disease, arteriosclerosis, ulcerative colitis, appendicitis, childhood lymphoma, liver disease; celiac disease and dental caries.

Psychological Benefits

- Breastfeeding promotes close physical and emotional bondage with the mother by frequent skin to skin contact, attention and interaction. It stimulates psychomotor and social development. It leads to better parent child adjustment, fewer behavioral disorders in children and less risk of child abuse and neglect.
- Breastfeeding promotes development of higher intelligence and feeling of security in infant.

Maternal Benefits

- Breastfeeding reduces the chance of postpartum hemorrhage and helps in better uterine involution.

Lactational amenorrhea promotes in recovery of iron stores. It can protect from pregnancy for first 6 months if exclusive breastfeeding is carried out.

- Breastfeeding improves metabolic efficiency and satisfaction with sense of fulfillment of the mother.
- It reduces the risk of breast and ovarian cancer of the mother.
- It improves slimming of the mother by consuming extra fat which accumulated during pregnancy.
- It is more convenient and time saving for the mother. Mother can provide fresh, pure, readymade, clean uncontaminated milk to her baby at right temperature without any preparations. Mother feels comfortable to feed the baby especially at night.

Family and Community Benefits

- Breastfeeding is economical in terms of saving of money, time and energy.
- Family has to spend less on milk, health care and illness.
- Community expenditure on health care and contraception are reduced. It is economic for the families, hospitals, communities and for countries.

Preparation for Breastfeeding

Preparation for breastfeeding must begin in the antenatal period. The idea of breastfeeding can be introduced in childhood period and during school education about its importance. Mothercraft training should be provided and includes benefits of breastfeeding which should be given in the prepregnant stage.

In the antenatal period, examination of breast and identification of problems, like retracted nipple, should be done with necessary advice for interventions. Adequate diet in prenatal period should be consumed in terms of energy and nutrients. Prevention of micronutrient deficiencies, rest, regular exercise, hygienic measures, etc. should be advised for better health in antenatal period. Antenatal counseling, family support, mother-support group also should be emphasized as the preparation of mothers for breastfeeding. Mother should be psychologically prepare to feed her baby immediate after birth.

Study of anatomy of breast helps nursing personnel during breastfeeding counseling (Fig. 5.1).

Initiation of Breastfeeding

Breastfeeding should be initiated within first half an hour to one hour of birth or as soon as possible. It should also be initiated within one hour even after cesarean section delivery, if the mother and baby, both are having no problem. Early suckling provides warmth, security and 'colostrum', the

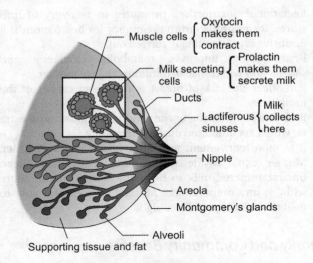

Fig. 5.1: Anatomy of the breast

baby's first immunization. Although little in amount, the first milk, colostrum, is most suitable and contains a high concentration of protein and other nutrients, the baby needs. It is rich in anti-infective factors and protects the baby from respiratory infections and diarrheal diseases.

Mothers should be demonstrated about the techniques of breastfeedings. Rooming-in or bedding-in should be done with infant and mother as soon as possible to prevent separation. Mother should be advised for exclusive breastfeeding up to 6 months and as demand feeding.

No food or drink other than breast milk should be given to neonates. No water, glucose water, animal milk, gripe water, indigenous medicines, vitamins and minerals drops or syrup should be given. No bottle and pacifier are allowed.

In case of preterm babies or sick babies, being in special care unit, they should be fed with expressed breast milk (EBM).

Nursing staff is responsible to ensure that nothing except breast milk is given. Mother should be instructed to assess the indicators of adequacy of breastfeeding and importance of increasing her own dietary intake with extra 550 cal and to drink fluids in response to her thirst. Rest and relaxation of mother are important for recovery from delivery and successful lactation in postnatal period.

Indicators of Adequacy of Breastfeeding

Adequacy of breastfeeding is indicated and established by the followings:

- Audible swallowing sound during the feed.
- Let down sensation in mother's breast.
- Breast is full before feed and softer afterward.
- Wet nappies 6 or more in 24 hours.

- Frequent soft bowel movements, 3 to 8 times in 24 hours.
- Average weight gain of 18 to 30 g/day.
- Baby sleeps well and does not cry frequently.
- Baby has good muscle tone and healthy skin.

Note: Passage of urine 6 to 8 times per day and average weight gain are considered as most important criterias.

Different Composition of Breast Milk

The composition of breast milk varies at different stages in the postnatal period to fulfil the needs of the baby.

Colostrum

It is secreted during first three days after delivery. It is thick, yellow and small in quantities. It contains more antibodies and cells with higher amount of proteins and fat soluble vitamin (A, D, E, K). It is sufficient and protective for the baby and should not be discarded.

Transitional Milk

It follows the colostrum and secretes during first two weeks of postnatal period. It has increased fat and sugar content and decreased protein and immunoglobulin content.

Mature Milk

It is secreted usually from 10 to 12 days after delivery. It is watery but contains all nutrients for optimal growth of the baby.

Preterm Milk

The breast milk secreted by a mother who has delivered a preterm baby is different from milk of a mother who has delivered a full term baby. This milk contains more proteins, sodium, iron, immunoglobulins and calories appropriate for the requirements of the preterm neonates.

Fore Milk

It is secreted at the starting of the regular breastfeeding. It is more watery to satisfy the baby's thirst and contains more proteins, sugar, vitamins and minerals.

Hind Milk

It is secreted towards the end of regular breastfeeding and contains more fat and energy. The mother should feed the baby allowing one breast to empty to provide both fore milk and hind milk, before offering other breast. For optimum growth and to fulfill adequate fluid and nutritional requirements, both fore milk and hind milk are needed for the baby.

Technique of Breastfeeding

Majority of mothers can feed their babies successfully. Some mothers need help in the technique of breastfeeding, specially the primi mother, mothers having breastfeeding problems in previous pregnancy, nonmotivated mothers about breastfeeding and the mother having retracted nipples. Nursing personnel should help the mother to follow the technique of breastfeeding as below:

- Mother should be comfortable and relaxed physically and mentally before giving breast feed. She should wash her hands and can have a glass of water or milk. Mother should have no due work in her hands. Baby should be cleaned and dried before feeding, otherwise baby may feel discomfort or may noncooperate during feeding.
- Correct positioning of mother and baby is an important aspect of successful breastfeeding. Mother can be in sitting or side lying position. Even mother can be lying flat with infant on top of the mother, especially following lower uterine cesarean section (LUCS) delivery. Baby should be supported by the mother's forearm in slight head elevated position and with head, neck and back in a straight line. Baby should be hold close to mother with trunk to trunk in touch and facing towards breast (Figs 5.2A to C).
- *Latching (Figs 5.3A and B):* After proper positioning, when baby's chin touches the breast, cheek touches the nipple, baby will open the mouth in 'rooting reflex'. Then the baby will be quickly move on to the breast with the lower lip below the nipple; so that the nipple and most of the areola go into the baby's mouth. The suckling of breast stimulates the 'milk secretion or prolactin reflex' (Fig. 5.4), which promotes the milk production and secretion. Then by the 'milk ejection or oxytocin reflex', (Fig. 5.5) milk flows out from the glands into the lactiferous sinuses and ducts and then to the baby's mouth. When

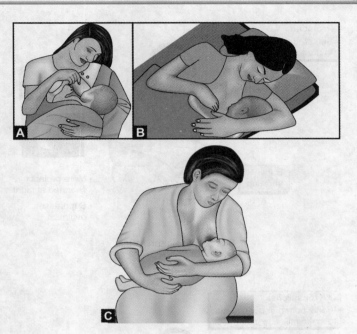

Figs 5.2A to C: (A and B) Positioning; (C) Correct positioning

baby suckles again and again in regular slow deep sucks with good 'sucking reflex', the adequate milk flows out and then baby's cheeks become full with milk. The mother may hear the swallowing sound and does not feel pain in the nipple. All these indicate favorable signs of good attachment or latching and breastfeeding. The baby should have good 'swallowing reflex' to take adequate feed with sufficient flow of milk. Baby's rooting, sucking and swallowing reflexes help the baby to take secreted milk from the breast successfully (Fig. 5.6). If the baby fall asleep after few sucks, mother should arouse the baby by gentle tap behind the ear or on the sole of the foot.

- Initially breastfeeding can be given at 1 to 2 hours interval and then on 'self-demand' by the baby. A baby usually cries when feel hungry and then must be put into the breast.

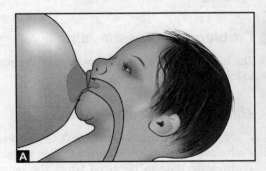
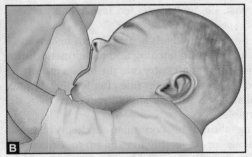

Figs 5.3A and B: (A) Latching; (B) Good attachment

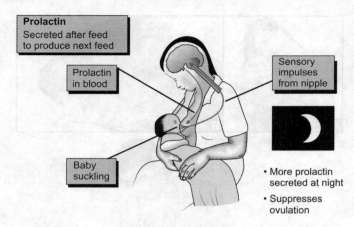

Fig. 5.4: Prolactin reflex

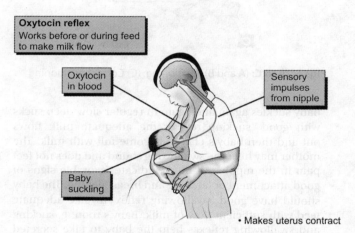

Fig. 5.5: Oxytocin reflex

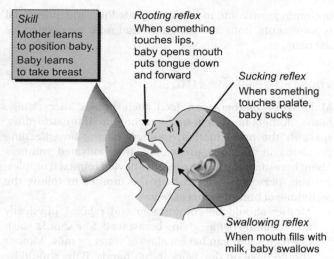

Fig. 5.6: Reflexes in the baby

- Duration of feeding should be continued till the baby is satisfied. The duration of sucking depends upon the vigour of the baby and on the 'let-down reflex'. One breast should be emptied completely before starting with another breast. Next feeding should be started with opposite breast, i.e. which was fed last in the previous feeding.
- Burping to be done gently. It is usually not necessary, if the baby is having good latching and attachment during feeding which prevent air entry into the baby's mouth.
- Baby should be placed on right side after feeding. Usually the baby falls asleep. Mother should make the baby dry and comfortable.
- Breastfeeding should be continued exclusively up to 4 months of age or preferably may be up to 6 months if adequate breast milk is available. The baby should be given only breast milk and nothing else, not even water for

first 4 months of life, even in summer months. Frequent suckling helps to have adequate amount of milk for the baby.
- Complementary foods can be started 6 months, exact age may vary, but breastfeeding should be continued up to 2 years of age or beyond and especially at night.
- Mother should maintain hygienic measures, take daily bath and wash her breast during bath and wear clean blouse during this period to prevent contamination of breast milk.

Contraindications of Breastfeeding

The true contraindications of breastfeeding are galactosemia and phenylketonuria. Maternal conditions which can be considered as 'REAL' contraindications are Radiotherapy, Ergot therapy, Antimetabolites therapy and Lithium therapy. Maternal illness should not result in interruption of breastfeeding. Expressed breast milk (EBM) can be given to the baby, whenever needed, from the mother or mother's substitute.

Problems of Breastfeeding

The measures to be taken to overcome the problems are as follows:

The Baby who does not Suckle

- No unneeded drugs to be given to breastfeeding mothers.
- No artificial food or water to be given to the baby.
- Breastfeeding to be given when the baby is alert and ready.

- Milk to be expressed into the nipple just prior to feed the baby.
- Nipple should be placed slightly upward towards the roof of the baby's mouth.
- Keeping the baby's nose free during breastfeeding.

The Baby who Refused on Breast

- Baby should be hold in comfortable position with good attachment to the breast and should be kept dry and warm.
- Avoiding pressure on potentially painful areas during feeding.
- Express breast milk to maintain lactation in both breast.
- Allowing the baby to feed only one breast.

Inverted Nipples

- Treatment should be started after birth of the baby.
- The nipple is manually stretched and rolled out several times a day.
- A pump or a plastic syringe (10 mL) is used to draw out the nipple and the baby is then put to the breast (Fig. 5.7). Precautions should be taken to prevent injury of breast and nipple during the traction with the syringe.

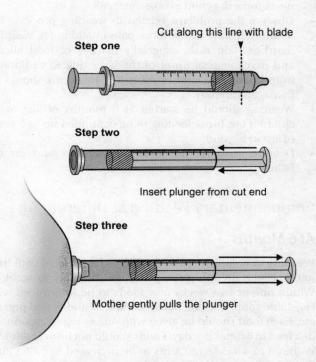

Fig. 5.7: Preparing and using a syringe for treatment of inverted nipples

Sore Nipple

- Correct positioning and latching of the baby to the breast.
- Frequent washing with soap and water should be avoided.
- Baby should not be pull off the breast while still sucking.
- Hind milk to be applied to the nipple after a feeding.
- Nipples should be aired and allowed to heal in between feeds.

Breast Engorgement

- Frequent feeding and correct attachment of the baby to the breast during feeding to be done to prevent engorgement.
- Treatment of this condition to be done with local warm packs and analgesics to the mother to relieve the pain.
- Milk should be expressed gently to soften the breast and then baby to be put to the breast with good latching.

Breast Abscess

- Treatment to be done with analgesics and antibiotics.
- Abscess may need incision and drainage.
- Breastfeeding must be continued.

Working Mother

- Mother should express her milk in a clean, wide mouthed container and this milk should be fed to her baby by the caretaker, in the absence of the mother.
- Express breast milk (EBM) can be stored at room temperature for 8 hours and in the refrigerator for 24 hours.
- EBM feeding should be given with cup/bati and spoon.
- Expression of milk should be done by hands which is more easier (Figs 5.8A and B).

Failure of Lactation

There are many factors which are responsible for failure of successful breastfeeding.

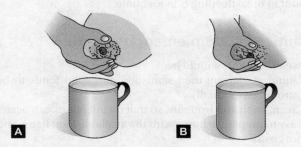

Figs 5.8A and B: Expression of breast milk: (A) Place the finger and thumb on the areola and press inward towards the chest wall; (B) Press the areola behind the nipple between the finger and thumb

- Prelacteal feeding, bottle feeding, incorrect technique of breastfeeding as poor attachment to breast and making the baby wait for breastfeeding or delayed feeding lessen the milk secretion.
- Medications like methergin or ergometrine, oral contraceptive also hinders the milk production.
- Maternal worry, anxiety, lack of interest, poor psychological bondage with baby, suppress the lactation and prevent successful lactation.
- Acute illness, chronic diseases, poor maternal health, breast engorgement, breast abscess, flat nipple, cracked nipple, sore nipple, painful breastfeeding inhibit the lactation.
- Faulty sucking, weak baby or sick baby are also important causes of lactation failure.
- Inadequate preparation for breastfeeding during antenatal care, mismanagement by elders in the family, advertisement of formula feeding or infant milk substitute, inadequate maternity leave for working mothers, are also contributing for lactation failure.

Most of the causes of lactation failure can be prevented by team approach and careful interventions to motivate the mother for breastfeeding and acceptance of the policy as stated by the Baby Friendly Hospital Initiative.

COMPLEMENTARY FEEDING OR WEANING

Breastfeeding alone is adequate and sufficient to maintain optimum growth and development of an infant up to the age of 6 months. It is therefore, necessary to introduce more concentrated energy riched nutritional supplements by this age. Infants also required iron containing food supplements after this age to prevent iron deficiency anemia.

Weaning or complementary feeding is the process of gradual and progressive transfer of the baby from the breastfeeding to the usual family diet. During this process the infant gets accustomed to foods other than mother's milk. Weaning does not mean discontinuity of breast feeding. Weaning foods are given in addition of breast feed when the amount of breastfeeding is inadequate.

Qualities of Complementary Foods

The weaning foods should be:
- Liquid at starting then semisolid and solid foods to be introduced gradually.
- Clean, fresh and hygienic, so that no infections can occur.
- Easy to prepare at home with the available food items and not costly.
- Easily digestible, easily acceptable and palatable for the infants.

- High in energy density and low in bulk viscosity and contains all nutrients necessary for the baby.
- Based on cultural practices and traditional beliefs.
- Well-balanced, nourishing and suitable for the infant.

Principles of Introduction of Weaning Foods

During introduction of weaning foods following principles to be remembered:
- Milk is the main food of infant, so additional feeds should provide extra requirements as per needs of the baby, that must be obtained from good quality food items and should be home made.
- A small amount of new foods to be given in the beginning and gradually the amount of food to be increased during the course of a week.
- New food to be placed over the tongue of the baby to get the taste of the food and to feel the consistency. The baby may spit the food out, but with patience the feed to be given again to get accustomed with it. A single weaning food is added at a time.
- Additional food can be given in the day time. Initially it can be given once, then twice or thrice.
- There should not be any strict rule for serving new foods, it may be modified. But the foods to be given regularly.
- New foods should be given when the infant is hungry, but never force the child to take the feeds.
- Observe the problems related to weaning process. The infant may have indigestion, pain in abdomen, weaning diarrhea, skin rash, especially in case of food allergy and psychological upset of the baby due to withdrawn from breast milk and sucking. The problems should be managed carefully.
- Weaning should be started at 6 months of age to all children but breastfeeding to be continued up to 2 years of age or beyond.
- Delayed weaning result in malnutrition and growth failure.

Complementary Feeding at Different Age

At 6 Months

Weaning or complementary feeding to be initiated with fruit juices, especially the grape juice, which is low in sorbitol. Within one or two weeks new foods to be introduced with vegetable soup, mashed banana, mashed and boiled potato, etc. Each food should be given with one or two teaspoons at first for 3 to 6 times per day. Foods should not be over diluted. Within 3 to 4 weeks amounts to be increased to half a cup. Breastfeeding must be continued.

6 to 9 Months

Food items to be given in this period include soft mixture of rice and dal, khichri, pulses, mashed and boiled potato, bread or roti soaked in milk or dal, mashed fruits like banana, mango, papaya, stewed apple, etc. Egg yolk can be given from 6 to 7 months onwards. Curd and khir can be introduced from 7 to 8 months onwards. By the age of 6 to 9 months the infant can enjoy to bite biscuits, piece of carrot and cucumber. The infant can have these foods 5 to 6 times per day and amount of food to be increased gradually. Breastfeeding should be continued.

9 to 12 Months

More variety of household foods can be added. New food items like fish, meat, chicken can be introduced during this period. The infant can eat everything cooked at home but spices and condiments to be avoided. Feeds need not to be mashed but should be soft and well-cooked. Breastfeeding to be continued.

12 to 18 Months

The child can take all food cooked in the family and needs half amount of mothers diet. Number of feeds can be 4 to 5 times or according to the child's need. Breastfeeding to be continued, especially at night.

The weaning period is most crucial period in child development. The appropriate weaning practices is an important aspect of child rearing and significant approach of preventive pediatrics towards healthy children.

ARTIFICIAL FEEDING

Artificial feeding means to feed the child other than breast milk. It involves the use of breast-milk-substitutes in the form of liquid milk, i.e. fresh cow's or buffalo's milk or commercially available dried whole milk. It is a form of supplementary feeding.

The main indications for artificial feeding are death or absence of mother, prolonged maternal illness and complete failure of breast milk production. Artificial feeding is given only, if there is no one available as mother surrogate to give breast feed to the infant or expressed breast milk is not available.

In spite of various attempts to promote the age old breastfeeding practices and superiority of human milk, today artificial feeding and bottle feeding are still in existence and practiced, where they are actually not needed.

The factors contributing to rising incidence of artificial feeding in India and other developing countries include: (a) lack of interest in breastfeeding by the health workers, mothers and family members, (b) wrong beliefs and ignorance related to breastfeeding, (c) increasing numbers of working mothers, (d) aping the Western countries, (e) changing lifestyle, (f) availability of alternatives to mothers milk, (g) urge to be sophisticated and (h) publicity and deceptively appealing advertisements.

The artificial feeding is a hazardous procedure in poor homes because of the dangers of contamination and over dilution of the feed. It is an expensive affair and having hazards as underfeeding, multiple nutritional deficiencies, gastroenteritis and other superadded infections. Long-term sequelae of exclusive artificial feeding include lactose intolerance, obesity, atherosclerosis, relatively poor learning abilities, poor parent-child relationship, frequent pregnancy, family disruption and population explosion.

Principles of Artificial Feeding

- The decision of giving artificial feeding must be taken after failure of all efforts to breastfeed the baby and non-availability of human milk.
- The aims of artificial feeding are similar to those of breastfeeding, i.e. it should (a) provide adequate nutrition to the infant, (b) be free from bacterial contamination, (c) be economical and (d) according to the needs of the child.
- The artificial feeding should be given by spoon and bowl or cup or glass. In sick and preterm infant, the feeding can be given with dropper and in hospitalized baby with orogastric or nasogastric tube.
- Bottle feeding must be avoided and mothers need explanation and information about the hazards of bottle feeding, especially about diarrhea, nipple confusion, etc.
- Strict cleanliness in the preparation and feeding procedure should be practiced. Milk left over from previous feed should not be used again.
- Feeding must be given with the calculated amount of fluid and calories according to the baby's expected weight. Actual weight may be less in malnourished child, so expected or average weight of the baby at the particular age should be considered to calculate the amount of feeds.
- Correct technique of feeding to be followed. The milk should be warm and not hot or cold.
- Time taken for feeds depends on the baby, but on an average 15 to 20 minutes may be needed to feed the total quantity, as required. Numbers of feeds can be 6 to 8 times in infant and 3 to 5 times in older babies or as needed by the child.
- Cow's milk is considered as cheaper alternative, which is well within the reach of many Indian families, which in fact is widely used for infant feeding as artificial feeds, other than human milk. Most health workers give very conflicting advice on the use of cow's milk for infant feeding. Some health care providers recommend undiluted cow's milk right from birth, forgetting the fact that human milk is made for human baby and cow's milk for the calf.

Most authorities in India and abroad including WHO have persistently recommended dilution of cow's milk during the first 2 months in order to reduce the solute load on neonatal kidneys. Afterwards undiluted boiled and cooled-warm milk should be given. Sugar can be added in diluted milk to provide required calories. Hygienic measures are very important.

- If dried milk is used, it should be reconstituted as per direction given by the manufacturer.
- During illness (e.g. fever) the calorie need is increased and it should be provided by frequent small quantity feeding.
- Burping may be needed to allow to push out the swallowed air and to prevent vomiting, abdominal discomfort and colic.
- Supplementation of vitamins and minerals may be needed for artificially fed babies to prevent deficiency conditions.

FEEDING PROBLEMS

Most infants have feeding problem as regurgitation, vomiting, suckling and swallowing difficulties, dehydration, fever, excessive crying, abdominal colic, underfeeding, overfeeding, change in bowel habits, etc.

Too little feed, too frequent feed, large amount feeding, wrong technique of feeding, bottle feeding, inexperienced mother are the responsible and prominent causes of feeding problems. These problems are preventable by simple measures.

Regurgitation

Regurgitation is a common problem related to infant feeding. It occurs as backward flowing of feeds from stomach along with swallowed air. It is also called as 'posseting'. In some babies, it becomes habit and they like to chew it (i.e. rumination). It is usually harmless unless the feeds are not inhaled.

The infant should be placed on right side after feeding and burping should be done by proper technique to remove the swallowed air. During feeding precautions to be taken to prevent excessive intake of air. The baby should not feed when crying.

Regurgitation of feeds need medical attention if the infant brings back the entire feeds and no weight gain is observed.

Vomiting

Vomiting may occur due to overfeeding, excessive swallowing of air, prolonged burping or may be due to pathological conditions like gastroenteritis, congenital pyloric stenosis, intestinal obstruction, etc.

The baby should be observed carefully to detect the cause. Faulty feeding technique can be corrected and pathological condition should be detected by specific investigations and management to be done accordingly.

Suckling and Swallowing Difficulties

Some neonates have suckling problem in first few days after birth. It may be normal in the process of adapting the breastfeeding technique. But the prolonged problem may be due to congenital malformations like cleft palate, cleft lip, large tongue, nasopharyngeal obstruction, choanal atresia, etc. This problem may be related to some conditions of the breast like cracked nipple, retracted nipple, big nipple, breast engorgement and breast abscess.

Preterm baby is more likely to have suckling and swallowing difficulties. Sick neonates, oral thrush, cardiac and respiratory diseases, neonatal jaundice and infections are among several causes related to these problems.

Careful assessment of the cause and specific management should be done quickly to prevent further complications and poor prognosis.

Dehydration Fever

Fever, drowsiness, lethargy and refusal of feed are common in neonates in first 3 to 4 days of life. It can be due to inadequate feeding or may be due to infections. The cause to be find out by details history and thorough examination. Mother should be advised to give breastfeeding frequently with patience to manage the dehydration. Antibiotics may be needed to treat the associated infection. Hygienic measures and adequate warmth to be maintained.

Excessive Crying

Excessive crying of the infant is usually related to hunger. It may be due to wet napkin, thirst, chilling, need for mothering, abdominal colic or any discomfort.

Mother should be made aware about the adequacy of breastfeeding and appropriate technique of it. Mother should take care of own diet to promote breast milk secretion. Other causes of crying should be detected and appropriate measures to be taken.

The infant may cry towards late afternoon or evening, especially in first three months of age and can be termed as 'three months colic' or 'evening colic'. It may be due to excessive intestinal activity. Mild antispasmodic therapy and prone position may help the infants to get relieve of the problem.

Underfeeding

Low breast milk production and early introduction of artificial feeding with highly diluted formula feed due to ignorance and economical problem are important causes of underfeeding and failure of weight gain. The infant may present with irritability, excessive crying and hunger.

Mother should be instructed to take measures for increasing breast milk production and appropriate technique of breastfeeding. Mother should offer both breasts at a feed and several times each. Feeding to be given frequently and longer, day and night, at least 10 to 12 times per day. Bottle feeding should be stopped. Mother should have increased amount of food and fluids with rest and relaxation. Locally available galactogogues or home-remedies to be used to increase milk secretion.

Overfeeding

Overfeeding is not a common problem in our country. But in affluent families and in overprotective mothers, the problem can be seen. Usually it is difficult to feed the infant forcibly and most infants refuse to take excess amount of feed. But some baby may have overfeeding which result in infantile obesity, excessive vomiting, fatty diarrhea, excessive crying, abdominal discomfort and emotional problem.

Mother and family members should be made aware about the problem. Required and calculated amount of feeds to be recommended according to the expected weight of the particular age of the child. Mother may need regular guidance from the health workers regarding infant feeding.

BALANCED DIET FOR CHILDREN

A balanced diet has become an accepted means to safeguard a population from nutritional deficiencies. It is defined as one which contains a variety of foods in such quantities and proportions that the need for energy, amino acids, vitamins, minerals, fats, carbohydrates and other nutrients are adequately met for maintaining health, vitality, and general well-being and also makes a small provision for extra nutrients to withstand short duration of leanness.

For planning a balanced diet, the following principles should be followed:

- At first, the daily requirement of protein to be met, i.e. 15 to 20 percent of the daily energy intake.
- Next, fat requirement should be limited to 20 to 30 percent of daily energy intake.
- Carbohydrates should constitute the remaining food energy and should contains natural fibers.
- Requirements of micronutrients should be met.
- Food habits, tastes, taboos, food culture, religion, economical capacity and climate should be considered during selection of food items.

Table 5.5 presents the balanced diets at low cost for children and adolescents.

Table 5.5 Balanced diets for children and adolescents

	Toddlers		Preschooler		School age children				Adolescents					
									Boys		Boys		Girls	
	1–3 years		4–6 years		7–9 years		10–12 years		13–15 years		16–18 years		13–18 years	
	Veg (g)	Non-veg (g)	Veg (g)	Non-veg (g)	Veg (g)	Non-veg (g)	Veg (g)	Non-veg (g)	Veg (g)	Non-veg (g)	Veg (g)	Non-veg (g)	Veg (g)	Non-veg (g)
Cereals	150	150	200	200	250	250	320	320	430	430	450	450	350	350
Pulses	50	40	60	50	70	60	70	60	70	50	70	50	70	50
Green leafy vegetables	50	50	75	75	75	75	100	100	100	100	100	100	150	150
Other vegetables, roots and tubers	30	30	50	50	50	50	75	75	150	150	175	175	150	150
Fruits	50	50	50	50	50	50	50	50	30	30	30	30	30	30
Milk	300	200	250	200	250	200	250	200	250	150	250	150	250	150
Fats and oils	20	20	25	25	30	30	35	35	35	40	45	50	35	40
Meat, fish and eggs	–	30	–	30	–	30	–	30	–	30	–	30	–	30
Sugar and jaggery	30	30	40	40	50	50	50	50	30	30	40	40	30	30
Roasted peanut	–	–	–	–	–	–	–	–	–	–	50	50	–	–

ASSESSMENT OF NUTRITIONAL STATUS

The nutritional status of an individual is influenced by the adequacy of food intake both in terms of quantity and quality and also by the physical health of the individual. The purpose of nutritional assessment is to detect nutritional problems and to develop the plan to meet the nutritional needs.

The assessment of nutritional status involves various techniques with different approaches. The assessment methods include: (a) dietary history, (b) clinical examination, (c) anthropometry, (d) biochemical evaluation, (e) functional assessment and (f) radiology.

Factors influencing the nutritional status like socio-economic factors, health care services, educational facilities and precipitating factors like parasitic, bacterial and viral infections also need to be assessed to have complete information regarding nutritional status.

Dietary History

The nutritional assessment must begin with dietary history. Detail information should be collected about the intake of food in terms of cereals, pulses, vegetables, fruits, milk, fish, eggs, oils, sugar, etc. Daily average consumption of proteins, calories and other nutrients should be estimated to assess the dietary inadequacies. Other than individual food consumption history, household dietary survey can also be done for direct assessment of food consumption.

Clinical Examination

It is the simplest and the most practical method for assessment of nutritional status of individuals. It is an essential aspect of nutritional assessment to detect the level of health status of the individual in relation to the food consumption. Head to toe examination should be performed to detect the signs of nutritional deficiency states such as hair changes, anemia, edema, xerosis, cheilosis, angular stomatitis, rachitic rosary, bleeding gums, dental caries, toad skin, enlarged thyroid gland, etc.

Anthropometry

Anthropometry is a very valuable index for evaluation of nutritional status. It includes measurement of height, weight, skinfold thickness, arm circumference, head circumference and chest circumference. These are valuable indicators of nutritional status as well as patterns of growth and development.

Biochemical Evaluation and Laboratory Tests

Biochemical tests include estimation of nutrients and their concentration in body fluids, assessment of enzyme level and detection of abnormal amount of metabolites. These tests are done for serum protein, serum retinol, serum iron, serum vitamins, urinary iodine, urinary creatinine, etc. Biochemical tests are time consuming and expensive and performed only in complicated conditions.

Laboratory investigations are done for the hemoglobin estimation, examination of stool for intestinal parasitosis, chronic dysentry, diarrhea, etc. and urine examination for sugar and albumin.

Functional Assessment

Functional indices of nutritional status are emerging as an important aspect of diagnostic tools. Some of these are—structural integrity of erythrocyte and capillary host defence, hemostasis, nerve function, work capacity of heart, vasopressor response and reproduction in later life.

Radiology

Radiology may help to detect retardation of bone age, osteoporosis, classical signs of scurvy or rickets which indicate the nutritional deficiency states.

A sample nutritional assessment schedule is given below:

Serial No :   Date :
Name   :   Age   :
Address   :   Sex   :
District   :   Village :
History - (Dietary and illness)

Clinical Assessment

1. General appearance : Normal built/thin built/sicky
2. Hair : Normal/lack of lustre/dyspigmented/thin and sparse/easily pluckable/flag sign
3. Face : Diffuse depigmentation/nasolabial dyssebacea/moon face
4. Eyes : Conjunctiva—normal/dry on exposure for ½ min/dry and wrinkled/Bitot's spots/brown pigmentation/angular conjunctivitis/pale conjunctiva, cornea—normal/dryness/hazy or opaque.
5. Lips : Normal/angular stomatitis/cheilosis
6. Tongue : Normal/pale and flabby/red and raw/fissured/geographic
7. Teeth : Mottled enamel/caries/attrition
8. Gums : Normal/spongy bleeding
9. Glands : Thyroid enlargement/parotid enlargement
10. Skin : Normal/dry and scaly/follicular hyperkeratosis/petechiae/pellagrous

		dermatosis/flanky paint dermatosis/ scrotal and vulval dermatosis
11.	Nails	: Koilonychia
12.	Edema	: In dependent parts
13.	Rachitic changes	: Knock-knees or bow legs/epiphyseal enlargement/beading of ribs/pigeon chest
14.	Internal systems	: Hepatomegaly/psychomotor change/ mental confusion/sensory loss/muscle wasting/motor weakness/loss of position/loss of vibration/dense/loss of ankle and knee jerks/calf tenderness/ cardiac enlargement/tachycardia

Anthropometric

Weight (kg) :

Head circumference (cm) :

Height (cm) :

Chest circumference (cm) :

Mid-upper-arm circumference (cm)

Skinfold thickness:

Laboratory

1. Hemoglobin (specify method)
2. Stool—negative/ascariasis/ancylostomiasis/giardiasis/ amoebiasis/strongyloides/others (state):
3. Blood smear—negative/MT/BT/filaria
4. Urine—albumin/sugar
5. Biochemical test (if any)
6. Radiology (if done)

Signature of Investigator

NUTRITIONAL COUNSELING AND GUIDANCE

The important responsibility of the pediatric nurse is to provide nutritional counseling and guidance to the parents and also to the children, with the goal of achieving optimum nutrition throughout the years of growth and development. The nutritional status of children is of vital importance in their growth and development, in the promotion and maintenance of health, in the prevention of disease and in the restoration of health following illness and injury. The adequacy of children's diets affects all aspects of their lives.

Nutritional counseling and guidance should be provided in all stages of growth and development considering the feeding patterns, dietary habits, food fads, culture, religion, availability of food, educational level and socioeconomic status of the family.

Nutritional Counseling during Infancy

Mother is the significant person during infancy and she is mainly responsible for maintenance of nutrition and for the promotion of health during this period. First 6 months of infancy depends upon breastfeeding and second half of infancy is the important period to become accustomed with family diet.

Mother needs guidance for breastfeeding. Information to be given regarding positioning, feeding schedule, timing, feeding technique, satisfaction of the infant and adequacy indicators. Other aspects include maternal diet, manual expression of breast milk, possible problems related to breastfeeding and remembering the importance of breast-feeding for nutritional and trusting relationship.

Mother should be encouraged to ask questions and her concern about breastfeeding. Family members should be explained about the continuous support from their end, to promote exclusive breastfeeding. Nurse or other health team members should discuss the questions asked by the parents and family members with scientific aspects of breastfeeding and help them to solve the problems and to promote the infants growth.

In later half of infancy, guidance and counseling should concern about different aspects of weaning which should be completed within one year of child's age. Weaning is an important transitional period in relation to child's nutrition. If weaning is not done appropriately, the child will present with malnutrition and growth failure which make the child prone to various infections and diseases.

The nurse should emphasize on calm, gentle relaxed and patience approach during weaning. Weaning foods to be selected with high nutrients content and cultural preferences. Forced feeding should be avoided. Principles of weaning, qualities of weaning foods and schedule of introduction of new food item in appropriate age should be informed, explained and discussed with parents and family members. Problems related to weaning should be handle carefully to help the infant to adapt gradually with family diet.

Nutritional Counseling for Toddler

Toddler is the period of increased autonomy and self-awareness which may cause refusals of food and assistance in feeding by which the toddler asserts himself or herself. In this period, the child may have decreased appetite due to slower growth rate and may be ritualistic in food preferences.

Parents and family members need guidance and counseling regarding balanced diet with full range of food items to supply the required nutrients. Though the child takes about one-half of the amount of foods that an adult consumes, the child should have breastfeeding especially up to 2 years of age and at night time.

Parents need guidance to encourage independence of the child during feeding but to provide assistance whenever necessary. Avoidance of force feeding and incentives during feeding may reinforce negative behavior and may lead to a dislike for mealtime. The child is required to maintain a regular mealtime schedule, attractive mealtime equipment and a variety of choiceable foods (eggs, meats, etc.)

The toddler and need Preschool children vitamin 'A' supplementation starting from 9 months of age up to 5 years. Iron-folic acid supplementation may also be needed to some child. The parents need information and explanation about the schedule of supplementations. They should be made aware about the deficiency conditions, their features, and preventive measures. Appropriate cooking process, food hygiene, food handling, hand washing and safe water consumption should also need attention. Maintenance of growth chart by regular weight measurement and nutritional assessment are also important aspects of nutritional counseling for all age groups especially the toddlers and preschoolers as they belongs to most vulnerable group for malnutrition and growth failure.

Nutritional Counseling for Preschooler

A preschooler usually develops to have complete independence at mealtime with increased imitation. Nutritional habits are developed in this period that become part of the child's lifetime practices. Mealtime promotes socialization and provides opportunities to learn appropriate mealtime behavior, language skills and understanding of family rituals. So mealtime requires special attention.

The child needs all food items as taken by adults but in smaller quantities with all nutritive values as required for the balanced diet. Emphasis should be placed on quality of food rather than quantity. Foods should be served attractively with good flavor.

The frequent causes of insufficient eating are, unhappy atmosphere at mealtime, overeating between meals, attention seeking, excessive parental expectations, inadequate variety or quantity of foods, tooth decay, physical illness, fatigue and emotional disturbances. Measures to be taken to increase food intake by maintaining calm environment with no distractions during mealtime and providing rest before meal. Food intake in between meal and threatening or giving incentives or punishment to the child who refuse to eat, should not be emphasized and must be avoided.

The nurse should guide the parents to provide balanced diet to their child and involves both parent and child during guidance and counseling session, whenever needed.

Nutritional Guidance to School Age Child

Nutrition education is useful for the school age children to help them to select food items wisely and to begin to plan and prepare for meals. Parental attitudes continue to be important as the child imitates parental behavior. There is gradual decline in food requirements per kg of body weight due to slower growth rate. The child becomes dependent on peer approval for the choice of foods and likes to eat away from home to experience more independence and increased socialization.

The parents, pediatric nurse and other health care providers should be well alert to maintain balanced and nutritious intake of foods with adequate calories, calcium and vitamin 'D' which are more important for preadolescent growth. These children may be required a nutritious heavy breakfast. Some companionship and conversation during meal and occasional invitation of peers for meals may be arranged. Mealtime should be relaxed and enjoyable without any diversion (such as television). Parents should not be over concerned about child's diet considering that the time and experience will improve the food habits. Regular health check-up is essential for the school children to assess the nutrition status and its deviations.

Nutritional Guidance to Adolescents

Nutrition education to be continued in the adolescents with special emphasis on nutritional need related to the growth, selection of iron-riched food items and preparing favorite adolescent foods for physical fitness. Dietary requirements may vary according to rate of physical growth, athletic and social activity and stage of sexual maturation. During rapid growth of puberty, increased energy requirement should be maintained. The menstruating teenage girls need more iron containing foods. Calcium and vitamin 'D' requirement should be fulfilled to promote bony growth.

Informal sessions for nutrition education are generally more effective than lecture on nutrition. Special nutritional interventions and guidance may be necessary in excessive eating, obesity, extreme food fads, anorexia nervosa or bulimia, constipation, iron-deficiency anemia, malnutrition, iodine deficiency and teenage pregnancy. The nurse is responsible for special counseling session to help the adolescents to solve their problems remembering that already learned dietary patterns are difficult to change. Emphasis should be given on nutritious foods relevant to the adolescent's lifestyle, maintenance of balanced diet and provision of nutritional supplementations (especially iron and folic acid for girls). Avoidance of cigarette smoking is essential which may contribute to poor nutritional status by decreasing appetite and increasing body's metabolic rate. Health supervision at regular interval should be emphasized for the early detection of problems.

Nutritional counseling and guidance are essential for all children during different stages of growth and development to promote optimum health and prevent deficiency states.

NATIONAL NUTRITIONAL POLICY

National Nutritional Policy was adopted in 1993, acknowledging that malnutrition, especially in infants and children is a major public health problem. The aims and objectives are:

- To identify vulnerable groups requiring immediate interventions
- To identify key areas for action in the field of food production, supply, information, nutrition education, rural development, health care, monitoring and surveillance.

In relation to National Nutritional Policy, Ministry of Human Resource Development has chalked out a National Plan of Action on Nutrition (NPAN). This plan helps as a guiding force and framework for implementation of multisectoral strategy to achieve the nutritional goals.

National Plan of Action on Nutrition

- Reduction in moderate and severe malnutrition among preschool children by half
- Reduction in incidence of low birth weight infants to less than 10 percent
- Reduction in chronic under nutrition and stunted growth in children
- Elimination of blindness due to vitamin 'A' deficiency
- Reduction in iron deficiency anemia in pregnant women by 25 percent
- Universal iodization of salt for reduction of iodine deficiency disorders to 10 percent
- Giving due emphasis to geriatric nutrition
- Production of 250 million tonnes of food grains
- Improving household food security through poverty alleviation programs
- Promoting appropriate diets and healthy lifestyle.

Short-term Measures

- Nutrition intervention for especially vulnerable groups in the form of:
  – expanding the safety net, particularly ICDS program
  – appropriate behavioral changes among mothers
  – reaching the adolescent girls
  – ensuring better coverage for expectant women for the better health and reducing the incidence of low birth weight infant.
- Fortification of essential foods with iron and iodine
- Popularization of low-cost nutritious food
- Control of micronutrient deficiencies amongst vulnerable groups.

Long-term Measures

- Food security
- Improvement of dietary pattern through production and demonstration
- Policies for affecting income transfer by improving the purchasing power and streamlining the public distribution system
- Land reforms
- Health and family welfare
- Basic health and nutrition knowledge
- Prevention of food adulteration
- Nutritional surveillance
- Monitoring of nutrition program
- Research into various aspects of nutrition
- Equal remuneration for men and women
- Better communication strategies
- Minimum wage administration
- Community participation.

NATIONAL PROGRAMS ON NUTRITION

The Government of India have initiated several nutrition programs throughout the country to prevent and control major nutritional problems. They include the followings:
- Vitamin 'A' prophylaxis program
- Prophylaxis against nutritional anemia
- Control of iodine deficiency disorders
- Applied nutrition program
- Special nutrition program
- Balwadi nutrition program
- Midday meal program for school children
- Integrated child development services scheme.

These nutritional programs are designed by the Government of India through various ministries, namely Ministry of Health and Family Welfare, Ministry of Social Welfare and Ministry of Education. The overall objectives of these programs are to improve nutritional status, to overcome specific deficiency conditions and malnutrition. In future, we can hope that improvement of nutritional status of Indian children can be achieved by the improvement of socioeconomic status of our community. So that each family will be able to afford balanced diets to their children towards optimum health.

Newborn Infant

6

- Healthy Newborn Infant
- Common Health Problems of the Newborn Baby
- High Risk Neonates
- Kangaroo Mother Care
- Grades of Neonatal Care
- Transport of Sick Neonates

HEALTHY NEWBORN INFANT

The healthy newborn infant born at term, between 38 to 42 weeks, cries immediately after birth, establishes independent rhythmic respiration, quickly adapts with the extrauterine environment, having an average birth weight and no congenital anomalies (Fig. 6.1).

The period from birth to 28 days of life is called neonatal period and the infant in this period is termed as neonate or newborn baby. The first week of life is known as early neonatal period and the late neonatal period extends from 7th to 28th days of age.

The neonates are 'at risk' for various health problems, even though they born with average birth weight. The morbidity and mortality rates in newborn infants are high. They need optimal care for improved survival. Neonatal care is highly cost-effective because saving the life of a newborn baby is associated with survival and productivity of the future adult. They constitute the foundation of life. So essential newborn care is emphasized to reduce the neonatal illness and deaths by preventing neonatal problems. Neonatal nurse is the key person for essential neonatal care. Assessment of neonates for early detection of problems and initiation of prompt management are the important responsibilities of nursing personnel. The nurse can provide essential neonatal care in all levels of health care facilities with simple and low-tech measures to save the infants and give them a chance to live a full span of healthy life.

Physical Characteristics of Healthy Neonates

A healthy newborn usually has the following physical characteristics:

Weight: The average weight of a normal full-term newborn infant is about 2.9 kg with a variation of 2.5 to 3.9 kg or more. The weight is very variable from country-to-country and in different socioeconomical status.

Length: At birth the average crown heel length of the term infant is 50 cm with the range of 48 to 53 cm. The length is a more reliable criterion of gestational age than the weight.

Head circumference: The head circumference is usually varies from 33 to 37 cm, with the average of 35 cm.

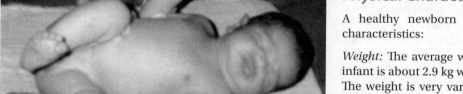

Fig. 6.1: Healthy neonates

Chest circumference: The chest circumference is about 3 cm less than head circumference. The chest is rounded rather than flattened anteroposteriorly.

Other Characteristics

The upper segment to lower segment ratio is 1.8:1. The midpoint of the length/stature of the neonate lies approximately at the level of the umbilicus, instead of the symphysis pubis as in grown up child and adults. The trunk is relatively larger and the extremities are short. Abdomen is prominent with short neck and large head.

The neonate lies in a posture of partial flexion attitude as *in utero.* The skin is pinkish but bluish hands and feet (acrocyanosis) may present for a short time after birth, even in normal infant. Skin may be covered with vernix caseosa and lanugo hair, especially at back. The head may show moulding and caput succedaneum. The ear cartilage is firm and fully curved, showing good elastic recoil. The eyes are largely covered with eye lids. The breast nodule is palpable, measuring over 5 mm in diameter. The scrotum shows adequate rugae with deep pigmentation and palpable testes (at least one). The labia majora covers the labia minora. The sole of foot shows prominent deep creases.

The external auditory canal is relatively short and straight. The eardrum is thick. The eustachian tube is short and broad. The maxillary and ethmoid sinuses are small. The frontal and sphenoidal sinuses are poorly developed. Kidney, liver and spleen may be palpable.

Physiological Characteristics of Healthy Neonates

The healthy neonates cries almost immediately after birth and establishes satisfactory and spontaneous respiration. The respiratory rate varies between 30 to 60 breaths per minutes, i.e. at resting state to crying, with an average 40 breaths per minute. The neonate can breathe both through nose and mouth. Respiration is usually periodic, shallow but irregular. It may be slow in some babies. It is usually thoracoabdominal without any retractions and grunting. The heart rate varies between 120 and 160 beats per minute, with an average of 140 beats per minute. It may be irregular and increased during crying and may be slow about 80 to 100 beats per minute during sleep. Blood pressure ranges from 60 to 80 mm Hg systolic and diastolic 25 to 40 mm Hg (average 60/40 mm Hg. The normal body temperature is 36.5 to 37.5°C which falls after birth but become normal within 4 to 8 hours.

The cry of the newborn baby is vigorous. Rooting, suckling and swallowing reflexes are well-developed. The newborn baby is able to take breastfeeding within one hour of birth and then fall asleep. A neonate spends about 80 percent of the time in sleeping (about 20 hours a day). Demand of feeding usually establishes every 3 to 4 hours after one week, initially feeding at irregular interval is seen. The energy requirement initially is 55 cal/kg/day which increase to about 120 cal/kg/day at the end of the first week of age. Protein and carbohydrates are efficiently digested by the newborn but the fat is not. Limitations of anatomical structure, slow peristalsis and imperfect control over cardiac sphincters can cause regurgitation and vomiting.

The neonate loses about 7 to 8 percent of body weight (may be up to 10%) during first week of life. The baby regains the birth weight by 10th day and then continues to gain weight about 20 to 30 g/day for the next 3 months of age.

The baby passes urine shortly after birth or within 24 hours. Some baby may pass within 48 hours. Limitations of renal function may lead to dehydration, acidosis and hyperkalemia. The first stool or meconium is usually passed within 24 hours. It is greenish-black colored thick and viscid. It is passed for first 3 to 4 days and 3 to 4 times a day. It is sterile and consists of cast off intestinal epithelial cells, lanugo hair, mucus, digestive juices, bile salts and bile pigments. Then the transitional stools, (greenish-brown) with milk curds passed for 3 to 4 days. The typical stools of a breastfeed baby may be passed after one week of age. It is golden yellow, soft, slight sour smell with acidic reaction.

The neonate has blood volume about 80 mL/kg of body weight with RBC—6 to 8 million/cmm, Hb%—18 g%, WBC—10000 to 17000/cmm, platelets—350000/cmm and nucleated red cells 500/cmm. ESR is markedly eleveted and poor clottings power are seen due to deficient vitamin-K. Blood sugar and calcium levels are relatively low. IgG level is high but IgM, IgA, IgE levels are negligible. IgM is near absent and T lymphocyte functions are reduced. RBCs are more vulnerable to hemolysis.

Neurological mechanisms are immature and not fully developed anatomically or physiologically. Reflexes are important indicator of neurological development. Due to immature neurological development, there is labile temperature regulation, poor muscular control and uncoordinated movement.

Temperature regulation is not fully developed, heat production is low and the infant responds readily to environmental heat and cold.

Limited hepatic function leads to decreased ability to conguate bilirubin, regulate blood glucose level and produce coagulation factors. Endocrine glands are better organized than other systems.

Assessment of Newborn Baby

Assessment of the newborn, as soon as possible after birth and subsequent assessment in the postnatal period are vital responsibility of the nurses working in hospital or in the community. The assessment should include details history of prenatal and intranatal period and genetic history of family along with head to foot examination and review of maternal investigations.

The purposes of initial assessment are mainly to assess the need for resuscitation, to ascertain the gestational age, to detect presence of any congenital anomalies or any disorders which may affect the well-being of the baby. It should be done at the place of birth by the trained birth attendant immediately after delivery of the neonate.

The assessment in the postnatal period should be done at least for three times, whether it may be in hospital or in home delivery. In the hospital/health center, first postnatal assessment should be done within 24 hours or next day and at the time of discharge and the second assessment within 2 weeks of age and third assessment within 4 to 6 weeks of age of the baby. In home delivery, the first postnatal assessment should be done within 3 days and others are same as institutional delivery. Mothers and family members should be informed about the times of postnatal assessment, because they have to take initiative for these subsequent procedures. They should also be explained about the danger signs, when the neonate needs medical attention during this period.

Initial Assessment

The initial assessment of neonate is a very important activity immediately after birth. The most essential assessment is the "first cry". Good cry helps in establishment of satisfactory breathing. The respiration, heart rate and skin color are the basic criterias which should be evaluated immediately to determine the need for life saving support, i.e. resuscitation. The physiological status including temperature, degree of consciousness, general level of activity, gross congenital anomalies, presence of birth injury, meconium staining and evidence of shock also need to be ascertained immediately and promptly after birth.

Another significant assessment of the neonate is 'Apgar scoring' as described by Dr Virginia Apgar. Despite its limitations, it is an useful quantitative assessment of neonate's condition at birth, especially for the respiratory, circulatory and neurological status. Five objective criterias are evaluated at one minute and 5 minutes, after the neonates body is completely born. The criterias are, respiration, heart rate/minute, muscle tone, reflex irritability and skin color (Table 6.1). Each of these criteria is an index of neonates depression or lack of it at birth and is given a score of 0, 1 or 2. The scores from each of the criteria are added to determine the total score. The neonate is in the best possible condition if the score is 10. Scores of 7 to 10 indicate no difficulty in adjustment in extrauterine life. Scores of 4 to 6 signify moderate difficulty and if the score is 3 or below, the neonate is in severe distress which must be treated immediately.

Usually, neonates have lower score at one minute, than the score at 5 minute due to the presence of depression

Table 6.1 Apgar scoring

Criteria	0	1	2
Respiration	Absent	Slow, irregular	Good, crying
Heart rate	Absent	Slow (Below 100)	More than 100
Muscle tone	Flaccid	Some flexion of extremities	Active body movements
Reflex response	No response	Grimace	Cry
Skin color	Blue, pale	Body pink, extremities blue	Completely pink

Total score = 10
- No depression: 7–10
- Mild depression: 4–6
- Severe depression: 0–3

immediate after birth. The 5 minute score has greater predictive value, since it correlates with neonatal morbidity and mortality. It also correlates more closely with the infants neurologic status at one year of age.

A significant aspect of neonatal assessment is the review of maternal and perinatal history. Details maternal history should include age, blood group, Rh type, chronic illness and infections, history of previous pregnancy and present pregnancy. Family history of illness and abnormal pregnancy also should be reviewed. The nurse must review the information of birth of this neonate including gestational age, duration of labor, color of amniotic fluid, type of delivery, use of sedation or anesthesia to the mother, resuscitation required, etc.

Thorough history provides useful clues to predict and anticipate problems in the newborn baby.

Initial assessment also should include assessment of gestational age, measurement of birth weight, length, head circumference, chest circumference and detailed head to foot examination to detect presence of congenital anomalies like anorectal malformations, cleft lip and palate. These assessment are usually done when the baby's condition is stable.

Assessment should be done in a comfortable warm room with good light. Safety measures should be followed especially, about prevention of infections. All information should be recorded immediately. If possible, mother should be allowed to be along with baby to promote bonding process.

Assessment of Gestational Age at Birth

Assessment of gestational age is mandatory for all neonates for further management. Last menstrual period is important clue

Table 6.2 Assessment of gestation age at birth

Physical characteristics	Preterm	Transitional	Term
• Hair texture and distribution on scalp	• Wooly, fuzzy and very fine	• Fine, wooly, fuzzy	• Silky, black coarse and individual strants
• Skin texture and opacity	• Shiny oily plethoric, plenty of lanugo, edema with visible veins and venules on abdomen	• Less shiny, peripheral cyanosis, less lanugo and veins are only found on abdomen	• Pink, scanty lanugo and only large veins are seen. Good elasticity or turgor
• Breast nodule and nipple formation	• Breast tissue less than 5 mm on one or both sides. No nipple present	• Breast tissue 5–10 mm Nipple present but not raised	• More than 10 mm diameter breast tissue and nipple raised above skin level
• Ear cartilage	• Pinna feels soft with no cartilage and no recoil	• Some cartilage present and some recoil	• Pinna is firm with definite cartilage and instant recoil
• Planter creases	• Faint red marks over anterior part of sole or may be absent	• Creases seen over anterior 1/3 to 1/2 of sole	• Entire sole covered with deep creases
• Genitalia - Male	• Scrotum small with no or few rugae and light pigmentation. Testis usually not descend or in inguinal canal	• Scrotum with some rugae and testis in the inguinal canal	• At least one testis descends in the scrotum. Prominent rugae and deep pigmentation
• Genitalia - Female	• Labia majora widely separated with prominent labia minora and clitoris	• Labia majora partially cover the labia minora	• Labia majora completely cover the labia minora and clitoris

for calculation of gestational age, but it may not be reliable in menstrual irregularities or mother may not remember the exact date. The clinical assessment is more practically significant. Physical and neurological examinations are done to detect the gestational maturity. Anthropometric measurement only are unreliable parameters because they may adversely affected by intrauterine growth retardation. Table 6.2 shows assessment of gestation age at birth.

Assessment of maturity of the neonates is fairly reliable on the basis of physical characterstics. But they are of limited value to assess the gestational age in less than 36 weeks of maturity. The neurological characteristics are more reliable for the precise assessment of maturity. The neurological assessment is performed based on four fundamental observations, i.e. muscle tone, joint mobility, certain automatic reflexes and fundus examination.

The *muscle tone* of the newborn baby is assessed by three parameters, i.e. posture or attitude, passive tone (popliteal angle and scarf sign) and active tone (traction response and recoil).

The *joint mobility* is less in preterm babies. A term baby has more flexible and relaxed joint. The degree of flexion at ankle and wrist (square-windows) is limited due to stiffness of joints in early gestation.

Certain *automatic reflexes* like Moro reflex, pupillary response to light, blink response to glabellar tap, grasp response, neck flexors, rooting reflex with coordinated suckling efforts are assessed to detect the specific age of gestational maturity based on appearance of these reflexes.

The *fundus examination* for disappearance of anterior vascular capsule of the lens is done to assess the gestational age. In infants less than 28 weeks, the anterior capsule is completely vascularized and after 34 weeks of gestational life, the vessels are almost atropied. This examination is difficult due to noncooperation and photophobia of the neonate.

With the scoring system of neurological assessment the accurate estimation of gestational age can be done. Presently, new Ballard score is widely used. Neuromuscular maturity is assessed by the test like posture, square window (wrist), arm recoil, popliteal angle, scarf sign and heel to ear, using the new Ballard scoring system. Physical maturity is assessed with this system by the characteristics like skin, lanugo, planter surface, breast, eye/ear and genitals (*see* Appendix XIX).

Assessment of gestational age should be performed carefully , because neonates of particular gestational age have particular and special problems. Therefore the early detection of problems and maturity of the neonates are useful guide for appropriate management and better prognosis of neonates.

Subsequent or Follow-up Assessment in the Neonatal Period

Subsequent assessment is usually done, in institutional delivery, on the first day of birth, i.e. within 24 hours and at the time of discharge. Daily clinical evaluation should be done, between first day examination and the day of discharge. But daily detailed examination is not necessary because it may introduce infections.

First day examination: It should include the followings:

Vital signs: Temperature should be recorded to detect cold stress or hypothermia. Skin temperature is measured usually by axillary method. Respiration, heart rate and blood pressure should also be recorded (when the baby is quiet) to detect the physiological status.

General behavior: Posture, position, general alertness, activity, movements of limbs, crying, response to stimulation, sleeping pattern, etc. should be assessed carefully.

Feeding behavior: Suckling and swallowing reflex, vomiting, regurgitation, chocking, frothiness (may be due to tracheo-esophageal fistula) should be evaluated to detect associated problems.

Pattern of elimination: Passage of meconium and urine should be observed and asked to assess presence of congenital anomalies especially anorectal malformations. The neonate passes urine and meconium within 24 hours. Afterwards for first few days, the baby voids 10 to 15 times and average six stools per day.

Measurements: Head circumference should preferably be measured after 24 hours when moulding or over-riding of sutures and caput succedaneum are disappeared. If chest circumference and length are not measured on the day of delivery, they should be recorded on the first day.

Gestational assessment: Assessment of gestational age can also be done on first day, if it is not done on the day of delivery or if the baby is having any problem on that day.

Skin: Skin color should be examined carefully to detect cyanosis, jaundice, pallor and plethora (reddish). Hair distribution (lanugo hair), vernix, skin turgor, edema, ecchymosis, petechiae, erythema toxicum (rash), dryness or peeling, hemangiomas, telangiectatic nevi (stork bites), milia, mongolian spots, port-wine nevus, etc. should be looked for. Presence of any abrasions and lacerations should be searched. Nails should be checked whether reached the end of fingertips and well-developed or absence (ectodermal dysplasia).

Head: Head should be examined for presence of caput succedaneum, cephalohematoma, moulding, forceps marks, any asymmetry, encephalocele, widely separated or closed sutures and abnormalities of fontanelles (enlarged, bulging, sunken). Hair is checked for wooly or fuzzy.

Face: Face should be observed for symmetry, paralysis, shape, swelling and abnormal movements.

Eyes: Eyes should be checked for edema, conjunctivitis or discharge, subconjunctival hemorrhages, color of sclera, (blue sclera is indicative of osteogenesis imperfecta and yellow discoloration of sclera indicates jaundice), Brushfield spots (Trisomy 21), strabismus, congenital cataract, pupillary size and reflex, abnormal placement of eyes (chromosomal anomalies) or abnormal distance between two eyes.

Nose: Nose is examined for patency, low nasal bridge, nasal discharge, nasal flaring, etc.

Ears: Ears should be examined for formation or size and shape, sufficient cartilage and position (low set ears indicate chromosomal anomalies), skin tags, preauricular sinus, etc.

Mouth: Mouth should be checked for cleft palate in hard palate or soft palate, size of mouth cavity and oral opening, size of the tongue, presence of natal teeth, Epstein's pearls, frenulum lingual, tongue tie, sucking callosities, blisters, oral infections, etc.

Neck: Neck should be examined for mobility, fracture clavicle, stiffness or rigidity, hyperextension, torticollis, any cyst or mass (thyroglossal cyst, cystic hygroma), excessive skin folds (trisomy 21) and webbing.

Chest: Abnormal shape and size of chest should be observed. Development of nipple and breast tissue should be checked to assess gestational age. Breast engorgement may present due to withdrawn of maternal hormones usually at day three. Rate and rhythm of respiration, chest retractions and abnormal respiratory sound should be examined. Heart sound should be ausculted for rate, rhythm and abnormal sounds.

Abdomen: Abdomen should be observed for its shape, distension (may be due to bowel obstruction, abdominal mass, enlargement of organ or infection) and synchronous movement with chest in respiration. Umbilical cord should be observed for signs of infection, discharge, redness around insertion, presence of hernia or any congenital anomalies (single artery). Abdomen should be palpated for any masses (liver edge usually felt 2 cm below costal margin and spleen tip). Occasionally lower poles of kidneys may be palpable. Auscultation of abdomen should be done in all four quadrants for bowel sounds.

Genitalia: Female baby should be examined to assess whether labia majora covers labia minora and clitoris. Hymenal tag or imperforate hymen may present. Vaginal white mucoid discharge or pink-red mucous discharge may be found due to withdrawal of maternal hormones.

Full term male baby usually have both testes in scrotal sac and scrotum appears pigmented and markedly wrinkled with rugae. Penis should be examined to detect hypospadias, epispadias, phimosis or abnormal length. Ambiguous genitalia, hydrocele, inguinal hernia should be looked for.

Back: Back should be checked for abnormal spinal curvature, tufts of hair or skin disruptions indicating spina bifida oculta. Meningocele, meningomyelocele, meningoencephalocele, anencephaly are usually detected at initial assessment.

Buttucks: It should be observed for any mass (sacrococcygeal teratoma). Perianal areas should be examined for anal opening, anal fissures or any other abnormalities.

Hips: Examination of hips to be done to detect congenital hip dislocation. Positive Ortolani's sign and asymmetrical gluteal folds are indicative of the condition.

Extremities: Extremities are examined for fractures, paralysis, range of motion and irregular position. Fingers and toes to be checked for missing digits, extra digits (polydactyly) or fused digits (syndactyly). Feet to be looked for structural or positional abnormalities mainly club foot (talipes equinovarus).

Neurological status: Assessment of neurological status is very important. In the neonates, neurological mechanisms are immature both anatomically and physiologically which result in disturbance of temperature regulation, uncoordinated movements and lack of control over musculature.

Examination of muscle tone, head control and reflexes are essential aspects. Two types of reflexes are present in the neonates, i.e. protective reflex (blinking, coughing, sneezing and gagging) and primitive reflex (rooting, sucking, moro or startle, tonic neck, stepping and palmer grasp). Table 6.3 shows various reflexes of the normal neonate.

Special senses: Neonates should be examined for special senses. Normal healthy neonate responds to various sensations. The sense of touch is the most highly developed special sense and mostly observed on the lips, tongue, ear and forehead. Failure to grasp the nipple indicates brain damage. Vision is difficult to assess. Hearing occurs after the first cry and the infant responds to sound with eye movements, cessation of activity, startle reflex or crying. Sense of taste is well-developed. Sweet fluids are accepted and sour or bitter are resisted. Neonates can smell breast milk and search for nipple and mother. The newborn baby appears to be highly sensitive to organic stimulation, since hunger and thirst are most common cause of crying.

The neonates are not likely to have abdominal colic, but in older infants it is common. The neonates react to

Table 6.3 Reflexes of the normal neonate

Reflex	Stimulation to elicit	Expected response	Age of disappearance
• Rooting	• Touching or stroking the cheek near the corner of the mouth	• Head turns towards the stimulation, mainly to find food	• 3–4 months when awake and 7–8 months when asleep
• Sucking	• Touching the lips with the nipple of the breast	• Suckling movements to take in food	• Begins to diminish at 6 months
• Swallowing	• Accompanies the sucking reflex	• Food, reaching the posterior of the mouth is swallowed	• Does not disappear
• Gagging	• When more food is taken into the mouth that can be successfully swallowed	• Immediate return of undigested food	• Does not disappear
• Sneezing and coughing	• Foreign substance entering the upper and lower airways	• Clearing of upper air passages by sneezing and lower air passage by coughing	• Does not disappear
• Blinking	• Exposure of eyes to bright light	• Protection of eyes by rapid eyelid closure	• Does not disappear
• Doll's eye	• Turn the neonate's head slowly to right or left side	• Normally eyes do not move	• When fixation develops
• Palmer grasp	• Object placed in neonate's palm	• Grasping of object by closing fingers around it	• Disappear in 6 weeks to 3 months
• Stepping or dancing	• Hold neonate in a vertical position with feet touching a flat and firm surface	• Rapid alternating flexion and extension of the legs as in stepping	• Disappear with 3 to 4 weeks
• Moro (startle)	• Startling the neonate with a loud voice or apparent loss of support due to change in equilibrium. The neonate is held in supine position supporting upper back and head with one hand and lower back with other. The neonate's head is suddenly allowed to drop down backward for an inch	• Generalized muscular activity. Symmetric abduction and extension of arms and legs with fanning of fingers. The thumb and index fingers form a 'c' shaped in both hand. The extremities then flex and adduct. The baby may cry	• Strong up to 2 months disappears by 3–4 months

both internal or external stimuli and manifest state related behavior. The newborn infant can exhibit at least five different states, i.e. quiet or regular sleep, rapid eye movement (REM) sleep, quiet alert, active alert and crying. Neonates respond to tactile, visual and auditory stimulation, which need to be examined.

Daily Observation of Neonates

Neonates should be observed daily during hospital stay. Detailed examination is not necessary but mother and baby should be approached two times daily and information should be collected from the mother (or caretaker) about the feeding behavior, vomiting, passage of stool and urine, sleep and presence of any problems. The neonates should also be assessed for hypothermia, respiratory distress, jaundice and superficial infections like conjunctivitis, umbilical sepsis, oral thrush and skin infection.

The neonates should be monitored for the danger signs. Presence of these features indicate special attention, re-evaluation and early interventions. The danger signs are:

- Poor feeding, sucking and swallowing reflex
- Cold to touch or having rise in body temperature
- Poor activity and poor response to stimulation
- Excessive crying and irritability
- Rapid respiration, more than 60 per minutes and presence of chest retractions
- Blue discoloration of lips or tongue (central cyanosis)
- Drooling of saliva or choking during feeding or frothiness
- Labored respiration or absence of respiration
- Jaundice appears within 24 hours or extending to palms or soles
- No urine within 48 hours and no meconium within 24 hours
- Convulsions or abnormal movements
- Bleeding from any site
- Umbilical discharge
- Superficial infections (pyoderma, abscess, oral thrush, conjunctivitis)
- Diarrhea, vomiting and abdominal distension.

Examination on Discharge

At the time of dicharge from the hospital all neonates should be examined detailed to detect any missed abnormalities. A neonate who is feeding well on the breast, has warm and pink palms and soles and having no danger signs, is essentially a healthy baby. Mother should be advised during discharge about essential care of the baby and informed about danger signs and need for follow-up regular interval.

Nursing Care of Healthy Neonates

Essential care of the normal healthy neonates can be best provided by the mothers under supervision of nursing personnel or basic/primary health care providers. About 80 percent of the newborn babies require minimal care. The normal term babies should be kept with their mothers rather than in a separate nursery. Bedding-in or rooming-in promotes better emotional bondage, prevents cross-infection and establishes breastfeeding easily. Mother participates in the nursing care of the baby and develops self-confidence in her. This also reduces the demand of nursing personnel.

Nursing care of healthy newborn baby after birth should be provided as immediate care of the neonates and daily routine care.

Immediate Basic Care of Neonates

Immediate basic care of the newborn at birth includes maintenance of temperature, establishment of open airway, initiation of breathing and maintenance of circulation. As majority babies cry at birth and take spontaneous respiration, no resuscitation requires at birth in about 95 to 98 percent neonates. These healthy normal neonates need only warmth, breastfeeding, close observation for early detection of problems and protection from infections and injuries. The baby should not be separated from the mother.

After cutting the umbilical cord aseptically, the baby should be kept dried, wrapped with dry warm cloths, examined thoroughly and quickly to assess normal characteristics, to detect congenital malformations or any signs of illness and then put to the mother's breast. Identification tag to be given to the mother and baby. The sex of the baby is shown to the mother. Recording to be done neatly and accurately about the event of birth of the baby (especially birth date, time, sex, examination findings or presence of any problems, etc.), in the delivery record sheet. The mother and baby should be transfered to lying-in-ward usually after one hour of observation in the delivery room or when the condition permits. Sick or at-risk neonates need special care in special setting.

Daily Routine Care of Neonates

The major goal of nursing care of the newborn infant is to establish and maintain homeostasis, i.e. stability in the normal physiological status. The continuous care to be provided immediately following birth, in the transition period and during the neonatal period. This care is performed involving mother and family members in the maternity unit of hospital or health centers and in the home, afterwards.

Majority of the complications of the normal neonates may occur during first 24 hours or within 7 days. So close observation and daily essential routine care are important for health and survival of the newborn baby. The *daily routine care* of the neonates are as follows:

Warmth: Warmth is provided by keeping the baby dry and wrapping the baby with adequate clothing in two layers, ensuring head and extremities are well-covered. Baby should be kept by the side of the mother, so that the mother's body temperature can keep the baby warm. Baby can be placed in skin to skin contact with mother (kangarooing) to maintain temperature of infant and facilitate breastfeeding.

Bathing is avoided to prevent hypothermia and infections. Ambient atmospheric temperature to be kept warm adequately (28–32°C). Temperature should be recorded (by axillary, skin or human touch method) frequently during initial postnatal period. Warmth to be maintained during transfer from hospital to home on discharge or whenever needed and unnecessary exposure or undressing to be avoided. The oil massage is both culturally and scientifically acceptable as it provides insulation against heat and prevents insensible water loss. But it can be avoided during hospital stay to prevent infections and better to postpone till the baby is 3 to 4 weeks old.

Breastfeeding: The baby should be put to the mother's breast within half an hour of birth or as soon as possible the mother has recovered from the exertion of labor. No prelacteal feeds to be given and colostrum feeding must be offered. All babies should invariably receive the colostrum during first three days of life. Mother should be informed about the importance and technique of breastfeeding. Initially the feeding should be given in short interval of 1 to 2 hours and then every 2 to 3 hours. Most babies regularize their feeding pattern by the end of first week and self-demand feeding is established in every 3 to 4 hours interval. Nurse should assist the mother to feed her baby adequately for the maintenance of hydration and optimum nutrition. Exclusive breastfeeding procedure should be explained to the mother and family members.

Skin care and baby bath: The baby must be cleaned off blood, mucus and meconium by gentle wiping before he/she is presented to the mother. No bath, especially dip baths, should be given till the umbilical cord has fallen off. In summer months, the baby can be sponged using unmedicated soap and clean lukewarm water. During hospital stay 'no bath' reduces the incidence of neonatal infections. No vigorous attempts should be made to remove the vernix caseosa, as it provides protection to the delicate skin. Each baby should have own separate clothing and articles for care to prevent cross-infection.

Baby bath: It can be given at hospital or home following the instructions for bathing. It should be given using warm water in a warm room gently and quickly. The baby should be dried swiftly and thoroughly from head to toe and wrapped in a dry warm towel or clothing. Bathing should be avoided in open place. Unnecessary exposure should be avoided. During winter months the baby should have sponge bath rather than dip bath to avoid cold stress or hypothermia. Use of olive oil or coconut oil can be allowed after 3 to 4 weeks of age. Oil massage improves circulation and muscle tone.

Most babies enjoy oil massage and feel comfortable. Oil can get absorbed from the thin skin of the baby and provides additional energy. It is better to avoid mustard oil for baby because it can cause irritation. Oil massage should be done before the bathing, in a warm place which is free from draughts. Exposure to sun rays is an important source of vitamin 'D' and warmth. But protection should be taken from exposure of U-V light of sunshine. The talcum powder can be used for aesthetic purposes and should be applied over the axillae, groins and buttocks. During bathing the baby should be observed for behavior and presence of any abnormalities or infections. Minor developmental peculiarities like mongolian spots, milia, toxic erythema, etc. are detected during bathing.

Care of the umbilical cord: The umbilical cord is cut about 2 to 3 cm from the naval with aseptic precautions during delivery and tied with sterile cotton thread or disposable plastic clip. The cord must be inspected afterwards for bleeding which commonly occurs due to shrinkage of cord and loosening of ligature. No dressing should be applied and the cord should be kept open and dry. Normally it falls off after 5 to 10 days but may take longer especially when infected. Application of gentian violet or triple dye is not advocated as a routine any more.

Care of the eyes: Eyes should be cleaned at birth and once every day using sterile cotton swabs soaked in sterile water or normal saline. Each eye should be cleaned using a separate swab. Application of 'kajal' in the eyes must be avoided to prevent infection or lead poisoning. The eyes should be observed for redness, sticky discharge or excessive tearing for early detection of problems and prompt management. The cultural practice of instillation of human colostrum in the eyes has been found to be useful to reduce the incidence of sticky eyes.

Clothing of the baby: The baby should be dressed with loose, soft and cotton cloths. The frock should be open on the front or back for easy wearing. Large buttons, synthetic frock and plastic or nylon napkin should be avoided. A triangle of square piece of thick, soft absorbent cloth should be used as napkin. The cloths should not be tight specially around the neck or abdomen. In winter, woollen or flannel clothing should be used. Woollen cloths should not be stored with moth balls, because there is chance of severe jaundice in the baby with G-6-PD deficiency. The cloths preserved with moth balls, should be exposed to bright sunlight for one or two days. Baby clothing should always be cleaned with light detergent, that will be washed properly and sun-dried to prevent skin irritation.

General care: The newborn baby should be kept with the mother for continuous mothering in hospital (bedding-in) or in home (rooming-in) in a well-ventilated room. Baby should be handle with gentle approach after proper hand washing.

No infected person should take care or touch the baby. Baby should be allow to sleep in supine position which can prevent sudden infant death syndrome. General cleanliness to be maintained and surroundings to be kept clean. Wet nappies should be changed immediately. Mother should be taught about art of mothering and to provide stimulation of touch and sound to the baby. Tender loving care should always be maintained and available for the baby.

Observation: The baby should be thoroughly observed twice daily for early detection of any abnormalities. Temperature, pulses/heart rate, respiration, feeding behaviors, stool, urine and sleeping pattern should be assessed. Mouth, eyes, cord and skin should be looked for any infections. Daily routine observation is essential to detect the presence of danger signs for early interventions.

Weight recording: The average daily weight gain in healthy term babies is about 30 g/day in the first month of life. It is about 20 g/day in the second month and 10 g/day afterwards during the first year of life. Most infants double their birth weight by 4 to 5 months. But in the first week of life there is physiological loss of body weight due to removal of vernix, mucus, blood, passage of meconium and reduction of extracellular blood volume. Delay and unsatisfactory feeding is also contributing to weight loss. With adequate breastfeeding, majority of the babies regain the weight within 7 to 10 days of birth.

There is no need of monitoring early weight changes in the healthy newborn because it can cause unnecessary anxiety to the mother and may lead to lactation failure. The adequacy of breastfeeding should be assessed. The babies with adequate breastfeeding should have good sleep and 5 to 6 times urination. They are satisfied and playful having no abnormal cry or irritability.

Immunizations: In institutional delivery, all neonates should be immunized with 'BCG' vaccine and 'O' dose 'OPV'. Hepatitis 'B' vaccine can be administered at birth as first dose and other two doses in one month and 6 months of age. In outside or home delivery, the BCG and OPV should be given within first week of life. The OPV may preferably be given after 3 days of age because colostrum may interfere with its uptake.

Mother should be informed about the recommended National Immunization Schedule and explanation to be given about importance of complete immunization and all possible reactions following vaccinations, especially about BCG vaccine, which is already given in case of institutional delivery.

Follow-up and advice: Each infant should be followed up, at least once every month for first 3 months and subsequently 3 months interval till one year of age. Follow-up is necessary for assessment of growth and development, early detection and management of health problems, and health education for prevention of childhood illnesses.

Health advice should be given during hospital stay and at the time of discharge regarding exclusive breast-feeding, warmth, hygienic measures, rooming-in, clothing, immunization and follow-up. Danger signs related to child-hood illnesses should be explained to the mother and family members. Preventive measures against various child health problems, like ARI and diarrhea, should be informed. Harmful cultural practices should be discouraged. Care at home should be discussed and demonstrated to the mother and family members so that care at hospital should be continued at home. Mother should be informed about her own lactational diet with extra 550 cal, hygienic measures and birth spacing. Community health nurse can help the mother and family about the neonatal care at home. Minimum three home visit should be done to assist and guide the mother and family members about baby care.

Harmful traditional practices for the care of neonates: A large number of customs and cultural practices are found for mothercraft and child rearing. Some of them are useful, but harmful practices are more in number. Some practices are uncertain and doubtful in utility. The common harmful traditional practices are:

- Not adopting measures for clean delivery at home and conducting delivery in a dirty place and cutting cord with dirty thing or blade.
- Harmful resuscitation practices.
- Use of unclean substance like cowdung, mud on umbilical cord.
- Immediate bathing of baby after birth.
- Unnecessary use of prelacteal feeds, discarding colostrum, delayed breastfeeding and giving water in between breast feeds.
- Neglecting newborn female baby emotionally and nutritionally.
- Application of kajal in the newborn's eyes.
- Instilation of oil drops into ears and nostrils during bathing the baby.
- Use of unhygienically prepared herbal preparations (ghutti) or gripe water orally.
- Use of pacifiers and introduction of artificial feeding with diluted milk.
- Giving opium and brandy to the neonates.
- Use of feeding bottles, and readymade expensive formula foods, use of costly baby care articles, early separation of neonates from mothers, lack of supports from the elderly women in family due to breaking up of joint families and less time for handling the neonates are harmful neocultural practices.

COMMON HEALTH PROBLEMS OF THE NEWBORN BABY

Neonatal health problems are frequently found ranging from minor physical or physiological peculiarities to the serious life-threatening illnesses. Minor problems should not be ignored lightly without adequate assessment of the conditions. Early diagnosis and management of the serious problems help to overcome life-long disability and to reduce neonatal morbidity and mortality. Nurses are responsible to manage the minor problems and to detect the serious problems for early and prompt management along with appropriate nursing interventions and support to the mother.

Minor Problems of Neonates

Neonates may have some physical or physiological peculiarities which are of no consequence. The conditions should be evaluated to detect any possible pathology. Mothers need adequate explanation and reassurance to remove her anxiety. Necessary advice to be given to overcome the minor problems. The common conditions which create anxiety to the mothers are as follows:

Vomiting

Vomiting is the most common problem of the neonates as complaint by the mothers. Mother needs explanation about the regurgitation of feeds and vomiting. Regurgitation of milk is never ejected forcefully, it just flows out of the mouth soon after feeding and usually due to faulty feeding technique and swallowed air while sucking. As the air is expelled, the part of the feed comes out.

Vomiting may occur in neonates due to various organic and nonorganic causes. Nonorganic causes are mainly irritation of the stomach due to swallowed amniotic fluid and blood, aerophagy and faulty feeding technique.

Organic causes can be mechanical, neurological, metabolic or infectious. Mechanical causes are due to hiatus hernia, gastroesophageal reflux, meconium plug, pyloric stenosis, intestinal obstruction, Hirschsprung's disease, etc. Neurological problems causing vomiting are related to increased intracranial pressure due to intracranial hemorrhage and birth asphyxia, kernicterus, birth injuries, congenital anomalies of CNS, hydrocephalus, etc. Infections are also important causes of vomiting mainly generalized septicemia, meningitis, encephalitis, gastroenteritis, etc. Metabolic causes of vomiting include hypoglycemia, galactosemia, phenylketonuria and congenital adrenal hyperplasia.

No management requires in case of regurgitation. Nonorganic causes should be managed by proper feeding technique, burping or holding the baby upright or made to sit up on the lap for 5 to 10 minutes after feeding along with reassurance and guidance to the mother. Stomach wash may be needed in persistent vomiting to remove swallowed amniotic fluid and blood which is given with 100 mL normal saline. Prolonged vomiting with associated symptoms, like projectile vomiting, bile stained, abdominal distension, fever, etc. need to be evaluated to exclude the exact cause and management.

Constipation

Constipation is common in artificial feeding especially with cow's milk. Other causes may be inadequate feeds or insufficient fluid intake. Organic causes may present especially congenital abnormalities of GIT, Hirschsprung's disease, cretinism, etc. need to be investigated. Nonorganic causes of constipation especially in artificial fed baby, can be managed by additional glucose water, extra sugar in the milk, honey and orange juice. No laxatives should be used. Lubricated stimulus of rectum often initiates reflex peristaltic activity. Mother should be advised to improve breastfeeding.

Diarrhea

Breastfed baby passes two to six times golden yellow, sticky, semi-loose stools due to high content of lactose. Mother should be explained about the breastfed stools. The intake of large quantities of glucose water or honey by the baby may cause diarrhea. Unhygienic feeding practices overfeeding, bottle feeding and serious underfeeding also can cause diarrhea in the neonates. The serious neonatal diarrhea may also occur in septicemia, necrotising enterocolitis, Hirschsprung's disease and phototherapy. Acute infective diarrheal diseases in neonates should preferably be treated with IV fluid therapy and systemic antibiotics. Breastfeeding should be continued exclusively to provide adequate nutrition and hygienic measures to be improved.

Excessive Crying

Cry is the only language of the babies. Crying of the baby should be considered as need for help or comfort or mothering. Crying of the baby usually causes maternal anxiety especially the night crying. The common causes of crying are hunger, discomfort, abdominal colic, unpleasant sensation of full bladder before passing urine, painful evacuation of hard stool, soiling by stool or urine and wet nappies, insect bite, hot or cold feeling, loneliness and lack of mothering. Pattern of crying may differ from one baby to other. An experienced mother or nurse or doctor can distinguish the cause of cry. The crying baby should be handled with patience, common sense and good humor. The cause of cry should be identified and eliminated.

The excessive crying may be found with various conditions like cerebral irritability, meningitis, abdominal colic, trauma, otitis media and other painful inflammatory conditions, narcotic withdrawal syndrome, thyrotoxicosis, etc. These conditions need specific management after detailed investigation.

Evening Colic or Three Months Colic

The attacks of sudden screaming with flexion of thighs and flushing of face with frowning may occur in the neonates in the evening regularly after few days of birth. This unexplained crying spells may present for minutes or hours. Apparently, it seems to be due to intestinal colic which leads to further swallowing of air and initiate vicious cycle of colic-crying-colic. Temporary relief may occur by holding the baby against skin, patting, kissing, prone position, etc. Home remedies can be used to relief colic and flatulence. This condition spontaneously subsides after 3 months.

Excessive Sleepiness

During first few days of life most babies sleep throughout the day and keep their eyes closed most of the time. This should not be the cause of anxiety. They should be kept aroused during feeding by tickling behind the ears or on the soles. Excessive sleepiness can be due to maternal sedation, metabolic disorders, septicemia or serious systemic diseases. These conditions should be evaluated and management should be done accordingly.

Dehydration Fever

The healthy neonates may develop transitory fever during second or third day of life especially in summer months due to inadequate feedings. The fever is usually about 38.5°C and the baby remains active. The condition is managed by adequate breastfeeding and lowering environmental temperature. Infections should be ruled out which is the most common cause of fever.

Sneezing and Nose Block

Sneezing is frequently seen in the healthy neonates due to nasal irritation by amoniotic fluid, blood, meconium, debris, etc. It should not be considered as sign of common cold. The nostril should be cleaned with sterile cotton swab, if sneezing is excessive.

Nose block is another common problem and can cause discomfort as the infant is an obligatory nose breather. There may not be any nasal discharge. It may also cause respiratory distress. This condition is managed by instilling one or two drops of normal saline into the nostrils 15 minutes before feeds. Medicated nasal drops are not indicated in newborn babies.

Hiccups

Hiccup after the feeds is normal in neonates. It occur due to irritation of the diaphragm caused by distended stomach. Mother should be reassured about the benign nature of hiccups which do not indicate any disease.

Napkin Rash

Napkin rash commonly found in artificially fed babies and also called as amonia dermatitis. It can occur in prolonged wet nappies or lack of cleanliness. Perianal skin may become red, indurated and excoriated. Perianal dermatitis often found following diarrhea or fungal infection or due to use of nylon or water tight plastic napkins. The condition can be prevented by immediate changing of soiled napkins and drying the area. Napkins should be washed adequately with antiseptic lotion. The perianal dermatitis can be managed by keeping the area dry and exposed to air or sunlight and application of coconut oil or bland ointment or antifungal cream.

Breath Holding Spells

Breath holding spells are rare in neonates but may found along with crying. The baby is over-reactive and lacks patience and demands immediate relief of minor discomfort. Parents become overindulgent and over-anxious as the baby may present with cyanosis. The condition should be evaluated to ruled out brain damage or congenital heart disease like Fallot's tetralogy.

Cradle Cap

Cradle cap is found as seborrheic crusting over the scalp and may cause seborrheic dermatitis in infancy which may be confused with atopic dermatitis. This problem can be managed by application of coconut oil over the affected part of scalp at night followed by shampoo with cetrimide or cetavlon. The gradual resolution usually occur, otherwise skin specialist should be consulted.

Obstructed Nasolacrimal Duct

It is characterized by persistent tearing from one or both the eyes without presence of any congestion or infection. Sometimes infection may be associated with watery discharge. It is usually due to simple congenital obstruction of the nasolacrimal duct which may open by the age of 3 to 4 months. Gentle massage should be done over the tear passage, between the eye and nose (the lacrimal sac area) from above downwards with inward pressure on the lacrimal sac for 15 to 20 times per day or whenever possible. Infection should be treated with antibiotic eye drops and cleaning with sterile eye swab. If the duct does not open by 3 to 4 months of age, probing and syringing is indicated to remove the obstruction.

Umbilical Granuloma

It presents as a small flesh-like pale nodule at the base of umbilicus with persistent discharge. It is usually associated with umbilical sepsis. The granuloma can be managed by cauterization with silver nitrate. Application of common salt can be done every 3 to 4 days till the base is dry. Sepsis should be treated with local antibiotics or if needed systemic antibiotic is administered.

Mastitis Neonatorum

Bilateral engorgement and swelling of breasts may occur in full term babies of both sex on third or fourth day due to sudden withdrawal of maternal hormones. Lack of inactivation of progesterone and estrogens after birth due to immaturity of neonatal liver leads to further increase in their levels thus resulting in hypertrophy of breasts. No management is needed, the condition recovers spontaneously by 2 to 3 weeks. Mother should be explained to avoid local massage, fomentation and squeezing to express the milk. Reassurance to the mother is important.

Vaginal Bleeding and Mucoid Secretions

In about one-fourth of female babies menstrual like vaginal bleeding (pseudomenstruation) may occur after 3 to 5 days of birth due to withdrawal of maternal hormone. This may last for 2 to 4 days and is mild and harmless. No therapy is required, only aseptic cleaning of genitals should be done.

Most female babies have thick, white viscid vaginal discharge in early neonatal period due to effect of trans-placental acquired estrogen on the vaginal mucosa. No treatment is required, cleaning of the area is advised.

Physiological Phimosis

In about 80 percent of newborn male babies may have a prepuce that is adherent to the underlying glans. The foreskin is usually nonretractable and urethral opening is often pinpoint without any difficulties of micturition. No effort should be made to retract this, as it is physiologic findings and disappears in due course. If the condition persists beyond 3 years of age and causes difficulty on passing urine, it should be considered as pathological and special attention should be paid.

Caput Succedaneum and Cephalhematoma

See Birth Injury (page no. 93).

Physiological Jaundice

See Neonatal Jaundice (page no. 96).

Superficial Infections

See Neonatal Infections (page no. 88).

Minor Developmental Peculiarities

Mongolian Blue Spots

These spots are found in babies of Asian and African origin. It has no relation with mongolism, i.e. Down's syndrome. Irregular blue patches of skin pigmentations are found on the buttocks, sacral area and sometimes over the back and extremities of the newborn babies. These spots usually disappear within 6 months to one year of age. It should not be confused with bruising in babies with breech delivery.

Milia

The multiple tiny raised white or yellow white spots or cysts may appear on the nose, nasolabial folds, cheeks and forehead of neonates due to retention of sebum in the sebaceous glands. These cysts or spots are disappear spontaneously in the first few weeks.

Erythema Toxicum or Urticaria Neonatorum

In full term neonates, an erythematous rash with central pallor may appear on second or third day on the face and spreads to the trunk and extremities. The rash disappears spontaneously after 2 to 3 days. The exact cause of this condition is unknown but may be due to irritation of vernix or by various agents like toilet articles, clothing or any allergy. There is no systemic manifestations. The condition should be differentiated from pyoderma and skin lesions of congenital syphilis.

Peeling Skin

This is usually found in post-term neonates due to less amniotic fluid and sometimes may found in term neonates also. Dry scaly skin with peeling and exaggerated transverse skin creases are seen after 2 to 3 days of birth. Nothing needs to do or care for, application of olive oil, emollient cream or liquid paraffin may be useful.

Harlequin Color Change

The neonates may become blanched and pale on one-half of the body while other half remains pink. It may be due to unexplained vasomotor phenomenon and last for few minutes. Mother's anxiety to be relieved by adequate explanation and reassurance.

Salmon Patches (Stork Bites or Nevus Simplex)

Pinkish-gray capillary hemangioma usually found on the nape of the neck, upper eyelids, forehead and root of the nose of neonates, which spontaneously disappear within few months.

Epstein Pearl

The whitish spots usually found lateral to the midline of the hard palate may be seen due to epithelial inclusion and are of no significance. It can also be found as prepucial spots in some neonates as round and 1 to 2 mm in diameter, which usually appeared on the tip of the prepuce at 6 o'clock position. No treatment required.

Sucking Callosities

Button like cornified plaque at the center of upper lip may found at birth. It indicates sucking attempts of the baby in the intrauterine life. It subsides spontaneously.

Predeciduous Teeth (Natal Teeth)

These may present at birth or may erupt soon after birth. These teeth may interfere with breastfeeding or may become loose with risk of spontaneous dislodgement and aspiration. These teeth usually found in the lower incisor position and may shed before primary dentition. They need to be extracted when create problem.

Tongue Tie

It is found as a thin broad membrane or thick fibrous frenulum with a notch at the tip of the tongue. It may interfere with sucking and later in speech development of the child. This condition is uncommon and is a source of parental anxiety. It may be managed by snipping after the age of 3 months.

Subconjunctival Hemorrhage

It may present as semilunar area of bleeding at the outer canthus and usually absorbed within a few days without any residual effect or pigmentation. It is common in normal babies

and produces anxiety to the mothers, who need explanation and reassurance.

Umbilical Hernia

It may found after the age of two weeks or later and associated with weakness or faulty closure of the umbilical ring. It spontaneously disappears by one or two years of age. The practice of strapping it, with or without coin and bandage over the hernia are not recommended as they may interfere with spontaneous regression. It rarely causes strangulation or incarcination.

Congenital Hydrocele

A small fluid containing sac may found in one of the scrotal sacs at birth or during first weeks of life. The small hydrocele of tunica vaginalis may extend upwards in the spermatic cord. It usually disappears by 3 to 6 months of life.

Bowed Legs

In normal babies, legs (when extended) form a concavity inwards due to genu varus giving an appearance of bowed legs. It does not indicate ricket or any deformity. Afterwards, the bowed legs is changed and replaced by physiological knock knees, in about one year of age.

Other developmental peculiarites include prominent xiphisternum, sacral dimple, hymenal tags, nonretractable prepuce, acne neonatorum, subcutaneous fat necrosis (pseudosclerema), cutis marmorata, craniotabes, asymmetric head shape and benign neonatal hemangiomatosis. No management needed for these conditions. Mothers need explanation and reassurance about the nature of these problems. Nurses who are working in the delivery room, lying-in-ward or neonatal care units or working as community health workers should identify these minor problems and developmental peculiarities and provide necessary support to the mothers and family members.

Birth Asphyxia or Asphyxia Neonatorum

Birth asphyxia is the leading cause of neonatal mortality and morbidity. It is also an important cause of developmental delay and neurological problems both in term and preterm infants. Approximately 5 to 10 percent neonates experience asphyxia at birth. In healthy neonates, first respiration usually takes place within 6 seconds, majority of the baby takes spontaneous first respiration within 20 seconds and some baby takes 90 seconds after birth to have normal respiration. Anticipatory preparation for resuscitation of all neonates at birth should be kept ready in the delivery room to prevent birth asphyxia.

Definition

Birth asphyxia is the nonestablishment of satisfactory pulmonary respiration at birth. It is failure of initiation and maintenance of spontaneous respiration with hypo-ventilation, anaerobic glycolysis and lactic acidosis. It is characterized by progressive hypoxia, hypercapnia, hypo-perfusion and metabolic acidosis. It may result in multiorgan system dysfunction including hypoxic-ischemic encephalopathy and long-term neuromotor sequelae.

National Neonatology Forum of India has suggested that birth asphyxia should be diagnosed when the baby has gasping and inadequate breathing or no breathing at one minute. It corresponds to one minute Apgar score of 3 or less.

Most of these babies do not require specialized care and they do not have enhanced neonatal morbidity or increased risk of neuromotor disability on follow-up, if by 5 minutes after birth, the neonate is stable and breathing normally. Specialized care and long-term follow-up for developmental assessment are indicated in babies who fail to establish effective respiration at 5 minutes or the Apgar score at 5 minute is 3 or less.

Perinatal Asphyxia

It is the term used to the state of decreased oxygen delivery (hypoxia) to the fetus or neonate resulting in inadequate tissue perfusion (ischemia). It is manifested by low Apgar score and metabolic acidosis. It is often develop as continuation of antepartum and intrapartum problems. Perinatal asphyxia may result in adverse effects on all major body systems including brain, heart, kidney and lungs. The clinical presentations in asphyxiated neonates range from mild to severe impairment. The perinatal asphyxia is diagnosed when the neonate is having all of the following clinical and biochemical features:

- Cord blood (umbilical artery) pH of less than 7.0 with a base deficit of more than 10 mEq/L.
- Neonatal neurological manifestations suggestive of hypoxic-ischemic-encephalopathy (HIE).
- Evidences of multisystem organ dysfunction (e.g. cardiovascular, renal, gastrointestinal, hematologic or pulmonary).

Etiological Factors of Perinatal Asphyxia

Approximately 90 percent of asphyxial events occur as a result of placental insufficiency due to antepartum and intrapartum factors. Postnatal factors account for the remaining. These factors are responsible for failure of respiratory center or failure of pulmonary expansion. They cause circulatory collapse and lead to asphyxia.

Antepartum factors: These include placental insufficiency due to pre-eclampsia, hypertension, anemia, diabetes mellitus and postmaturity. Other factors include antepartum hemorrhage, malpresentation or abnormal lie, multifetal pregnancy, poor fetal growth, Rh-isoimmunization, bad obstetrical history, maternal systemic diseases (asthma, heart disease), poly- or oligohydramnios, maternal drug therapy (with lithium, reserpine, magnesium, etc.) or maternal drug abuse, placental malformations, vascular anomalies of the cord and congenital anomalies of fetus.

Intrapartum factors: The important intrapartum factors are fetal distress, preterm labor, antepartum hemorrhage (placenta previa, abruptio placentae), cord prolapse, tight umbilical cord around the fetal neck, premature rupture of membrane, meconium stained liquor, prolonged labor more than 24 hours, prolonged second stage more than 2 hours, maternal distress (dehydration, hypotension, acidosis), use of anesthesia and narcotics to the mother, birth trauma (increased intracranial pressure due to hemorrhage), difficult delivery in malpresentation and instrumental or operative delivery.

Postnatal factors: These are mainly related to pulmonary, cardiovascular and neurological abnormalities of the neonate. Aspiration causing obstruction of air passages, is an important factor of postnatal asphyxia. Circulatory collapse due to blood loss and shock may also lead to birth asphyxia. Preterm babies are more prone to birth asphyxia due to weak respiratory muscle, poor pulmonary expansion, low alveolar surfactant and inefficient respiratory center.

Pathophysiology of Asphyxia

Birth asphyxia is related with reduction in the arterial oxygen tension, accumulation of carbon dioxide and fall in blood pH. Acidosis occurs due to the anaerobic utilization of glucose, production of lactic acid and accumulation of carbon dioxide. These biochemical changes result in constriction of muscular pulmonary arterioles and raise pulmonary arterial pressure which lead to reduced filling of left heart and right to left shunts and heart failure. Hypoglycemia occurs due to utilization of glucose and depletion of glycogen stores. Petechial hemorrhage occur due to anoxic capillary changes. Cerebral edema develops due to intracellular collection of sodium and inappropriate release of ADH. In prolonged asphyxia, myocardial function and cardiac output deteriorate. Blood flow to all organs is reduced and progressive organ damage result.

Initial deprivation of oxygen results in rapid breathing, if asphyxia continues, the respiratory movements stop and the heart rate begins to fall with gradual diminution of neuromuscular tone. Then the baby enters into a period of apnea known as primary apnea. In this stage stimulation and exposure to oxygen may induce respiration.

But if the asphyxia continues, the neonate develops deep gasping respiration, the heart continues to decrease, the blood pressure begin to fall, the baby becomes nearly flaccid, the respiration becomes weaker and weaker until the neonate takes last gasp and enters into a period of secondary apnea. The baby becomes unresponsive to stimulation and will not spontaneously resume respiratory efforts unless resuscitation with assisted ventilation and oxygenation is initiated promptly.

Primary and secondary apnea is difficult to distinguish. All apnea at birth should be considered as secondary apnea and resuscitation should be initiated immediately to prevent brain damage and multiorgan system dysfunction.

Clinical Features

The clinical manifestations depends upon the etiology, intensity, duration of oxygen lack, plasma carbon dioxide level and acidosis. According to the intensity of clinical features the condition have been classified previously as: (a) asphyxia livida or stage of cyanosis, primarily due to respiratory failure with Apgar score 4 to 6 and (b) asphyxia pallida or stage of shock due to combined respiratory and vasomotor failure with Apgar score 0 to 3.

Depending upon the Apgar scoring system the score 0 to 3 indicate severe depression, the score 4 to 6 indicates moderate depression and the score 7 to 10 indicates no depression.

The most severely asphyxiated neonates may present with coma or stupor, hypotonia, periodic or irregular breathing, loss of reflexes, apnea and seizures. The survived infants may have permanent neurodevelopmental sequelae.

The Apgar scoring system is not used to determine when to initiate resuscitation or to make decisions about the course of resuscitation. The evaluation is based on three important signs, i.e. respiration, heart rate and skin color. Based on the assessment of these signs prompt initiation of resuscitation can be done, not delaying one minute for Apgar scoring. A delay could result critical problem specially in severely depressed baby. While the Apgar score is not helpful for decision-making at the starting of a resuscitation, it may be useful for assessing the baby's condition and effectiveness of the resuscitative measures at 5 minutes. The scoring can be done every 5 minutes for up to 20 minutes to assess the baby's condition.

Preparation for Resuscitation

Considering every birth as a high risk, all resuscitation arrangement and essentials to be kept ready. At least one health personnel should be skilled in neonatal resuscitation, who should present at the delivery room. Heat source should be kept ready for use.

The resuscitation room/area in the delivery room must be well-lighted, warm with all arrangement for resuscitation. The essential articles should be in good working condition and must be checked by the nursing personnel in every duty shift. Resuscitation procedure should be performed with full aseptic precautions. Universal precautions against HIV infection should also be maintained.

The essential equipment and supplies of neonatal resuscitation are as follows:

1. **Suction equipment:** Mucous aspirator (disposable DeLee's type), meconium aspirator, mechanical suction apparatus (slow sucker machine), suction catheters, feeding tube and 10 or 20 mL syringe.
2. **Bag and mask** for neonatal resuscitation and oxygen source with flowmeter, oxygen reservoir and tubing. Face mask should be of appropriate size for both term and preterm babies.
3. **Intubation equipment:** Neonatal laryngoscope with straight blade (No-00, 0 for preterm and No-1 for term babies), extra bulb and batteries, endotracheal tubes (size—2.5, 3.0, 3.5, 4.0 mm ID), stylet, scissors.
4. **Medications:** Epinephrine, naloxone hydrochloride, normal saline, Ringer's lactate solution, sodium bicarbonate, albumin, dextrose (5%, 10%), sterile water ampule for injection, dopamine, slow infusion pump.
5. **Miscellaneous:** Watch with seconds' hand, prewarmed linen, towel shoulder roll, radiant warmer or heat source (bulb–200 W), stethoscope, syringes (1, 2, 3, 5, 10, 20, 50 mL), needles, umbilical catheters (3.5F, 5F), three-way stopcocks, gloves, gauze, adhesive tape, room thermometer, low reading thermometer or telethermometer, scalp vein set or IV canula, neonatal feeding tube, airway tube and spot light.

TABCs of Resuscitation

The components of the neonatal resuscitation procedure are described as the acronym TABCs of resuscitation.

T - Maintenance of temperature
- Provision of radiant heat source
- Drying the baby
- Removing wet linen

A - Establishment of an open airway
- Position the infant
- Suction the mouth, nose and in some instances the trachea (in meconium stained liquor)
- If necessary, insert an ET tube to ensure open airway.

B - Initiation of breathing
- Tactile stimulation to initiate respirations
- Positive pressure ventilation (PPV), using either bag and mask or bag and ET tube.

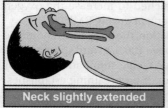 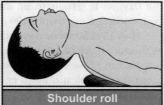

Fig. 6.2: Positioning

C - Maintenance of circulation
- Stimulate and maintain the blood circulation by chest compression and/or medications.

Initial Steps of Resuscitation
[See NRP-Guideline (Appendix XVII)]

a. Receiving the newborn baby in a prewarmed towel and placing the baby on the preheated radiant warmer. If warmer is not available, room heater or a bulb of 200W can be used, which should be fixed in a suitable place. Never allow the baby to become hypothermic.
b. Positioning the baby on the back with the neck slightly extended sniffing position. Hyperextension or underextension should be prevented which may decrease air entry. To maintain correct position, shoulder roll may be useful, elevating the shoulder 3/4 to 1 inch off the mattress (Fig. 6.2). If the neonate has copious secretions, head should be turned to one side. Never keep the baby's head too low for too long time.
c. Suctioning of the mouth should be done first then the nose, otherwise there is chance of aspiration of secretions from mouth. Suctioning should be done carefully to prevent stimulation of posterior pharynx which can lead to bradycardia and apnea. Vigorous and continuous suction to be avoided. Suction pressure to be kept around 80 to 100 mm Hg (100–130 cm water). Tracheal suctioning may be needed through endotracheal (ET) intubation in meconium stained liquor.
d. Drying the baby's whole body and head quickly and removing the wet linen immediately. The baby is then placed further on a prewarmed towel to reduce heat loss. Drying the baby prevent evaporative heat loss and provide gentle stimulation which may help to initiate respiration.
e. *Providing tactile stimulation* by slapping or flicking the soles of the feet or rubbing the infant's back once or twice to stimulate breathing (Fig. 6.3). Continued use of tactile stimulation in an infant who does not respond, may be harmful and wastage of valuable time. The baby who is not taking respiration spontaneously, may breathe after one or two tactile stimulation only.
f. *Using free flow oxygen* by blowing over the infant's nose so that the baby breaths oxygen enriched air. This can be given by using oxygen mask or cupped hand at the flow rate of 5 liters per minute (Fig. 6.4).

After these initial steps of resuscitation the baby should be evaluated for respiration, heart rate and skin color. Evaluation may be done before tactile stimulation.

If the baby is having spontaneous respiration and heart rate above 100 beats per minute with skin color pink or acrocyanosis then the baby needs observation and monitoring only.

If the baby is breathing spontaneously and heart rate is more than 100 beats per minute, with cyanosis at lips or tongue (central) then free flow oxygen is administered.

When the infant has no spontaneous breathing then positive pressure ventilation (PPV) should be started with bag and mask. If the baby is taking respiration spontaneously but heart rate is below 100 beats per minute, at that condition also PPV should be started immediately.

Bag and Mask Ventilation

Bag and mask ventilation should be started if after tactile stimulation, (a) the infant is still apneic or gasping or (b) having spontaneous respiration but heart rate is below 100 beats per minute. It is contraindicated in diaphragmatic hernia. It should be done after tracheal suction in thick meconium stained liquor.

For bag and mask ventilation, the baby's neck should be slightly extended to ensure open airway. Mask to be placed in position and seal to be checked by 2 to 3 ventilation. Place the mask covering tip of the chin, the mouth and the nose.

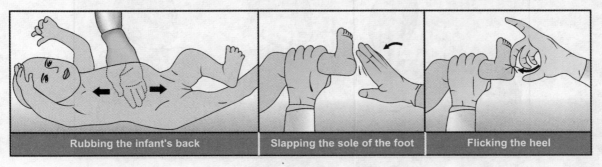

Fig. 6.3: Tectile stimulation

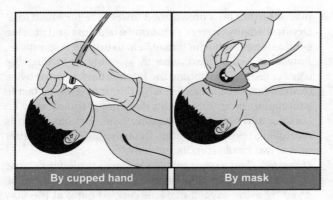

Fig. 6.4: Free flow oxygen therapy

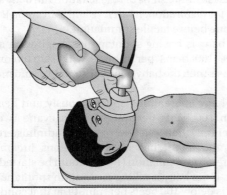

Fig. 6.5: Bag mask ventilation

Rise of chest to be observed and if chest does not rise then reapply mask, reposition baby's head, suction if needed and ventilate with slightly open mouth and increased pressure. Ventilation should be done at the rate of 40 to 60 breaths per minute. Follow a "squeeze", "two", "three", "squeeze" sequence (Fig. 6.5).

Bag and mask ventilation (BMV) should be initiated with air only. Then oxygen tubing from the oxygen source and the oxygen reservoir to be attached to increase the oxygen concentration even upto 100 percent during BMV.

After 15 to 30 seconds ventilation, the baby again should be evaluated. If the heart rate is above 100 b/m and spontaneous respiration present then provide tactile stimulation, monitor heart rate, respiration and color. If no breathing establishes, continue ventilation.

If heart rate is between 60 and 100 b/m and increasing then ventilation to be continued. If heart rate not increasing with ventilation then check adequacy of ventilation and start chest compression. When heart rate is below 60 b/m then ventilation to be continued and chest compression to be started.

When bag and mask ventilation is continued more then 2 minutes then an orogastric feeding tube should be inserted and left open to decompress the abdomen. For giving bag and mask ventilation full palmer grasp should not be used.

Chest Compression

Chest compression must always be performed along with ventilation and 100 percent oxygen. It is indicated if after 15 to 30 seconds of PPV with 100 percent oxygen, the heart rate is below 60 beats per minute and not increasing. Chest compression or external cardiac massage is given to increase the intrathoracic pressure and to circulate blood to the vital organs of the body. It is done by thumb technique or two fingers technique (Fig. 6.6). The pressure is applied to the lower third of the sternum to depress it 1/2 to 3/4 inches. The rate of chest compressions in one minute should be 90 along with 30 PPVs, (3:1), a total of 120 events. One ventilation should follow every third chest compressions. Follow "one and two and three and breath and" sequence. Person 1 will do chest compression and person 2 will do PPV with bag and mask. Three chest compression in 1.5 seconds and 1/2 second for ventilation. To determine the effectiveness of chest compression brachial or femoral pulse should be checked. There is risk of trauma (broken ribs, pneumothorax) during chest compression,

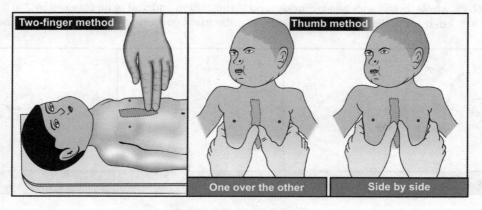

Fig. 6.6: Chest compression

so it should be done with correct position of fingers and appropriate pressure.

Chest compression should be continued along with ventilation till the heart rate is 60 b/m or above. Medications may be required. When heart rate is 60 b/m or above, chest compression should be discontinued and when 100 b/m and have spontaneous breathing, ventilation should be discontinued.

Endotracheal Intubation

Endotracheal (ET) intubation is a specialized and skilled procedure. It is indicated when, (a) prolonged PPV is required, (b) bag and mask ventilation is ineffective, (c) tracheal suction is needed and (d) diaphragmatic hernia is suspected.

Appropriate size of the tubes should be selected and must have vocal cord guide. It is cut at 13 cm and the connector to be replaced. Laryngoscope should be in working condition and of appropriate size. Infant should be positioned on a flat surface with the neck slightly extended. The procedure is usually performed by skilled neonatologist or anesthesiologist or any doctor skilled with this technique. Preparation of the essentials, positioning, assisting during the procedure are the important responsibilities of the nursing personnel. Only a small number of neonates required ET intubation.

Medications (See NRP Protocol 2010)

All essential medications should be kept in the resuscitation room and should be administered aseptically. Umbilical vein is preferred route via a catheter, because scalp veins and extremities are difficult to approach. No intracardiac injections are recommended in neonates. Direct injection in to umbilical cord should not be attempted. Some medication can be given directly through ET tube. Epinephrine and normal saline are commonly used in recommended doses. Recommended dose of epinephrine is 0.01 to 0.03 mg/kg/dose intravenous and 0.05 mg to 0.1 mg/kg/dose intratracheal. The concentration of epinephrine for either route should be 1:10,000 (0.1 mg/mL). Normal saline should be given with 10 mL/kg body weight. Sodium bicarbonate should not be administered till the ventilation is established. No respiratory stimulants is needed. Metabolic acidosis should be managed by oxygen and volume expander and not with sodium bicarbonate. If indicated in case of diagnosed acidosis, sodi-bi-carb should be diluted 1:1 with water for injection and administered slowly (*See* Neonatal Resuscitation Guidelines in Appendix XVII).

Systemic Manifestations of Severe Birth Asphyxia

Hypoxia can cause damage to almost every tissue and organ of the baby. A variety of clinical problems are found in severe birth asphyxia in early neonatal period. Long-term sequelae are found as neurological problems, mental retardation and multiorgan system dysfunction.

Brain: Hypoxic-ischemic encephalopathy, intracranial hemorrhage, apneic attacks, convulsions.

Heart: Persistent fetal circulation, hypoxic cardiomyopathy, cardiac dysrrhythmias, congestive cardiac failure, tricuspid regurgitation, shock.

Lungs: Meconium aspiration syndrome, hyaline membrane disease, pulmonary hemorrhage, pneumonia, pnemothorax.

Kidneys: Hematuria, renal failure, acute tubular necrosis, renal vein thrombosis.

Gastrointestinal: Necrotizing enterocolitis, paralytic ileus and obstruction.

Hematologic: Disseminated intravascular coagulopathy (DIC), hyperbilirubinemia and sepsis.

Endocrine: Adrenal hemorrhage, syndrome of inappropriate antidiuretic hormone and transient hypoparathyroidism.

Immunologic: Septicemia.

Prognosis of birth asphyxia depends upon the associated factors, maturity of the baby, duration and intensity of hypoxia and acidosis and initiation of resuscitative measures in the delivery room. Subsequent competent care and available facilities also influence the outcome following birth asphyxia.

Preventive measures of neonatal asphyxia are very important. Intensive antenatal care to detect risk factors and adequate interventions or referal are vital aspects of prevention. Intranatal assessment of fetal hypoxia and management of fetal distress should be done promptly. Careful and intelligent use of anesthetic agents and depressant drugs in labor along with efficient management of delivery and care of neonates at birth are the essentials for the prevention of birth asphyxia. Special attention should be paid for avoidance of preterm delivery, care of preterm and low birth weight infant to prevent birth asphyxia.

Nursing personnel should work in all levels of care to prevent this life-threatening condition. Appropriate management following intelligent assessment by the nursing personnel in the antenatal and intranatal period can help to save the neonatal life and prevent the long-term sequela of the problem.

Postasphyxia Management of Neonates

After effective resuscitation and initial stabilization of the asphyxiated neonates at the delivery room, these infants need supportive and symptomatic management with continuous monitoring for their better prognosis. It is necessary to prevent permanent neurological sequel resulting from extension of cerebral injury.

Supportive management of asphyxiated neonates includes maintenance of temperature, oxygenation, tissue perfusion and normal metabolic state along with early detection of complications by clinical and biochemical monitoring.

The following supportive care must be provided to the asphyxiated neonates in the special neonatal care units (SNCUs) or in neonatal intensive care units (NICU):

- Care under radiant warmer with thermoneutral state of the baby. Hyperthermia should be avoided. Presently, evidence shows that hypothermia is neuroprotective for asphyxiated neonates.
- Provision of oxygen therapy with maintenance of oxygen saturation (SpO_2) in between 88 to 92 percent in preterm and 88 to 93 percent in term neonates by pulse oximetry. Both hypoxia and hyperoxia should be avoided as they can damage the neurons. PaO_2 should be kept in normal range. Baby may require CPAP or invasive ventilator support.
- Clinical monitoring should be done for respiratory status, heart rate, color, SpO_2, CRT, BP, skin temperature, urine output, abdominal circumference to rule out any ileus, level of consciousness, muscle tone, convulsions, features of sepsis, etc.
- Biochemical monitoring and maintenance of normal blood glucose (75–100 mg/dL), serum calcium (9–11 mg/dL), hematocrit, urea, creatinine and electrolyte (Na, K) level are very important along with IV fluid therapy as per daily requirement.
- Maintenance of systemic mean arterial blood pressure (Mean BP) is very important to maintain cerebral perfusion. Mean BP should be 45 to 50 mm Hg for term infants, 35 to 40 for infants weighing 1000 to 2000 gm and 30 to 35 mm Hg for infants less than 1000 gm.
- Capillary refilling time (CRT), pulse volume and urine output should be assessed frequently and maintained within normal range. Normal value of CRT is less than 3 seconds and urine output is 1–3 mL/kg/hour.
- If the neonate is having prolonged CRT due to poor tissue perfusion and features of shock, then fluid resuscitation is done by IV normal saline bolus of 10 mL/kg over 20 to 30 minutes. Repeat bolus can be given if there is no improvement. If the signs of poor perfusion persist despite two fluid boluses, then vasopressors (Dopamine, Dobutamine) should be administered as per recommended dose.
- Injection vitamin 'K' must be given, if not received at birth.
- If the neonate is having seizures in presence of normal blood glucose then anticonvulsant drug (ACD), Injection Phenoberbitone should be administered in a loading dose of 20 mg/kg, slowly IV at the rate of 1 mg/kg/minute. Additional boluses of 10 mg/kg can be given if seizures continue or recur. Maximum loading dose can be given up to 40 mg/kg. Maintenance dose followed by bolus should be administered with 3 to 4 mg/kg/day. If seizures persist despite of above treatment, then phenytoin may be administered as loading dose with 20 mg/kg IV, followed by 4 to 8 mg/kg/day as maintenance dose. ACD should be discontinued before discharge from hospital, if neurological examination is normal. There is no need to taper the ACD.

- Feeding should be started when the neonate is hemodynamically stable, there is no abdominal distension and the baby has passed meconium. Feeding should be given with expressed breast milk (EBM) 20 to 30 mL/kg and increasing the amount of feed as the baby tolerates. Initially gavage feeding is given with EBM. Then gradually shifted to paladai or katori-spoon feeding with EBM and to breast feeding. Asepsis must be maintained for feeding procedures. Intake output chart should be maintained strictly. Neonates should be monitored for the features of sepsis.
- Baby friendly environment should be provided with soft sound, soothing light, thermoneutral environment, infection free environment, nesting as boundaries, appropriate positioning, clustering of care activities, gentle handling with soft touch and involvement of mother in routine care.
- Developmental supportive care with humanized approach and therapeutic stimulation are important to prevent neurological complications and muscular deformities. Humanized care is very significant in the highly technological environment of intensive care.
- Symptomatic treatment should be provided with necessary diagnostic investigations. Screening for ROP and hearing should be arranged. Regular communication and counseling to be done with family members for management of neonates.
- Discharge planning with mother's teaching for home care and follow-up care is important for prevention of long term complications.

Poor Prognostic Factors

Poor prognosis as poor neurodevelopmental outcome may be anticipated in the presence of one or more of the following features:

- Failure to establish respiration by 5 minutes of life
- Apgar score of 3 or less at 5 minutes
- Onset of seizure within 12 hours of birth and refractory seizure
- Severe hypoxic ischemic encephalopathy (stage-III)
- Persistant oliguria (less than 1 mL/kg/hour) for 36 hours of life
- Inability to establish oral feeds by one week.

Neonatal Hypothermia

Hypothermia is considered as silent killer in neonates. It increases the neonatal morbidity and mortality. Maintenance of warmth of the neonates enhances their survival.

Piere Budin (1900) first drew attention to the high neonatal mortality due to cold. Optimum thermal environment for neonates was identified in mid 1960s, as they are easily influenced by the extremes of environmental temperature. Thermal protection of the newborn babies is considered as one of important essential neonatal care.

Definition

Hypothermia is a common alteration of thermoregulatory state of the neonates. Neonatal hypothermia occurs when the body temperature drops below 36.5°C or 97.7°F in the newborn infant (WHO). Normal body temperature is between 36.5 to 37.5°C.

Stages of Neonatal Hypothermia

The thermoneutral state of the neonates is considered within the normal range of 36.5 to 37.5°C.

The *stages of hypothermia* are as follows:
a. *Cold stress:* When the body temperature of the newborn baby is between 36 to 36.4°C (96.8–97.6°F) then the baby is under cold stress.
b. *Moderate hypothermia:* An infant with temperature of 32 to 35.9°C (89.6–96.6°F) has moderate hypothermia, which is a danger to the baby.
c. *Severe hypothermia:* An infant with a temperature of below 32°C or 89.6°F is suffering from severe hypothermia, which need urgent skilled care.

A skin temperature change is the initial indicator of cold stress. A decreased core temperature (rectal) is a late warning sign indicating that the neonate is already compromised.

Factors Responsible for Neonatal Hypothermia

Lack of awareness and attention, about the importance of warmth for neonates, among health care providers.

Inappropriate care of the baby immediately after birth by inadequate drying and wrapping.
- Separation of baby from the mother.
- Cold environment at the place of delivery and baby care areas.
- Change of temperature from womb to cooler extrauterine environment.
- Inadequate warming procedure before and during transport of the baby.
- Excessive heat loss by evaporation, conduction, convection and radiation from wet baby to the cold linen, cold room and cold air.
- Certain characteristics of neonates, i.e. large body surface area per unit of body weight, large head, developmental immaturity of heat regulation center, poor insulation due to less subcutaneous fat in LBW baby and reduced brown adipose tissue (BAT) as heat source.
- High risk neonates—LBW baby, birth asphyxia, congenital malformations and mother having anesthetic drugs.

Process of Thermoregulation

Neonates are easily affected by temperature variation (thermolabile). Thermoregulation is important for both term and preterm neonates because they have to adapt from intrauterine life to extrauterine life during transition.

In fetal life, placenta acts as heat exchanger from mother. But after birth, the baby has to maintain and produce heat for his own. At birth, the infant adapts from warm womb's temperature (approx 37°C) to external environment which can be 10 to 20°C cooler and evaporative heat loss is about 200 cal/kg per minute with fall of skin temperature about 0.3°C per minute. Neonates have limited energy source for temperature regulation.

Thermoregulation is maintained by the process of heat production or gain and heat loss.

The mechanism of heat production in neonates is known as nonshivering thermogenesis (NST) and the site of heat production is brown adipose tissue (BAT). When heat loss begins, thermoreceptors of subcutenous tissue, spinal cord and hypothalamus are stimulated and NST is triggered. The noradrenaline released from sympathetic nervous system which acts on brown fat and helps in heat production. In full-term neonates BAT accounts for 4 percent of total fat, which is less in LBW infants. BAT is located in the axillary, neck, interscapular region, mediastinum, around kidney and adrenal glands. It helps in chemical thermogenesis.

Heat loss in neonates occur by evaporation, conduction, convection and radiation. Heat loss by evaporation occurs immediately after birth if the baby is not dried and not covered adequately. If humidity of the room is less, then evaporative heat loss increased from exposed areas. Neonate may loss heat by conduction, i.e. direct contact with cooler object or surface (e.g. cold table, mackintosh, towel, tray, hands, weighing scale, etc.). Heat loss by convection takes place, when the baby is placed in the cooler air and air movement is present there, (e.g. open window, fans). By radiation the infant loses heat to cooler object. Colder the object and closer it is to the neonate, the greater the loss of heat by radiation.

Clinical Features of Neonatal Hypothermia

Early clinical signs
- Skin temperature of the neonate is below 36.5°C
- Hands, feet, abdomen are cold to touch
- Weak sucking ability, weak cry and lethergy
- Blue hands and feet due to peripheral vasoconstriction.

Late signs due to persistent hypothermia
- Gradual fall of body temperature
- Slow, shallow and irregular respiration
- Slow heart rate
- Lethargy and poor response
- Pale body with face and extremities of bright red color
- Central cyanosis may present
- Edema and sclerema (localized hardening of the tissue) may be present
- Weight loss.

Consequence of Neonatal Hypothermia

Neonatal hypothermia has a number of serious consequences. It has both immediate and long-term effects. The effects are hypoxia (due to more oxygen consumption), hypoglycemia (due to increased metabolism), metabolic acidosis (due to BAT hydrolysis), respiratory distress, neonatal sepsis, neonatal jaundice, sclerema, pulmonary hemorrhage, impaired cardiac function, coagulopathy, sudden infant death syndrome, delayed growth and development, mental retardation, etc.

Concept of "Warm Chain"

The concept of warm chain was introduced to describe a set of interlinked procedures to minimize the likelihood of hypothermia in all neonates. The links of warm chain are warmth at birth place, warmth during transportation and warmth at hospital or home. These should be maintained by the following activities:

a. Warm delivery room (more than 25°C) which should be free from draught.
  - Warm reception and resuscitation of all neonates
  - Immediate drying and wrapping
  - Skin to skin contact between the mother and neonate (kangaroo mother care)
  - Putting in mother's breast within half an hour of birth.
  - Postponing bathing
  - Appropriate clothing, and bedding and covering head properly
  - Mother and baby nursed together (bedding-in or rooming-in) in the delivery room or in lying-in ward.
b. Warm and safe transportation.
c. Warmth in special neonatal care unit.
  - Training of all health care providers who are involved in birth and subsequent care of the neonates, especially on prevention of hypothermia, for improvement of awareness about the silent killer.

Prevention of Neonatal Hypothermia

The following measures should be taken for the prevention of neonatal hypothermia (Fig. 6.7):

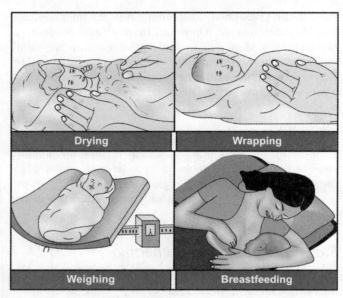

Fig. 6.7: Prevention of hypothermia

At the time of birth in delivery room
- Delivery room should be warm and free from draught.
- Immediate drying and wrapping of the neonate in layers of soft cloths or prewarm towel. Ensuring that head is well-covered. Wet cloth to be changed immediately.
- Provision of extrawarmth by radiant warmer or room heater or 200 W bulb, as available.
- Baby should be kept by skin to skin contact or by the side of the mother so that mother's warmth will keep the baby warm.
- Fans to be kept off to prevent air movement, windows to be kept closed to prevent draught. Room temperature to be maintain 28 + 2°C or according to baby's weight and postnatal age.
- Baby bath should be postponed. Cleaning of blood and meconium should be done with lukewarm water. Undue exposure of the baby should be avoided during nursing procedures.
- Allowing breastfeeding with half an hour of birth or as early as possible to provide warmth, nutrition and protection.
- Continuous observation of thermal state and other vital signs.
- Keeping the baby in skin to skin contact with mother in kangaroo method to maintain temperature, facilitate breastfeeding and improve mother-infant bonding.

During transportation: Transportation is the potential weakest link of warm chain. Temperature maintenance during transport is an important aspect of prevention of neonatal hypothermia.

- Baby should be transferred after establishment of thermal stability.
- Assess the baby's condition and temperature. Baby's hands and feet should be as warm as abdomen.
- Baby can be transferred in skin to skin contact with mother in kangaroo method or mother can keep the baby close to her chest. Baby should be wrapped in prewarmed cloth. Baby's head, and extremities should be covered properly avoid undressing the baby unnecessarily.
- Baby can be transferred within thermocol box with prewarmed linen, plastic bubble sheet or silver swaddler.
- Simple open transport trolley should be avoided.

At neonatal care unit: When mother is sick and unable to take care of her baby then neonates are kept in the neonatal care unit. Precautions should be taken to prevent hypothermia along with other essential care.

- Receiving the neonate in prewarmed cot.
- Covering the baby with adequate clothing including head and extremities and avoiding undue exposure.
- Keeping the ambient atmospheric temperature warm for baby's weight and age (28–32°C).
- Maintaining humidity around 50 percent.
- Early feeding with breast milk.
- Avoiding dip bath during hospital stay, till the umbilical cord has fallen off. Sponge bath can be given with warm water in warm room quickly and gently then wrapping promptly.
- Monitoring baby's temperature 3 hourly, during initial postnatal days considering axillary temperature is as good as core temperature.
- Gradual rewarming of the baby if she or he is cold. Using extra warming devices whenever needed like radiant warmer, room heater, heated water filled mattress, isolette or incubator. Avoiding direct use of hot water bottles.
- Decrease heat loss by convection, conduction and radiation.

At home: Nurse should teach the mother and family members about neonatal care at home especially for maintenance of warmth and breastfeeding. Warmth to be maintained by warm room (rooming-in), skin to skin contact (kangarooing), adequate clothing, exclusive breastfeeding, bathing with warm water in warm room, oil massage and use of solar heat. Mother should be taught to assess the thermal state by touch. The warm and pink feet of the baby indicate that the baby is in thermal comfort. But when feet are cold and abdomen is warm to touch, the baby is in cold stress. In hypothermia both feet and abdomen are cold to touch.

Assessment of Temperature in Neonates

Low reading thermometer should be used to measure the neonate's body temperature. Same thermometer should be used in an individual neonate at the same site.

Axillary temperature is preferable as it is safe and hygienic. It reflects rectal temperature if taken properly. For accurate results, the neonate's arm should be adducted with the thermometer bulb deep in the axillary pit. Axillary temperature is as good as core temperature, provided thermometer kept for 3 to 5 minutes. Normal axillary temperature range is 36.3 to 37°C.

Skin temperature is measured by thermistor (telethermometer) taped to skin of abdomen. The normal skin temperature for term babies is 36 to 36.5°C and in preterm babies 36.2 to 37.2°C.

Rectal temperature is not recorded in neonates for routine monitoring. It is used only for a sick hypothermic newborns. Normal rectal temperature in neonates is 36.6 to 37.2°C. Rectal thermometer to be inserted with precaution in backward and downward direction. The depth of insertion should be 3 cm for term babies and 2 cm for preterm babies.

Baby's temperature can be assessed with reasonable precision by human touch. Abdominal temperature is representative of the core temperature and reliable in the diagnosis of hypothermia.

Management of Neonatal Hypothermia

A hypothermic neonate should be rewarmed as quickly as possible. Rewarming procedure depends upon the severity of hypothermia and available facilities.

In moderate hypothermia (32–35.9°C), the neonate should be placed with mother in skin to skin contact in a warm room and warm bed. Radiant warmer or incubator can be used if available. Rewarming should be continued till the temperature reaches normal range. Monitor temperature every 15 to 30 minutes.

In severe hypothermia, rewarming should be done with air heated incubator (air temperature 35–36°C) or manually operated radiant warmer or thermostatically controlled heated mattress set at 37 to 38°C. When body temperature reaches 34°C, the rewarming process should be slowed down. Room heater, or 200 W bulb or infrared bulb can also be used. Monitor blood pressure, heart rate, temperature and blood glucose level. Preventive measures to reduce heat losses from the baby should be followed. IV infusion with 10 percent dextrose, oxygen therapy and vitamin 'K' injection (1 mg for term baby and 0.5 mg for preterm baby) should be administered along with routine and supportive care.

Preventive measures should be implemented against neonatal hypothermia to reduce morbidity and improved survival of newborn babies, which are more easier than the curative management and rewarming for neonatal hypothermia. Good quality obstetrical and neonatal care services and attention of concerned health care providers are essential for prevention of this health hazards. The health worker and mother should have knowledge and skill for assessment and prevention of hypothermia with use of common sense, which is more important than the availability of expensive equipment to keep the baby warm.

Respiratory Distress in Neonates

Respiratory distress in neonates is a common emergency life threatening condition. It is identified with the presence of tachypnea (respiration rate more than 60 breaths/minute), chest indrawing (subcostal, substernal, intercostal retractions) and expiratory grunting. Cyanosis, nasal flaring along with alteration of air entry may also found in this problem.

Common Causes

- *Pulmonary causes:* Respiratory distress syndrome (RDS) or hyaline membrane disease (HMD) due to surfactant deficiency, meconium aspiration syndrome (MAS), transient tachypnea of newborn (TTNB), persistant pulmonary hypertension (PPHN), pneumonia, milk aspiration, pneumothorax, pleural effusion and congenital malformations like tracheoesophageal fistula with esophageal atresia (TEF with EA), congenital diaphragmatic hernia (CDH), lobar emphysema, pulmonary hypoplasia and bilateral choanal atresia.
- *Nonpulmonary causes:* Perinatal asphyxia, hypothermia, hypoglycemia, metabolic acidosis, cerebral edema, neurological disorders, congenital heart disease, congestive heart failure, hemorrhage, severe anemia, etc.

Diagnostic Evaluation

- Details relevant antenatal and perinatal history should be collected which include gestational age, age of onset of respiratory distress, prolonged rupture of membrane more than 24 hours, intrapartum fever of mother, meconium stained liquor, presence of asphyxia, maternal diabetes mellitus etc.
- Examination should be done to assess severity of respiratory distress, air entry, neurological status, capillary refill time, cyanosis, features of sepsis and presence of malformations.
- Assessment of severity of respiratory distress to be done using Silverman – Anderson Scoring and Downe's scoring system (Fig. 6.8, Tables 6.4 and 6.5).
- Chest X-ray, sepsis screen and blood culture are very important to confirm the diagnosis and cause of respiratory distress.

Management

1. Maintaining of thermoneutral environment to keep the baby warm with normal body temperature.
2. Providing clear airway by positioning and removal of secretions by suctioning.
3. Administering oxygen by oxygen hood or nasal prongs to maintain target saturations. SpO_2 level should be

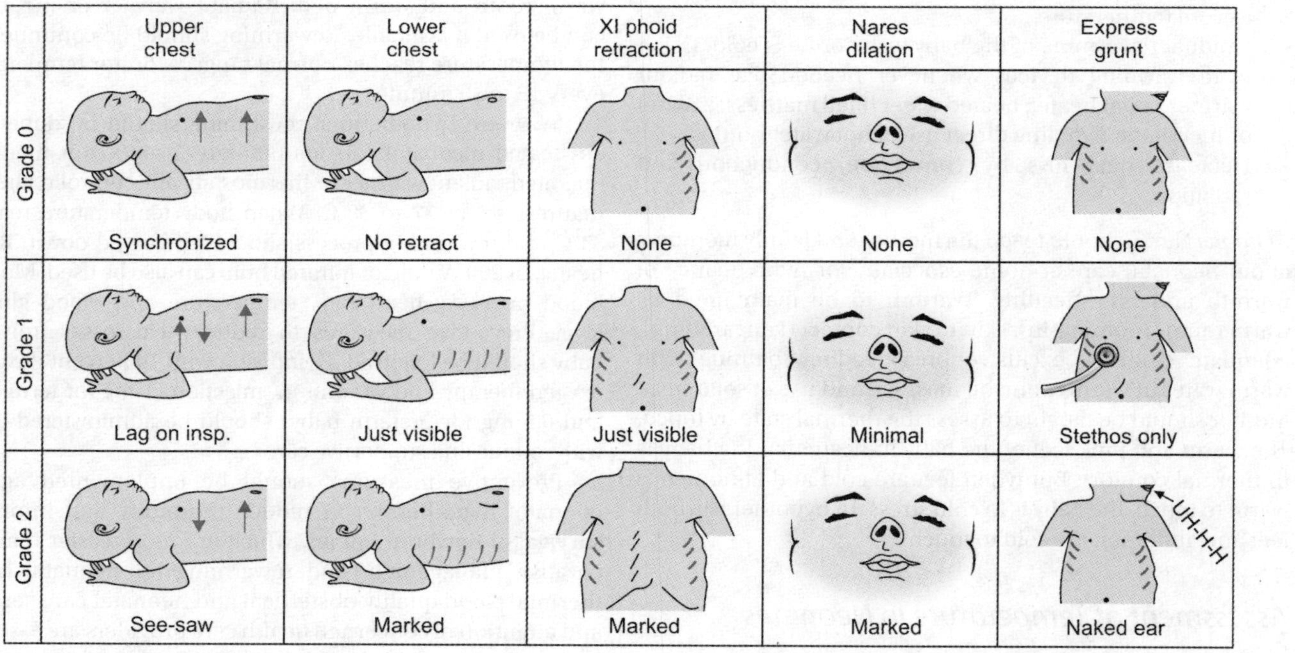

	Upper chest	Lower chest	Xl phoid retraction	Nares dilation	Express grunt
Grade 0	Synchronized	No retract	None	None	None
Grade 1	Lag on insp.	Just visible	Just visible	Minimal	Stethos only
Grade 2	See-saw	Marked	Marked	Marked	Naked ear

Fig. 6.8: The Silverman score for assessing the magnitude of respiratory distress (From Avery ME, Fletcher BD. The lung and its disorders in the newborn. Philadelphia, WB Saunders Company, 1974) (*Courtesy:* WA Silverman)

Table 6.4 Silverman Anderson score and its interpretation

Score	Upper chest retraction	Lower chest retraction	Xiphoid retraction	Nasal flaring	Grunt
0	Synchronized	None	None	None	None
1	Lag during inspiration	Just visible	Just visible	Minimal	Audible with stethoscope
2	See-saw	Marked	Marked	Marked	Audible with unaided ear

Interpretation
Score 0–3 = Mild respiratory distress—O_2 by hood
Score 4–6 = Moderate respiratory distress—CPAP
Score > 6 = Impending respiratory failure

Table 6.5 Downe's score and its interpretation

Score	Respiratory rate	Cyanosis	Air entry	Grunt	Retraction
0	< 60/min	Nil	Normal	None	Nil
1	60–80/min	In room air	Mild decrease	Audible with stethoscope	Mild
2	>80/min	In >40% FiO_2	Marked decrease	Audible with unaided ear	Moderate

Interpretation
Score < 6 = Respiratory distress
Score > 6 = Impending respiratory failure

maintained for term neonates 90 to 93 percent and for preterm neonates 88 to 92 percent. Arrangement to be kept ready for respiratory support by CPAP (Continuous Positive Pressure Ventilation) or by invasive mechanical ventilation in case of impending respiratory failure.

4. Continuous monitoring of neonates general condition, respiratory status (respiration rate, retractions, grunting, cyanosis, nasal flaring), heart rate, body temperature, SpO_2, CRT, BP, blood gas, and other parameters.
5. Giving IV fluid therapy and maintaining normal blood glucose and calcium level.
6. Treating apnea, if present, with PPV (Positive Pressure Ventilation) using resuscitation bag and mask or endotracheal tube and resuscitation bag. Drugs (Aminophylline or Caffeine Citrate) may be required to treat apnea in some cases.
7. Antibiotic therapy may be needed to treat sepsis, if present.
8. Surfactant therapy is now recommended as the treatment of choice in preterm neonates with moderate to severe RDS.
9. Insertion of orogastric tube to be done to decompress the stomach during respiratory distress.
10. Initiation of gavage feeding to be done with minimal amount of EBM, when the respiratory distress subsides. Gradually paladai or katori-spoon feeding to be started and then to be shifted to breast feeding when the baby is comfortable to suck and swallow.

11. Providing routine care and practicing infection control measures.
12. Arrangement of cause-specific management to be done to promote better prognosis. Surgical interventions should be planned as emergency or elective operations depending upon the nature of problems.
13. Details records and reports to be maintained.
14. Discharge planning and teaching to the mother and family members should be done for home care and follow-up.

Prognosis

Prognosis of this condition depends upon early identification of problems, cause of respiratory distress and the time of initiation of treatment.

Prevention of Respiratory Distress Syndrome in Preterm Neonates

Antenatal corticosteroid therapy should be given in preterm labor or APH before 34 weeks of pregnancy for prevention of respiratory distress syndrome (RDS) in preterm neonates. Optimal effect is observed, if delivery occurs after 24 hours of starting this therapy. Recommended dose is injection Betamethasone 12 mg IM every 24 hours with two doses or injection Dexamethasone 6 mg IM every 12 hours with four doses.

Neonatal Infections

Perinatal infections, especially neonatal bacterial infections, is the most common cause of neonatal mortality in India. Infections can occur in intrauterine life, or during delivery or in the neonatal period. The neonates are more susceptible to infections because they lack in natural immunity and take some time for the development of acquired immunity. In the newborn, the deficient complement activity, lack of immunoglobulin content and defective phagocytic response leading to diminished inflammatory reactions. Damage by infective agents in the period of rapid growth may leave lasting effects on the various organs of the survivors.

Sources of Infections

Infections can occur in antenatal, intranatal and postnatal period due to various conditions:

Antenatal period
a. Intrauterine infections may occur due to various microorganisms and described with an acronym of STORCH where in 'S' for syphilis, 'T' for toxoplasmosis, 'O' for others (e.g. gonococcal infection, tuberculosis, malaria, varicella, hepatitis B, HIV, etc), 'R' for rubella, 'C' for cytomegalovirus and 'H' for herpes simplex hominis. These infections can develop due to direct transplacental transfer or following placental infection.
b. Ascending infections with contaminated liquor amnii and amnionitis related to infected birth passage and premature rupture of membrane may also lead to intrauterine infection of the fetus.

Intranatal period: A neonate can be infected during delivery due to:
a. Aspiration of infected liquor in prolonged labor following early rupture of membrane which may lead to neonatal aspiration pneumonia.
b. Infection may occur due to repeated vaginal examination by the delivery assistant especially when the membrane is ruptured.
c. Infected birth passage (vagina) may infect the eyes and mouth of the neonates leading to ophthalmia neonatorum and oral thrush.
d. Improper aseptic technique during care of umbilical cord may cause umbilical sepsis.

Postnatal period: The followings are important causes of neonatal infections in postnatal period:
a. Transmission of infection from human contact or care givers especially from infected hands of mother, family members and health care providers (doctor, nurses, other staff).
b. Cross-infection from other baby who is infected and no barrier nursing is practiced and universal precautions are not followed.
c. Infected articles for baby care and contaminated clothing.
d. Invasive procedures without aseptic technique.
e. Infected environment around the neonates at hospital/health center or home.

Factors Responsible for Neonatal Infections

The predisposing factors of neonatal infections are:
- Low birth weight infants.
- Contaminated intrauterine environment like prolonged rupture of membrane, unhygienic and multiple vaginal examination, meconium-stained liquor, etc.
- Infected birth passage and infection at birth in delivery room or neonatal care units.
- Birth asphyxia and resuscitations.
- Congenital anomalies.
- Various neonatal procedures with inadequate asepsis during IV infusion, parenteral medications, endotracheal intubation, assisted ventilation, exchange blood transfusion, etc.
- Sex of the baby—male babies are more prone to neonatal infections than female in two times. The exact explanation is not known, but may be due to possible locus of gene for synthesis of immunoglobulins at X-chromosomes, which provide more resistance to the female babies to infections.
- Artificial feeding other than human breast milk.

Common Infections in Neonates

The neonatal infections may occur as superficial and localized or systemic. The common sites of superficial infections are eyes, skin, umbilicus and oral cavity. The systemic infections include septicemia, meningitis, pneumonia, necrotizing enterocolitis, tetanus neonatorum, systemic candidiasis, sclerema, DIC (disseminated intravascular coagulopathy), pyelonephritis, osteoarthritis, etc.

Intrauterine infections may be manifested at birth or delayed for a few days to several weeks. Viral infections *in utero* may lead to fetal death, congenital malformations or severe systemic manifestations of the disease. The presence of any three of the following features should make alert to the possibility of intrauterine infections: (a) maternal history of infection, (b) intrauterine growth retardation, (c) hepatosplenomegaly, (d) jaundice, (e) petechiae and purpura, (f) meningoencephalitis (with microcephaly, hydrocephaly, cerebral calcification, retinopathy, cataract, etc.), (g) osteochondritis and (h) raised IgM in cord blood.

Neonatal Conjunctivitis (Ophthalmia Neonatorum)

Inflammation of conjunctiva during first three weeks of life is termed as ophthalmia neonatorum. Sticky eyes without purulent discharge are common during first 2 to 3 days after birth. Unilateral conjunctivitis after 5 days of life is often due to *Chlamydia trachomatis*. Purulent conjunctivitis with profuse discharge is usually due to gonococcus which may affect one or both eyes within 48 hours of age. Other microorganism causing neonatal conjunctivitis are *Streptococcus, Staphylococcus, Pneumococcus, E. coli*, herpes simplex virus, etc. Chemical conjunctivitis may occur due to irritation of silver nitrate, soap and local antibiotic drops.

Mode of infections are infected hands of caregivers, infected birth canal and cross-infection from other infected infants. Infection can occur directly from other sites of infections like skin and umbilicus.

The *clinical features* varies with mode of infection and causative organism. The neonate may present with sticky eyes with or without discharge ranging from watery or purulent or mucopurulent in one or both eyes. The eyelids may be markedly swollen and stuck together with redness of eyes. Closed eyelids may present due to spasm of orbicularis oculi muscle.

Management is done with specific antibiotic therapy (as eye drops or in parenteral route), after identification of causative organism. The baby should be kept isolated to prevent cross-infection. Sulfacetamide or framycetin or gentamycin or chloramphenicol drops or erythromycin ointment can be used. For gonococcal infection penicillin therapy (local and parenteral) should be initiated promptly. If organisms are resistant to penicillin, then cefotaxime or ceftriaxone are used. Cleaning of the infected eyes with sterile cotton swabs soaked in saline should be done after hand washing. Instillation of eye drops to be done with proper aseptic precautions.

Preventive management include treatment of maternal infection, aseptic technique during delivery, special care and attention in face and breech presentation, isolation of infected baby and maintenance of general cleanliness.

Prognosis of this infection is good if detected and treated promptly. In neglected cases, orbital cellulitis and dacrocystitis with obstruction of nasolacrimal duct may develop. In gonococcal infection, corneal ulceration may occur leading to corneal opacity. In rare cases blindness may occur if no treatment done.

Umbilical Sepsis (Omphalitis)

The incidence of umbilical sepsis is reduced due to aseptic technique and clean practices at birth. The source of infection may be unhygienic environment of delivery, umbilical catheterization, exchange transfusion, contaminated cord cutting instrument, infected hands of care giver or infected clothing. The causative organisms are mainly *Staphylococcus, E. coli* or any pyogenic organism. *Clostridium tetani* can also infect umbilical cord and produces tetanus neonatorum. The incidence of tetanus neonatorum is also reduced due to administration of tetanus toxoid to antenatal mothers. But till it is found in rural areas in home delivery and delivery in very unhygienic condition.

The *clinical features* of umbilical sepsis are mainly swollen and moist periumbilical tissue with redness, foul smelling and serous or seropurulent discharge, delayed falling off umbilical cord and fever. Jaundice and features of septicemia may appear in complicated cases. The clinical manifestations of tetanus are found in *Clostridium tetani* infection (See page 236).

Management of this condition is done with dressing of the infected cord with spirit and antibiotic ointment, powder or lotion. Umbilical cord should left uncovered rather than application of dressing. Systemic antibiotic is given in complicated cases. The infected baby should be kept in isolation. Special management required in tetanus neonatorum. Culture and sensitivity test of umbilical swab may be needed in some cases who are not responding to the routine treatment.

Umbilical sepsis can be complicated with thrombo-phlebitis of umbilical vein, umbilical granuloma, hepatitis, liver abscess, peritonitis and portal hypertension. Prognosis depends upon nature of infection, initiation of management and nursing care. Prevention of umbilical infection is more easy and important in neonates.

Oral Thrush

It is fungal infection of the oral cavity and tongue by *Candida albicans* in the late first week or second week of age. Infection occurs from infected birth canal, infected feeding bottles and teats or contaminated feeding articles, mother's hands and breast nipples. It may develop due to prolonged antibiotic therapy.

The neonate usually presents with milky-white elevated patches on the buccal mucosa, lips, tongue and gums, which cannot be easily wiped off with gauze and oozes blood on attempt to scrap the patches. Swallowing difficulties may present due to posterior oropharyngeal white patches. Sucking reflex may be normal. Infection may cause monilial diarrhea, perineal moniliasis and lung infections.

Oral thrush is managed by oral application 0.5 percent aqueous solution of gentian violet after each feed, which gives prompt response. Nystatin and ketoconazole or cotrimazole lotion are effectively used 4 times per day for

5 to 7 days. Parenteral antifungal drugs can be administered in disseminated candidiasis.

This condition can be prevented by the treatment of maternal fungal infection, adequate cleaning of utensils and maintenance of general cleanliness and hygienic measures.

Pyoderma

Pyoderma is the superficial skin infection usually caused by *Staphylococcus aureus*. The skin eruptions and pastules are commonly seen on scalp, neck, groin and axillae. These are more commonly found in summer months. This infection occurs from contaminated hands of the personnel responsible for care of the neonate. Unhygienic environment, spread from other infected baby and contaminated baby clothing can also result in this infections.

The infection may spread to cause abscess, osteomyelitis, parotitis and septicemia. The life-threatening staphylococcal infection may result in pemphigus neonatorum, that is manifested as marked erythema, bullous lesions and exfoliation which give an appearance of scalded skin syndrome.

Treatment of these lesions include puncturing, cleaning with hexachlorophene, antiseptic skin care and application of antibiotic ointment over the punctured lesions. Pus should be sent for culture and sensitivity test. In case of spread of infection, erythromycin 50 mg/kg per day orally in 3 divided doses should be administered. In complicated cases and presence of 10 pustules parenteral administration of antibiotic should be done. The baby to be kept in isolation.

This condition can be prevented by avoidance of dip baby bath in hospital delivery and during hospital stay, isolation of infected baby, maintenance of general cleanliness (including clean clothing) and treatment of source of infection.

Prognosis is usually good if treated promptly and good nursing care is provided.

Neonatal Sepsis

Neonatal sepsis is a serious problem causing high mortality in neonates. Early recognition and treatment of the condition can reduce the fatal outcome.

When pathogenic bacteria gain access in the blood stream, they may cause an overwhelming infections. The systemic bacterial infections of neonates are termed as neonatal sepsis which incorporates septicemia, pneumonia and meningitis of the newborn. In most cases it is caused by *Klebsiella pneumoniae, Staphylococcus aureus, E. coli, Pseudomonas aeruginosa, Acinetobacter*, etc.

The *predisposing factors* of neonatal sepsis are intrauterine infections, premature and prolonged rupture of membrane, meconium stained liquor, repeated vaginal examination, maternal infections, lack of aseptic practices, birth asphyxia, resuscitation without aseptic precautions, low birth weight, invasive procedures, needle pricks, superficial infections, aspiration of feeds and lack of breastfeeding.

The *sources of infection* include, infusion sets, IV sites, face masks, feeding bottles, catheters, ventilators, resuscitators, incubators (especially humidity tank), baby care contaminated articles, infected care givers and unhygienic environment.

Types of Neonatal Sepsis

a. *Early onset neonatal sepsis:* It develops before 72 hours of life due to intrauterine infections, maternal conditions and intranatal causes. It manifests frequently as pneumonia and less commonly as septicemia and meningitis.

b. *Late-onset neonatal sepsis:* It develops after 72 hours may be at the end of first week or in second week. It acquired as nosocomial infections from baby care area or due to inappropriate neonatal care. The clinical presentations are those of septicemia, pneumonia or meningitis. Various factors enhances the chances of entry of organisms into the body systems of neonates who are much less immunocompetent as compared to older children.

Clinical manifestations: The manifestations of neonatal sepsis are often vague, nonspecific and therefore demand a high index of suspicion for its early diagnosis. The infection may manifest without much localization as septicemia or may get predominantly localized to the lungs in pneumonia and in the meninges in meningitis. Early onset neonatal sepsis may present as perinatal hypoxia, resuscitation difficulties and congenital pneumonia in the form of respiratory distress. The late onset neonatal sepsis in a very small baby may be silent who may die suddenly without presenting any signs and symptoms.

The baby "does not look well" may sound vague but is a most useful clue to an experienced doctor and nurse. The baby who had been active and sucking normally, become lethergic, inactive, pale or unresponsive and refuses to suck. The most important feature is an alteration of the established feeding behavior. Hypothemia is common than fever, in neonatal sepsis. Poor cry, vacant look, comatosed and not arousable baby with distension of abdomen, diarrhea, vomiting, less weight gain or loss of weight and poor neonatal reflexes are other associated features. Episodes of apnea or gasping may be the only feature of the condition. In sick neonates, skin may becomes tight giving a hide bound feel (sclerema) and poor perfusion (capillary refill time of over 3 seconds) are found. In critical neonates circumoral cyanosis, shock, bleeding, excessive jaundice and renal failure may develop.

The evidence of penumonia include fast breathing, chest retractions, grunting, early cyanosis, apneic spells in addition to inactivity and poor feeding, Cough is unusual.

Meningitis is often silent, the clinical features are dominated by manifestations of septicemia. But the presence of high pitched cry, fever, irritability, convulsions, twitching, blank look, neck retraction and bulging fontanelle are highly suggestive of meningitis.

The neonatal sepsis may present with hypoglycemia, urinary tract infection, coagulopathy (DIC), necrotizing enterocolitis (NEC), etc.

Investigations: No investigation is required as a prerequisite to start management in a clinically obvious case. The early treatment is of critical importance.

The recommended investigations are sepsis screen, blood culture, swab culture from septic umbilicus or from any other location of superficial infections and lumber puncture for CSF study. Other useful investigations are urine for routine examination and culture, chest X-ray, blood sugar, serum bilirubin, leukocyte count, ESR, C-reactive protein, etc. for sepsis screening procedures.

Management: Initiation of prompt treatment is essential for optimum outcome of neonates with sepsis. Early recognition of problems, administration of effective and appropriate antibiotic therapy with optimal supportive care are mandatory to improve the survival of this neonates. Initial supportive care makes the difference between life and death in the early hospital days. Antibiotics take at least 12 to 24 hours to show any effect.

The *supportive care* is provided to maintain normal body temperature, to stabilize the cardiopulmonary status, to correct hypoglycemia and to prevent bleeding tendency.

The *supportive care* of sick septic neonates include the followings:

a. Maintenance of warmth to ensure consistently normal temperature. Baby should be nursed in warm environment. Heat sources to be used to keep the baby warm. Body temperature should be monitored frequently.
b. Intravenous fluid to be administered. If the neonate is having poor perfusion, then normal saline bolus to be infused with 10 mL/kg over 5 to 10 minutes. It can be repeated with same dose 1 to 2 times over the next 30 to 45 minutes, if perfusion continues to be poor.

    Dextrose (10%) 2 mL/kg bolus can be infused to correct hypoglycemia which is usually present in neonatal sepsis and to be continued for 2 days or till the baby can have oral feeds.

    Intravenous fluid can be continued with electrolytes or N/5 saline (one-fifth saline) in 10 percent dextrose from third day onward. Potassium is added as KCl, 1/100 mL of fluid after 2 to 3 days of age provided the infant is passing urine normally.
c. Oxygen therapy should be provided if the neonate is having respiratory distress or cyanosis.
d. Bag and mask ventilation with oxygen may be required if the infant is apneic or breathing is inadequate.
e. Vitamin 'K' 1 mg intramuscularly should be given to prevent bleeding disorders.
f. Enteral feed is avoided if the neonate is very sick or has abdominal distension. Maintenance of fluid should be done by IV infusion.
g. Other supportive measures include gentle physical stimulation, nasogastric aspiration, close and constant monitoring of infant's condition and expert nursing care.

Antibiotic therapy should be administered considering the common causative organisms. A combination of ampicillin and gentamycin/amikacin is recommended for treatment of sepsis and pneumonia. In case of suspected meningitis, chloramphenical should be added. Duration of antibiotic therapy should be individualized. In general, antibiotics should be given 10 to 14 days in septicemia and pneumonia, 14 days for urinary tract infection and 21 days for meningitis.

*   Other antibiotics which are used for neonatal sepsis include amoxycillin, cloxacillin, ceftriaxone, ceftazidime, ciprofloxacin, cefotaxime, etc.
*   Other durg therapy includes anticonvulsive (diazepam or phenobarbitone) in case of convulsions, and corticosteroids in severely sick neonates with endotoxic shock, sclerema and adrenal insufficiency. Dopamine is used to treat shock and mannitol can be used in raised intracranial pressure.
*   Phototherapy and exchange blood transfusion may be necessary in hyperbilirubinemia. Blood transfusion may be required in anemia and bleeding disorders. Immunoglobulin preparation containing type-specific antibodies to group—'B' streptococci have been shown to be beneficial. Treatment of superficial infections like umbilical sepsis, pyoderma, oral thrush, conjunctivitis, should be done appropriately.

Prognosis: Despite availability of newer broadspectrum antimicrobial agents, almost 25 to 30 percent neonates die in case of neonatal sepsis. Extremely high mortality is associated with endotoxic shock, sclerema, NEC, DIC, etc. Associated congenital malformations like meningomyelocele, TEF, LBW and surgical procedure adversely effect the prognosis. The early onset sepsis due to group—'B' streptococci, nosocomial infections due to *Klebseilla* and *Pseudomonas aeruginosa* are also associated with adverse outcome.

Early initiation of specific antimicrobial therapy with the help of sepsis screen, excellent supportive care and close monitoring are likely to improve the outcome of neonatal sepsis.

Necrotizing Enterocolitis

Necrotizing enterocolitis (NEC) is a severe inflammatory condition and damage of intestinal mucosa affecting small and large bowel of preterm infants due to ischemia resulting from asphyxia or prolonged hypoxia.

The NEC is found in preterm neonates in first week of life with stressful condition. Clinical manifestations of this condition resemble with neonatal septicemia.

It usually occurs due to mucosal injury caused by ischemic damage of the intestinal mucosal barrier as a result of fetal distress, perinatal asphyxia, respiratory distress syndrome (RDS), hypothermia, and exchange blood transfusion for hyperbilirubinemia. Bacterial infection of the injured gut (with *E. coli*, *Klebsiella*, or *Pseudomonas*), diarrhea or stasis of intestinal contents due to poor peristalsis may also result in NEC. Another most important contributing factor for NEC is formula feeding. Breast milk is protective for this condition. Almost all neonates with NEC are artificially fed before onset of this problem.

Clinical Manifestations

Clinical features of NEC may be described in three stages.

Stage I or suspected NEC: Neonates usually present with lethargy, abdominal distension, vomiting, blood in stool, instability of body temperature, bradycardia, apnea and cyanosis. X-ray abdomen shows mild intestinal distension.

Stage II: In this stage, neonates present with features of stage I along with diminished bowel sound, metabolic acidosis and mild thrombocytopenia. X-ray abdomen shows gas in the intestine (Pneumatosis intestinalis) and dilatation of intestine.

Stage III: In this stage of NEC, neonates present with all features of stage I and II along with low blood pressure, disseminated intravascular coagulation (DIC), anuria and peritonitis.

Diagnostic Evaluation

Physical examination, history of illness, X-ray abdomen, blood count, sepsis screening, culture and sensitivity (blood, urine, stool, CSF) should be done to confirm the diagnosis.

Management

Warmth, fluid therapy for maintenance of fluid and electrolyte balance, management of shock with fluid resuscitation and vasopressors, no oral feeding, insertion of gastric tube to relieve abdominal distension and to aspirate gastric contents and continuous monitoring should be provided. Parenteral nutrition to maintain nutritional requirement, plasma and platelet transfusion for bleeding and antibiotic therapy may be needed in some neonates. Surgical intervention is required in case of intestinal perforation. Surgery is done after initial stabilization of the sick neonate. Supportive nursing care is important with need based individualized approach.

Prevention of this problem can be done by reducing incidence of asphyxia, quick management of hypoxia, and early initiation of feeding with breast milk, avoidance of formula feeding and meticulous infection control measures with continuous monitoring of preterm neonates.

Prognosis

Mortality rate due to NEC is about 40 to 50 percent. Death may occur within a few hours. Survived neonates may have complications like intestinal strictures and malabsorption.

Prevention of Neonatal Infections

It is far more cost-effective to prevent infections rather than treat them with expensive antibiotics and high cost supportive care. The following practices promote prevention of infections in neonates and should be strictly followed:

- Strict aseptic management of institutional delivery.
- Five clean practices in home delivery—clean surface clean hands, clean cord tie, clean blade and clean cord stump. Sixth clean practice include clean clothing for mother and baby.
- Hand washing before and after handling the babies.
- Use of sterile gown before entering the baby care unit/ neonatal nursery and changing of shoes.
- Minimum handling of the newborn baby.
- Exclusion of infected persons or carriers from the neonatal care areas.
- Maintenance of cleanliness of the environment, i.e. delivery room, neonatal care unit, postnatal area and separate area for mother and baby at home.
- Use of separate and disposable belongings for each baby, e.g. clothing, feeding equipment, etc.
- Aseptic cleaning of baby-cot, incubators, warmer, photo-therapy machine, weighing machine etc.
- Strict asepsis for all invasive procedures.
- Maintenance of general cleanliness of baby and mother. Teaching the mother to maintain the hygienic measures.
- Separate accommodation of infected baby and outside confined babies.
- Avoid unnecessary IV fluid, injections, needle pricks and no sharing of needles and syringes.
- Visitors to be restricted in postnatal ward.
- Encouraging exclusive breastfeeding and no prelacteal feeding. Strict aseptic measures for expressed breast milk feeding or artificial feeding.
- Prevention and treatment of maternal infections in antenatal and postnatal period. Active immunization to the mothers.
- Any baby showing features, suggestive of infections should be isolated immediately.
- Prophylactic antibiotic therapy to be given, if any three of the following factors are present, considering the baby as infected (presumed early sepsis) and should be treated with antibiotics (ampicillin and gentamicin) immediately after birth. The factors are: (a) preterm babies less than

36 weeks or birth weight less than 2 kg, (b) maternal fever in the preceding 2 weeks, (c) foul smelling liquor, (d) prolonged rupture of membranes more than 24 hours, (e) more than three vaginal examinations in labor, (f) birth asphyxia, Apgar score less than 4 at 5 minutes, (g) prolonged or difficult delivery with instrumentation and in case of chorioamnionitis.

Birth Injuries

Birth injury is the trauma during the process of delivery. It includes both avoidable and unavoidable trauma during birth process. It is one of the important cause of perinatal morbidity and mortality and reflects the standard of obstetrical services of the place or center. It can be prevented by adequate antenatal check-up and skilled management of labor. Incidence of birth injuries varies from one health care institution to other.

The common site of birth injury is head, because 96 percent babies are delivered by cephalic presentations. Other parts of the body may also be injured, i.e. nerves, bones, muscles and superficial tissue. Preventive measures to be followed to reduce the incidence of this condition.

Injuries of the Head

The common injuries of head include caput succedaneum, cephalhematoma, intracranial injury, intracranial hemorrhage, fracture of skull bones and scalp injuries.

Caput succedaneum (Fig. 6.9): It is edematous swelling on the babies scalp due to infiltration of serosanguinous fluid by the pressure of girdle of contact, i.e. the cervix, bony pelvis or vulval ring. The swelling develops due to reduced venous blood supply and lymphatic drainage from the unsupported part of scalp that is lying over the cervical os. The area becomes congested and edematous and present as caput at birth.

It may cross the sutureline and tends to grow less. It pits on pressure, nonfluctuant and diffuse in nature. No management requires of the condition because it usually disappear within 36 hours. It should be differentiated from cephalhematoma. Maternal anxiety should be reduced by reassurance.

Cephalhematoma (Fig. 6.10): It is collection of blood in between the periosteum and the flat bone of the skull. It occurs due to rupture of small emissary veins from the skull resulting from the friction between the fetal skull and pelvis. It may found in complicated or forceps delivery but may also be seen following normal delivery. It may be associated with fracture of the skull bone.

Cephalhematoma is never present at birth but gradually develops a few hours after birth or on the second day. It is found as incompressible, cystic, circumscribed, fluctuant swelling limited by suture lines and usually unilateral over parietal bone. It tends to grow larger and may persist for weeks. The

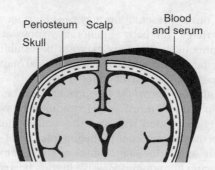

Fig. 6.9: Caput succedaneum

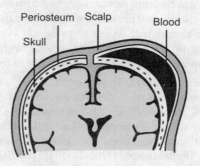

Fig. 6.10: Cephalhematoma

edges of the swelling may give a false impression of depressed skull fracture due to organized rim of cephalhematoma. The overlying scalp may show discoloration. The condition should not be confused with caput or meningocele or encephalocele. Meningocele always lies over a suture line or fontanelle and there is impulse on crying. Encephalocele usually located on occipital region.

Most cephalhematomas disappear spontaneously after few days or weeks. No active treatment is necessary unless it becomes complicated or infected. Vitamin K 1 to 2 mg intramuscularly should be given to correct any co-existent coagulation defect. In case of infected hematoma, the condition is treated with incision and drainage, systemic antibiotics and monitoring of hematocrit and bilirubin level. Mother should be explained about the condition and its prognosis. Prognosis is usually good with appropriate management.

Intracranial Injury

The differentiation between the isolated perinatal hypoxia and intracranial injury is difficult and is guided by the nature of events during delivery rather than any specific syndrome of neurological manifestations.

The improved obstetrical management has reduced the incidence of birth trauma including intracranial injury. Precipitate labor or difficult forceps delivery, vacuum extraction of a large baby, extraction of breech and other abnormal (brow) presentation may cause intracranial injury and hemorrhage. The baby is generally asphyxiated at birth and spontaneous respirations may not be established even after resuscitation. The abnormal neurological manifestations usually appear within first 48 hours of life.

i. *Traumatic intracranial hemorrhage* can be extradural or subdural hemorrhage. Extradural hemorrhage is usually associated with fracture skull bone. Subdural hemorrhage may occur following fracture of skull bone, rupture of inferior sagital sinus or small veins of cortex producing hematoma. Massive hemorrhage result from tear of the tentorium cerebelli and injury to the superior sagittal sinus.

ii. *Anoxic intracranial hemorrhage* can be intraventricular, subarachnoid and intracerebral. It occurs due to rupture of sub-ependymal vessels, bridging veins between leptomeningeal arteries or superficial or major vessels. The important predisposing factors are as follows:

Immaturity, hypoxia, hypercapnia, precipitate delivery, RDS, rapid injection of hyperosmolar sodium bicarbonate, hypothermia, acidosis, shock, Rh-incompatibility, trauma, etc.

Clinically it may be impossible to differentiate between neurological manifestations of perinatal hypoxia and intracranial hemorrhage. Hypoxia may predispose to the development of intracranial bleeding and vice versa.

Clinical features include convulsions, apneic attack, hypotonia, bulging anterior fontanelle, vomiting, high pitched cry, in coordinate movement, twitching, flaccid limbs, paresis, etc. Age of onset of clinical features may vary. Baby may be still born or may have severe respiratory depression at birth with Apgar score below 3.

Management: Mostly the symptomatic and supportive management are done with intensive care. Oxygen therapy, warmth, clear airway, ventilatory support, fluid therapy, anticonvulsive drugs, tapping of CSF, vitamin 'K' and antibiotic therapy are essential. Supportive measures like monitoring of vital signs, gentle handling, quite environment, physical stimulation should be provided.

Prognosis: It depends upon nature of hemorrhage. Intracranial hemorrhage is having poor prognosis with high mortality. Survivors may develop mental retardation and neurological disorders in later life.

Fracture skull: It is common in frontal bone or at the anterior part of the parietal bone. It may be linear skull fracture or depressed fracture. It occurs due to difficult forceps delivery or due to projected sacral promontory of the flat pelvis.

Fracture of skull may be associated with cephalhematoma, extradural or subdural hemorrhage. No management needed for linear or fissure fracture. But for depressed fracture, associated with neurological manifestations, surgical elevation may be required. Subdural hematoma may have to be aspirated or excised surgically.

Scalp injuries: This may occur due to abrasion by the tip of the forceps blades in forceps delivery or by the incised wound in LUCS delivery or during episiotomy. The wound should be dressed with antiseptic lotion and should be observed for hemorrhage or infection. Occasionally the incised wound may cause brisk hemorrhage and requires stiches aseptically.

Injuries to the Nerves

Nerve injury is common in neonates during the process of delivery. They include the followings:

Facial palsy (Fig. 6.11): It is also known as Bell's palsy. The facial nerve may injured by direct pressure of the forceps blades or by hemorrhage or edema around the nerve. It may occur in normal delivery with much pressure on the ramus of mandible where the nerve crosses superficially. Facial nerve gets injury as it remains unprotected after its exit through the stylomastoid foramen.

The diagnostic features of facial palsy are facial asymmetry, inability to close the eye and absent of rooting reflex on the affected side. On crying, the angle of the mouth is drawn over the unaffected side. Sucking reflex remains unaffected. Prognosis is excellent and complete. The condition usually recovers within weeks, because of greater regenerative power and short length of the nerves. Eyes should be protected with antiseptic ointment, as they remains open, even during sleep.

Facial palsy can be found bilateral or in association with intracranial lesions. Partial facial palsy or congenital absence of depressor anguli oris muscle is a relatively frequent condition.

Brachial palsy: The damage occurs in the brachial nerve roots or in the trunk of the brachial plexus due to stretching or effusion or hemorrhage inside the nerve sheath or tearing of the fibers. The causes are hyperextension of neck during attempted delivery of shoulder dystocia or even in spontaneous vaginal delivery or during difficult breech extraction. Unilateral involvement is common. The two common clinical types are:

i. *Erb's palsy:* This is the most common type when upper cervical roots (C5, C6) are involved. The paralysis causes the arm hangs limply, adducted and internally rotated with elbow extended. Pronation of the forearm and flexion of the wrist (waiter's tip) also developed. Arm recoil is lost. Moro reflex and biceps jerks are absent on the affected side. Respiratory distress occurs in associated diaphragmatic paralysis. It may be associated with fracture clavicle or involvement of lower cervical roots (Fig. 6.12).

Management of the condition is done with use of splint to hold the arm abducted to a right angle and externally rotated. Massage and passive movement are also helpful. Usually complete recovery takes place

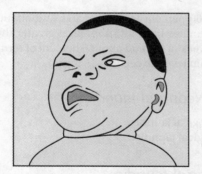

Fig. 6.11: Facial palsy (left)

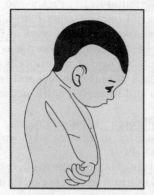

Fig. 6.12: Erb's palsy

Long bone fractures are mainly found following breech extraction or shoulder impaction. The forcible manipulation and pulling may result in fractures of humerus and femur. The clinical features include limitation of movements, asymmetric moro response and crepitus at the site of fracture along with pain. The fracture may be greenstick or complete type. Management is done usually by immobilization. Prognosis is good and rapid union occurs with callus formation. Deformity is a rare condition and found when the fracture bone end are not in a good alignment.

Spinal fracture: It may occur due to acute bending of spine during delivery of after coming head in breech. Fracture of odontoid process or fracture dislocation of cervical vertebra may occur and result instant death of the baby due to compression of medulla.

The neonate may present with flaccid paraplegia with retention of urine and overflow incontinence. Respiratory failure due to diaphragmatic paralysis may dominate the clinical picture. There may be dull or absent of sensations below the site of lesion. The prognosis in this condition is grave.

Dislocation of joints: The common sites of dislocation are shoulder, hip, jaw and cervical vertebra. The condition is diagnosed during neonatal examination and confirmed by radiology. Management is done by immobilization and consultation with orthopedic surgeon. Surgical correction may be required in few cases (like congenital dislocation of hip).

within weeks or months, but in severe injury permanent disability may develop.

ii. *Klumpke's palsy*: It occurs due to damage of 7th or 8th cervical or 1st thoracic nerve roots. The features are paralysis of the muscles of the forearm with wrist drop and flaccid digits. The arm is flexed at the elbow, the wrist extended with flaccid hands and flexed fingers. Miosis, ptosis and anhidrosis may present due to damage of cervical sympathetic chain of the first thoracic root.

Management consists of splinting of arm and placing of cotton ball in the baby's hand to avoid contractures. Gentle massage and passive movement are also helpful. The prognosis is usually good, but the permanent deformity may persist in severe laceration of nerves and hemorrhage. The lesions of the upper brachial plexus have a better prognosis than those of lower or total plexus. If paralysis persists more than 3 months, neuroplasty is indicated.

Injuries to the Bones

Other than the skull bones, the common sites of fracture or injury to the bones in neonates are mainly femur, humerus and clavicle. Occasionally spinal fracture may occur.

Injuries to the Muscles

The sternomastoid muscles are commonly injured in neonates due to difficult breech delivery, attempted delivery following shoulder dystocia or excessive lateral flexion of the neck in normal delivery. There is ruptured of muscle fibers and blood vessels followed by formation of hematoma, cicatrical contraction and transient torticolis. Hematoma appears commonly at the junction of upper and middle third of the muscles about 7 to 10 days after birth.

No management usually needed. It disappears by six months to one year of age. Mother should be advised to overextend the affected muscle by turning the infant's head in the opposite direction and flexing the neck towards unaffected side. Surgical correction may be indicated, if torticolis persists beyond one to two years of age.

Injuries to the Skin and Subcutaneous Tissue

Superficial abrasions, petechiae and bruising may be found following forceps delivery or prolonged labor. Spontaneous recovery occurs within 2 to 3 days. Local application of antiseptic lotion can prevent infection of the area.

Visceral Injuries

Visceral injuries may occur following difficult breech extraction or unskilled external cardiac massage. Capsular laceration of liver and spleen and adrenal hemorrhage may develop. The hemorrhage may remain concealed as subcapsular hematoma or capsule may rupture with blood flowing into the peritoneal cavity.

The neonate may present with pallor, tachycardia and evidences of shock. The condition may be managed by correction of hypovolemia and anemia. Surgical management may be needed to repair the injured viscera. Prognosis is usually poor.

Prevention of Birth Injuries

The incidence of birth injuries can be reduced by comprehensive antenatal and intranatal care. During antenatal period identification of high-risk cases, (especially which may cause traumatic delivery) is very important for early and subsequent management. Skilled antenatal examination is the essential part of the preventive measures.

During intranatal period, following practices can reduce the incidence of birth injuries:

- In spontaneous vaginal delivery, the neck should not be unduly stretched during delivery of shoulder to prevent injuries to brachial plexus or sternomastoid muscle.
- Episiotomy should be given carefully to prevent scalp injury.
- Continuous fetal monitoring to be done to prevent cerebral anoxia.
- Special care to be taken in preterm delivery to prevent anoxia or traumatic delivery.
- Precautions to be followed during forceps delivery to prevent injuries, as it causes majority of the birth injuries.
- Vaginal breech delivery should be done by the skilled personnel with gentle and careful approach to prevent intracranial injuries, spinal injury and other injuries.
- Prolonged labor should be managed carefully.

Preventive measures should be emphasized to minimize birth injuries and permanent disabilities, thus reducing the number of handicapped citizen in future.

Neonatal Jaundice

Jaundice is the visible manifestation of hyperbilirubinemia. The clinical jaundice in neonates appear on the face at a serum bilirubin level of 5 mg/dL, whereas in adults, it is diagnosed as little as 2 mg/dL. The yellowish discoloration is first seen on the skin of face, nasolabial folds and tip of nose in the neonates. It is detected by blanching the skin with digital pressure in the natural light. Neonatal jaundice is also termed as icterus neonatorum or as neonatal hyperbilirubinemia.

Almost 60 percent term neonates and about 80 percent preterm neonates have bilirubin level greater than 5 mg/dL in the first week of life and about 6 percent of term babies will have bilirubin levels exceeding 15 mg/dL.

Types of Neonatal Jaundice

a. Physiological jaundice
b. Pathological jaundice.

Physiological Jaundice

Multiple factors are responsible for the physiological jaundice, which commonly found in both term and preterm babies. There is elevation of unconjugated bilirubin concentration due to various reasons in the first week of life. The possible mechanisms of physiological jaundice are as follows:

a. Increased bilirubin load on hepatic cells due to increased volume of RBCs in polycythemia and reduced life span of fetal RBCs and increased enterohepatic circulation of bilirubin.
b. Defective bilirubin conjugation due to decreased enzymatic activity of uridine diphosphate glucuronyl transferase (UDPG-T).
c. Defective uptake of bilirubin by the liver from plasma due to decreased ligandin and increased ligandin-binding by other anions.
d. Defective bilirubin excretion due to congenital infection.

Characteristics of physiological jaundice
- It appears in between 30 to 72 hours of age in term babies and in preterm babies may appear earlier but not before 24 hours of age.
- Maximum intensity of jaundice is found on the 4th day in term babies and 5th to 6th day in preterm babies.
- Serum bilirubin dose not exceed 15 mg/dL.
- Usually disappears by 7th to 10th day in term babies and by 14th day in preterm babies.
- Subsides spontaneously and no treatment is needed.
- Mother needs encouragement for exclusive breastfeeding for adequate hydration and reassurance.
- Careful observation for signs of complications along with essential neonatal care are important.
- May aggravated by prematurity, asphyxia, hypothermia, infections and drugs.

Pathological Jaundice

About 5 percent of neonates develop pathological jaundice. Appearance of jaundice within 24 hours of age is always pathological. Some causes of this condition may appear after 72 hours, though age of appearance of jaundice may overlap. Investigations should be done to ruled out the exact cause of pathological jaundice.

Causes of pathological jaundice

a. *Excessive destruction of RBCs* due to hemolytic diseases of newborn, e.g. Rh-incompatibility (most common), ABO-incompatibility, congenital spherocytosis, G-6 PD-deficiency, neonatal septicemia and cytomegalic diseases, etc.

b. *Defective conjugation of bilirubin* due to diminished production of enzyme glucuronyl transferase by the immature liver cells and inhibition of enzymatic activity by breast milk or in congenital familial nonhemolytic jaundice (Crigler-Najjar syndrome).

c. *Failure to excrete the conjugated bilirubin* following umbilical sepsis, congenital obstruction by absence or stricture of common bile duct (extrahepatic biliary atresia), syphilis and galactosemia.

d. *Miscellaneous:* Viral hepatitis, toxoplasmosis, malaria, intrauterine infections, hypothyroidism, alpha thalassemia, durg therapy (vitamin K, salicylates), maternal diabetes, anoxia, concealed hemorrhage (intracranial hemorrhage, cephalhematoma), etc.

Types of pathological jaundice

a. *Prolonged unconjugated hyperbilirubinemia* due to Rh-incompatibility, ABO-incompatibility, hereditary spherocytosis, G-6-PD-deficiency, pyruvate kinase deficiency, alpha-thalassemia, vitamin K_3 induced hemolysis, sepsis, increased enterohepatic circulation in pyloric stenosis or large bowel obstruction, inborn errors of metabolism in Criglar-Najjar syndrome, hypothyroidism and breast milk jaundice.

b. *Prolonged conjugated hyperbilirubinemia* due to biliary atresia (extra- and intrahepatic), neonatal hepatitis, generalized sepsis, urinary tract infections (*E. coli*), choledochal cyst, galactosemia, total parenteral nutrition, Down syndrome, etc.

Characteristics of pathological jaundice: Any of the following features indicate pathological jaundice and needs to be investigated:

- Clinical jaundice appears within 24 hours of birth and persist more than one week in term babies and more than 2 weeks in preterm babies.
- Bilirubin level is increasing by more than 5 mg/dL per day or 0.5 mg/dL per hour.
- Total bilirubin level is more than 15 mg/dL (hyperbilirubinemia)
- Direct bilirubin more than 2 mg/dL (conjugated hyperbilirubinemia).
- Palms and soles are yellow.
- Stool clay or white colored and urine is staining clothes.

Sequelae of unconjugated hyperbilirubinemia: Unconjugated bilirubin may penetrate brain cells by crossing blood brain barrier in some circumstances and result in neurological dysfunction and death. Bilirubin level should be monitored to prevent the following complications in neonates:

1. *Transient encephalopathy:* It is a reversible neurologic complication suspected in increasing lethargy along with rising bilirubin levels. Recovery is possible with prompt initiation of management and exchange blood transfusion.

2. *Kernicterus:* It is a pathological condition of the brain due to toxicity by unconjugated bilirubin. It occurs as a result of necrosis of neurons in basal ganglia, hippocampal cortex, subthalamic nuclei and cerebellum followed by gliosis of the areas. The cerebral cortex usually is not affected. Other lesions include necrosis of renal tubular cells, intestinal mucosa and pancreatic cells which may present as GI bleeding or hematuria.

The neonate with kernicterus presents with poor sucking, lethargy, hypotonia, poor or absent Moro reflex, alteration of consciousness, fever, high pitched cry, convulsions, twitching, nystagmus, progressing hypertonia and opisthotonus position and death. If the baby survives various complications may develop which include cerebral palsy, hearing loss, mental retardation, etc.

Assessment of a neonate with jaundice: To evaluate the clinical condition of the neonate and to distinguish physiological jaundice from pathological jaundice the following assessments should be performed:

1. *History collection:* The important history includes the followings:
   a. Family history of jaundice and anemia.
   b. Previous babies with neonatal jaundice, exchange blood transfusion, neonatal or early infant death due to liver disease.
   c. Maternal illness with viral infections, maternal drug intake like antimalarial, sulphonamides, etc.
   d. Maternal blood group and Rh factor, time of onset of jaundice, use of oxytocin in labor, birth asphyxia, feeding of neonate, etc.

2. *Physical examination:* The baby should be examined for yellowish discoloration of skin and mucous membrane. It should be done in natural light by blanching the skin, i.e. pressing the finger on the baby's skin till it blanches and skin is noted for yellow color.

   Clinical criteria is used to assess the extent of jaundice and rough estimation of serum bilirubin. Jaundice proceeds downward to the trunk and extremities when it increases in intensity. A baby, with jaundice restricted to the face, is having bilirubin about 5 mg/dL and when palms and soles are yellow then it is over 15 mg/dL. Clinical assessment of neonatal jaundice is done by the use of Krammer's Rule (Fig. 6.13). Clinical judgement is equally reliable with laboratory value, if done by experienced person.

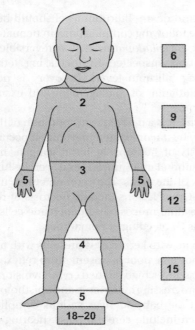

Fig. 6.13: Krammer's rule for assessment of cutaneous levels of jaundice

The neonate should be examined for presence of IUGR and cephalhematoma, features of intraventricular hemorrhage, intrauterine infections and kernicterus. The baby should be assessed for gestational age and general condition.

3. *Noninvasive assessment of jaundice:* It is done with ingram icterometer and transcutaneous bilirubinometer. These methods are more accurate and less subjective in estimating jaundice.

Ingram icterometer is a piece of transparent plastic, which is painted with five transverse strips of graded yellow lines. This instrument is pressed over the nose of the baby and the color of the blanched skin is matched with the appropriate yellow strip and the level of jaundice is assessed by the marked level of bilirubin.

Transcutaneous bilirubinometer is a costly and sophisticated equipment used to measure the intensity of jaundice by reflecting light rays on the blanched skin.

4. *Laboratory investigations:* Serum bilirubin level, (total, conjugated and unconjugated), Hb%, serum albumin, RBC morphology, direct Coombs' test, blood culture, acid-base level, hematocrit value, reticulocyte count, sepsis screen, liver and thyroid function tests, TORCH titers, G6PD deficiency, etc. can be done.

Hemolytic Disease of the Newborn

Hemolytic disease of the newborn is the most common cause of hyperbilirubinemia in the neonates. It occurs due to blood group incompatibility between the mother and fetus. The common incompatibilities are Rh, ABO and minor groups. Normally fetal and maternal blood vessels do not communicate with each other. But in some cases, during labor, there is fetomaternal bleeding, when fetal blood crosses the placenta into maternal circulation that produces antibodies against the fetal RBCs. These antibodies are IgG type and cross the placental barrier to produce hemolysis of fetal RBCs in subsequent pregnancy. Depending upon the extent of the isoimmunization, the neonates may develop severe anemia and jaundice.

Rh-incompatibility: Rh-isoimmunization is also called as erythroblastosis fetalis, a major cause of severe hyperbilirubinemia. It occurs in Rh-negative mother, who is carrying an Rh-positive fetus. The antigen of fetal RBCs may invoke antibody response in the maternal immunologic system. Enough antibodies may not be present during first pregnancy but each subsequent pregnancy with an Rh-positive fetus results in increase antibody response. The disease can be assessed in antenatal period by blood group test and estimation of antibody titer (anti-D antibodies) by indirect Coombs' test. Severity of hemolysis can be detected by amniotic fluid bilirubin and optical density measurements.

The clinical manifestations of Rh-hemolytic disease of newborn may vary from stillborn baby with hydrops fetalis or icterus gravis neonatorum or congenital hemolytic anemia. Normal baby without any features may also be found in some cases.

In severe hemolysis, the baby is born with severe anemia, gross hepatosplenomegaly, and generalized anasarca (hydrops fetalis). The baby may also die in intrauterine life. Jaundice (icterus gravis neonatorum) may appear as early as 30 minutes after birth or usually within 24 hours of age. The jaundice is not present at birth because the bilirubin produced in intrauterine life, is cleared by the maternal circulation. These neonates may have birth asphyxia, hypothermia, hypoglycemia, acidosis and coagulopathy.

ABO-incompatibility: It occurs commonly in 'O' group mother and 'A' or 'B' group fetus. It is milder than Rh-hemolytic disease and may occur even in first born baby. The history of increasing severity of disease in subsequent pregnancies is generally not present.

The neonate with ABO-hemolytic disease may present with jaundice and mild splenomegaly. Anemia is usually absent. The disease can be diagnosed by examining cord blood for elevation of serum bilirubin and presence of maternal IgG anti-'A' or anti-'B' antibodies. Direct Coombs' test generally negative or weakly positive. The jaundice may reach critical levels and requires management with phototherapy and exchange blood transfusion.

Minor groups-incompatibility: Isoimmunization can occur for minor groups like the Kell, Duffy M and N, etc.

Management of Neonatal Jaundice

Management of neonatal jaundice is aimed at reduction of serum bilirubin level within safe limit and prevention of CNS toxicity as kernicterus and brain damage. The management include:

- Prevention of Rh-isoimmunization by anti-D gamma-globulin to Rh-negative mother in case of birth of Rh-positive baby or abortion.
- Reduction of bilirubin level by phototherapy and exchange blood transfusion and prevention of hyperbilirubinemia.
- Reduction of enterohepatic circulation by drug therapy.
- Intensive neonatal nursing.

Phototherapy: It is noninvasive, inexpensive and easy method of degradation of unconjugated bilirubin by configurational isomerization, structural isomerization and photo-oxidation. The light waves convert the toxic bilirubin into water soluble nontoxic form which is easily excreted from the blood in the bile, stool and urine. Phototherapy also enhances hepatic excretion of unconjugated bilirubin into the intestinal lumen.

It is recommended that phototherapy may be started early when serum bilirubin approaches 15 mg/dL. A full term healthy infant with hyperbilirubinemia, in the absence of hemolysis or sepsis can be managed by phototherapy alone and there is no need of exchange blood transfusion (EBT) for such an infant. In preterm babies, phototherapy is started at a serum bilirubin level of 5 mg/dL or more to prevent to need for exchange blood transfusion. Prophylactic phototherapy may be indicated in very special circumstances such as extremely low birth weight or severly bruised babies. Phototherapy can be given continuously or intermittently using fluorescence or halogen light. CFL or LED light source used presently for effective phototherapy.

Technique of phototherapy: Blue light is most effective for phototherapy. White day light lamps are also effective. The wavelength of the light should have in the range of 420 to 600 nm for maximum absorption by the bilirubin. Blue light interferes with observation of skin color of the baby. A combination of white and blue lamps are preferred. A baby care unit with 6 to 8 light source or tube lights can be used which should be covered with plastic sheet or plexiglas. Light source is fixed over crib or incubator or it can be portable type.

A naked infant is placed under single or double light source at a distance of about 45 cm from the skin of the baby. It can be reduced to 15 to 20 cm for intensive phototherapy. Baby's eyes should be covered to prevent retinal damage and a diaper to be kept on to cover the genitals especially in male baby to prevent gonadal damage. Position should be changed every two hours or after each feed for maximum exposure to light. Temperature to be recorded two hourly to detect hypothermia or hyperthermia. More frequent (2 hourly) breastfeeding to be given or extra fluid to be provided by IV infusion or NG tube feeding to prevent dehydration. Baby's weight to be recorded once a day. Constant observation should be made for urine, green or loose stool, skin rash, behavior change, convulsions and features of any complications. Serum bilirubin level to be estimated at least every 12 hours.

Double surface phototherapy can be given for more effective management. The infant can be placed on a fiber optic cool biliblanket. For effective phototherapy, minimum spectral irradiance or flux of 6 to 9 $\mu W/cm^2/nm$ to be maintained at the level of infant's skin. Flux should be checked with fluxmeter after every 100 to 200 hours.

Phototherapy is discontinued when serum bilirubin level are less than 10 mg/dL for two times. Intensive phototherapy usually reduce 1 to 2 mg/dL of serum bilirubin within 4 to 6 hours of exposure.

Complications of phototherapy: Though phototherapy is safe, there are some side effects found immediately or later in life. The immediate problems are dehydration hypothermia, hyperthermia, loose stool or green stool, bronze-baby-syndrome, electric shock, skin rash, hypocalcemia, etc. Long-term problems may be found as disturbances of endocrine or sexual maturation, retinal damage and skin cancer (rare).

Drug therapy in neonatal jaundice: The drugs have very little role in the treatment of neonatal jaundice. They act by interfering with heme-degradation, accelerating normal pathway of bilirubin clearance and by inhibiting enterohepatic circulation.

The drugs which can be used to bind unconjugated bilirubin in the gut and to prevent its recirculation are charcoal, agar, polyvinyl pyrrolidone and cholestyramine.

Other drugs like orotic acid, metabolic precursor of UDPG acid, can be used to promote conjugation of bilirubin. Tin-mesoporphyrin can be used to inhibit heme-oxygenase, which diminish the production of bile pigments. Albumin infusion can be given before EBT to facilitate more effective removal of bilirubin and to improve the bilirubin binding capacity.

Combining phenobarbitone with phototherapy is no more effective than phototherapy alone and hence is not used in routine clinical practice.

Exchange blood transfusion (EBT): It is the most effective and reliable method for reduction of bilirubin level in case of severe hyperbilirubinemia to prevent kernicterus and to correct anemia. It is done in seriously affected Rh-isoimmunized erythroblastic babies to remove anti-'D' antibodies and Rh-positive RBCs coated with antibodies. Early exchange reduces the need for subsequent exchange and improve congestive cardiac failure in hydropic infants. It also helps to stop hemolysis in the affected baby. It is given when phototherapy fails to prevent a rise in bilirubin to toxic levels.

Early indications for EBT in infants with Rh-hemolytic desease of the newborn are:

- Cord blood hemoglobin level—10 g/dL or less.
- Cord blood bilirubin level—5 mg/dL or more.

- Unconjugated serum bilirubin level—10 mg/dL within 24 hours or 15 mg/dL within 48 hours or rate of rise of more than 0.5 mg/dL per hour.

High risk neonates with perinatal hypoxia, hypothermia, acidosis, hypoglycemia, sepsis, etc. should have exchange transfusion at relatively lower serum bilirubin levels. Preterm infants should be exchanged at lower level of bilirubin (10–18 mg/dL). EBT may be necessary is ABO incompatibility or in severe hyperbilirubinemia due to other causes when indirect serum bilirubin level is 20 mg/dL or more or bilirubin protein ratio is more than 3.5 during neonatal period.

Nature and amount of blood for EBT
- In Rh-isoimmunization—Rh-negative, ABO compatible blood is used.
- In ABO—incompatibility—O group, Rh-compatible blood is used.

Fresh blood collected less than 72 hours is preferred. The quantity of blood used is 160 to 180 mL/kg for one exchange transfusion to replace 80 to 90 percent of fetal blood.

Procedure of EBT: Exchange blood transfusion is done in strict aseptic technique by the expert team members in a well-equipped set-up. The process is very slow and continued over an hour. The baby must be kept warm and well-restraint. The stomach contents should be aspirated. Baby's cardiac status and temperature should be monitored continuously. Umbilical vein or artery is used and cannulated for the procedure. Peripheral vein or artery can also be used. Venous pressure to be measured before and in between exchange. Air-tight blood transfusion set with four way stopcock are required which should be rinsed with heparinized saline (10 units of heparin/mL). The donor blood should be at normal body temperature (37°C).

The blood is withdrawn with gentle suction and donor's blood is injected slowly in aliquots of 10 to 20 mL depending upon the size of the baby. The aliquots can be 5 to 10 mL during each push or pull. This push and pull method can be repeated for 30 to 40 cycle with same amount of withdrawn and replacement. Accurate record of in and out amount of blood should be maintained strictly. Calcium gluconate should be injected slowly after every 50 mL of exchange to prevent tetany, if CPD (citrate phosphate dextrose) blood is transfused. NaHCO$_3$ may be needed to prevent acidosis.

Exchange blood transfusion chart to be maintained with the following information: in and out volume of blood exchanged, heart rate, respiratory rate, oxygen saturation, temperature and color of the baby, venous pressure and any problems arise or any drugs administered. Hb% and bilirubin estimation to be done before and after exchange transfusion.

Postexchange care should include close monitoring of baby's condition, phototherapy, antibiotics (if asepsis is at suspect), warmth, routine essential care, bilirubin estimation, follow-up to detect complications and emotional support to the parents and family members.

Complications of EBT: Immediate complications are cardiac failure, air embolism, acidosis, tetany, sepsis, hyperkalemia, umbilical or portal vein perforation, hypoglycemia, thrombocytopenia, etc.
- Delayed complications include extrahepatic portal hypertension, portal vein thrombisis, HIV, hepatitis B and C infection, ulcerative colitis, etc.

Prevention of pathological jaundice in neonates
- Administration of anti-D immunoglobulin to the Rh-negative mother having Rh-positive baby to prevent Rh-isoimmunization.
- Minimizing fetomaternal bleeding during delivery.
- Prevention of perinatal distress—like hypoxia, hypothermia, hypoglycemia, etc.
- Adequate and early feeding to prevent dehydration and hypoglycemia to reduce enterohepatic recirculation.
- Avoidance of jaundice aggravating drugs like vitamin 'K' in large dose.
- Aspiration of cephalhematoma, if present with jaundice.
- Treatment of sepsis and hepatitis.
- Administration of phenobarbitone to improve uptake, conjugation and excretion of bilirubin by liver.
- Management of Rh-sensitized mother during antenatal period with rising titer of indirect Coombs' test.

Neonatal Hypoglycemia

Neonatal hypoglycemia is a common metabolic disorder which can cause unexplained death and high mortality. Incidence and severity of the condition can be reduced by initiating appropriate feeding regimen and timely administration of supplements. Prompt intervention and therapy have dramatic response in the improvement of the neonatal condition.

Hypoglycemia in the newborn baby is termed when the blood glucose level is less than 40 mg/dL, irrespective of period of gestational age. At bedside, when blood glucose level by glucometer is found less than 45 mg/dL, it is also considered as hypoglycemia. It may be asymptomatic or symptomatic.

Causes of Neonatal Hypoglycemia

Neonatal hypoglycemia is found soon after birth in low birth weight infants and infants of diabetic mothers. It may seen as secondary problem to perinatal stresses like asphyxia, hypothermia, infection, polycythemia, respiratory distress and neurological disturbances. It may also be found in IUGR, smaller twins, babies born to mother with PIH, Rh-incompatibility and maternal tocolytic therapy like isoxsuprine, salbutamol, etc. Intractable hypoglycemia may occur due to number of metabolic and developmental disorders like glycogen storage disease, galactosemia, fructosemia, maple syrup urine disease, organic acidemia, adrenal insufficiency, etc.

Clinical Manifestations

The clinical features are associated with release of epinephrine and activation of autonomic nervous systems which may altered due to anoxia and intracranial injury.

The neonates may present with refusal of feeds, sweating, tachycardia, limpness, jitteriness, tremors, twitching, pallor, hypothermia, lethargy or irritability, restlessness, convulsions and coma. Apnea with cyanosis, tachypnea with irregular breathing may also occur in preterm babies.

Management

Hypoglycemia should be prevented by early initiation of breastfeeding within first hour of birth. The baby should be nursed in warm or thermoneutral environment with careful observation of 'at-risk' situations and prevention of hypoxia and hypothermia .

In symptomatic infant with convulsions, 10 percent dextrose 2 mL/kg intravenously is given as a bolus. If there is no convulsions, 10 percent dextrose 2 mL/kg/IV bolus is given followed by continuous infusion of 10 percent dextrose at a rate of 6 to 8 mg/kg/minute. Blood glucose level to be checked every 1/2 hourly. Infusion rate to be reduced only if last two glucose estimation is more than 60 mg/dL. Oral feeds are introduced gradually and glucose infusion is tapered off.

If blood glucose level is not corrected then bolus administration of dextrose can be repeated and serum cortisol and insulin levels to be checked. Hydrocortisone therapy is given 5 mg/kg/IV every 12 hours in intractable case. Glucagon and/or epinephrine, diaoxide may be given to the babies with maternal diabetes mellitus or erythroblastosis.

Asymptomatic cases with low blood sugar level should be treated as symptomatic cases.

Prognosis

The prognosis of hypoglycemia is generally poor. Untreated symptomatic neonates usually have fatal outcome. Among survivors of symptomatic cases, about 50 percent neonates may have mental retardation or cerebral palsy with convulsions. In asymptomatic hypoglycemic babies of diabetic mothers the prognosis is usually excellent.

Neonatal Convulsions/Seizures

Neonatal convulsions are common life-threatening emergency in the newborn due to cerebral or biochemic abnormality. Preterm and LBW babies are more prone to this problem. Newborn babies do not manifest febrile convulsions. Common causes of neonatal convulsions are hypoxic-ischemic encephelopathy (HIE), hypocalcemia, hypoglycemia, septicemia with meningitis and polycythemia.

Etiology of Neonatal Convulsions

1. *Developmental neurological problems:*
   - Congenital hydrocephalus, microcephaly, cerebral dysgenesis, porencephaly, polymicrogyria, hydranencephaly, lissencephaly, agenesis of corpus callosum, etc.
2. *Perinatal complications:* HIE, birth asphyxia, birth injuries, intracranial hemorrhage.
3. *Perinatal infections:* Meningitis, septicemia, intrauterine infections (STORCH).
4. *Metabolic problems:* Hypocalcemia, hypoglycemia, hypomagnesemia, hypo- or hypernatremia, severe hyperbilirubinemia with kernicterus, inborn errors of metabolism, pyridoxine dependency.
5. *Drugs:* Neonates born to narcotic addicted mothers (Narcotic withdrawal syndrome), theophylline, phenothiazine (used in eclampsia), inadvertent injection of local anesthesia into fetal scalp.

Types of Neonatal Convulsions

Five major types of seizures are seen in neonates, i.e. subtle, generalized tonic, multifocal clonic, focal clonic and myoclonic seizures. About 50 percent of all neonatal seizures are subtle type, which may manifest as eye movements (blinking, fluttering, deviation with jerking, eye opening sustained with ocular fixation), orobuccolingual movements, screaming, rowing and pedalling movements, apneic spells and bradycardia.

Pure tonic and clonic convulsions are not seen in neonates as neonatal seizures are mainly subcortical in origin. Twitching, rolling of eyes, generalized tonic stiffness without clonic phase with apnea and respiratory irregularity or only a change in baby's skin color and vacant look may indicate convulsive disorders and should be investigated.

Jitteriness should be differentiated from seizures. It is initiated by stimulation and aborted by gentle restraint. Prolonged jitteriness can be pathological.

Investigations

Blood examination for calcium, sugar, phosphorus, electrolytes, amino acids, organic acid, pH, ammonia, etc. and lumber puncture for CSF study help in diagnosis the cause. Electroencephalogram (EEG), USG brain, CT scan, MRI, ECG sepsis screen and serology for STORCH infections help to exclude the exact etiology of neonatal convulsions. Time of onset of convulsions, family history of convulsions, history of maternal drug addiction and infections are important aspect of investigations.

Management

The neonate needs special care with airway clearance, oxygen, IV line, thermal protection, prevention of aspiration and injury, respiratory support and anticonvulsive therapy (phenobarbitone, phenytoin, sodium valproate, etc.). The exact cause of convulsions should be detected and treated appropriately, e.g. hypoglycemia, hypocalcemia HIE, meningitis, kernicterus, IVH, etc. Follow-up care and re-evaluation are important for future outcome of the child.

Prognosis

The prognosis is good in hypocalcemic convulsions. About one-fourth to 40 percent of neonates with neonatal convulsions die. Birth trauma and hypoxia are having bad prognosis. Among survivors, about 25 percent suffer from recurrent convulsions and neurodevelopmental defects.

HIGH RISK NEONATES

Identification of high risk neonates is very important responsibility of the nursing personnel at delivery room. Careful assessment should be done to detect the problems and to initiate prompt management in better health care facilities or in special care neonatal units.

The following babies are transferred to the special care nursery for better supervision and management without unnecessary delay:
- Birth weight less than 2000 g
- Gestational age less than 36 weeks
- Severe birth asphyxia with 5 minutes Apgar score of 3 or less
- Rh-incompatibility
- Gross congenital malformations
- Maternal diabetes mellitus
- Respiratory distress or any other systematic problems of the neonates
- Unwell or unwed or unwilling mother.

In the community, the health workers or community health nurse should identify the high risk and sick baby without delay and referred the neonate to level-II neonatal care facilities.

Common Indications for Referral

- Birth weight less than 1800 g or gestation age less than 34 weeks
- Delayed passage of meconium (more than 24 hours) and urine (more than 48 hours)
- Inability to suck or swallow
- Reduced activity or excessive crying
- Marked changes in skin color—pale, blue or yellow
- Cold baby or febrile baby
- Rapid breathing more than 60 breaths per minutes, chest retractions and alae nasi movements
- Superficial infections with purulent conjunctivitis, oral thrush, umbilical sepsis, pyoderma, abscess
- Persistent vomiting or watery diarrhea
- Abdominal distension
- Bleeding from any site and any features of injury
- Convulsions and abnormal movements
- Delayed capillary refill time
- Fontanel bulging or depressed
- Sudden loss of weight
- Presence of any congenital anomalies.

Community health workers and nurses should be aware about the identification of high risk and sick newborn babies. They can provide basic and essential neonatal care to enhance the survival of the neonates in the community.

Low Birth Weight Babies

A neonate with a birth weight of less than 2500 g irrespective of the gestational age are termed as low birth weight (LBW) baby. They include both preterm and small-for-dates (SFD) babies. These two groups have different clinical problems and prognosis. In India about 30 to 40 percent neonates are born LBW. Approximately 80 percent of all neonatal deaths and 50 percent of infant death are related to LBW. These LBW babies are more prone to malnutrition, infections and neurodevelopmental handicapped conditions. They are more vulnerable to develop hypertension, diabetes mellitus, coronary artery disease in adult life.

High incidence of LBW babies in our country is due to higher number of babies with intrauterine growth retardation (small for dates) rather than preterm babies. It is not possible to provide special care to all LBW babies, especially in India. The baby with a birth weight of less than 2000 g is more vulnerable and need special care. About 10 percent of all LBW babies require admission to the special care neonatal units.

Terminology

Very low birth weight (VLBW) babies: Babies with a birth weight of less than 1500 g (up to and including 1499 g)

Extremely low birth weight (ELBW) babies: Babies with a birth weight of less than 1000 g (up to and including 999 g).

Small for dates (SFD) babies: Babies with a birth weight of less than 10th percentile for their gestational age. They are also termed as small for gestational age (SGA) or light-for-dates or intrauterine growth retardation. Dysmaturity refers to the marasmic appearance of a baby indicating placental dysfunciton. The term dysmaturity should be avoided.

Appropriate for dates (AFD) babies: Babies with a birth weight between 10th to 90th percentile for the period of their gestational age. They are also termed as appropriate for gestational age (AGA).

Large for dates (LFD) babies: Babies with a birth weight more than 90th percentile for the period of their gestational age. The neonate with a birth weight more than 97 percentile for their gestation are at high risk and should be monitored for hypoglycemia. They are also termed as heavy-for-dates or large for gestation age (LGA).

Preterm baby: A baby born with a gestational age of less than 37 completed weeks (or less than 259 days) is termed as preterm baby. These babies are also termed as immature, born early or premature.

Term baby: A baby born with a gestational age between 37 to 41 weeks (259 to 293 days) is called as term baby.

Post-term baby: A baby born with a gestational age of 42 weeks or more (294 days or more) is called post-term baby.

By combining classification of the babies on the basis of gestational age alone and gestational age with birth weight, the neonates can be divided into 9 subgroups:

- Preterm
  1. Small for date
  2. Appropriate for date
  3. Large for date
- Term
  1. Small for date
  2. Appropriate for date
  3. Large for date
- Post-term
  1. Small for date
  2. Appropriate for date
  3. Large for date

(*See* Appendix XVIII for details).

Prevention of LBW Babies

Prevention and reduction in incidence of low birth weight (LBW) babies is the most important strategy to reduce perinatal and infant mortality rates and improve the quality of life among those who survive. Causes of preterm birth and SFD babies should be eliminated to fulfill the objectives.

Preterm Infants

Approximately 10 to 12 percent of Indian neonates are born before 37 completed weeks of gestation. These infants are vulnerable to various physiological handicapped conditions with high mortality rate due to their anatomical and functional immaturity.

Subcategories of preterm infants are:
  a. Extremely preterm (less than 28 weeks of gestation)
  b. Very preterm (28 to 32 weeks of gestation)

  c. Moderate to late preterm (32 to less than 37 weeks of gestation)

Causes of Preterm Birth

Spontaneous causes: There may be spontaneous onset of preterm labor leading to preterm birth. The causes may be:
- Antepartum hemorrhage, cervical incompetence and bicornuate uterus
- Chronic and systemic maternal diseases or infections
- Threatened abortion, acute emotional stress, physical exertion, sexual activity and trauma
- Low maternal weight gain and poor socioeconomic condition
- Maternal malnutrition L-carnitine deficiency and anemia
- Cigarette smoking during pregnancy and drug addiction
- Multiple pregnancy and congenital malformations
- Very young and unmarried mother
- Too frequent child birth and history of previous preterm delivery.

Induced causes: The preterm labor may be induced to safeguard the interests of the mother or fetus, when there is impending danger for them. The conditions are:
- Maternal diabetes mellitus and severe heart diseases
- Placental dysfunction with unsatisfactory fetal growth
- Eclampsia, severe pre-eclampsia and hypertension.
- Fetal hypoxia and fetal distress.
- Antepartum hemorrhage.
- Severe Rh-isoimmunization.
- Iatrogenic—improper diagnosis of maturity in elective deliveries.

Characteristics of Preterm Infants

Physical characteristics (Figs 6.14A to C)
- A preterm baby is small in size with relatively large head. Crown-heel length is less than 47 cm and head circumference is less than 33 cm but exceeds the chest circumference by more than 3 cm.
- General activity of the baby is poor with sluggish or incomplete neonatal reflexes such as Moro, sucking and swallowing reflex. Limbs are extended due to hypotonia with poor recoil of flexed forearm when it is extended.
- Head is larger than body, skull bones are soft, sutures are widely separated and fontanelles are large. Face is small with small chin and less or absent buccal fat. Scalp hairs are scanty, wooly and fuzzy with separate individual hair fibers.
- Eyes remain closed and protruding due to shallow orbits. Ears are soft, flat and cartilage is not fully developed.
- Skin is shiny, thin, delicate and pink with little vernix caseosa and plenty lanugo hair. There is less subcutaneous fat. Edema may present.

- Breast nodules are absent or less than 5 mm. Nipples and areola are flat. Abdomen is full, soft and round with prominent veins.
- Nails are short and not grown up to finger tips. Deep creases over soles and palms are absent or less.
- Genitalia—in male baby, testes are undescended and scrotum is poorly pigmented with few rugosities. In female baby, labia minora is exposed due to poorly developed and widely separated labia majora. Clitoris is hypertropied and prominent.

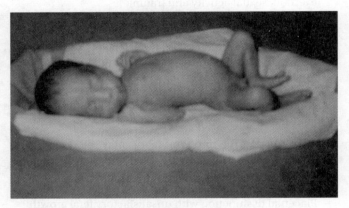

Fig. 6.14A: Preterm baby (34 weeks). Birth weight 1120 g, present weight 1350 g at 3 weeks of age

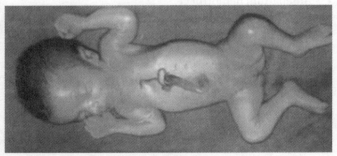

Fig. 6.14B: A preterm baby at birth of 1300 g, 35 weeks

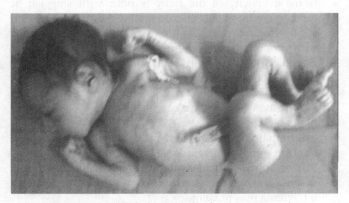

Fig. 6.14C: IUGR baby at birth of 1800 g, 38 weeks

Physiological handicaps: Various clinical hazards are found in preterm neonates due to functional immaturity of different systems.

1. *Alteration of respiratory functions:* Respiration of preterm neonates are rapid, shallow irregular with periods of apnea and cyanosis. Breathing is mostly diaphragmatic, periodic and associated with intercostal recessions due to soft ribs. Cough and gag reflex are weak or absent. Pulmonary aspiration and atelectasis are common problems. Hyaline membrane disease may develop in these babies. They are vulnerable to develop chronic pulmonary insufficiency due to bronchopulmonary dysplasia. Weak respiratory muscle, poor development and expansion of lungs, inefficient respiratory center and deficiency of surfactant in the alveoli are responsible for respiratory problems and resuscitation difficulties at birth.

2. *Immaturity of central nervous system:* The preterm infants are inactive, lethargic and having poor cough reflex. Sucking and swallowing reflexes are in cordinated leading to feeding difficulties. Oxygen toxicity causing retinopathy of prematurity (ROP) or retrolental fibroplasia is found in preterm babies (less than 35 weeks). These babies are prone to kernicterus and brain damage at lower serum bilirubin level due to inefficient blood-brain barrier. They are also vulnerable to intraventricular or periventricular hemorrhage due to deficient coagulation factors and increased capillary fragility.

3. *Disturbances of circulatory functions:* In preterm neonates, the closure of ductus arteriosus may be delayed. The peripheral circulation is inadequate. Thromboembolic complications may develop. Intracranial hemorrhage may occur due to poor autoregulation of cerebral blood flow. Weak and fragile blood vessels and hypofunction of bone marrow may result hemorrhagic problems.

4. *Impaired thermoregulation:* The preterm babies are more prone to develop hypothermia due to poorly developed heat regulating center, large body surface area in relation to body weight, poor insulating subcutaneous fat and less brown adipose tissue. Inadequate thermic response are seen due to poor food intake, poor muscular activity and less oxygen consumption. In these babies heat production is less, whereas more heat loss occur due to poor control over thermoregulation and various environmental factors.

5. *Inefficient gastrointestinal and hepatic functions:* Sucking and swallowing reflexes are poor leading to poor intake of feeds. Capacity of the stomach is less and cardioesophageal sphincter is incompetent resulting in regurgitation and aspiration. Gastroesophageal reflux and associated problems are common. Digestion of protein and carbohydrate is adequate but fat is pooly absorbed. Abdominal distension and functional intestinal obstruction are found due to hypotonia. Necrotizing enterocolitis may occur. Immaturity of liver and its poor enzymatic action leads to hyperbilirubinemia.

Hypoglycemia is common due to poor hepatic glycogen stores, delayed feeding, birth asphyxia and respiratory distress syndrome. These neonates are prone to malnutrition, iron deficiency anemia and deficiency of Vitamin A, D, E, K due to poor absorption of nutrients. Poor vitamin 'K' synthesis in liver and poor prothrombin production leads to hemorrhagic disease.

6. *Metabolic disturbances:* Due to poor metabolic functions, the preterm neonates are prone to develop hypoglycemia, hypocalcemia, hypoxia, acidosis and hypoproteinemia.

7. *Increased susceptibility to infections:* Preterm neonates are 3 to 10 times more vulnerable to infections than normal neonates. Inefficient cellular immunity and low IgG antibody level make them more susceptible to infections. Excessive handling, humid and warm environment, resuscitation and other invasive procedures are responsible for high incidence of infections.

8. *Impaired renal functions:* Due to low glomerular filtration rate and reduced concentrating ability of renal tubules, the preterm neonates are more prone to develop acidosis. They may be dehydrated due to inability to conserve water. Urination may be delayed. Edema may develop due to solute retention and low serum proteins. Renal failure may develop as complication.

9. *Drugs toxicity:* Poor hepatic detoxification and reduced renal clearance lead to toxic effects of drugs unless precautions are followed during administration. Oxygen toxicity may lead to retinopathy of prematurity due to higher concentration of oxygen which constrict the retinal arteries resulting anoxic damage and retinal detachment. This condition is also termed as retrolental fibroplasia which can cause blindness in future life.

Management of Preterm Babies

Prevention of preterm birth is important by early detection and management of high risk antenatal mothers. Preterm labor should be managed efficiently by appropriate referral to well-equipped obstetrical and neonatal care facilities for better management of the preterm babies.

Delivery of preterm baby must be attended by neonatologist for prompt management. Expert nursing care is essential for better recovery from various problems due to physiological handicaps.

Care of preterm babies at birth: Efficient resuscitation and prevention of hypothermia are important aspect of care at birth. Delayed cord clamping may improve the iron stores and reduce the incidence of hyaline membrane disease. It should be done according to baby's condition. Continuous breathing support may be necessary. Warmth should be maintained by heat source, vitamin 'K' 0.5 mg should be administered intramuscularly. Then after stabilization of condition, the baby should be transferred to neonatal intensive care unit (NICU) for special care with all precautions.

Care at neonatal intensive care unit: Neonatal intensive care unit (NICU) should provide as like as intrauterine environment for the preterm neonates. The NICU should be warm, free from excessive sound and have smoothing light. Protection from infections should be ensured by aseptic measures and effective hand washing. Rough handling and painful procedures should be avoided. Baby should be placed on a soft-comfortable, 'nestled' and cushioned bed. Continuous monitoring of the baby's clinical status are vital aspect of management which depends upon the gestational age of the baby.

Baby can be placed in prone position during care. Prone posture makes the neonates comfortable, less cry and reduced chance of aspiration. This position relieves abdominal discomfort, improve ventilation and enhances arterial oxygenation. Unsupervised prone position may cause sudden infant death syndrome (SIDS).

Maintenance of breathing: Respiratory distress is the most common problem in preterm baby. Baby should be positioned with neck slightly extended and air passage to be cleared by gentle suctioning to remove the secretion, if needed. Precautions should be taken to prevent aspiration of secretions and feeds. Oxygen therapy should be administered only when indicated. Head box to be used for oxygen therapy. Concentration of oxygen to be maintained to have SPO_2 between 90 and 92 percent and PaO_2 between 60 and 80 mm Hg.

Baby's respiration rate, rhythm, signs of distress, chest retraction, nasal flaring, apnea, cyanosis, oxygen saturation, etc. to be monitored at frequent interval.

Tactile stimulation by sole flicking can be provided to stimulate respiratory effort. Chest physiotherapy by percussion, vibration and postural drainage may be needed to loosen and remove respiratory secretions.

Maintenance of stable body temperature: Baby should be received in a prewarmed radiant warmer or incubator. Environmental temperature should be maintained according to baby's weight and age (as recommended by neutral thermal environmental temperature). Baby's skin temperature should be maintained 36.5 to 37.5°C. Baby with birth weight of less than 1200 g should be cared in the intensive care incubator with 60 to 65 percent humidity, oxygen (if needed) and thermoneutral environment for better thermal control and prevent heat loss. Kangaroo-mother care can be provided when the baby's condition stabilizes. Baby should be clothed with frock, cap, socks and mittens. Constant monitoring of temperature is essential with low reading thermometer. Bathing should be delayed. All measures to be taken to prevent heat loss. External heat sources to be used for thermal protection of these neonates, whenever needed.

Maintenance of nutrition and hydration: Caloric needs of nongrowing LBW babies during first week of life are 60 kcal/kg/day. After first 1 to 2 weeks of life most preterm babies

Table 6.6 Fluid requirements of LBW infants (mL/kg/day)

Day	< 1000 g	1000-1500 g	> 1500 g
1st and 2nd	100–120	80–100	60–80
3rd and 4th	130–140	110–120	90–100
5th and 6th	150–160	130–140	110–120
7th and 8th	170–180	150–160	130–140
9th onwards	190–200	170–180	150–160

require 120 to 150 kcal/kg/day to maintain satisfactory growth. Fluid requirements of LBW babies are given in Table 6.6. Requirements of all nutrients should be maintained with adequate feeding. Nutritional supplementation should be given.

Additional allowances are recommended in some neonatal conditions for:

- Phototherapy — 20 to 30 mL/kg/day
- Radiant warmer—20 to 30 mL/kg/day

Feeding should be initiated early. Those babies who have good sucking and swallowing reflexes should start breastfeeding as early as possible. Expressed breast milk (EBM) can be given with spoon and bowl at 2 hours interval. Katoris-spoon or palady can also be used for feeding the preterm babies. Gavage or nasogastric tube feeding can be given with EBM to all babies with poor sucking reflex. Intravenous dextrose solution should be started for the babies weighing less than 1200 g or sick babies. Starvation to be avoided and early enteral feeding should be started as soon as the baby is stable.

Prevention of infections: Preterm babies are prone to infections due to poor immunity. Measures to be taken to prevent nosocomial infections. Thorough hand washing, separate baby care articles, changing of shoes and wearing of sterile gown and mask by the caregivers, restriction of visitors and avoidance of infected person inside the neonatal care unit should be followed. Infected babies should be kept separate. Antiseptic cleaning of all equipment, gadgets, nursery floors and walls are essential aspects. Baby bath should be withheld and general cleanliness to be maintained. Strict aseptic technique to be followed for all invasive procedures.

Gentle rhythmic stimulation: Sensory stimulation to be provided to the preterm babies by talking, singing, cuddling, gentle touching during care. Visual and auditory stimulation also can be provided. Kissing the baby should be avoided.

Prevention, early detection and prompt management of complications: The baby should be observed for respiration, skin temperature, heart rate, skin color, activity, cry, feeding behavior, passage of meconium or stool and urine, condition of umbilical cord, eyes and oral cavity, any abnormal signs like edema, bleeding, vomiting, etc. Biochemical and electronic monitoring to be done if needed. Weight recording should be done daily in sick babies otherwise alternate days. Position to be changed frequently at 2 hours interval. Baby should be placed on right side after feeding to prevent regurgitation and aspiration. Mother should be allowed to take care of the baby whenever condition permits. Any problem identified should be managed immediately.

Family support discharge planning, follow-up and home care: Baby's condition and progress to be explained to the parents to reduce their anxiety. Treatment plan to be discussed. Parents should be informed about the care of the baby, after discharge at home. Need for warmth, breast- feeding, general cleanliness, infection prevention measures, environmental hygiene, follow-up plan, immunization, etc. should be explained to the parents.

Before discharge all high risk neonates should have ROP and hearing screening with plan for future management. During follow-up visit developmental assessment with hearing and vision assessment should be done to detect problems and initiate early interventions. Early intervention services can be provided as physiotherapy, stimulation for hearing, vision, speech and language and cognition. Play therapy, special education and parental counseling also include in this services.

Most healthy infants with a birth weight of 1800 g or more and gestational maturity of 35 weeks or more can be managed at home. Mother should be mentally prepared and trained to provide essential care to the preterm baby at home. At the time of discharge the baby should have daily steady weight gain with good vigour and able to suck and maintain warmth. Ultimate survival of the baby depends upon continuity of care. The community health nurse should visit the family every week for a month and provide necessary guidance and support.

Prognosis for survival is directly related to the birth weight and quality of neonatal care. Long-term complications may be found as neurological handicaps in the form of cerebral palsy, seizures, hydrocephalus, microcephaly, blindness (due to ROP), deafness and mental retardation. Minor neurological disabilities are found as language disorder, learning disabilities, behavior problems, attention deficit and hyperactivity disorders. Physical growth correlates with the conceptional age. Preterm AFD babies catch up in their physical growth with term counterparts by the age of 1 to 2 years.

Small for Dates Babies/Intrauterine Growth Retardation

The babies with intrauterine growth retardation (IUGR) are found as three different types:

1. *Malnourished small for dates (SFD) babies (asymmetric IUGR):* They appear long, thin, marasmic and alert. They have less subcutaneous fat, poor muscle mass and excess

skin folds on the buttocks and thighs. Back of the hands and feet are wrinkled. Head circumference is generally more than 3 cm than chest circumference. Internal organs (liver, lungs) are shrunken. The growth retardation is due to reduction in the size of the cells but not the cell number and probably occurred during latter part of gestation due to placental dysfunction. Prognosis is better with appropriate nutritional rehabilitation. This type is the most common variety.

2. *Hypoplastic SFD babies (symmetric IUGR):* These babies are small in all parameters including head size. The number of body cells are reduced. The growth retardation occurs in early part of gestation due to intrauterine infections, certain genetic and chromosomal disorders. Prognosis is poor with permanent mental and physical growth retardation.
3. *Mixed group:* These babies neither look obviously malnourished nor grossly hypoplastic. There is reduction in the cell number and the cell size. They are the outcome of adverse factors of early or mid pregnancy.

Ponderal Index

Ponderal index (PI) is calculated by multiplying the weight in gram by hundred then dividing by the cube of length in cm i.e. by the formula—weight in g × 100/ (length in cm)³. If the PI is less than 2, it indicates asymmetric IUGR, and when it is more than 2, it indicates symmetric IUGR. PI more than 2.5 indicates term AGA neonate.

$$\text{Ponderal index} = \frac{\text{Weight in grams}}{(\text{Length in cm})^3} \times 100$$

If Ponderal index is <2 = Asymmetric IUGR
It Ponderal index is >2 = Symmetric IUGR (Also in term AGA)

Causes of Small for Dates Babies

1. *Maternal factors:* Short stature mother, primi or grand multipara, teenage pregnancy, low prepregnant weight, maternal illness (anemia, heart disease, malaria), complications of pregnancy (PIH, hypertension), smoking, alcoholism or drug abuse by mother and poor weight gain during pregnancy.
2. *Placental factors:* Disorders of placental implantation, abruptio placenta, structural and functional abnormalities of placenta and umbilical cord.
3. *Fetal factors:* First born babies, twin or multiple pregnancy, intrauterine infections, genetic or chromosomal aberration.
4. *Environmental factors:* Poor socioeconomic status, nutritional habits, cultural practices, ethnic, racial and geographic influence.

Common Problems of Small for Dates Babies

The clinical problems and prognosis are different in SFD babies as compared to preterm babies. The clinical problems may be found in these babies are:
- Fetal hypoxia and intrapartum death due to placental dysfunction
- Severe birth asphyxia, meconium aspiration syndrome
- Congenital malformation
- Symptomatic hypoglycemia and hypocalcemia
- Inappropriate thermoregulation
- Hyperbilirubinemia
- Pulmonary hemorrhage, polycythemia due to unknown cause
- Increased risk of infections
- Poor growth potential
- Development of diabetes mellitus, hypertension and coronary artery disease in adult life.

Management

Although the preterm and SFD babies have physiological differences, the principles of management of all LBW infants are common. The prognosis is much better than preterm babies. The important aspect of management are—efficient resuscitation, prevention of hypothermia and thermal protection, adequate fluids and feeds, monitoring and early detection of complications with appropriate management of specific conditions. Appropriate place of care for these babies are as follows:
- Birth weight more than 1800 g—Home care, if the baby is well.
- Birth weight 1500 to 1800 g—Secondary level neonatal care unit (level-II).
- Birth weight less than 1500 g—Tertiary level newborn care unit (level-III of care).

KANGAROO MOTHER CARE

Introduction

Caring low birth weight baby is a great challenge for the neonatal care unit and the family. Number of low birth weight baby is still far beyond the expected target in our country. The cost of quality management of these babies is increasing day by day. Kangaroo mother care is a low cost approach for the care of low birth weight baby. This method of care was introduced and popularized by Dr Edger Rey, in 1978. It was then developed by Dr Martinez and Dr Charpak.

Definition

Kangaroo mother care (KMC) is a special way of caring low birth weight (LBW) infants by skin-to-skin contact.

It promotes their health and welling by effective thermal control, breastfeeding and bonding. KMC is initiated in hospital and continued at home. Three important aspects of KMC are kangaroo position, nutrition and follow-up.

Components of KMC

In KMC, the infant is continuously kept in skin-to-skin contact by the mother and breastfed exclusively to the utmost extent. The two components of KMC are:

1. *Skin-to-skin contact:* Direct, continuous and prolonged skin-to-skin contact is provided between the mother and her baby to promote thermal control.
2. *Exclusive breastfeeding:* Skin-to-skin contact promotes lactation and feeding interaction with exclusive breast-feeding for adequate nutrition and to improve desired weight gain.

Prerequisites of KMC

A. *Support to the mother:* Mother needs support in hospital and home from care-givers and family members. Counseling and supervision should be provided to the mother by the health personnel in hospital, whereas mother requires assistance and co-operation from her family members at home.
B. *Postdischarge follow-up:* KMC should be continued at home after discharge from hospital. For safe and successful KMC at home, a regular follow-up should be arranged to solve problem and to evaluate health status of the infant.

Benefits of KMC

1. KMC helps in thermal control and metabolism. Prolonged, continuous and direct skin-to-skin contact between mother and neonate provides effective thermal control and reduces risk of hypothermia.
2. KMC results in increased duration and rate of breastfeeding.
3. KMC satisfies all five senses of the infant. Baby feels warmth of the mother through skin-to-skin contact (touch), listen to mothers voice and heart beat (hearing), sucks the breast to feed (taste), smells the mother's odor (olfaction) and makes eye contact with mother's (vision).
4. During KMC, the baby has more regular breathing and less predisposition to apnea.
5. KMC protects against nosocomial infection and reduces incidence of severe illness including pneumonia during infancy.
6. Daily weight gain is slightly better with KMC, thus duration of hospital stay may be reduced. LBW baby

receiving KMC could be discharged from the hospital earlier than conventional care.
7. KMC facilitates better mother-infant bondage due to significantly less stress during kangarooing than the incubator care of the baby.
8. KMC is one of the best methods of transporting small babies by keeping them in continuous skin-to-skin contact with mother or family members.
9. Mother feels increased confidence, self-esteem, sense of fulfillment and deep satisfaction with KMC. Father feels more relaxed, comfortable and better bonded.
10. KMC does not require additional staff compared to incubator care.

According to the Cochrane Review in 2011, KMC was found to reduce infant mortality and lower rates of severe infection/sepsis, nosocomial infections, hypothermia, lower-respiratory-tract diseases and severe illness in neonates. It also found that there is reduction of length of hospital stay in sick and preterm neonates. The review also revealed that KMC resulted in improved weight gain, increase in length and head circumference, improved breast feeding, mother infant bonding and maternal satisfaction. Other studies on KMC show that there is almost no fluctuation of temperature among KMC babies. There is reduced response to painful stimuli in neonates and decreased postpartum depression among mothers by practice of KMC. In a meta-analysis in 2010, it is found that KMC significantly reduced neonatal mortality.

Requirements for KMC Implementation

- Training of nurses, doctors and other staff on KMC, specially who are involved in care of mother and baby.
- Educational materials like information booklet, pamphlets, poster, video film, etc. on KMC in local language.
- Reclining chairs or beds with adjustable backrest or pillow or ordinary chair.
- KMC does not require extra staff. Once KMC is implemented, care-givers appreciate it because of health benefits to the babies and the satisfaction expressed by the mothers.

Eligibility Criteria for KMC

For Baby

- All stable LBW babies are eligible for KMC. It is particularly useful for caring LBW infants weighing below 2000 gm.
- In a stable baby, KMC can be initiated soon after birth.
- KMC should be started after the baby is hemodynamically stable.
- Sick LBW infants may take a few days to initiate KMC. So the sick baby needs transfer to a proper facility immediately.

- Infants of birth weight less than 1200 g with serious prematurity related morbidity may take days to weeks to allow initiation of KMC.
- KMC can be initiated who is otherwise stable but may still be on IV fluid therapy, tube feeding and/or O$_2$ therapy.

For Mothers

- All mothers can provide KMC irrespective of age, parity, education, culture and religion.
- Mother should be free of serious illness and able to take adequate diet and supplements recommended by her doctor.
- She must be willing to provide KMC to her baby.
- She should maintain good hygiene, daily bath/sponge, change of clothes, hand hygiene, short and clean finger nails, etc.
- She should have supportive family and community to be encouraged to continue KMC to her baby.

Preparation for KMC

Counseling

- Explain the benefits of KMC to the mother and the family members.
- Demonstrate the procedure to the mother gently with patience.
- Answer the questions as asked by the mother and the family members to remove anxiety.
- Allow the mother to interact with someone who have already practicing KMC for her baby.
- Discuss about the procedure to the mother-in-law, husband or any other members of the family.

Mother's Clothing

Mother should wear front-open, light dress, as per local culture. Mother can wear sari-blouse, gown, shawl, etc.

Baby's Clothing

Baby should be dressed with front-open sleeveless shirt, cap, socks, nappy and hand gloves.

KMC Procedure

Kangaroo Positioning

- The baby should be placed between the mother's breast in an upright position.
- Baby's head should be turned to one side and in a slightly extended position which helps to keep the

airway open and allow eye to eye contact between mother and baby.
- Baby's hip should be flexed and abducted in a froglike position. The arms should also be flexed and placed on mother's chest.
- Baby's abdomen should be placed at the level of mother's epigastrium.

This position helps to reduce the occurrence of apnea, as mother's breathing and heartbeat stimulate the baby. Baby can be supported with a sling or binder or especially prepared KMC bag.

Monitoring during KMC

- During initial stage of KMC the baby should be monitored for airway, breathing, color and temperature. Hands and feet should be examined to assess the warmth. Airway must be kept clear with regular breathing, normal skin color and temperature.
- Baby's neck position should be neither too flexed nor too extended.

Feeding

- Mother needs help to breastfeed her baby during KMC. Holding the baby near the breast stimulates milk production and the Kangaroo position makes the breastfeeding easier.
- Baby could be fed with paladai, spoon and tube depending upon the baby's condition.

Psychological Support to Mother

- Mother needs motivation to continue KMC
- She should be encouraged to ask questions to remove anxieties.

Privacy

Privacy should be maintained to avoid unnecessary exposure on the part of the mother which makes her nervous and de-motivating.

Time of Initiation of KMC

- KMC should be initiated gradually with a smooth transition from conventional care to continuous KMC.
- KMC can be started as soon as the baby is stable in the neonatal care unit.
- Short KMC sessions can be initiated during recovery with ongoing medical treatment, i.e. IV fluid, O$_2$ therapy, etc.

- KMC can be provided while the baby is with gavage feeding.

Duration of KMC

- Duration of KMC should not be less than one hour to avoid frequent handling which may be stressful to the baby.
- Gradually the length of KMC sessions should be increased up to 24 hours a day. Interruption only can be done for changing of diapers.
- KMC should be continued in postnatal ward and home.
- It may not be possible for mother to provide KMC prolonged period in the beginning. Encourage her to increase the duration each time to provide KMC as long as possible.
- When mother is not available then other family members such as father, grandmother, aunty can provide KMC.

Can the Mother Continue KMC during Sleep and Resting?

- Mother can sleep with baby in KMC position in a reclined or semi-recumbent position about 15 to 30° from above the ground.
- A comfortable chair with adjustable back may be useful to provide KMC during sleep and rest at ward or home.
- Adjustable bed or several pillows or an ordinary bed can be used to maintain the position, which usually decreased the risk of apnea of the baby.
- Supporting garment can be used to carry the baby in kangaroo position during sleep and rest.
- Father and family members can provide KMC to relieve mother during and rest.

Discharging Criteria

The baby should be transferred from the Neonatal Care Unit to the postnatal ward, when the baby is stable and gaining weight and the mother is confident to look after the baby.

The baby should be discharged from hospital when the baby is having the following conditions:

- General health is good and there is no evidence of infection and apnea.
- Feeding well exclusively with breast milk.
- Gaining weight 15 to 20 g/kg/day for atleast three consecutive days.
- Maintaining normal body temperature satisfactorily for atleast three consecutive days in room temperature.
- Mother and family members are confident to take care of the baby at home and would be able to come regularly for follow-up visits.

- Home environment should be suitable and congenial for continuation of KMC.

Discontinuation of KMC

- KMC can be continued until the baby gains weight around 2500 g or reaches 40 weeks of postconception age.
- KMC can be discontinued if the baby starts wriggling to show discomfort or pulls limbs out, cries and fusses every time, when mother tries to put the baby back into skin contact.
- When mother and baby are comfortable, KMC can be continued as long as possible at health facility or at home.
- Mother can provide skin-to-skin contact occasionally after the baby bath and during cold nights.

Postdischarge Follow-up

Each neonatal care unit should formulate its own policy for follow-up.

- In general a baby is followed up once or twice a week till 37 to 40 weeks of gestation or till the baby reaches 2.5 to 3 kg of weight.
- There after a follow-up once in 2 to 4 weeks may be sufficient till 3 months of postconceptional age. After that 1 to 2 months during first year of life. The baby should gain adequate weight 15 to 20 g/kg/day up to 40 weeks of post-conceptional age and 10 g/kg/day subsequently.
- More frequent visits should be made, if the baby is not growing well or the condition demands.
  Adopted from: KMC India Network

Infants of Diabetic Mothers

Maternal diabetes mellitus may cause various problems to the infants. These neonates are usually remarkably heavy, plump, full-faced, plethoric and covered with lot of vervix caseosa. Maternal hypoglycemia leads to fetal hypoglycemia and it is the most common cause of large for dates (LFD) babies. Large fetal size is due to accumulation of fat.

- Perinatal complications related to maternal diabetes mellitus include the followings:
  - Sudden fetal death in last trimester of pregnancy.
  - Preterm delivery may be induced to prevent unexplained fetal death in last trimester.
  - Macrosomia or large fetal size may result birth trauma, birth asphyxia and operative delivery (LUCS).
  - Neonatal respiratory destress syndrome due to hyaline membrane disease (HMD).
  - Hypoglycemia due to diminished production of glucose and increased removal by insulin.
  - Hypocalcemia may occur due to diminished production of parathormone.

- Hyperbilirubinemia may be due to breakdown of hemoglobin in cephalohematoma.
- Polycythemia and increased viscosity of blood.
- Higher risk of congenital anomalies (congenital heart disease).
- Cardiomyopathy and persistent pulmonary hypertension.
- Lazy left colon syndrome.
- Hypertrichosis and hairy pinna.

Management of infants of diabetic mothers should be done same way as a preterm or small for dates babies. Oral feeding should be started as early as possible. Intravenous glucose drip may be needed. Respiratory distress syndrome should be managed promptly by early detection. Other clinical problems should be paid due attention for appropriate management. Infants of diabetic mothers have one to nine percent incidence of diabetes in later life.

Infants of HIV Positive Mothers

Children are innocent victims of HIV (human immunodeficiency virus) infection through vertical transmission. Approximately 90 percent of pediatric HIV infections are acquired from infected mother resulting in vertical transmission to her infant. Mother to child transmission may occur passively *in utero* (30–35%), during delivery (60–65%) and also through breastfeeding (10–15%). Rate of vertical transmission ranges from 13 to 40 percent.

The factors responsible to increase the rate of mother to child transmission include high levels of viremia and lack of matching antibody in the pregnant women, advanced maternal HIV disease, low maternal CD_4 counts, maternal p24 antigenemia, placental membrane inflammation, high CD_8 counts, preterm infants, first born twins, lack of antiviral therapy to infected pregnant woman and breastfeeding.

Asymptomatic HIV positive mother can transmit infection to her offspring. The infection in the pregnant woman can be suspected by high risk behavior (promiscuous sexual behavior, drug addiction) which should be confirmed by positive serological test during antenatal visit as a measure of prevention of parent-to-child transmission.

Perinatal HIV Disease

HIV infected child: A child less than 18 months of age who is HIV seropositive or born to HIV infected mother and has positive results on two separate determinations from one or more of the following tests—(i) HIV culture (ii) HIV specific PCR and (iii) HIV antigen (p24) or meets clinical criteria for AIDS diagnosis.

Perinatally exposed: A child who does not meet the criteria above but is seropositive by ELISA and confirmatory test (Western blot) and is less than 18 months of age at the time of the test or has known antibody status, but was born to a mother known to be infected with HIV.

Seroreverter: A child who is born to an HIV infected mother and who has been documented as HIV antibody negative (two or more negative ELISA test performed at 6–18 months of age or one negative ELISA test after 18 months of age) and has had no other laboratory evidence of infection and has not had an AIDS defining condition.

Diagnosis

The definite diagnosis of HIV infection in neonates born to HIV infected mothers is difficult due to various reasons. An HIV infected mother transmits her IgG antibodies to the newborn transplacentally. These neonates are usually antibody positive at birth, but only 15 to 30 percent are actually infected. Maternal antibodies usually undetectable in 9 months but occasionally remain at significant levels until 18 months, hence IgG antibody tests are not reliable indicators of infection status in a child before 18 months of age. Therefore presence of antibody beyond this period is necessary to consider the child infected especially in an asymptomatic child.

The definite diagnostic test for HIV infection in the newborn include: (a) detection of p24 antigen, (b) ELISA for, detection of IgA and IgM, (c) PCR to detect viral nucleic acid in the peripheral blood.

Prevention and Treatment

Vertical transmission can be prevented by zidovudine prophylaxis to HIV-infected pregnant women with a CD_4^+ cell count of less than 200 per mL. It is given from 14 weeks of gestation to till delivery. The infant of an HIV positive mother should be given zidovudine till 6 weeks of life.

The infant should have good nutrition, with symptomatic and supportive care. Withholding of breastfeeding can lead to infections and nutritional problems. The decision of breastfeeding should be individualized.

The symptomatic HIV infected infant should not be given OPV and BCG vaccines. But DPT, HBV, MMR and inactivated polio vaccines can be given. The asymptomatic HIV infected infant should receive BCG and other vaccines.

Parents need emotional support with necessary guidance and counseling. Universal precautions to be followed by the health care providers (doctors, nurses and other staff) for the prevention of transmission. Extraordinary isolation procedures are unwarranted. Information to be given to increase awareness about nature of the disease.

Prevention of HIV infection is more approachable by improvement of healthy lifestyle and following the precautions regarding HIV infection by any mode of transmission. Children are infected mainly from their parents as an innocent victims. Health workers especially the nurses are responsible to create awareness by the preventive measures to protect the children.

GRADES OF NEONATAL CARE

Based on birth weight and gestational age, a three tier system of neonatal care is proposed for developing countries.

Level-I Care

About 80 to 90 percent of neonates require minimal care which can be provided by their mothers with support from family members and under supervision of basic health professionals. The neonates weighing above 2000 g or having gestational age of 37 weeks or more belong to this category. This care can be given at home, subcenter and primary health centers. Essential perinatal care should be provided as basic care at birth, provision of warmth, maintenance of asepsis and promotion of breastfeeding.

Level-II Care

Neonates weighing between 1500 to 2000 g or having gestational age of 32 to 36 weeks need specialized neonatal care supervised by trained nursing staff and pediatricians. This intermediate neonatal care should be provided by the equipped district hospitals, teaching institutions and nursing homes. There should be arrangement of resuscitation procedures, maintenance of thermoneutral environment, intravenous infusion, gavage feeding, photo therapy and exchange blood transfusions. Only 10 to 15 percent of all neonates require this care. It should be available at all hospitals where 1000 to 1500 deliveries take place per year.

Level-III Care

Neonates weighing less than 1500 g or born before 32 weeks of gestation require intensive neonatal care. Only 3 to 5 percent of all newborn babies need this care by skilled nurses and neonatologists especially trained in neonatal intensive care. Apex institutions or regional perinatal centers equipped with centralized oxygen and suction facilities, incubators, ventilators, monitors and infusion pump, etc. are best suited to provide intensive neonatal care.

High-risk pregnancies which are associated with birth of high risk neonates must be identified during pregnancy and referred to an appropriate center for skilled management and better outcome. At birth, detection of high risk neonates should be done at all levels of health care delivery system and appropriate referral is essential to different level of neonatal care for prevention and reduction of neonatal mortality and morbidity.

TRANSPORT OF SICK NEONATES

Neonates are usually transported from labor room to nursery with level II or III facilities or NICU. Neonatal transport may be required from home to level I centers, level I to level II centers or level II to level III centers.

In utero transfer or referral may be needed, if the birth of an 'at-risk' neonate is anticipated, then mother is transported to the facility with optimum maternal and neonatal care.

Transport of the sick neonates is a difficult job and should be done when unavoidable with danger signs and definite indications.

Principles for Transporting Neonates

- Correct assessment of the baby should be done to justify the indication of transport and referral.
- Explain the condition of the baby and reasons for referral.
- Baby's condition to be stabilized and hypothermia should be corrected before transporting.
- Record case history, need for referral and treatment given in the referral card or sheet.
- Mother should accompany the baby at the time of transport or at the earliest time.
- A doctor or nurse or health worker or dai should accompany the neonate to provide necessary care on the way to referral center.
- Provide instructions and guidelines to the attendants/ health worker for care during transport (IV infusion, clearing air passage, position, observation, etc.).
- Ensure warmth of the baby on the way to maintain 'warm chain'. Baby should be covered fully with cloths including head and extremities. The best method to keep the baby warm is skin to skin contact with mother (or another adult) as kangaroo mother care. Transport incubator can also be used if available.
- Mother should be instructed to give breastfeeding if possible, otherwise expressed breast milk to be given with bowl and spoon. Gavage feeding also can be given on the way by the nurses if they accompany the baby.
- Nearest referral facilities to be availed by the shortest route and using fastest, possible and available mode of transport.
- Reverse transport should also be communicated with feedback information, e.g. from NICU to postnatal ward and to rural hospital or home. Follow-up should be done to evaluate the outcome.

Growth, Development and the Healthy Child

7

- Growth and Development
- Needs of the Healthy Child

- Health Promotion of Children and Guidance to Parent for Child Care

GROWTH AND DEVELOPMENT

The process of growth and development starts before the baby born, i.e. from the conception in the mother's womb. The period extends throughout the lifecycle. But the principal changes occurs from the conception to the end of adolescence. Growth and development are closely inter-related. Each child has individualized pattern of growth and development. Promotion of child health and care of children depend upon understanding of growth and development.

Importance of Learning Growth and Development

The study of growth and development is essential to the nurse to provide appropriate care to the children. It helps the nurses in the following aspects:

- To learn what to expect from a particular child at a particular age.
- To assess the normal growth and development of children.
- To detect deviations from normal growth and development, i.e. physical and psychological abnormalities and to understand the reasons of particular conditions and illnesses.
- To ascertain the needs of the child according to the level of growth and development.
- To plan and provide holistic nursing management to the child, based on developmental stages.
- To teach and guide the parents and caregivers to anticipate the problems and to render tender loving care to their children.

- To develop a rapport with the child to enhance the provision of health care and to help to build healthy life-style for optimum health for the future.

Definitions of Terms

Growth

It is the process of physical maturation resulting an increase in size of the body and various organs. It occurs by multiplication of cells and an increase in intracellular substance. It is quantitative changes of the body which can be measured in inches/centimeters and pounds/kilograms. It is progressive and measurable phenomenon.

Development

It is the process of functional and physiological maturation of the individual. It is progressive increase in skill and capacity to function. It is related to maturation and myelination of the nervous system. It includes psychological, emotional and social changes. It is qualitative aspect of maturation and difficult to measure. It is orderly, not haphazard and having direct relation between each stage and the next.

Maturation

It is an increase in competence and change in behavior and ability to function at a higher level depending upon the genetic inheritance.

Characteristics of Growth and Development

Growth and development depend upon each other and in normal child they are parallel and proceed concurrently. Though these terms are used interchangeably but they are not the same. They are used together but not synonymous.

The characteristics and principles which regulates growth and development in children are as follows:

- Growth and development is continuous and orderly process with individual difference and is unique to each child.
- It proceeds by stages and its sequence is predictable and same in all children but there may be difference in the time of achievement.
- There is coordination between increase in size and maturation.
- They proceed in cephalocaudal (i.e. from the head down to the tail) and proximodistal (i.e. from the center or midline to periphery) direction.
- Initial mass activities and movements are replaced by specific response or actions by the complex process of individualized changes.
- Rate of growth and development is inter-related and rapid in infancy and in puberty but slow in preschool and school age.
- Growth and development depend on combination of many interdependent factors especially by heredity and environment.

Stages of Growth and Development

Stages of growth and development can be studied as intra-uterine life or prenatal period and extrauterine life or postnatal period.

Prenatal Period

- *Ovum:* 0 to 14 days after conception
- *Embryo:* 14 days to 8 weeks
- *Fetus:* 8 weeks to birth.

Postnatal Period

- *Neonate:* From birth to four weeks of life
- *Infancy:* First year of life
- *Toddler:* One to 3 years
- *Preschool child (early childhood):* 3 to 6 years
- *School going child (middle childhood)*
  - 6 to 10 years (girls)
  - 6 to 12 years (boys)
- *Adolescent:* From puberty to adulthood
  - Prepubescent (early adolescent/late childhood)
    - 10 to 12 years (girls)
    - 12 to 14 years (boys)
  - Pubescent (middle adolescent)
    - 12 to 14 years (girls)
    - 14 to 16 years (boys)
  - Postpubescent (late adolescent)
    - 14 to 18 years (girls)
    - 16 to 20 years (boys).

Factors Influencing Growth and Development

Growth and development depend upon multiple factors or determinants. They influence directly or indirectly by promoting or hindering the process. The determinants can be grouped as heredity and environment. Heredity determines the extent of growth and development that is possible but environment determines the degree to which the potential is achieved.

Heredity or genetic factors are also related to sex, race and nationality. Environment includes both prenatal and postnatal factors. Postnatal environment can be internal or external. All these factors determine constitution of the body.

Genetic Factors

Each child has a different genetic potential. Genetic predisposition is the important factor which influence the growth and development of children. Different characteristics such as height, body structure, color of skin, eyes and hair, etc. depend upon inherited gene from parents. Thus, tall parents have tall children and parents with high intelligence are more likely to have children with high level of inherent intelligence.

Abnormal genes from ancestors may produce different familial diseases which usually hinders the growth and development, e.g. thalassemia, hemophilia, galactosemia, etc. The process of growth and development is also affected in children with chromosomal abnormalities, e.g. in Down's syndrome, Turner's syndrome, Klinefelter syndrome.

Sex: The sex of children influences their physical attributes and patterns of growth. Sex is determined at conception. At birth, male babies are heavier and longer than the female babies. Boys maintain this superiority until about 11 years of age. Girls mature earlier than boys and bone development is more advanced in girls. But mean hight and weight are usually less in girls than boys at the time of full maturity.

Race and Nationality: Growth potential of different racial groups is different in varying extent. Physical characteristics of different national groups also vary. Height and stature of Americans and Indians are usually differ because of the differences in growth patterns.

Prenatal Factors

Intrauterine environment is an important predominant factor of growth and development. Various conditions influence the fetal *growth in utero*.

Maternal malnutrition: Dietary insufficiency and anemia lead to intrauterine growth retardation. Low birth weight and preterm babies have poor growth potentials. In later life, those children are usually having disturbances of growth and development.

Maternal infections: Different intrauterine infections like HIV, HBV, STORCH, etc. may transmit to the fetus via placenta and affect the fetal growth. Various complications may occur like congenital anomalies, congenital infections etc. which ultimately affect the growth and development in extrauterine life.

Maternal substance abuse: Intake of teratogenic drugs (thalidomide, phenytoin etc.) by the pregnant women in the first trimester affects the organogenesis and lead to congenital malformations which hinder fetal growth. Presence of congenital anomalies in later life influence childhood growth and development. Maternal tobacco intake (smoking and chewing) and alcohol abuse also produce fetal growth restriction.

Maternal illness: Pregnancy-induced hypertension, anemia, heart disease, hypothyroidism, diabetes mellitus, chronic renal failure, hyperpyrexia, etc. have adverse effect on fetal growth. Iodine deficiency of the mother may lead to mental retardation of the baby in later life.

Hormones: Hormones like thyroxine and insulin influence the fetal growth. Thyroxine deficiency retards the skeletal maturation of the fetus. Maternal myxedema results in fetal hypothyroidism. Antithyroid drug therapy and iodides during last trimester of pregnancy may lead to fetal goiter and hypothyroidism. Excess insulin stimulates fetal growth leading to large size fetus with excessive birth weight due to macrosomia.

Miscellaneous: Various prenatal conditions, which may also influence fetal growth include: uterine malformations (septate uterus, bicornuate uterus), malpositions of the fetus, oligohydramnios, polyhydramnios, faulty placental implantation or malfunction, maternal emotion during pregnancy, inadequate prenatal care, etc.

Postnatal Factors

Postnatal environment which influences growth and development are as follows:

Growth potential: Growth potential is indicated by the child's size at birth. The smaller the child at birth, the smaller she/he is likely to be in subsequent years. The larger the child at birth, the larger she/he is likely to be in later years. Low birth weight babies have various complications in later life which retard child's growth.

Nutrition: Balanced amounts of essential nutrients have great significant role in growth and development of children. Both quantitative and qualitative supply of nutrition (i.e. protein, fat, carbohydrates, vitamins and minerals) in the daily diet are necessary for promotion of growth and development. Adequate food intake helps the child in body building, energy production and protection from infections. Well-nourished child has positive physical and mental growth, whereas undernourished child usually suffers from growth retardation and various health problems. The nutritional requirements during growth period depend upon age, sex, growth rate, level of activity and health status of the child.

Childhood illness: Chronic childhood diseases of heart, (congenital heart disease, rheumatic heart disease), chest (tuberculosis, asthma), kidneys (nephrotic syndrome), liver (cirrhosis), malignancy, malabsorption syndrome, digestive disorders, endocrinal abnormalities, blood disorders, worm infestations, metabolic disorders, etc. generally lead to growth impairment.

Acute illnesses like ARI, diarrhea, repeated attack of infections result in malnutrition and growth retardation.

Congenital anomalies, accidental injury and prolong hospitalization usually have adverse effect on growth and development.

Physical environment: Housing, living conditions, safety measures, environmental sanitation, sunshine, ventilation and fresh air, hygiene, safe water supply, etc. are having direct influence on child's growth and development. Drought, famine and disaster also influence the child's growth.

Psychological environment: Healthy family, good parent-child relationship and healthy interaction with other family members, neighbors, friends, peers and teachers are important factors for promoting emotional, social and intellectual development. Lack of love, affection and security leads to emotional disturbances which hinders emotional maturity and personality development. Broken family, sibling jealousy and inappropriate school environment has poor effect on psychological development.

Cultural influences: Growth and development of an individual child are influenced by the culture in which he or she is growing up. The childrearing practices, food habit, traditional beliefs, social taboos, attitude towards health, standard of living, educational level, etc. influence the child's growth and development. The child learns standard of traits like honesty, discipline, intellectual inquiry, manners, aggression, individual industry and achievement from the culture of the family and society.

Socioeconomic status: Poor socioeconomic groups may have less favorable environment for growth and development than the middle and upper groups. Parents of unfortunate financial conditions are less likely to understand and adopt modern scientific child care. They lack money to buy essentials for diet and health care and even unable to accept medical or hospital services.

Climate and season: Climatic variation and seasonal changes influence the child health. Weight gain is more in late summer, rainy season and autumn. Maximum gains in height among children occur in the spring. These variations may be due to difference in activity level.

Play and exercise: Play and exercise promote physiological activity and stimulate muscular development. Physical, physiological, social, moral, intellectual and emotional developments are enhanced by play and exercise.

Birth order of the child: Birth order alone does not determine intelligence, personality traits or method of coping but it has a significant influence on all of these. The first born child gets full attention until the second child born. They learn from adult, whereas the second born child learns mainly from elder one. Middle born child gets less attention during rearing.

The first born child is usually intelligent, achievement oriented, conforming, perfectionistic and anxious. The only child is likely to develop more rapidly and intellectual with higher self-esteem but may be more dependent. The middle born is more adaptable, less achievement oriented less aggressive towards goals and learns how to compromise. The youngest child receives a great deal of love and attention, and tends to develop a good natured, friendly, warm personality and with high self-esteem. However, each child is different and need total attention and care from parents to develop their personality to the fullest extent possible.

Intelligence: Intelligence of the child influences mental and social development. A child with higher intelligence adjusts with environment promptly and fulfil own needs and demands, whereas a child with low level of intelligence fails to do that. Intelligence is correlated to some degree with physical development.

Hormonal influence: Hormones are the important aspects of internal environment which have vital role in growth and development of the children. All hormones in the body affect growth in some manner. The important three influencing hormones are somatotropic hormone, thyroid hormone and adrenocorticotropic hormone that stimulate to secrete gonadotropic hormones. Other hormones that less directly influence the process of growth and development include insulin, parathormone, cortisol and calcitonin.

Thus, growth and development is a complex process with the influence of various factors. Favorable conditions promote growth and development. Whereas unfavorable factors inhibits the process leading the growth retardation or growth failure and developmental delays. Pediatric nurse is the unique person to detect the deviations at the earliest time and initiate prompt interventions to overcome the problems and deprivations of children.

Postnatal Growth Patterns

Different tissues of the body grow at different rates in the postnatal period. Major four types of growth are studied, i.e. general body growth, neural growth, genital growth and lymphoid growth.

General Body Growth

It is increased in size of the body as a whole externally, including the total growth of muscles, skeleton and various internal organs. This growth occurs slowly and steadily but marked acceleration as growth spurt is found in infancy and during puberty.

Neural Growth

It includes the growth of brain, spinal cord, meninges and optic apparatus. At birth, head size is about 65 to 70 percent of adult's size which grows to about 90 percent by the age of two years. At 8 years, it is close to the adult size which is maintained without regression.

Genital Growth

The growth of genital structures like testes, ovaries, epididymis, uterine tube, prostate, prostatic urethro and seminal vesicle, remain dormant during childhood. But at puberty, they grow faster causing various changes with appearance of secondary sex characteristics.

Lymphoid Growth

The growth of lymphoid tissue is rapid in infancy and highly accelerated during mid-childhood. It reaches the peak of development at about the age of 12 years and stop growing or regress.

The major types of postnatal growth curves are shown in the Figure 7.1.

There are variations in body proportions as the body growth is not uniform at different ages. During infancy size of the head is larger in relation to the size of the body. Gradually this proportion changes to assume adult shape. In younger children, the limbs are short, but in later life, they continue to grow rapidly.

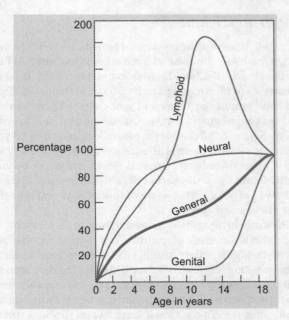

Fig. 7.1: Major types of postnatal growth curves

The changes in body proportion from birth to physical maturity is shown in Figures 7.2A to E.

Types of Body Build

The physical growth of the body may differ from one individual to other during the process of maturation and at the time of full maturity. Sheldon classified the human physique into three categories.

Ectomorph

Having linear structure with light bone, small musculature and less subcutaneous tissue in relation to body length.

Endomorph

Having large amount of soft tissue with stocky body build. Maturity is earlier than the ectomorphs.

Mesomorph

Having hard heavy rectangular structure with more muscle, connective tissue and bone. Mixed features of ectomorphs and endomorphs are found.

Assessment of Growth

Assessment of physical growth can be done by anthropometric measurements and the study of velocity of physical growth. Measurement of different growth parameters is the important nursing responsibility in child care. The criteria for assessment of physical growth are mainly weight, length or height, head circumference, chest circumference and mid upper arm circumference.

Assessment of body mass index, body ratio, fontanelle closure, skinfold thickness, dentition and bone age also used as parameters for evaluation of physical growth.

Technique of Assessment of Growth

Weight

Weight is one of the best criteria for assessment of growth and a good indicator of health and nutritional status of child.

Among Indian children, weight of the full-term neonate at birth is approximately 2.5 to 3.8 kg. There are about 10 percent loss of weight during first week of life, which regains by 10 days of age. Then, weight gain is about 25 to 30 g per day for the first 3 months and 400 g per month till one year of age. After that, the weight gain follows an average pattern. The infants doubled their birthweight by 5 months of age, trebled

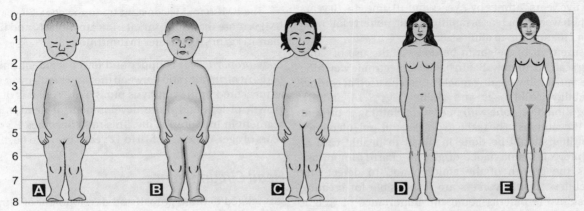

Figs 7.2A to E: Changes in body preparation from birth to adolescence. (A) Newborn infant; (B) 18 months old child; (C) 3 years old child; (D) 11 years old child; (E) 18 years old adolescence

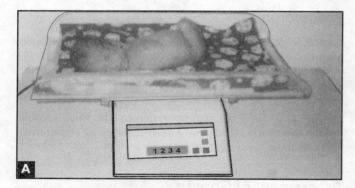

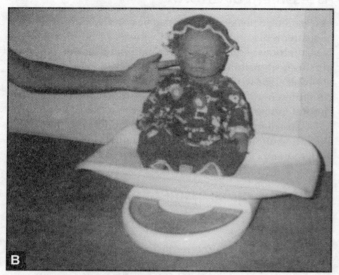

Figs 7.3A and B: Measurement of weight. (A) Weighing baby in digital machine; (B) Weighing infant in baby weighing machine (dial type)

Length and Height

Increase in height indicates skeletal growth. Yearly increments in high gradually diminished from birth to maturity. At birth, average length of a healthy Indian newborn baby is 50 cm. It increases to 60 cm at 3 months, 70 cm at 9 months and 75 cm at one year of age. In second year, there is 12 cm increase, third year, it is 9 cm, fourth year, it is 7 cm and in fifth year, it is 6 cm. So, the child doubles the birth length by 4 to 4.5 years of age. Afterwards, there is about 5 cm increase in every year till the onset of puberty. Gradual slow increase in height is usually found up to the period of postpubescence. *Appendix IV* shows the height and weight of Indian boys and girls from one to 18 years of age.

Recumbent length is measured up to 2 years of age. Infantometer or simple tape measure is used for assessing the crown-heel length by placing the child on hard surface in supine position with extended legs. In older children standing height is measured by vertical height scale or stadeometer or with tape-measure. Standing height can be measured against a wall, while the child stands in bare feet on the floor surface, arms hang by the side and occiput, upper back, buttocks and heels touch the wall along with straight head in parallel vision. A flat object is placed top of the head and the height is then marked and measured accurately using simple tape measure. Measurement of length of a baby lying on a mattress with cloth tape is inaccurate and not recommended (Fig. 7.5).

Recording of length/height and comparing them with weight, as indicator of growth, are important aspect of assessment.

Body Mass Index (BMI)

It is an important criteria which helps to assess the normal growth or its deviations, i.e. malnutrition or obesity.

$$BMI = \frac{Weight\ in\ kg}{(Height\ in\ meter)^2}$$

The BMI remains constant up to the age of 5 years. If the BMI is more than 30 kg/m², it indicates obesity and if it is less than 15 kg/m², it indicates malnutrition.

Body proportion: It is upper and lower segment ratio of the body. At birth, the ratio between the upper and lower segment as measured from symphysis pubis, is 1.7:1.0. It is due to low growth of legs and more development of head and upper segment in intrauterine life. This ratio becomes 1.3 : 1.0 at 3 years of age. At the age of 10 to 12 years, the ratio becomes 1:1.

Head Circumference

It is related to brain growth and development of intracranial volume. Average head circumference measures about 35 cm

by one year, four times by two years, five times by 3 years, six times by five years, 7 times by 7 years and 10 times by 10 years of age. Then weight increases rapidly during puberty followed by gradual maturation to adult size.

Measurement of weight to be done by the use of same weighing scale accurately. Beam balance, electronic weighing machine and adult weighing machine can be used according to availability, child's age and ability (Figs 7.3A and B). Weighing should be done with minimum clothing to prevent chilling. Precautions to be taken to prevent fall and infections.

Recording should be done in 'Road to health' card at regular interval. Maintenance of growth chart is important to assess the growth of the children and to detect any abnormalities. Health workers are responsible for creating awareness in the parents about the importance of weight recording (Fig. 7.4).

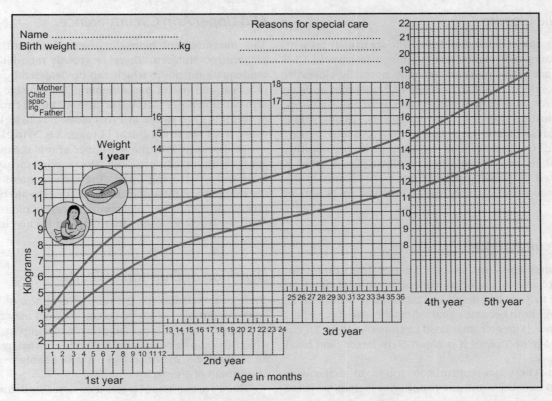

Fig. 7.4: Growth curve, road to health card

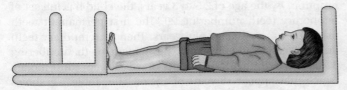

Fig. 7.5: Measurement of length by infantometer

at birth. At 3 months, it is about 40 cm, at 6 months; 43 cm, at one year; 45 cm, at 2 years; 48 cm, at 7 years; 50 cm and at 12 years of age; it is about 52 cm, almost same as adult.

If head circumference increases more than 1 cm in two weeks during the first 3 months of age, then hydrocephalus should be suspected. Abnormal growth may be found as abnormal shape and size of head. Large size head may be found in hydrocephalus, rickets, chondrodystrophy or syphilis. Familial large head or macrocephaly is harmless. Small size head or microcephaly is usually associated with premature closure of skull sutures and found in Down's syndrome and mental retardation. Abnormal growth may be seen as tomb shaped (oxycephaly), boat shaped (scaphocephaly) and asymmetrical (plagiocephaly).

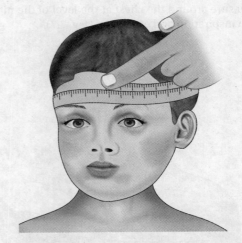

Fig. 7.6: Measurement of head circumference

Head circumference is measured by ordinary tape measure, placing it over the occipital protuberance at the back, above the ears on the sides and just over the supra-orbital ridges in front and measuring the point of highest circumference (Fig. 7.6).

Fontanelle Closure

At birth, anterior and posterior fontanelle are usually present. Posterior fontanelle closes early within a few weeks (6–8 weeks) of age. The anterior fontanelle normally closes by 12 to 18 months of age. Early closure of fontanelles indicate craniostenosis due to premature closure of skull sutures. Delayed closure may be due to rickets, malnutrition, hydrocephalus, cretinism, congenital cyanotic heart disease, etc. Craniotabes may be present in prematurity, rickets, syphilis, or osteogenesis imperfecta. Craniotabes is demonstrated by pressing the occipito parietal area of the skull with the thumb which results indentation (a sort of 'give').

Chest Circumference

Chest circumference or thoracic diameter is an important parameter of assessment of growth and nutritional status. At birth, it is 2 to 3 cm less than head circumference. At 6 to 12 months of age both become equal. After first year of age, chest circumference is greater than head circumference by 2.5 cm and by the age of 5 years, it is about 5 cm larger than head circumference.

At birth, chest is approximately round in shape with nearly equal transverse and anteroposterior diameters. There after, the width of chest becomes greater than depth due to rapid increase in transverse diameter. Abnormal shape of chest is found in rickets, malnutrition and congenital heart disease. Chest circumference is measured by placing the tape measure around the chest at the level of the nipples, in between inspiration and expiration (Fig. 7.7).

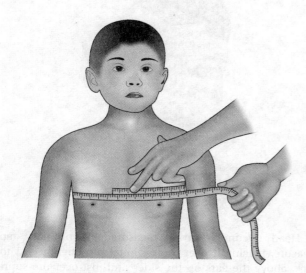

Fig. 7.7: Measurement of chest circumference

Mid Upper Arm Circumference

This measurement helps to assess the nutritional status of younger children. There is growth retardation due to inadequate nutrition, which can be detected by this simple practical and useful measurement. The average mid upper arm circumference (MUAC) at birth is 11 to 12 cm, at one year of age, it is 12 to 16 cm, at 1 to 5 years; it is 16 to 17 cm, at 12 years; it is 17 to 18 cm and at 15 years; it is 20 to 21 cm.

To assess MUAC, the left upper arm is measured firmly gently without compressing. The arm is measured while the hand is left hang freely. The measurement is taken at the midpoint of the upper arm between the tip of acromion process of scapula and olecranon process of ulna. The simple tape measures are used. There should be no cloths on the arm.

Dentition or Eruption of Teeth

There is a variation for the time of eruption of teeth. First teeth commonly the lower central incisors may appear in 6 to 7 months of age. It can be delayed even up to 15 months, which also can be considered within the normal range of time for teething. So, dentition is not a dependable parameter for assessment of growth.

There are two sets of teeth, temporary teeth for small face in small size and permanent teeth, bigger in size for growing face. There is a phase of mixed dentition with two sets of teeth.

Temporary or milk teeth also called as deciduous teeth which erupt at the rate of one tooth every month after first eruption. By the age of 2.5 to 3 years, the child has full set of temporary teeth numbering 20. The first permanent teeth usually erupt at the age of 6 years. Then all temporary teeth are replaced gradually. Total permanent teeth numbering 32 usually erupt within 12 years of age. Except third molars which may appear 18 years of age or later. Table 7.1. shows the number of temporary and permanent teeth according to child's age.

Rarely, baby may born with natal tooth at birth, which is usually harmless. It may interfere with breastfeeding. Delayed dentition may be found due to familial tendency, poor nutritional status, rickets and osteogenesis imperfecta. Malocclusion of teeth may occur due to thumb sucking. No teeth or anodentia may occur as congenital anomalies. No dentition beyond 1.5 years needs special attention.

Osseous Growth

Bony growth follows a definite pattern and time schedule from birth to maturation. It is calculated by the appearance of ossification center by X-ray study. Skeletal maturation or bone growth is an indicator of physiological development and is

Table 7.1 Eruption of teeth

Age	Type	Total number of teeth
Temporary teethings		
6–12 months	Incisors (central and lateral)	2–8
12–15 months	First molars	8–12
15–24 months	Canines (cuspids)	12–16
24–30 months	Second molars	16–20
Permanent teething		
6–7 years	First permanent molars	- 24
7–10 years	Replacement of temporary incisors and canines	
10–12 years	Replacement of temporary molars by premolars	
12–15 years	Second permanent molars	- 28
- 16 years onwards	Third permanent molars	- 32

distinct from the chronological age. Skeletal maturation starts from intrauterine life and continue up to 25 years of age.

A full-term neonate has five ossification centers namely, at distal end of femur, proximal end of tibia, talus, calcaneus and cuboid. By 6 months of age two more ossification centers appear in carpal bones, i.e. capitate and hamate. A child of 2 years will have 3 ossification centers at wrist. It will be a useful guide to remember that number of ossification centers at wrist is equal to age in years plus one. Twenty ossification centers are generally used for determining bone age. These include carpal and metacarpal bones, patella, phalanges and toes.

Advanced bone age may be found, is precocious puberty, thyrotoxicosis and adrenal hyperplasia. Retardation of bony growth is found in cretinism.

Stem Stature Index

It refers to the sitting height (crown-rump length) as a percentage of total height or recumbent length. It is 70 at birth, 66 at 6 months, 64 at one year, 61 at 2 years, 58 at 3 years, 55 at 5 years, 52 at puberty and 53 to 54 at 20 years.

Span

It is the distance between tips of middle fingers when the arms are outstretched. In young children, it is 1 to 2 cm less than the length or height. At 10 years of age, it is equal and after 12 years, it is 1 to 2 cm more than the height.

Systemic Changes during Growth and Development

Respiratory Changes

Respiratory rate in neonates is about 36 to 40 breaths per minutes and gradually it diminished to 16 to 20 breaths per minutes at 15 years. In newborn baby the breathing is diaphragmatic and breath sound is bronchovesicular. In infancy, it is mainly thoracic and breath sound is vesicular.

Sinuses gradually developed which complete within 7 years of age. In young children, larynx is 1/3rd of adult size and maximum growth occurs at puberty.

Cardiovascular Changes

Functional closure of temporary structures of fetal circulation occurs soon after birth and anatomical closure occurs whithin 2 to 3 months. Apex beat shifted from 4th intercostal space to 5th intercostal space. There is a gradual change in pulse and blood pressure as the age increases.

Pulse rate in newborn is in between 120 and 160 beats per minutes, at one year it is about 100 to 160 b/m, at 4 years it is 80 to 120 b/m, 8 years it is 70 to 100 b/m, at 15 years it is 70 to 90 b/m and at 18 years it is 70 to 80 b/m.

Blood pressue in neonates is 80/46 mm Hg (average), at one year it is about 96/66 mm Hg, at 4 years it is 99/65 mm Hg, at 8 years it is 102/56 mm Hg, at 12 years 113/59 mm Hg and at 14 years it is about 118/60 mm Hg.

Hb level in new born baby is about 17 (14-20) g/dL, at 3 months to 6 years it is about 12 (10.5-14) g/dL and in older children about 14 to 16 g/dL. The size of RBCs, number of RBCs and WBCs and hematocrit values are gradually reduced as age increases.

Brain Growth

Brain growth occurs 2/3rd in first years, 4/5th in second year and fully developed within 5 years.

Gastrointestinal System

The secretary enzymes of the digestive tract are usually adequate for the newborn baby. Fat is handleless. Liver in neonates is usually 4 percent of bodyweight and increases gradually to 10 times in puberty from 120 to 160 g to 1500 to 2300 g at 15 years. Liver is palpable throughout the childhood usually up to 18 months of age.

Urinary System

The kidneys are large at birth. The urine amount gradually increases from 250 mL per day in neonates to 1200 mL per day in 14 years. The amount of creatinine is low in infants about 10 to 20 mg/kg/day which gradually changed to 5 to 40 mg/kg/day in older children.

Lymphoid Tissue and Immunity

The growth of lymphoid tissue (spleen, tonsils, thymus) reaches its peak at 6 to 7 years which becomes about double of adult size. Then gradually regresses up to puberty.

Synthesis of gamma globulin antibodies ordinarily begin after 2 to 4 weeks of age. Then depending upon the antigenic stimuli the gamma globulin level increased and usually reached the adult range (700 to 1200 mg/100 mL) by the 3 to 4 years of age.

Hormonal Changes

Thyroid is well developed at birth and islets cells of pancreas are relatively large. The adrenal glands are large and become proportionate within one year. Testicular and ovarian hormones appear at puberty.

Sexual Development

Preparatory changes of adolescence may be detectable as early as 7 to 8 years of age. The process of maturation of adolescence continues till the attainment of physical, emotional and mental maturity of adulthood.

Changes in Puberty (Adolescence)

Adolescence begins with the onset of puberty. It is defined by the UNICEF as "The sequence of events by which the individual is transformed into a young adult by a series of biological changes". It is the period of development of secondary sex characteristics. Adolescence period extends from the onset of puberty till the time sexual maturation is completed. Somatic growth is also almost completed during this period and the individual is psychologically mature to be able to contribute to the society.

The ages of onset of puberty and sexual maturation vary widely in different individual depending on the genetic and environmental factors. According to WHO, adolescence is the period of life that extends from 10 years to 19 years. It is divided into three phases as early, middle and late adolescence. Early adolescence refers to age 10 to 13 years, middle adolescence to 14 to 16 years and late adolescence to 17 to 19 years. (see stages of growth and development).

In girls, preadolescent growth spurt begins at about 10 to 12 years of age and in boys it is 12 to 14 years of age. Structural growth usually extends up 16 to 17 years in girls and 18 to 19 years in boys.

During prepubescent period, rapid physical growth and appearance of secondary sex characteristics occur. In puberty, the girls begin to menstruate and the boys produce spermatozoa. Menarche refers to the time of first menstrual bleeding. Puberty changes in boys and girls follow an order of appearance of various characteristics toward physical development. Puberty is basically the organic phenomenon of adolescence when they become mature in psychosexual aspect.

Common Order of Puberty Changes in Girls

- Accelerated growth in weight and height gain
- Breast changes like pigmentation of areola and enlargement of breast tissue and nipple
- Increase in pelvic girth mainly the transverse diameter
- Appearance of pubic hair and change in vaginal secretion
- Activation of axillary sweat glands
- Appearance of axillary hair
- Onset of menstruation (menarche). First bleed occurs usually 2 years after the first manifestation of puberty
- Abrupt slowing of gain in height.

Common Order of Puberty Changes in Boys

- Accelerated increase in weight and hight gain.
- Increase in the size of external genitalia.
- Appearance of pubic hair followed by hair in axilla, upper lip, groin, thigh and between symphysis pubis and umbilicus.
- Appearance of facial hair two years after the pubic hair.
- Changes in voice as cracking then deepening.
- Nocturnal discharge of semen during sleep.
- Abrupt slowing in height gain.

Adolescents need special attention during this period of transition. There are numbers of problem found in this age group. But adolescence health is till neglected. They are not considered as adult nor as children. There problems need to be handled with care. The child health care services should include the prevention and management of adolescent problems. According to the Indian Academy of pediatrics (IAP), health problems of children up to 18 years should be the responsibility of pediatricians. The new medical specialities, *Ephebiatrics,* is now in practice to help the teenagers to solve their problems and to fulfil their special needs. (Ephebos—means youth and puberty). A world wide compaign has also begun to focus attention on adolescence health by concerted efforts of the WHO and the UNICEF.

Different Aspects of Development

Development of children has different aspects which can be described in four important areas, viz gross motor, fine motor-adaptive, language and personal-social behavior. Other aspects are sensory, intellectual, emotional, sexual, moral and spiritual. These divisions of development are arbitrary. They all usually progress together in the process of maturation and learning.

Motor Development

Motor development depends upon maturation of muscular, skeletal and nervous system. It is usually termed as gross and fine motor development.

Gross motor development involves control of the child over his/her body by increasing mobility. It is assessed by ventral suspension, supine position, prone position, turning, reaching the object, etc. The important gross motor developmental milestones include head holding, sitting, standing, walking, running, climbing upstairs, riding tricycle, etc. It promotes independent locomotion and proceeds fine motor activities.

Fine motor development depends upon neural tract maturation. Initial neurological reflexes are replaced by purposeful activities. Fine motor development promotes adaptive activities with fine sensory motor adjustments and include eye-coordination, hand eye co-ordination, hand to mouth co-ordination, hand skill as finger-thumb apposition, grasping, dressing, etc. It develops as the reflexes give way to the acquisition of motor dexterity.

Motor development is not affected by sex or geographical area or parental education. It is mostly affected by nutritional status and adverse environmental influence. It varies widely in young children.

Language Development

Language development is the sensory motor development. It depends upon hearing, level of understanding, power of imitation and encouragement. It is skill of communication with development of true speech.

Personal and Social Development

Personal and social development includes personal reactions to his own social and cultural situations with neuromotor maturity and environmental stimulation. It is related to interpersonal and social skill as social smile, recognition of mother, use of toys, play and mimicry.

Sensory Development

Sensory development depends upon myelinization of nevous system and responds to specific stimuli. Taste, smell, touch and hearing are initial senses present in newborn babies. The visual system is the last to mature at about 6 to 7 years.

Emotional Development and Personality Development

Emotional development and personality development is a continuous process. It is the sumtotal (sumtotal indicates total resulting from addition of items) of physiologic, psychological and sociological qualities of the individual. Adequate guidance and problem solving at different stages help for the healthy progress to next stage of personality development which promotes emotional maturation in adulthood. The emotional needs also considered as emotional foods, are essentials for healthy development of personality. The emotional needs include effective mothering, love, affection, safety, security, protection, play, faith, achievement of potentialities, guidance and counseling, independence, acceptance with positive approach, approval, etc.

According to Erik Erikson the stages of psychosocial development and Freud's psychosexual stages are shown in Table 7.2.

Psychosexual Development

The sex of a child is determined genetically at the time of conception. Development of sexuality after birth is influenced

Table 7.2 Stages of psychosocial and psychosexual development

Stage	Approximate age	Erikson's psychosocial stage		Freud's Psycho-sexual stages	Significant persons
		Task	Counterpart		
Infancy	0–1year	Sense of trust	Mistrust	Oral	Maternal person or substitute
Toddler	1–3 years	Sense of autonomy	Shame and doubt	Anal	Parental persons
Preschool age	3–6 years	Sense of initiative	Guilt	Phallic	Basic family
School age	6–12 years	Sense of industry	Inferiority	Latency	Neighborhood, school
Early adolescence	12–? years	Sense of identity	Identity diffusion	Puberty	Peer groups, outgroups, models of leadership
Late adolescence and young adult	––	Sense of intimacy and solidarity	Isolation	Genitality	Partners in friendship, sex competition, co-operation

by the development of physical, mental, emotional and sociocultural aspect of living. Human sexuality is expressed in everyday life. It refers to the total quality of an individual, not just to the genitals and their functions. It is normal human process that expresses itself in a vast range of individual variability. It is related to many aspects of total personality functions. It is concerned with cultural beliefs, attitudes, feeling like loving and caring, sex-role, stereotypes, self-image, body image and spiritual values. Open communication improves human sexual functioning.

According to *Sigmund Freud* the development of sexuality proceeds in different stages, i.e. oral, anal, phallic, latency, puberty and genitality. Freud believed that sexual feelings do not suddenly emerge during puberty and adolescence. They are present from infancy and gradually change from one form to another until adult sexual life is achieved. Freudian psychoanalytic theory with its stages of psychosexual development has greatly influenced modern psychiatric thinking. In each stages, instinctual sexual energy (libido) is invested in different biologic areas of body. These areas determine how the child interacts with other people. *Freud's* phases of psychosexual development include the followings:

The *oral stage* includes roughly the period of infancy, the first year of life. The greatest sensual satisfaction is obtained through stimulation of oral region or sensory area of mouth as in breastfeeding and sucking.

The *anal stage* includes the toddler period, the second and third years of life. Gratification is obtained from the anal and urethral areas through holding or expelling feces or urine.

The *phallic stage* includes the preschool period, the 4th and 5th years of life. The greatest sensual enjoyment is obtained from the genital region by fondling the genitals. The oedipal complex develops in this stage. The child loves and feels attraction to the parent of opposite sex and the parent of same sex is considered as rival.

The *latency stage* includes the school age from 6th to 12th year of life (roughly). In this stage sexual interests are repressed and lie dormant. The child develops close relationship with others of same sex and same age. This is period of gang formation, gang loyalties and fierce. Oedipal conflict resolved in this stage.

The *pubescent stage* and *adolescence* include the period from 12 years of age to adulthood. In this period of puberty and genitality, the secondary sexual characteristics appear in both sexes with experience of romanticism and emotional changes. The psychosexual conflict of oedipal period revived in the phase. With the resolve of that conflicts, the child develops normal heterosexual relationship and feels attraction with opposite sex. The normal heterosexual relationship is determined by family relationship and social experiences of the child rather than biologic factors alone. Early learning of gender role or sexual identity is very important in determining gender identity of human beings in later life.

Other important aspects of development are social development, intellectual development, moral development, development of body image, and spiritual development.

Social development or socialization is achieved through the training of the child by meeting and communicating with people and participating in the group activities.

Intellectual development depends upon genetic inheritance and environmental influences through mental maturation and achievement of intelligence. It occurs as a result of maturation of innate abilities, learning by association of stimulus response, reinforcement of appropriate behaviors and insight.

Moral development helps in formation of value system. It is not acquired by simply following rules of society but through an internal and personal series of changes in attitudes. Moral development parallels mental development and consists of two stages, i.e. respect for rules and a sense of justice.

Development of body image occurs as a mental picture of what the body is like along with certain attitudes toward it and its parts. It includes both conscious and unconscious feeling about the body. It is closely related with ideas of self-worth and acceptance by family and peers.

Spiritual development is closely related to cultural background and influences the family relationship and responsibilities. It is expressed through religious belief, rituals, symbols specific to religious traditions and faith. It is multidimensional and a way of learning about life as an ongoing process.

Developmental Milestones

Development is the functional maturation of organs. It depends upon neuromuscular maturity, genetic determinants and environmental influences. Developmental milestones are accomplished by the children at an anticipated age. There may be great variations of time in achievement of different levels of development with extreme ranges. Indian infants attain their developmental milestones earlier than the Europeans.

The average achievement levels in different age group of children up to 12 years are as follows:

Infants (Fig. 7.8)

1 to 2 months: Able to lift the chin momentarily on prone position. Able to regard bright colored object at 20 cm distance. Cries when hungry or at discomfort. Able to turn head toward sound and smiles back to mother or caregiver.

2 to 3 months: Able to lift head and front part of chest by supporting weight on extended arms. Can follow moving object with steady eye movement and able to focus eyes.

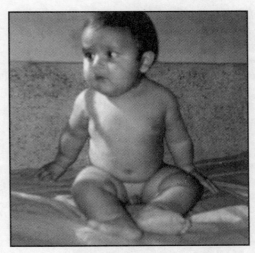

Fig. 7.8: Healthy infants of 7 months

Produce 'cooing' sound and enjoy people talking with her/him. Able to recognize mother and turn head to sound.

4 to 5 months: Can hold head steadily in upright position. Able to hold a rattle and bring to mouth. Can reach a thing and grasp it crudely with palm. Make coos, gurgles and respond by making sounds. Join hands together in play, enjoy people and laugh out loudly.

5 to 6 months: Able to sit with support, can hold a cube and transfer from one hand to other. Try to imitate sound and enjoy own mirror image.

7 to 8 months: Can sit without support and roll in bed from back to side then back to abdomen. Produce bubbles and say '*aam*', '*da*', '*la*'. Recognize unknown person and show anxiety. Resist toys to be taken from him/her.

8 to 9 months: Able to crawl on abdomen. Speak '*Da-Da*' and '*Ma-Ma*' combining syllables without meaning.

9 to 10 months: Able to creep on hands and knees. Can stand with support and cruises around furniture. Able to pick up a pellet with thumb and index finger. Understand emotions like anger, anxiety. Wave 'bye-bye' and want to please caregiver, say *ba-ba, da-da, ma-ma* with meaning.

10 to 12 months: Can stand without support and walk holding furniture. Able to feed himself/herself with spilling. Pick up small bits of food and take to mouth. Able to push toy car alone and play simple ball game. Can speak 3 to 5 meaningful words and understand meaning of several words. Respond for affection by kiss.

Toddlers (Fig. 7.9)

15 months: Able to walk alone, can walk several steps sidewise and few steps backward. Can feed himself or herself without spilling. Able to turn 2 to 3 pages at a time.

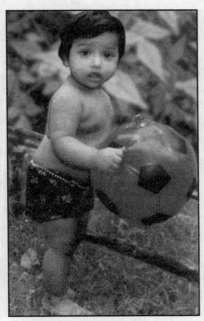

Fig. 7.9: Healthy toddler

18 months: Can creep upstairs. Able to feed from cup. Take shoes and socks off. Want potty, point the parts of body, if asked. Build tower of two blocks and stop taking toys to mouth. Use 6 to 20 words. Copy mother's action.

2 years: Able to run and try to climb upstairs by resting on each step and then climbing up on next. Put shoes and socks on. Can remove pants. Build tower of six to seven blocks. Can copy and draw a horizontal and vertical line. Control bladder at day time (dry by dry). Speak simple sentences without use of verb.

3 years: Can walk on tip-toes and stand on one leg for seconds. Jump with both feet. Climb upstairs by coordinated manner. Ride tricycle. Can dress and undress. Brush teeth with help. Can draw a circle. Build tower of nine blocks. Has vocabulary of about 250 words. Repeat three numbers (once in three times). Know own name and sex. Achieve bladder control at night (dry by night). Fear dark interact and play simple games with peers.

Preschooler

3 to 6 years: Can jump and hop. Able to draw a cross ('+') by 4 years and tilted cross ('x') by 5 years of age. Can draw a rectangle by 4 years and a triangle by 5 years. Able to copy letters. Can tell stories and describe recent experience. Become independent, impatient, aggressive physically and verbally. Jealous of sibling but gradually improve in behavior and manner.

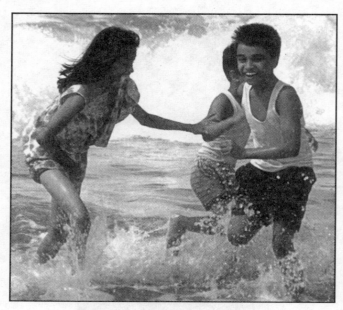

Fig. 7.10: Healthy school children

School Age (Fig. 7.10)

6 to 8 years: Able to run, jump, hop and climb with better co-ordination. Develop better hand-eye coordination. Able to write better and take self-care. Able to use complete sentences to express feelings and follow commands. Play in group. Learn discipline. Appreciate praise and recognition.

8 to 10 years: Play actively with different physical skill. Improved writing skill and speed. Use short and compact sentences. Participate in family discussion. Peer group involvement and increased awareness about sex role.

10 to 12 years Develop more coordinated, skilful manipulative activities and games. Able to use parts of speech correctly. Accepts suggestions and instruction obediently. May show short burst of anger.

Important Developmental Milestones at a Glance up to 3 Years

- *Social smile:* 6 to 8 weeks
- *Head holding:* 3 months
- *Sitting with support:* 5 to 6 months
- *Sitting without support:* 7 to 8 months
- *Reaches out to an object and holds it:* 5 to 6 months
- *Transfers object from one hand to other:* 6 to 7 months
- Holding small object between index finger and thumb: 9 months
- *Creeping:* 10 to 11 months
- *Standing with support:* 9 months
- *Standing without support:* 10 to 12 months.

- *Walking without support:* 13 to 15 months
- *Feeding self with spoon:* 12 to 15 months
- *Running:* 18 months
- *Climbing upstairs:* 20 to 24 months
- *Says bisyllables words (da-da, ba-ba):* 8 to 9 months
- *Says two words with meaning:* 12 months
- *Says ten words with meaning:* 18 months
- *Says simple sentence:* 24 months
- *Tells story:* 36 months
- *Takes shoes and socks off:* 15 to 18 months
- *Puts shoes and socks on:* 24 months
- *Dresses ownself fully:* 3 to 4 years
- *Controls bladder and bowel at day time:* 2 years
- *Controls bladder and bowel at night time:* 3 years
- *Knows full name and sex:* 3 years
- *Riding tricycle:* 3 years.

Assessment of Development

Assessment of development is essential to detect abnormal developmental delays. The most widely used screening test for detecting developmental delays in infancy and preschool years is known as Denver Developmental Screening Test (DDST). It is a worldwide popular test developed in 1967, for the assessment of development in four areas, i.e. gross motor, fine motor-adaptive, language and personal-social behavior. There are 105 items, some of which are indeed difficult to administer. It is inappropriate for children with mothers having poor education. It has less items related to language. DDST was modified in 1992 in the form of Denver II or modified DDST with 125 items.

Other developmental screening tests include DASII Scale (Developmental Assessment Scale of Indian Infant). Baroda DST, Trivandrum DST, Gessell DST, Bayley DST, Woodside DST, cognitive adaptive test, Early language milestones scale, etc.

For older children 3 to 15 years, the development chart can be used. Assessment of development should not be confused with assessment of general intelligence using such tests as Stanford-Binet intelligence scale, Welchsler intelligence scale, etc.

In India, *Baroda screening Test* was developed by Dr. Promila Phatak with 25 test items primarily for psychological aspects. The test is relevant for age 0 to 30 months. Gross motor, fine motor and cognitive aspects are evaluated in 10 minutes mainly by the psychologists.

Trivandrum development screening test is the simplified version of Baroda DST that can be used by the health workers, nurses and pediatricians/physicians. It has 17 test items relevant for 0 to 2 years of age. The children are evaluated in three domains, i.e. gross motor, fine motors and cognitive for 5 minutes only. Figure 7.11. presents Trivandrum Development Screening Test (TDST).

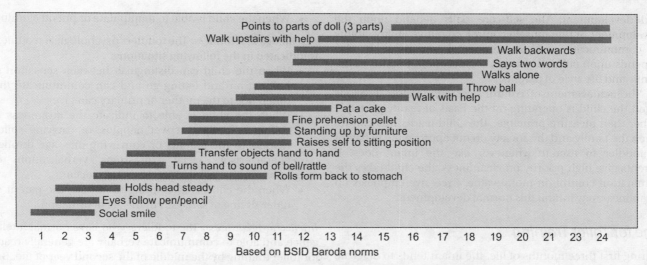

Fig. 7.11: Trivandrum developmental screening chart (TDSC)

Approaches of Development Screening

- Informal screening during routine pediatric check up and collecting history from parents.
- Routine formal screening in systematic developmental screening of all children with the help of standardized screening instruments.
- Focused screening in suspected developmental problems and in high-risk neonates with potential developmental delay.

NEEDS OF THE HEALTHY CHILD

Each child has basic human needs like adults to fulfill the essentials of life and to promote growth and development. The physical, social, emotional and intellectual needs are the motivating force behind human behavior. According to Maslow (1954), the physiologic needs are primary needs and nonphysiologic or secondary needs are higher needs.

The physiologic needs are essential for survival and stimulation. Water, air, food, warmth, hygiene, elimination, rest, sleep, comfort, sexual pleasure, activity and avoidance of pain are the predominant needs in the motivation of behavior and maintenance of homeostasis of the internal environment of the body.

The nonphysiologic and higher needs are: (a) safety and security needs for the protection from environmental hazards, (b) need for love and affection, closeness and intimacy with family and friends for emotional maturation (c) need for recognition and self-esteem to become independent (d) need for creativity and self-actualization for ultimate use of individual abilities. (e) cognitive needs for knowledge, comprehension, understanding of new ideas and learning. (f) aesthetic needs as desire for beauty in its various forms.

All these needs are important, but their total fulfillment is impossible, whether the child is well or ill. The responsibility of the nursing personnel is to help the parents and child to adjust to the problem situation in the best way possible. To assist the children and their families to achieve the highest level of possible wellness, the nurse should promote self-care or provide compensatory care when they cannot fulfill their needs for health care. The major aspects of child care should be emphasized through promotion of health, prevention of illness, maintenance of health and restoration of health.

Health promotion during different stages of childhood and prevention of illness can be enhanced by nutritional counseling, weaning, immunization, toilet training, provision of play and toys, safety measures with prevention of accidents, sex education, etc.

Nutritional Counseling and Weaning (*See* Chapter 5)

Nutritional Counseling Weaning and Immunization are important needs of the healthy child.

Immunization

(*See* Chapter 4).

Toilet Training

The children begin to learn independence in self-care, by the time they reach 3 years of age. Initially, the children imitate the actions of parents and siblings for self-care skills in feeding, dressing, toileting and grooming. Achievement of control of the bodily functions of defecation and urination is one of the major tasks of the toddler period during growth and development. The self-care skills depend upon the development of fine muscle control, cognitive ability, ability to communicate and environmental situations. It also depends upon cultural pattern, socioeconomic status of the family and life style of parents.

The achievement of control over elimination develops when the child is operating on the basis of reality principle rather than pleasure principle. The child learns this control when the family and the society do not approve the behavior of toddler to excrete whenever like the infant does. If parents give high priority on cleanliness, the child takes the elimination control on moral value. Excessive emphasis on cleanliness may inhibit this normal development.

Age for Toilet Training

During first three months of life, the infant tends to defecate after each feed due to gastrocolic reflex. This reflex becomes weak by the age of 4 months. Bowel movement becomes regular without any relation to feed at about 7 months of age. The infant can be placed on potty chair or toilet seat at the age of 10 months, as sitting without support usually achieved within this age. By the age of 15 to 18 months toddler can walk to toilet and ready for starting toilet training and should be encouraged to go to toilet. At 2 years the child is trainable. By the age of 3 years the child can withhold and postpone bowel movement.

For bladder control, the child is able to indicate wet pant by the age of 18 months. At 2 years, the child is generally toilet trained in the daytime and remains dry by day. The 2.5 years old child may have begun to master night time bladder control and usually by the age of 3 years becomes dry by night. Bladder control may not be completed until the child is 4 to 5 years of age.

Indications of Toddler's Readiness for Toilet Training

An important responsibility of the nurse is to help parents to determine the readiness of their toddlers for toilet training. The actual age of readiness can be determined on evidences of their physiological, psychological and intellectual levels of maturity.

Physiological readiness: Children are physiologically ready for toilet training in the following situations:
- When neuromuscular systems are sufficiently mature, i.e. when myelination of nerves has occurred to the urinary and anal sphincter and the child is able to walk.
- When the bladder size has increased sufficiently so that the child can hold urine for two hours or awaken from sleep to keep the napkin dry. Toilet training is most successful during this stage.

- When the child is able to manipulate or put off clothing.

Psychological readiness: The toddlers psychological readiness is indicated in the following situations:
- When the child can distinguish between sensation of holding on and letting go and can communicate this difference to the mother or primary caregiver.
- When the child is able to indicate the awareness of soiling or pulling at wet nappies, or carrying soiled diapers to the parents or conveying message through characteristics facial expressions, verbalizations or behavior that elimination is about to occur.
- When the child is attempting to imitate, the parent or older sibling of same sex in the act of urination.

Intellectual readiness: The toddlers, who have normal intelligence and able to communicate verbally are generally ready for toilet training by the middle of the second year of life. But those who are intellectually impaired may not be ready for a variable period after that time.

Learning a new skill is difficult before the critical period at which the child is able and motivated to learn. Unfavorable attitudes may develop, if the child is pressured to learn before this stage occurs. Even if toilet training is not done at proper time, the children may develop unfavorable response as they miss the pleasure of learning new skill and self-image may be damaged.

Process of Toilet Training

The approach of parents are more important in the process of toilet training rather than actual procedure. Positive attitude of the parents towards toilet training, relaxed parental behavior without undue anxiety and healthy parent-child relationship are essentials for successful toilet training. Bowel training is easier than bladder training due to less number of stools in a day than the number of times of urination. Parents should be made aware about the following aspects during toilet training:
- Comfortable child size toilet seat or potty chair to be provided at suitable area as the child likes.
- Feeding at same time each day both at day and night.
- Parents should stay with the child and explain in simple language about what to be done during urination and defecation.
- The child should not be permitted to play with toys during toilet training to avoid distraction of attention.
- Wiping immediately and drying the child after toilet to promote comfort.
- Changing the pant as positive reinforcement and putting attractive panties for the child.
- Rewarding the child with praise and cuddling on desired behavior to get cooperation. Punishment and negative

approach by forcing on potty may lead to unsuccessful training.

- Child's illness, accidents and hospitalization during toilet training may cause regression and ineffective training. Unsuccessful training may also occur in new home, broken family, parental divorce, etc.
- Patience and persistence behavior are necessary in helping the child during toilet training.

Problems of Toilet Training

Delay in achieving the bladder and bowel control is common problem. Fecal smearing may be found as the children may think of their warm feces as gifts and enjoy manipulating and smearing them upon wall or floor or furniture or themselves. It occurs between the age of 15 and 18 months. After the child has learned to use the potty chair, smearing is usually not found. Parents should accept their child's feeling and problems and not express strong disapproval.

Nursing responsibility includes to help the parents to understand the readiness for toilet training and appropriate approach during the process of training. Adequate information about different aspects of toilet training should be provided to the parents with necessary guidance.

Play and Play Materials

Play is universal for all children. It is work for them and ways of their living . It is pleasurable and enjoyable aspect of child's life and essential to promote growth and development.

Play is the activity that has no serious motive and from which there is no material gain. The distinction between work and play however lies in the mental attitude. Football can be play for children or can be work and means of earnings for the professional footballer.

Importance of Play

Play helps in development of children in various aspects, i.e. physical, intellectual or educational, emotional, moral and social.

Physical development enhanced during play. Muscular and sensory abilities developed at the time of running, climbing, riding cycle and in other active play. These activities help to strengthen muscle and to learn coordinated movements and skills. The young children learn to differentiate the sensations by visual, auditory and tactile stimulations through the use of play materials.

Intellectual and educational development promote during play. Children learn color, size, shape, number, distance, height, speed, name of the objects, etc. while playing with various toys and play things. Creative activity, problem solving, abstract thinking, imagination, communication and speech development occur during play. Children improve their attention span and concentration by playing. They can make difference of reality and fantasy through play. It helps them to experience thrill of achievement.

Emotional development: Play improves emotional development. Children express their fear, anxiety, anger, joy, etc. during play. It reduces stress and strain and removes irritability and destructiveness, thus enhances the coping abilities. It helps to communicate with others and outside world. Play acts as outlet of negative feeling and considered as safety valve to release emotional tension and reduce emotional trauma. It is recreation and diversion for the children. Play helps in socialization. Children become a social being through play. They learn interaction with playmates by sharing, understanding others and communicating. Play improves social relationship and working capacity with other people. It helps to learn rules of social living and cultural activities.

Moral development: Play is the means of moral development. Children learn morality from parents, teachers and other adults. During play with peers, child's behavior will reflect the right and wrong things, honesty, sportsmanship, and value system. Children show awareness about the needs and wishes of others and give importance to the friendship and cooperation. They learn norms of moral behavior and responsibility. They become creative and independent through play. They learn sex-role behavior in play.

Types of Play

Play is natural and spontaneous. It depends upon age, sex, interest, personality, ability, cultural pattern and socioeconomic status of the child's family. Play, playtime and playmates decrease as the age increase. Play is a social behavior which differs in various age groups and depends upon the level of development. It is an individualized behavior.

Infants: Usually engage in social affective play, sense-pleasure play and skill play. In social affective play infants response by smiling, cooing to the interacting adult. In sense pleasure play, they learn and explore environment through various sensory experience. They develop skill through imitation. Young children also engage in sense pleasure play and skill play.

Preschool children enjoy dramatic play through which they identify themself with adult and dramatize adult's behavior. Structured formal play begins to be played during later preschool years.

School children enjoy competitive sports, games and they develop hobbies for recreation and diversion. School age children imitate and dramatize more complex activities even acting out stories in books.

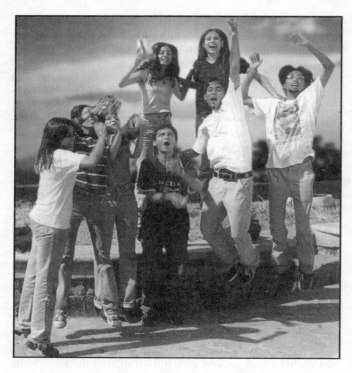

Fig. 7.12: Healthy adolescents in play

- *In associative play* social interactions occur between children. This is common in preschool age group. They play with same thing and do similar activity. Conversation and association with peers are main interest.
- *Cooperative play* behavior is found in preschool and school children. They engage in formal game in group like football or dramatic play of life situation.

Selection and Care of Play Materials

Selection of play materials and toys depends upon age, abilities, interests, likes and dislikes, culture, experience, personality and level of intelligence of the child. The play materials should have the following characteristics:

- Safe, washable, light weight, simple, durable, easy to handle and nonbreakable.
- Realistic, attractive, constructive and offer problem-solving opportunities.
- No sharp edges and no small removable parts which may be swallowed or inhaled.
- Not over stimulating and frustrating.
- No toxic paints, not costly, not inflammable and not excessive noisy.
- Play things with electrical plugs should be avoided, only children over 8 years of age should be permitted to use them.

Parents should avoid impulse of buying toys because of advertisement in the mass media. Toys can be purchased on the basis of the above mentioned criteria and safety measures to be followed. Supervision during play is important to prevent accidental injury. There is no substitute for being with children when they are playing.

Children must be taught the followings:

- *Correct use of toys:* Parent should explain the directions for use and the caution labels.
- Safe storing of toys in a space with easy reach and away from busy areas.
- Keeping the playthings in good conditions. Parents should repair or discard damaged and broken toys.
- Keeping the play materials of older brothers and sisters away from younger children. The wrong toys for the wrong ages can be injurious to children.
- Electronic toys and games can also be shared by the adults in the children's play time. Parents may interact and initiate the use with precautions.

The nurse should encourage and motivate the children and parents for play and make them aware about the importance of play. Parent should allow the child to play and arrange the play things. The important nursing responsibility is to teach the parent about safety measures and observation, interaction and supervision of the children during play. Nurse should initiate play at home, hospital or in health care agency

Adolescents and older school age children engage in a more sophisticated type of fantasy activity called daydreaming. They spent their leisure time in competitive sports, operating computers, watching television, listening to the radio, hobbies, reading, etc. (Fig. 7.12).

According to Parten and Newhall (1943), play behavior can be described as—unoccupied, solitary, onlooking, parallel, associative and cooperative.

- *In unoccupied play* behavior, the child is not involved in play activity but may move around randomly, crawl under a table, climb on and off a chair or follow another person or just stand alone with least social involvement.
- *Solitary independent play* indicates when the child plays alone independently. Toddlers and pretoddlers engage in this type of concentrating play with less interaction with others.
- *Onlooker play* behavior found when the child watches others play but does not become engaged in their play. The child may sit nearby or hear or see what others are doing or talking as she/he feels interest. Young children usually do not exhibit this form.
- *Parallel play* is an independent play activity when the child plays alongside other children but not with them. They play similar or identical play as other children play nearby. Toddlers typically play in this manner.

depending upon the individual choice with high flexibility. Nurse should inform about the modern concept of play to the parents and family. Traditionally, girls are expected to play with dolls and boys with the toys required greater muscular activity. Presently, children of both sexes engage in dolls play as well as play of muscular effort and learn the roles of sexual equality.

Suitable Play Material According to Age

Infant: Infant learns motor skill, bodily control and co-ordination by various means. They need stimulation with toys for visual, auditory and tactile sensations. The play materials suitable for them can be as follows:

4 weeks to 4 months: Bright and moving objects, hanging cradle toys, musical toys, balloons, rattles, etc.

4 to 6 months: Soft squeeze toys, rattles, toy animal, balloons, etc.

7 to 9 months: Squeeze and sound toys, blocks, cubes, plastic ring, rattles, etc.

10 to 12 months: Motion toys, water play, blocks, doll, ball, musical toys, picture books or stiff cards, rocking horse walker, transporting objects, pull and push toys.

Toddlers: Like informal free spontaneous, constructive and parallel play. They should be provided with fitting toys, pull-push toys, pyramid toys, blocks, vehicles, ball, doll, pots and pans, household articles, mud or clay, crayons, picture books or cards, play telephone, doll's house, etc.

Preschool children: Like cooperative, imitative, creative and imaginative play. Suitable playthings for this group are puppets, animals, dolls, doll's house, carpentry tools, large blocks, paint materials, colored picture books, doctor set toys, hospital equipment (like plastic syringe, blunt scissors), housekeeping toys, paper-modeling clay, cooking materials, tricycles, etc.

School-age children: Prefer competitive formal organized and cooperative play. They like imitation and self-direction. They like games rather than toys. Toys are popular up to 8 years of age. Children of this group enjoy games of muscular activity, running, climbing, swinging, etc. They like carpentory tools, painting materials, chess, chinese-checkers, cards, balls, crafts, music, puzzles, aquarium, maps, animals to make zoo or farm or pets, gardening, etc. They become interested in exploring matters.

Playing is the natural medium of development and expression of children. Play can keep the child away from boredom, bad temper, irritability and destructiveness. It is better to encourage a child to play in a group to make him social. Children should be allowed to play without much interference, so that they become more independent.

Safety Measures and Prevention of Accidents

Safety measures are important aspect of child care to minimize the accidental hazards. Children are by nature accident prone. They are curious, investigative, impulsive, impatient and less careful to listen warning. Accidental injuries are the leading cause of hospitalization, disability and death of children. It is expensive aspect of community health. Greatest number of accidental injuries occur in 2 to 3 years and 5 to 6 years of age. Most frequently young children are injured at home and older children are injured outside the home.

According to WHO, an accident is an event, independent of human will caused by an outside force acting rapidly and resulting in physical or mental injury. The occurrence of injury is unintended. About 90 percent of all accidents are preventable by safety measures.

Certain Situations may Predispose the Accidental Injury in Children

- Curious, interested, hyperactive, and daring child has more chance of accidents than lethargic and uninterested one.
- Boys are more daring and having risk of more accidents than girls.
- Accidents are more common in aggressive, stubborn poor concentration and unsupervised children.
- Single child and oldest child of the family are having less chance of accidents than others.
- Accidents increased in overcrowded home, when the child is hungry and tired and parents are busy or if mother is pregnant and the child is cared in unfamiliar environment or cared by unfamiliar person or by the too young to assume this responsibility.
- Change in daily routine of the child or parent may cause accidents.
- Lack of outside play facilities is responsible for more home accidents.
- Accidents may occur frequently if the parent is having poor knowledge, ignorance, carelessness or lack of awareness about safety measures for accident prevention or lack of supervision of children.

Causes and types of accidents depend upon level of growth and development. Types of accidents are related to age sex, intelligence, social circumstances or personality of the child. Newborn baby is relatively safe from accidents. But infants and toddlers are more prone to accidental injury due to their innate curiosity, mobility with poor physical co-ordination, lack of experience and inability. Preschoolers, school-age children and adolescents may victimized in danger thoughtlessly. Accidents may happen in any place—indoor or outdoor. Home accidents are more common in younger children.

Common Accidental Injury in Different Age Groups

Infant: Falls, burns, cuts and injury, suffocation, foreign body (aspiration, ingestion, in the ear, nose, etc.)

Toddlers and preschoolers: Falls, burns, cuts and injuries, ingestion and aspiration foreign bodies, drowning and near drowning, poisoning, electrocution, suffocation and strangulation, bites and stings, vehicle or road-traffic accidents, sports injury, etc.

School-age children and adolescents: Sports injury, falls, electrical or instrumental injury, road-traffic accidents, bites and stings, drowning, etc.

Major Types of Accidents

Accidents can be classified, according to the required health intervention into five categories:

1. *Accidents requiring medical interventions:* Drowning, burns (especially in homes), falls, cuts and wounds, agroindustrial injuries, animal bites (dogs, snakes), poisoning (insecticides, rodenticides, kerosene oil, drugs, acids, etc.)
2. *Accidents requiring surgical interventions or observations:* Head injuries, burns, soft tissue injury (faciomaxillary injuries) fractures, trauma to abdominal organs, etc.
3. *Accidents involving eyes:* Bow and arrow play, gulli-danda play, fire works, stone throwing, broom stick injury, sharp-edged toys, balls, shuttle cocks, fist fighting, fall from height, knife or scissors or needle injury, chemical or thermal injury.
4. *Accidents involving ENTL:* Foreign bodies, roadside accidents, corrosive poisoning (K. oil), sudden exposure to noise causing sudden deafness, physical injuries (slap), mechanical injuries with sharp objects, strangulation from cloths being entangled in rotary machines, and automobiles, kite -flying causing laryngotracheal cut, loss of pinna, etc.
5. *Road Traffic Accidents (RTA):* Careless road crossing, reversing car, playing in streets with vehicular traffic, allowing children to stand in a car or to sit in driver's lap.

Prevention of Accidents and Safety Precautions

Prevention of accidents requires three things. That is forethought, time and discipline. First is the forethought, i.e. the anticipation of possible risk of accidents to the child. Second is time, which is needed sufficiently to supervise and watch the child and his activities. Third is the discipline, which need to be well balanced to prevent the accidental hazards.

Parents play a major role in prevention of accidents and safety precautions. Family members also need to contribute to follow the safety measures to prevent this hazards. In hospital, nursing personnel are responsible to maintain safety precautions to prevent accidents.

The *safety precautions* according to various age groups are as follows:

For infants:
- Never leave an infant alone on cot or table or in unprotected place to prevent fall.
- Never give very small things to the child.
- Toys should not have removable small parts which can be aspirated or put into the ear or nose.
- Never feed solids which are difficult to chew, e.g. ground nut.
- Coins, buttons, beads, marbles must not be left within child's reach.
- Keep the stove or fire source and hot things far away from the child.
- Electrical appliances should be kept out of reach.
- Never leave the infant near water tub or pond and never allow to go out alone.

For toddlers and preschoolers:
- Never use negative statement for any activities, i.e. 'don't do that', 'don't go there', etc.
- Give proper directions for activity.
- Provide constant supervision.
- Protect stairs by gate and keep doors closed.
- Keep harmful substances like hot things, drugs, poisons, kerosine oil, electrical appliances, sharp objects, etc. out of child's reach.
- Give adequate instructions to the caretaker to look after the child and to follow the precautions.
- Provide safe play materials and toys.
- Floor should not be slippery.
- Furniture should be placed firmly to prevent fall and the child should not be allowed to climb over it.
- The child must not be allowed to wear inflammable synthetic materials which may catch fire easily.
- Mother should not hold the baby in lap when drinking tea or coffee or during cooking.
- Children should not be allowed to play with cord, plastic bags or pillow which may cause suffocation.
- Batteries of the torch must not be left free to avoid risk or lead poisoning.
- Children must not be allowed to stand in a car when in motion.
- Electric switch should be out of child's reach.

For school children and adolescents:
- Teach safety precautions with fire, fire works, match box, electricity, sharp instruments, etc.
- The child should be taught swimming as soon as he / she is old enough.
- Encourage playing in safe places and supervise game whenever needed to prevent sports injury.

- Discourage the children from kite flying from rooftops and playing door banging games and from closing the doors with a lot of force.
- Children must not be allowed to play on streets, they should be taught about road safety, use of zebra crossing and cautions in bicycles or tricycles riding.
- Never left the child alone in the car unless it has been ensured that the keys are not 'in'.

Nursing Responsibilities in Prevention of Accidents

- Health education is considered as vaccination for prevention of accidents. The significant role of nursing personnel is to improve the level of knowledge and awareness about the safety precautions. Parents should be taught to anticipate the risk to maintain discipline and to provide time to supervise children. Anticipatory guidance should be provided to the parents, family members, school teacher, grown up children and general public about prevention of accidents.
- Provision of safe environment to eliminate or reduce the hazardous conditions for the children. It should be arranged at home, school, community and hospitals.
- Safe child care should be organized and provided to prevent accidental hazards. Assessment of child's characteristics for accidental liability is important. Parents should be involved in safety program of child care. Elimination of causative factors need to be emphasized through health education.
- Assisting in medical care to prevent disabilities and handicapped condition is an important responsibility of the nurse.
- Emergency care at comprehensive trauma care unit improves the survival rate. Rehabilitation facilities should be organized with necessary referral.
- Public health measures regarding prevention of accidents should be implemented. Traffic rules, restriction of speed, use of helmets, avoidance of alcohol while driving, regular checking of vehicles, etc. must be strictly enforced. Nurse should make the people aware about the strict implementation of rules.
- Participate in policy making and research activities related to accidents prevention and changing of behavior for controlling accidents.

Sex Education

Sex education is the significant need of the adolescent and preadolescent boys and girls.

Adolescence is the period of transition from childhood to maturation. It is concerned mainly with rapid physical, physiological and sexual development. This sudden transformation along with exposure to influences of peers and print and electronic media makes the adolescent confused on knowledge, attitude and behavior regarding sex.

The adolescent is often anxious about nocturnal discharge of seminal fluid, size of the penis or its shape and erection, size shape of breasts, menstruation, puberty changes and appearance to influence the opposite sex. In the absence of appropriate information about sex and barrier of communication with parents enhance adolescent's worry and anxiety.

Most adolescents practice masturbation for gratification of sexual desire and to obtain pleasure. This practice leads to intense guilt feeling and anxiety which make them run to quacks who induce treatment without any scientific and psychological approaches. So, the adolescents need emotional support and information regarding sexual concerns.

Common Sexual Problems of Adolescents

The sexual concerns of adolescents leads to various problems like homosexuality, promiscuous sexual behavior, unprotected and unsafe sex, unwanted pregnancies, illegal abortion and its complications (like septicemia, maternal death), unwanted child or orphanage, sexually transmitted diseases including HIV/AIDS and psychological problems related to sexuality and sexual concerns.

Need for Sex Education

Sex education is an important preventive and continuing approach to the care of preadolescents and adolescents. They have great need of appropriate and adequate orientation about sex and sexual concerns. They need guidance regarding sexual development, sexual hygiene, sexual impulse, curiosities, and reactions to opposite sex.

In the absence of sex education at home and schools, the preadolescents and adolescents learn about sex from peers, magazines, TV, movies, etc. which may confuse their sexual behavior. So, sex education should be started early in school age. The time and process of sex education are both vitally important.

Sex education helps to induce safe sex practices thus to control unwanted pregnancy and STDs/RTIs. It also helps and motivates the young people to prepare for responsibility of married life and parenthood by a healthy and responsible sex behvior. It protects from sexual abuse, exploitation and molestation. It prevents sexual calamities and promotes positive attitude toward sex in a socially approved and desired means.

Organizing Sex Education

Sex education should be given based on age, interest and level of understanding of the children. It should be simple and clear discussion on questions related to sex and sexuality.

The content of sex education should include anatomy and physiology of reproductive system, changes during puberty, sex hygiene, sexlife, marriage counseling and socially accepted sexual patterns. Safer sex practices by use of contraceptives and consequences of risk behavior also to be included. Discussion can be done on ovulation, menstruation, fertilization, pregnancy, masturbation, nocturnal emission of seminal fluid, STDs/RTIs and about the sexual feelings with related problems.

Sex education can be given by the parents, teachers, school health nurse or any health team members like doctor and social worker. Psychologist and sexual counselor can also help the preadolescents and adolescents in sexual concerns. Sex educator may have special training. Parents can answer the questions from own experience. Sex education can be given informally by the parents and other significant family members or it can be given at school as formal program.

During preadolescence period, the source of sex information is mainly family based. It may lead to misconceptions and misinformation. Peer discussion about sex may misguide and produce intense curiosity which prevents emotional control. So, formal sex education should be organized at the school by health team members and teachers.

Parents should provide basic informations about puberty changes and sex. They need to answer questions without any hesitation. Some parents may not have enough idea to answer all questions. They should identify the concern and problems in the children and consult the appropriate person for help, whenever necessary.

School health nurses can help them by answering questions and initiating discussion whenever needed. The nurse is considered by the most parents and their children as nonjudgmental and not having a disciplinary role as do the teachers. Nurses should have special training on sex education. They should examine the feelings, fantasies and misconceptions about reproductive functions and sex behavior in the preadolescents and adolescents. Need for sexual counseling and guidance should be identified and necessary steps should be taken. Nurse should not attempt to identify problems concerning sexuality during the adolescent years, unless they are also willing to discuss it. Nurse should keep in mind that unsolicited advice is seldom welcomed at any age but during adolescence it may be very disruptive.

HEALTH PROMOTION OF CHILDREN AND GUIDANCE TO PARENT FOR CHILD CARE

Nurses are responsible for health promotion of children in different stages of development and to guide the parent for child care. They are the significant health care providers to assist the parent to understand different aspects of growth and development and to meet the needs of children during development stages.

Health problems and needs of the children vary during various stages of development. The areas of health care activities also changed in different stages to promote holistic development of the child. Role of the parents in child health care requires adequate explanation and guidance from health care team members.

Health Promotion during Infancy

Health promotion of the infants is best done by the fulfillment of physical and physiological needs, through essential neonatal care, breastfeeding, weaning, immunization, safety precautions for prevention of accidents, play stimulation and health supervision at regular interval. Emotional social needs should be fulfilled by parent-infant interactions and trusting relationship through love, security and satisfaction. Mother is the significant person for the promotion of psychosocial development. The changes in the infant between birth and the age of one year are dramatic. The care of infant also be altered during this period. Health care providers should assist the parents to make decisions and to take care of their children according to their individual child's needs.

Parents need Guidance on the Following Aspects

- Early detection of problems of the infant and seeking consultancy from health professionals. Warning signs and danger signs should be explained to the parents for anticipation of 'at risk' or 'high-risk conditions.'
- Maintenance of nutritional requirements, hygiene, gentle handling, safety measures, should be emphasized.
- Importance of immunizations, play stimulation and healthy environment need to be informed.
- Avoidance of emotional deprivation, and trauma due to separation anxiety from mother.
- Promotion of self-care activities in late infancy for the improvement of independence by self-feeding, self-directed play, etc.
- Maintenance of health and immunization record along-with special events in the first year of life (My childhood).
- Acceptance of the infants as they are with their different characteristics especially avoiding gender bias and providing equal opportunities with love, affection, safety and security.

Health Promotion during Toddlerhood

Health maintenance and health promotion of toddlers should include the important areas like nutritional counseling, accident prevention, toilet training, provision of play and play materials, immunization and health supervision. Meeting the emotional needs through love and affection, avoiding separation anxiety, from parents promoting discipline and developing self-esteem through sense of autonomy are important aspect of psychosocial development.

Nurses are responsible for guiding and assisting parents to meet their children's need. The different areas of guidance are as follows:

- Provision of balanced diet, nutrition supplementation, hygienic measures especially dental care, immunizations and play facilities.
- Prevention of accidents and safety measures.
- Toilet training according to readiness of the toddlers.
- Characteristic behaviors of toddlers like imitation of domestic activities, sharing with family meal, beginning of reading and writing, short attention span, negativistic attitude and independence, ritualistic, behavior likings—disliking, parallel play, etc.
- Consistency in discipline and control of temper tantrums.
- Regular health check up for early detection of problems.

Health Promotion during Preschool Age

Nurses are responsible for helping the parents in understanding the developmental changes occur in the appearance, skills and behavior of preschoolers. They should guide the parents in health maintenance, health promotion, accident prevention and health supervision.

Parents are still responsible for the health care and health supervision of their preschool children. The health care providers should share information on the developmental needs of preschooler as well as respond to the concerns of parents. Active involving of parents, their children and family members must be ensured.

Important Areas of Guidance

- Food preference, likes and dislikes should be approved to maintain nutritional requirements.
- Acceptance of the children by their parents within the individual limitations of the child.
- Provide limited frustration from environment to assist the child in better coping.
- Allowing some work to do with promotion of self-care ability and safety measures for prevention of accident.
- Allow and accept friends of the child during play and lunch.
- Expands child's world with social interaction, trips to zoo, restaurant, market, relatives house, etc.
- Provide brief nonthreatening separation from parents and home by sending out to nursery school, play school, relatives house, etc.
- Health check-up at regular interval, immunization, nutritional supplementation (if needed), maintenance of health record and information about possible health hazards need to be provided to the parents.

Supplying verbal and written information in response to the parents questions encourage them to share and follow the instructions in the care of their children.

Health Promotion during School Age

School age children become increasingly capable to take self-care. They follow the values, belief and habits of the parents. Parents are still responsible for information giving and explaining physiologic changes that occur during the school years. Anticipatory guidance is needed for parents and their children for maintenance and promotion of health. The areas of health information are nutrition, eating habit, dental health, rest and sleep, prevention of accidents, emotional support, sexual abuse, drug abuse, smoking, etc. Both physical and mental health need to be emphasized for optimum development.

The optimum health of the school child is influenced by the health supervision and care received from school health nurse, family doctors and dentists. Health instructions to be given to the child by parents, teachers, school health nurse/community nurse at home and school. The responsibility for a child's health however rests with parents. The areas of guidance to the parents and their children are as follows:

- Emotional support and guidance to the child by parents, family members and teachers.
- Promoting coping ability in home and school.
- No humiliation to be done by punishment.
- Promoting self-esteem by reward and approval within the child's limitation.
- Behavioral problems should not be handled negatively, but to be solved constructively.
- Encourage peer activities, exercise and home responsibilities.
- Explore unique talents of the child and unfamiliar experiences to promote creativity.
- Allowing recreation and play activities.
- Answering and discussing questions about physical and physiological changes.
- Explaining about sexual concerns and sexuality in simple language and organizing sex education.
- Understanding and guiding to resolve conflict between dependence and independence.
- Regular health check-up and physical examination for height, weight, posture, hearing, vision, etc. to detect problems. Dental examination is recommended twice a year. Immunization should be completed. Health education to be given to promote self-care ability. Participation in health fair, health camp should be promoted and emphasized.

The school health program is an important part of national health programs. The purpose is to maintain, improve and promote the health of every school child. Adequate supervision of physical, mental, emotional and social aspects of school life are included in the program. All children should receive routine health appraisals, follow-up care along with health education and counseling to the children and also to their parents, as necessary.

Health Promotion during Adolescence

Adolescents have special needs for optimum growth and development towards maturation. They require special help regardless of their complaints. In addition to the usual health problems, the characteristics of adolescence, predispose young people to a wide range of experience including sexual problems, emotional disorders, experimentation with drugs and alcohol, suicidal ideation, etc. Their problems are usually handled by the physician and sometimes by the pediatrician when they are younger. Adolescent health now considered as special area of growing medical speciality and known as 'Ephebiatrics' (from the Greek 'ephebos' meaning youth, puberty). Main objectives of this super speciality is to help teenagers to solve their problem with special consideration.

As adolescents mature, they are able to accept increasing responsibility for their own health care. Supervision and guidance is needed from parents, teachers, nurses, doctors, social workers, psychologists, etc. for health maintenance and health promotion. Role of the parents is vital in all aspects of health promotions towards optimum development.

The important areas of health information and guidance to the adolescents and their parents include regular physical examination, promotion of self-care by balanced diet, eating habit regulation, hygienic measures, dental health, breast self-examination, prevention of accidents, prevention of addictive behaviors, emotional control, prevention of suicidal ideation, education for parenthood and prevention of sexual abuse and sexual calamities.

Parents should provide guidance and supervision to the adolescents with the help of health team members. They should emphasize on the following aspect:

- Promotion of self-care by rest, sleep, exercise, hygiene, balanced diet with adequate energy consumption and healthy eating habit.
- Arrangement of regular health check-up and breast-self-examination and dental examination (mouth-self examination).
- Preventive education on accidents, addictive behavior, adolescents problems, sexually transmitted diseases, unwanted pregnancy, etc.
- Allowing recreations sports, dancing, reading novel, hobbies, television, talking on telephone for emotional need to prevent boredom.
- Encouraging independence and allowing to handle own affairs and problems and financial independence by earning own money.
- Supporting to control emotions, frustration, depression and preventing self-destruction (suicide) and antisocial activities.
- Understanding the conflicts of the adolescents and helping them for crisis intervention and resolution of conflicts.
- Helping them to accept body image and changes during puberty.
- Promoting adjustment with wide range of experiences. Parent should limit rules and regulation and induce realistic consistent behavior in the context of present value system.
- Arranging sex education to assist for development of universally approved heterosexual relationship and to prevent sexual problems thus to promote respectful healthy sexual behavior towards healthy parenthood. Adolescent may need counseling on sexual experimentation, contraceptive use, sexual problems, STDs, sexual role, special sexual concerns and reproductive health.

Parental attitude, healthy parent-child interaction, socio-economical status, environmental influences, sex and family position of the children have important contributions towards health promotion and optimum development of the positive health of the children.

Sick Child

8

- Setting of Pediatric Illness Care Delivery
- Hospitalization of Sick Child
- Child's Reaction to Hospitalization and Prolonged Illness
- Effects of Hospitalization on the Family of the Child
- Role of Nurse to Help to Cope with Stress of Illness and Hospitalization of Children
- Nursing Interventions and Adaptations in Nursing Care of Sick Child

INTRODUCTION

The sick child is different from sick adult. The differences of illness in children and adults are based on anatomic, physiologic and psychologic differences between the immature child and the mature adult. Many illnesses are common both in children and adults like pneumonia, diarrhea, appendicitis, etc. But their consequences may be different. Other than the common conditions, the children are prone to acquire conditions not seen in adult medical care. The types of illnesses peculiar to children are congenital anomalies, perinatal and neonatal problems, nutritional disorders, accidental injuries, various infections, malignancies (like leukemia, brain tumor, Wilms' tumor, bone tumor, etc.) emotional disturbances (conduct disorders, psychosomatic disorders, etc.) and disorders of growth and development (failure to thrive, acne vulgaris, obesity, dwarfism, etc.).

The older a child becomes, the greater the chances of survival. The risk of mortality is greater in younger infants. Each age group of children is particularly affected by certain factors of an unfavorable environment and susceptible to certain diseases and exposed to various accidental hazards.

Parents can usually recognize the early features of illness in their child. The age of the child, the severity of the signs and symptoms of illness and duration of illness help to determine whether or not the child requires immediate care. Several facilities and sources of care for children are available today. These sources and facilities are available both in community and in hospital settings. Hospitalization often needed for the sick child.

SETTING OF PEDIATRIC ILLNESS CARE DELIVERY

The sick child prefers and benefits from being at home or in a home like environment. Many additional factors influence the increase use of nonhospitalized care of sick children. Length of hospital stays is shortened even in seriously ill children due to family-preference and community health services provided by the public and private sectors of health care delivery systems.

The pediatric health care facilities include home-based care involving the parents, health centers, clinic services, out-patient services in hospital setting, day-care services, school health services, health camps and hospital or extended care facility. General practitioners or pediatrician can provide private care in home or hospital setting.

Several kinds of facilities are available for the care of the sick children within the hospital. These include pediatric unit in a general hospital, a children hospital, pediatric or neonatal intensive care units, neonatal units or baby nursery and pediatric research center. In the pediatric unit or pediatric hospital separate departments are available as medical unit, surgical unit or special care unit like pediatric oncology, pediatric orthopedic unit, infectious diseases, pediatric emergency unit, postoperative recovery room or intermediate care unit. Pediatric extended care facility in hospital include laboratory services, diagnostic imaging, physical therapy, etc.

Pediatric Unit in a Hospital

The pediatric unit must have the facilities for adequate provision of care of the children and protection for physical dangers, i.e. accidents and infections along with protection from psychologically threatening environment. A pediatric unit should be happy and attractive place with cheerful and home like surroundings. It should have colorful walls with suitable pictures. Furniture should be of attractive and fast color without any poisonous paints, any projections and sharp edges. Floor should not be slippery and safety measures to be maintained.

A pediatric unit should have facilities of separate areas for different types of ill child, treatment room, examination room, play room, dining room and pantry, waiting room for visitors and parents, consultation room, teaching room, store room, bathroom for children and adults, nurses station, doctors room, etc.

The pediatric unit must meet the needs of children and their parents. The nurses are responsible for creating a healthy physical and psychological environment and preventing spread of infection, accidents and emotional trauma.

The physical environment of the pediatric unit should be pleasing by the maintenance of cleanliness and orderliness of furniture and equipment. There should have good lighting, plenty or fresh air and good ventilation without any draughts. Comfortable temperature (about 22-25°C) and humidity (about 65%) should be maintained. The spacing between two beds should be 6 to 8 feet with adequate cleaning facilities. The unit should be free from fly, mosquitoes, bed bugs, cats and dogs. There should have facilities for isolation of infectious patients, disinfections of articles and other methods of prevention of cross infections. Provision of safety measures for prevention of accidents should be available in the pediatric unit. There should be recreation facilities like toys, music and television, to reduce fear and anxiety of the children.

HOSPITALIZATION OF SICK CHILD

In spite of best preventive and promotive health care, some children become sick and need hospitalization. Preparation for hospitalization is important to prevent psychologic or emotional trauma of hospitalization. Older children can be explained about the need for admission to the hospital especially in case of planned admission. For emergency hospitalization also, sick children should be prepared by the parents, health team members and nurses, to promote coping with the traumatic event.

Admission to the hospital can be a positive psychologic experience for children, if prepared properly. It helps to develop confidence in dealing with stressful situation in future. Consistent support to the children and their parents can only bring this positive outcome. The following concepts help to minimize the emotional trauma to the children and their parents for better adjustment during hospital stay.

- Family integrity and the child's relationship should be maintained. Family interactions must be understood to follow the child's behavior and reaction during health and disease.
- The sick child should be supported and guided to learn to handle new experiences and feelings by family participation to provide love and security during illness and hospital stay.
- Needs of each child are different based on individual differences, family background, level of growth and development and degree of illness. Assessment of these needs as well as those of family members forms the basis of nursing interventions.
- The pediatric nurse seeks to promote, maintain and restore health in both children and their parents by health counseling and teaching about the needs.
- Hospitalized child should be cared by the professional nurses following scientific principles of disease process and nursing process with appropriate therapeutic and nursing interventions.
- Family participation for planning, implementation and evaluating plan of care is essential for optimal outcome by continuity of care.
- Within a safe environment, the sick child needs expert physical care, emotional support, expression of feelings (through play) and continuation of school education, to promote continued growth, both in acute and chronic illness.
- Parents should have trusting relationship with nurses and health team members and permission for expression of feelings and emotions in the hospital environment.
- Family members and their child, who are under great stress, when a child is terminally ill or dying must be supported emotionally, so the child can die with dignity and with a feeling of being loved.
- Hospitalization is the break in the unity of the family. So, the emotional effects should be considered first, because it is often mistakenly accorded less importance than the physical care given to the sick child.

CHILD'S REACTION TO HOSPITALIZATION AND PROLONGED ILLNESS

Illness threatens both the physical and psychological development of children. Sickness causes pain, restraint of movement, long sleepless periods, restriction of feeds, separation from parents and home environment which may result emotional trauma. Hospitalization and prolonged illness can retard growth and development and cause adverse reactions in the child, based on stage of development.

Reactions of Neonates

Hospitalization and prolonged illness in neonatal period interrupt in the early stages of development of a healthy mother-child relationship and family integration. Impairment of bonding and trusting relationship, inability of the parents to love and care for the baby and inability of the baby to respond to parents and family members are common reactions of the neonates.

Reactions of Infants

Infant's reactions are mainly separation anxiety and disturbance of development of basic trust, when the infant is separated from mother and when illness and hospitalization interfere with meeting the infant needs. Emotional withdrawal and depression are found in the infants of 4 to 8 months of age. Interference of growth and delayed developments also found. Older infants (8 to 12 months of age) may have limited tolerance due to separation anxiety which is found as fear of strangers, excessive crying, clinging and overdependence on mother.

Reactions of Toddlers

Toddlers reactions due to hospitalization are found as protest, despair, denial and regression.

The toddler protests by frequent crying, shaking crib, rejecting nurses attention, urgent desire to find mother and showing signs of distrust with anger and tears, especially when with mothers.

In despair, the toddler becomes hopeless, apathetic, anorectic, listless, looks sad, cry continuously or intermittently and use comfort measures like thumb sucking, fingering lip and tightly clutching a toy.

In denial, the child reacts by accepting care without protest and represses all feelings. The child does not cry in the absence of mother and may seem more attached to nurses.

The toddlers may react by regression in an attempt to regain control of a stressful situation. They are found to stop using newly acquired skills and may return to the behavior of an infant during illness and hospitalization.

Reactions of Preschool Child

The preschool children adopt various mental mechanisms (defense mechanisms) to adjust with the stressful experiences of hospitalization and prolonged illness. They react by exhibiting regression, repression, projection, displacement, identification, aggression, denial, withdrawal and fantasy. The preschooler may simply show similar behaviors of the toddlers, i.e. protest, despair and denial. The stage of protest in preschool children is usually less aggressive and direct.

Reactions of School-aged Children

During hospitalization and prolonged illness, the school-aged children are concerned with fear, worry, mutilation, fantasies, modesty and privacy. They react with defense mechanisms like regression, separation anxiety, negativism, depression, phobia, unrealistic fear, suppression or denial of symptoms and conscious attempts of mature behavior.

Reactions of Adolescents

Adolescents are concerned with lack of privacy, separation from peers or family and school, interference with body image or independence or self concept and sexuality. They react with anxiety related to loss of control and insecurity in strange environment. They may show anger and demanding or uncooperative behavior or increased dependency on parents and staff. They may adopt mental mechanism like intellectualization about disease, rejection of treatment, depression, denial or withdrawal.

EFFECTS OF HOSPITALIZATION ON THE FAMILY OF THE CHILD

Hospitalization of child is the break in the unity of the family. Emotional reactions of each member of the family must be considered to help them to adjust with stress due to the hospital situation and illness.

Parents whose children have been admitted to the hospital feel not only separation from their children but also they may have feeling of inadequacy as others (nurses, doctors) provide care for their children. They feel anxiety, anger, fear, disappointment, self-blame and possible guilt feeling due to lack of confidence and competence for caring the child in illness and wellness.

The specific causes of parental anxiety related to hospitalization of their children are the fear of the followings:
- Strange environment in the hospital
- Separation from the child
- Unknown events and outcome
- The suffering of the child
- Spread of infections of other members of the family.
- Unbearable financial obligations incurred through the illness.
- Society will look upon the illness as a reflection of something wrong with the parents.

There are so many factors which may increase the parental anxiety. The anxious parent can be recognized by the trembling, coarse or wavery voice, restlessness, irritability, withdrawal or erratic body movements. Hostile and aggressive behavior may be evident toward those caring for the child.

The reactions of the parents and family members can be influenced by cultural and spiritual beliefs which may affect the rate of recovery of the child. They may feel that the illness is due to any fault in child rearing and considered as punishment by the God or curse of any Goddess. Some families hesitate to discuss their concern about illness of the child where as some families want long discussions.

ROLE OF NURSE TO HELP TO COPE WITH STRESS OF ILLNESS AND HOSPITALIZATION OF CHILDREN

The role of nurse in helping child and family members for coping with stress of hospitalization and illness is complementary and supportive. Parents and their children want nurses as a helping people for the adjustment with the stress and as a source of comfort, strength and knowledge. The nurse should earn sufficient confidence to develop positive relationship with the children and their parents. The pediatric nurse must be aware about the feelings of both parents and children to help them to handle their problems. The nurse should avoid criticizing parent's attitude, however unreasonable it may appear. Nurse should have patience, tenderness and great emotional strength in times of stress. In addition to the provision of rest and physical care to acutely ill children, the nurse must recognize anxiety and provide relief from it by patiently listening to complaints and showing concern about them. Parents usually who care for the child may be more in need of the nurse's sympathetic understanding and permissive guidance.

The nurse may help the parents and children to feel more secure and calm in the hospital and less anxious by the following means:

1. *Provide family centered care* with different approach to specific age group.
2. *In neonates:* Provide continual contact between baby and parents with active involvement by rooming-in and sensory-motor stimulation as appropriate.
3. *In infants:* Encourage mother to balance her responsibilities and minimize separation with confidence and competence. Basic needs of the infant should be fulfilled promptly with attention and appropriate handling from a limited number of personnel. Mother can be allowed during procedure. Tension and loneliness can be relieved by toys.
4. *In toddlers:* Provide rooming-in and unlimited visiting hours to express child's feeling. No punishment to the child. Home routine can be continued especially regarding sleeping, eating, bathing, etc. Familiar toys and articles can reinforce the child's sense of security. Allow play and choice whenever possible and arrange physical setting to encourage independence. Parents should provide love and understanding to help the child to restore trusting relationship. Hostility and withdrawal of love can cause the child's loss of trust, self-esteem and independence.
5. *In preschool children:* Minimize stress of separation by providing parental presence and participation in care. Plan to shorten the hospital stay, as possible. Help the child to accept the stressful situation by love and concern. Set limits for the child and provide opportunity to verbalize the feelings. Careful preparation for all procedures by privacy and explanation according to level of understanding. Encourage the child to participate in self-care and hygiene as appropriate. Remove fears (especially castration and mutilation) by adequate explanation. Reassure the child that no one is to blame for the illness and hospitalization. Discourage parents from reinforcing negative feelings to the child, e.g. "If you are not listening to me, I shall leave you here".
6. *In school children:* Help the parent to prepare the child for elective hospitalization. Respect the child's need for privacy and modesty during examination. Thorough nursing history should be obtained to plan the care. Help the child to identify problems and to ask questions. Use treatment rooms whenever possible to perform painful and invasive procedures. Explain the procedure and its purpose with reassurance. Encourage the child in self-care, play and to continue school work when the condition permits. Assist the family members to understand child's reaction to illness and hospitalization. Help parents to deal with their own anxieties and to assist their child to cope with the situation. Encourage parental participation in child care and consistent visiting pattern especially with peers and siblings. Parents may be introduced to other parents of the same unit.
7. *In adolescent:* Help parents to prepare the adolescent for planned hospital admission. Assess the impact of illness and hospitalization and presence of misconceptions. Hospital staff, hospital routines and facilities available in the hospital unit should be explained soon after admission. Obtain thorough nursing history about illness, habits, recreation, hobbies, etc. Respect the need for privacy, recreation, personal preferences on self-care and food habit. Involve the adolescent patients in planning of care and help them to accept restrictions and health teaching. Explain all procedures and reassure to accept the plan of care and to co-operate. Provide opportunities for recreation, peer relationships, interaction with other adolescent patients and expression of feelings. Assist parents to deal effectively, adolescent's response related to stress of illness and hospitalization.

Nurse guide the hospitalized child in health promotion and restoration activities. It is important for nurses to recognize and respond to the needs of hospitalized child with the help of parents and family members.

NURSING INTERVENTIONS AND ADAPTATIONS IN NURSING CARE OF SICK CHILD

The nursing interventions involve doing something for, doing something with or doing something that allows the child or family to take actions that resolves the problems or needs. These are the actions taken to help the patient and/or family to move from their present state to a condition described as a projected goal or outcome. The types of intervention selected depends on the nursing diagnosis and the projected goals. The specific interventions depends on the illness, capabilities, choices and resources of the child and family. It is also important for the nurse to select interventions that are socially, culturally and economically appropriate for the child and the family.

Various members of the health team help to plan and implement nursing interventions. Setting precise goals and making decisions about specific measures to be used to resolve problems or needs through appropriate planning. The planning must also involve continuous interaction between the child and family and the nurse.

Adaptation in Nursing Care of the Sick Child

Hospitalization may have positive psychologic outcomes for children who have been well prepared for their experiences. However, even with the best preparation some children and their parents may still feel severe stress during illness and admission to hospital. The sources of stress included the five following categories:

Psychological stress: Due to separation from home, parents, other family members and friends, change in role, anxiety, fear and pain.

Physiologic stress: Due to loss of sleep, diagnostic and treatment procedures, trauma, burns, surgery, immobilization and physical restraint.

Environmental stress: Due to loss of daily routine, unfamiliar noise, strange odor and stimuli and various gadgets especially in intensive care unit.

Biological stress: Due to pathological organisms and cross infections.

Chemical stress: Due to drugs, toxic substances, reactions to blood transfusions, anesthesia, etc.

Stress is the nonspecific response to stressors or demands made on the body. The ability of children to cope with stresses of the growth and development as well as those of hospitalization depends upon their present developmental stage, their parents reaction and their cultural and religious backgrounds. The way an individual, either child or adult, copes depends on those direct actions aimed at eliminating or minimizing stressful situation. Coping is the way an individual deals with a situation and adapts to it. The nurse can assist the child and parents in coping efforts in regard to hospitalization by using reality oriented and task oriented coping strategies. Trusting relationship with the child, parents and family members helps in maximum co-operation and reduction of stress.

Strategies for Adaptation in Nursing Care

- Welcome the child and parents heartily during each nursing interventions.
- Call by name and touch the child gently with love.
- Explain the interventions in simple sentence according to the level of understanding and tell about the event, what will exactly happens.
- Ask for co-operation and its benefit.
- Encourage to express the feelings, allow to verbalize and answer questions.
- Demonstrate the interest and empathy to the child and family members.
- Explain and reason out any unpleasant experience of the past which will reduce anxiety level and help to obtain co-operation.
- Discuss about cultural and religious belief of the family, never condemned those belief.
- Allow parent or significant other during any treatment or nursing procedures or ask to wait nearby.
- Maintain privacy, minimize exposure and gentle handling of the child during nursing care.
- Provide physical comfort by appropriate positioning, warmth, bladder evacuation, etc. before and during the interventions.
- Take opinion of the parents and the child during any decision making regarding the treatment plan, diagnostic procedures and nursing interventions.
- Maintain eye level contact during conversation.
- Divert the child's attention by toys or telling story or simply talking with him/her. Show the articles use in procedure and allow the child to manipulate the equipment, if possible, e.g. stethoscope, torch, hammer, plastic syringe, etc.
- Restraints should be used only if there is no alternative.
- Skillful and confident approach to be practiced throughout the procedures.
- Protect the child from physical injury and infections.

- Assure about the confidentiality of the information whenever required especially for older children.
- Patience, tenderness and emotional strength are essential during nursing care to the children.
- Never tell lie and negative statement to the child, honest explanation is important for positive approach.
- Praise the child for co-operation, never threat or blame the child for noncooperation.
- Establishment of rapport and friendly approach are the key points to gain co-operation. A genuine expression of liking and warmth sets the tone for the parents and child and help them to relax.

Pediatric Nursing History

Obtaining history is an important aspect of health assessment and to evaluate the health status of an individual. History regarding the child's health condition can be collected from the parents or significant others or from grown up child. Skilled communication process with effective interview technique helps to get relevant information. Leading questions to be asked, avoiding embarrassing questions. The success of interview depends primarily in the nurses ability to establish and maintain sound interpersonal relationship. Questions should be asked in friendly approach according to the level of understanding. The nurse should observe nonverbal clues and allows freedom of expression. Responses to the questions should be recorded clearly, orderly, factually and objectively. The nurse also should record immediate impressions, thoughts and feeling of the interviewees. Strategies for gaining co-operation to be followed during collection of history.

The purposes of health history of a child is to obtain data to help in diagnosis and treatment and to formulate individualized plan for care. It helps to establish relationship with the child and family and to assess the understanding of the family members about their child's health. It helps to correct misconceptions and misinformation of the family regarding the child rearing practices based on their cultural and socioeconomic patterns.

The following information to be collected and recorded:

1. *Identifying information:* Child's name, age, sex, address, name of the informant and relation with the child, date and time of history collection and in case of hospitalized child, name of unit, bed numbers, registration number, date and time of admission to the hospital, etc.
2. *Chief complaints:* Reasons for hospital admission or seeking medical care along with duration of complaints and any treatment taken prior to hospitalization for the present problems.
3. *History of present illness:* Quality, quantity and severity of complaints, time sequence, degree of symptoms, aggravating and alleviating factors, associated symptoms, etc.
4. *Past history of illness:* Medical illness and surgical illness other than the present illness, accidents and injuries, hospitalization and operations (with date, indications, complications and reactions), medications, blood transfusion, radiation, allergy and diagnostic screening procedures.
5. *Birth history:* Details of prenatal, intranatal, perinatal, neonatal/postnatal information.
6. *History of growth and development:* Previous weights, lengths, dentition, important developmental milestones, toilet training, social behavior, language, motor skills and sexual development.
7. *Immunization history:* Complete or incomplete schedule, defaulter.
8. *Dietary history:* Duration of breastfeeding, weaning, feeding problems, dietary pattern (frequency and content of meal), weight gain, amount of food consumption, food preferences, allergies, etc.
9. *Personal history:* Hygiene, sleep, eliminations habit, exercise and rest, play, hobbies, special talents, relationship with others (sibling and parent), expressions of emotions (temper tantrum), behavioral problems (thumb sucking, nail biting, pica, etc.) and schooling (age of school admission, performance, school behavior).
10. *Family history of illness:* Any history of illness in the family members, presence of hereditary diseases and congenital anomalies.
11. *Socioeconomic history:* Residence (rural, urban or slum), housing (type, location), water supply, waste disposal, communication facilities, recreational facilities, financial condition with family income, source of income, total number of family members, family relationship, cultural belief especially regarding child care, etc.

At the completion of history collection "*review of systems*" should be done to exclude any missing problems of any system. The following information to be collected by *systems review* alongwith details history.

General: Activity, appetite, sleep, weight change, edema, fever, behavior pattern, affect/mood, hygiene and self-care.

Allergy: Eczema, asthma, drug allergy, food allergy, sinus disorders, hay fever.

Skin: Rash, eruptions, nodules, pigmentations, sweating, itching, infection, hair growth, texture change.

Head: Headache, head trauma, dizziness.

Eyes: Vision, corrective lenses, strabismus, lacrimation, discharge, itching, redness, photophobia.

Ears: Hearing, infection, drainage, pain.

Nose: Cold, running nose, infection, drainage.

Teeth: Hygiene, cavities, malocclusions.

Throat: Sore throat, tonsillitis, difficulty in swallowing.

Speech: Change in voice, hoarseness, stammering.

Respiratory: Breathing difficulty, shortness of breath, chest pain, cough, wheezing, pneumonia, tuberculosis.

Cardiovascular: Cyanosis, fainting, exercise intolerance, palpitations.

Hematologic: Pallor, anemia, bruises, bleeding.

Gastrointestinal: Appetite, nausea, vomiting, abdominal pain and abnormal size, bowel habit, nature of stools, passage of parasite, encopresis, colic, etc.

Genitourinary: Age of toilet training, frequency of urination, dysuria, hematuria, previous urinary tract infection, enuresis, urethral or vaginal discharge, menstruation in adolescents.

Musculoskeletal system: Deformities, fracture, sprains, joint pain or swelling, limitation of motion, abnormality of nails.

Neurologic: Weakness or clumsiness, co-ordination, balance, gait, tremor, convulsions, personality changes.

Physical Examination of Children

Pediatric nurse plays an important role in carrying out the physical examination of the child in hospital and community. Head to foot examination is done along with examination of different system to evaluate the general condition of the child and to exclude the presence of any abnormality. It also includes anthropometric examination of the child.

Physical examination is done by inspection, manipulation, percussion, palpation and auscultation. The findings of physical examination help in diagnosis of the problem and to plan and provide best possible management. It promotes secondary prevention by early detection of deviations from normal health status and by preventing complications. It also helps to assess the recovery rate during follow-up care and to teach the child and the parents on child health measures.

General Principles

- Examination should be done according to the needs of the patient in an orderly manner.
- Gentle handling of the child with minimum exposure is very important.
- Examination should be done informally with a friendly approach, appreciating the co-operation and assistance.
- Attempt to develop rapport with the child should be made from the moment of first meet.
- Explanation about the procedure should be useful in older children for gaining co-operation.

- Restraints should be used only whenever necessary.
- Remember that the safest place for a young child is on parent's lap.
- Privacy and warmth to be maintained, as much as possible.
- Positioning of the child to be done according to the body parts to be examined. For examination of the back, the child should be placed in prone position. For examination of chest and abdomen, supine position with modified mummy restraint can be used exposing the parts as necessary. The child may be allowed to sit or stand during examination, whenever needed. Parental presence reassures the young child. Older children prefer to have their parents wait outside the examination room.
- Recording should be done immediately and accurately.

Approach to the Child

- The older child can be asked to choice to be examined on parent's lap or special examination table.
- The chest is a good part of the body to begin the examination, then already exposed parts can be examined, i.e. hands, legs, etc.
- Head to toes examination should be done thoroughly and systematically but strict sequence may not be followed.
- The child's clothing should be removed gradually and observing the parts carefully during examination.
- Show the procedure to the child by demonstrating on the doll or parent before the procedure.
- Some children are less frightened, if allowed to hold the examining equipment first.
- Diaper area of the infants and genital area of the older children should be examined until last.
- Uncomfortable and irritating procedures such as examination of throat, ear, rectum should be left towards the end.
- The sequence of examination depends upon the co-operation received from the child. No rigid sequence may be followed.
- In irritated and panicky child, prolonged examination to be avoided.
- Useful distractions to be adopted to gain co-operation during physical examination, e.g. talking with the infants or giving toys or having the parents play with them.
- Obtain as much information as possible while the child is calm and not feeling threatened.

Technique of Physical Examination

Vital signs: Obtain temperature, pulses, heart sound, respiration and blood pressure, as often as thought necessary, based on child's condition.

Anthropometry: Record anthropometric measurements, i.e. child's weight, length/height, head circumference, chest circumference mid-upper arm circumference, skin-fold thickness, etc. Growth chart to be maintained by plotting the findings especially weight.

General appearance: Observe general appearance like—body position, posture, evidence of pain, crying, hygiene, nutritional status, mental alertness, restlessness, behavior pattern, presence of developmental abnormalities, or any abnormal features.

Skin: Examine skin for color, pigmentation, lesions, jaundice, cyanosis, pallor, scar, superficial vascularity, moisture, edema, condition of mucous membrane, presence of birthmarks, tenderness, masses, texture, turgor, elasticity, rash, petechiae, subcutaneous nodules, etc.

Lymph nodes: Observe and palpate for lymph node enlargement in lymph chain areas i.e. neck, axilla, inguinal region, etc.

Hair: Observe color and distribution of hair on head, back and any other parts of the body.

Head and neck: Examine head for shape, and size, fontanelle, sutures, hair color and texture, presence of infection or any lesions, dandruff or lice, movement of head, head holding, webbing of neck, torticolis, enlarged thyroid or neck swelling, etc.

Face: Examine face for expression, asymmetry, paralysis, nose bridge, size of maxilla and mandible, tenderness over sinuses, etc.

Eyes: Observe eyes for infection, periorbital edema, photophobia, distance between the eyes, distribution of eyebrows, mongoloid slant, epicanthal fold, Brushfield spots, exophthalmos, condition of pupils, cataract, corneal opacities, squint, nystagmus, xerophthalmia and vision. Ophthalmoscopic examination also can be done.

Ears: Examine ears for shape, size, position, low-set ear, deformities, discharge, tenderness over mastoid bone, and hearing abilities. Otoscopic examination can be done to inspect the condition of ear drum.

Nose: Examine nose for patency, discharge, bleeding, deviated septum, depressed nasal bridge, nasal polyp, foreign body, flaring of nostrils, condition of nasal mucous membrane, etc. Paranasal sinuses to be examined for tenderness and order of development.

Mouth and throat: Examine the color of lips, lesions at the corners of mouth, cleft lip or cleft palate, number of teeth, evidence of dental caries, staining on the teeth, malocclusion and extra or missing teeth, gum bleeding, swelling and lesions of buccal mucosa, tongue and pharynx, presence of any infections, tonsillitis, presence of any spot, ulcer and swelling, tongue tie or short tongue, etc.

Chest: Observe the size, shape and symmetry of chest, presence of chest retractions (suprasternal, substernal, intercostal, subcostal, supraclavicular), pigeon chest deformity, funnel chest, rachitic rosary, condition of breast and nipples, breath sounds, heart sounds, etc.

Abdomen: Examine abdomen for size and shape, distension, any swelling or enlargement, presence of infection or scar, cleanliness, condition of umbilical cord in neonate, presence of any congenital anomalies or development problems (hernias).

Limbs: Limbs to be examined for any deformity, asymmetry, hemihypertrophy, bow legs, knock-knees, edema, any swelling or limitation of movements of the joints, paralysis, clubbing of fingers, number of fingers and toes (syndactyly, polydactyly), creases on the palms and soles, changes in the nails (koilonychia), deformity of the feet (talipes, flat feet), any infections, tenderness, swelling, general cleanliness, etc.

Spine and back: Note the signs of abnormal spinal curvature, (kyphosis, scoliosis, lordosis), dimples, sinuses, tufts of hair, spina bifida, meningocele or meningomyelocele, dislocation of hip, neck stiffness, any swelling at the back or tenderness.

Genitalia: Male genitalia to be examined for urethral opening and its abnormalities, hypospadias, epispadias, phimosis, paraphimosis, hydrocele, hernia, undescended testes, size of penis and ambiguous genitalia.

Female genitalia to be observed for hypertrophy of clitoris, labia majora and minora, vaginal and urethral openings, any vaginal discharge, cleanliness, infections, swelling of periurethral or greater vestibular (Bartholin's) glands in adolescents.

Anus and rectum: Observe for patency of anus, presence of fissures or fistula, rectal prolapse, perinanal erythema, etc.

Neurological examination: Note characteristics of cry, posture of head, neck and extremities, neurological reflexes (like sucking and swallowing reflex, grasp reflex, blinking reflex, stepping reflex) motor co-ordination, muscle tone, sense of touch or pain, presence of meningeal irritation, paresis or paralysis, etc.

Behavioral pattern: Note the behavior of the child (whether irritable, depressed, nervous, apathetic, excited, aggressive and disobedient) ability to respond, aptitude to the situation, attitude towards health team members, habit disorders, emotional problems, and mental status.

Abnormal signs and symptoms: Examine for presence of cough and cold, bleeding from any site, vomitus, loose motion, lack of hygiene, convulsions, oliguria, full bladder, anemia, edema, wound, ulcer, etc.

Safety Measures during Pediatric Techniques

Safety, security and protection are the basic needs to be fulfilled for each individual. These needs are important next to physiological needs of survival and stimulation. The persons who are taking care for the child in illness or wellness must be concerned about safety and security measures.

The safety precautions to be followed for hospitalized sick child during all procedures. Preventive measures of accidental injuries, infections and psychological trauma should be emphasized and strictly followed during hospital stay. The safety of hospitalized children is an important nursing responsibility. The following principles of safety should be observed in the pediatric units during various procedures.

Adequate explanation and informed consent for child care: Consent of the parent or guardian or other adult, responsible for the child's care, is required, as written or oral consent for some specific diagnostic procedures as well as for medical and surgical treatment. Parents, older children and guardian have rights of all information of making decisions with possible risks and complications of any illness and its treatment.

Safety precautions to be adopted in the hospitals for prevention of accidents: Emphasis should be given on the safety measures with practical demonstrations, for avoidance of accidental hazards, to the parents.

The restraint of children is necessary for the safety: It is used at the time of examination and to facilitate treatment procedures by protecting the children from any harm.

Aseptic techniques to be followed to prevent transmission of infections: Universal precautions of infections control should be strictly followed. Isolation of infected cases are important. Sterilization, disinfection, waste disposal and cleanliness to be practiced meticulously.

Prevention of aspiration of feeds during feeding and prevention of aspiration of oropharyngeal secretions in unconscious or postoperative patients are important safety measures.

Safety measures in the administration of drugs are most important aspect. Principles of six rights to be followed which include—the right patient, the right drug, the right dose, the right route, the right time and right of the parents and the child "to know" the necessary information (right information).

Recording of all procedures and findings are significant aspect of safety principle to prevent duplication of procedure and for follow-up.

Constant supervision of the child is a vital aspect of safety principles to prevent complications and hazards.

Gentle approach and special attention to emotional reactions of the hospitalized child help to prevent psychological trauma.

Guidelines or procedure manual of particular pediatric unit to be followed during procedures for legal safety and necessary informations to be given to the parent.

Protection of the Child from Accidents in Hospitals

Children in the pediatric unit may have accidents because of their lack of understanding of the many potential dangers inherent in the hospital setting. Safety precautions to be adopted to protect the children from those potential dangers of accidents. Practical demonstrations to be given to the parents or caregivers regarding prevention of accidents at hospitals, which may also occur in the home. The following safety measures should be practiced.

Buildings: The pediatric unit should be well ventilated without draught or suffocation. Windows should be protected with net or bar. Varandahs should not be open and wire netting should be provided for protection. Doors should open one way. Staircase should be railed and grilled. Floor should not be slippery. Toilets and bathroom should be cleaned daily and not slippery. No cats and dogs should be allowed inside the ward.

Furniture: All furniture in the pediatric unit should be cleaned and without poisonous painting. The cribs should be removable with easily operable side rails. Railing of the cribs or baby cot should be kept up to prevent fall. Space between two crib should be 6 and 8 feets.

Electrical appliances: Electric points in the walls should be high enough for the children reach. Electrical equipment must be kept unplugged when not in use. Electrical extension cords should not lying across the floor. Electrical appliances should be checked at regular interval for working condition without any leakage.

Medicine cabinets: Medicine cabinets must be locked when not in use and medications should never be given without adequate identification of child. Oily medications should never be given orally when the child is crying because of the danger of aspiration. Medicines should never left on the bedside table.

Instruments and solutions: These things should be kept in cabinets or on shelves where children cannot reach them. Utility and procedure room doors should be kept closed and children should not be allowed in those areas.

Toys: Play materials should be unbreakable, washable and without any sharp edges or small removable parts or poisonous painting. Toys should never be left on the floor. The children should not allow to run in the wards because of danger of falling. Supervision should be made during play to prevent any hazards.

Disposal of waste: Empty containers, bottles, broken glass syringes, needles, tubing, etc. should be out of reach of the children. Any spillage of blood or body fluids or solutions on the floor should be immediately cleaned to prevent fall. Cleanliness to be maintained to prevent flies, mosquitos, cockroaches and bed bugs.

Clothing: Clothing should not be too long that can cause a child to slip and fall. Safety pins should be closed at once when taken from a child's clothing and should be put out of reach.

Feeding: Small children should be fed with precautions to prevent aspirations. Forced feeding to be avoided. Children to be taught to chew food well, before swallowing. Warmth of the food to be checked before putting it in the child's mouth.

Nursing care: Precautions to be taken during application of hot water bottles by tightly stoppered and covered before being placed near the child's body. Glass thermometer to be checked for crack and should be used with precautions. The small children should never be carried off the unit or transport by hand because of danger of falling. A baby carriage, crib, stretcher, trolley or wheelchair can be safely used. In the dining space or pantry, heated substances should be kept out of reach of the children. Spouts of kettles or handles of saucepans should be kept away from the edge of table. Table cloth should not be hanging from the sides of the tables. Inflammable substances and matchbox should be kept away from the young children. Handwashing, isolation techniques and universal precautions to be followed to prevent nosocomial infections. Parents or any other family members should be allowed with the child for constant supervision and prevention of accidental hazards. Health team members should anticipate the potential dangers, take precautions to prevent the accidents and initiate prompt management whenever necessary.

Restraints

Restraints are protective measures to limit movements. There can be a short-term restraint to facilitate examination and minimize the child's discomfort during special tests, procedures and specimen collections. Restraints can also be used for a longer period of time to maintain the child's safety and protection from injury.

Restraints should be used only when it is absolutely necessary. The nurse should give the child a choice between trying to be still when asked for, or to be restrained. If the child fails to keep himself or herself to keep still, then restraints may be used with proper explanation about its purpose, depending upon the level of understanding of the child. Restraints should be removed as early as possible and then the child should be rewarded by any means to make a happier mood.

General Principles for Use of Restraints

1. Appropriate, safe and comfortable restraints should be selected.
2. Restraints should be loose as possible, tight restraint prevents normal circulation.
3. Nurse should talk soothingly to the child to provide stimulation and diversion and to relieve the sense of helplessness and loneliness of the child.
4. Sufficient padding must be used for extremity restraints to prevent skin irritation.
5. Restraints must be checked every 15 to 30 minutes for constrictions or any hazards. It can be removed periodically, at least every 2 hours, when used for long-time. It should be removed one at a time and reapplied so that the child can gain some degree of activity, especially when all extremities are restrained. Before the reapplication of restraints, the child's position to be changed to improve physiological functioning.
6. Child's comfort and body alignment to be maintained.
7. Any required knots should be tied in a manner that permits their quick release.
8. Provide range of motion and skin care routinely. When one arm is restraints, another arm and legs to be moved.
9. Do not secure the restraints to the side rails which may cause traction on the restraint or injury to the child, when the side rail is raised or lowered.
10. Proper documentation is required when restraints are in use.
11. Application of restraint can be demonstrated first on the child's doll, to get co-operation of the child and to prevent emotional trauma.

Types of Restraints

Commonly used restraints for children are mummy restraint, elbow restraint, extremity restraint, abdominal restraint, jacket restraint, finger restraint, crib-top restraint, etc. (Figs 8.1A to C).

1. *Mummy restraint:* It is a short-term type of restraint used on infants and small children during examinations and treatment of head and neck. It is used to immobilize the arms and legs of the child for a brief period of time. This involves securing a sheet or blanket around the child's body in such a way the arms are held to the sides and leg movements are restricted. It is also used during scalp vein puncture, gastric gavage and gastric lavage. A modified

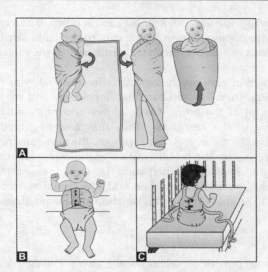

Figs 8.1A to C: Types of restraint: (A) Mummy restraints; (B) Belt restraints; (C) Jacket restraints

mummy restraint may be used when the child's chest and abdomen are to be examined.

2. *Elbow restraint:* This restraint is used to prevent flexion of the elbow and to hold the elbow in an extended position so that the infant cannot reach the face. It is especially useful for infants receiving scalp vein infusion, nasogastric tube feeding, surgery of face or head, repair of cleft lip or cleft palate or having eczema or other skin disorders in those areas. Commercial plastic elbow restraint can be used, otherwise elbow cuff and well padded wooden splint can also be used to wrap around and immobilize the child's arm.

3. *Extremity restraint:* This may be used to restrain infants and young children for the procedures such as IV therapies and urine collection. It is used to immobilize one or more extremities. One type of extremity restraint is *clove-hitch restraint* which is done with gauze bandage strip (2 inches wide) making figure-of-eight. The end of the gauze to be tied to the frame of the crib. This restraint should be used with padding of wrist or ankle. Precautions to be taken to prevent tightening of the bandage and disturbances of circulation. The knot should not be too loose, which may slip over the infant's hand or foot. The fingers and toes of the restrained extremities should be checked for coldness, discoloration and signs of skin irritation. Commercial type of elbow restraints is also available, but the precautions must be taken when they are used.

4. *Abdominal restraint:* This restraint helps to hold the infant in a supine position on the bed. It should be applied with precautions so that respiratory movements of the abdomen are not inhibited. It operates exactly like the restraints of extremity. The strip of material is wider and

has only one wide flap for fastening around the child's abdomen.

5. *Jacket restraint:* It can be used to help the child remain flat in bed in a supine position or to prevent the child from falling from crib, highchair, wheelchair or other conveyance. The jacket is put on with the strings and opening in the back and tied securely. The long tapes are secured appropriately, i.e. to the frame of the crib, or arm supports of a chair or around the back of the wheelchair or high chair. The child should be observed frequently to make certain that strangulation does not occur, and restraint has not slipped out of place.

6. *Mitten or finger restraint:* Mitts are used for infants to prevent self-injury by hands in case of burns, facial injury or operations, eczema of the face or body. Mitten can be made wrapping the child's hands in gauze or with a little bag putting over the baby's hand and tie it on at the wrist.

Hazards of Restraints

Inappropriate use of restraints may cause injury to the brachial plexus, sore or gangrene, exhaustion and loss of energy, dislike for the hospital and health team members, etc. Prolonged immobility of children may result in physiologic loss of muscular strength and flexibility which influence the respiratory volume and peripheral circulation. Long periods of restraints may result psychological hazards and inability to develop motor and psychosocial skills in children. There may be difficulty in developing own body image.

The nurse should use restraint only when it is absolutely necessary, remembering that all infants and children have physiologic and psychologic needs to be mobile.

Medical Aseptic Technique

In the pediatric units, the nurse should maintain medical asepsis to prevent transmission of infection from one child to another or to the caregivers. All the health team members are responsible to maintain asepsis during the procedures and techniques.

Medical aseptic technique is necessary when the patient and care-articles are considered as contaminated. The person who care for the child are considered to be clean when they enter the unit but become contaminated when they touch the patient or handle the articles of the isolation unit.

The following practices are important for medical asepsis:
- Infected patients are kept in isolation unit, which can be an area or cubicle or room or part of a unit.
- Furniture of the isolation unit should be simple and easily cleaned. The floor to be washed daily and the furniture to be cleaned at regular interval.
- There should be facilities for handwashing, place for cleaning used equipment, covered container for soiled

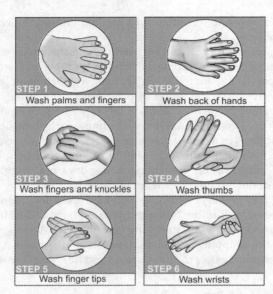

Fig. 8.2: Steps of effective handwashing

linen, disposal of contaminated waste and wet mopping of the areas.

- Facilities for sterilization should be available and sufficient equipment depending upon the child's age, kind of infection and number of isolated patients, should be arranged.
- Bedside equipment should be sterilized at regular interval, while the patient is in an isolation unit. Personal equipment (thermometer, bathing articles, mouth care articles, syringe, needles, etc.) to be provided separately for each child. Toys brought to the hospital with the child should not be dropped to the floor and to be easily cleaned whenever necessary.
- Gown and handwashing techniques are time consuming but are important factors in medical asepsis (Fig. 8.2).
- Mask technique is also important aspect, since some infections are commonly spread through droplet spray from the nose and mouth. A mask should be worn once and then discarded. It should never be dropped loosely around the neck and then drawn up into position over the nose and mouth.
- Techniques of concurrent and terminal disinfection to be followed according to hospital policy.
- Visitors are allowed to preserve parent-child or family relationship. Visitors need explanation about the safety precautions to prevent spread of infections. Limited numbers of visitors are permitted.

Newer equipment is now developed and used to provide more effective care to the children in isolation units with less emotional disturbances to them and their parents. Such devices can provide sterile environment of the bed or crib,

covered completely with a plastic canopy much like an oxygen tent with opening for providing care to the child. Air-borne infections can be prevented by 'air-filtered' at the intake and outlet areas.

Isolation may psychologically affect the behavior of the children. They feel separateness, loneliness and may also be fearful of the gown, mask, gloves and repeated handwashing of the caregivers. They may feel neglected and disturbed by the strange environment. The nurse and parents must recognize the problem when giving explanation about isolation. Parental participation in child care activities, physical contact, reassurance and play facilities can help better to be able to cope with isolation and hospitalization.

Therapeutic Play

Play can provide a release from stress and tension for individuals of all ages. Play is as essential for the sick child as for the healthy one. The sick child needs play to fill lonely hours and for expressing feeling and aggression through it, to reduce the trauma caused by hospitalization. The idea of providing play facilities is certainly not a recent one in hospitals, but the practice of providing this need is new in many hospitals considering as social and emotional welfare programs. Such programs are called as 'child life programs', 'play therapy' and 'recreational therapy'.

Therapeutic play is the specialized play activity by which a child acts out or expresses his unconscious feelings. It is a central mechanism in which children cope, communicate, learn and master a traumatic experience such as hospitalization. It is guided by health team members. It can be provided to the convalescent and immobilized bedridden children when they passed over acute illness at hospital or at home. Play in hospital setting can occur only when children are less threatened. When no play is permitted, it indicates psychological abuse.

Importance of Play for Hospitalized Children

Play in hospital helps the child and health team members or caregivers as follows:

A. It helps the child
   1. To enhance coping abilities in hospital environment.
   2. To express fear, anxiety, tension, anger and fantasies.
   3. To understand and comprehend the hospital procedures.
   4. To communicate with others and to reduce emotional trauma due to hospital experiences.
   5. To continue growth and development in physical, psychological, social, moral and educational aspects.
   6. To get rid of boredom due to prolong illness and to release hostile feelings.

B. It helps the health team members

1. To gain co-operation and trusting relationship of the hospitalized children and their family members.
2. To diagnose the child's feeling and behavior, and plan for psychological approach during care.
3. To find out and correct the misconceptions and beliefs regarding hospitalized care.
4. To reassure the anxious parent and to promote their participation in child care during illness and wellness.

Types of Play for Hospitalized Children

Therapeutic play differs from normative play in its design and intent. Specialized techniques, strategies and play environment are created for sick children by the health team members to enhance emotional and physical well-being. It can be *three* types:

1. *Emotional outlet or dramatic play:* It is used to express the child's anxiety, to solve conflict and as a diagnostic tool to identify child's concern about the illness and hospitalization, e.g. playing with doll being a nurse and caring sick doll with expression of own feeling, storytelling, etc.
2. *Instructional play:* Instruction is given for therapeutic play to the children according to their past experiences, coping abilities and physiological status. Instructional play should be well-planned, e.g. use of color in drawing, drawing in blank paper, learning the instructions on health habit from TV or teaching films, etc.
3. *Physiological enhancing play:* It is used to maintain and improve physical health and body functions. It can be selected to treat pathological condition, e.g. breathing exercise to treat respiratory problems by blowing bubbles, whistling and laughing. Squeezing the bath sponge or ball improves neurological functions.

Nursing Responsibilities for Therapeutic Play

1. Organize play facilities for the sick children. Every pediatric unit should have some space for play or play room with facilities for storage of play materials. Age-appropriate play things to be arranged for the children in adequate numbers. Individual play materials can also be permitted. There should not be any fixed period of time of play for hospitalized children. Any time should be play time for them.
2. Involve other members of health team, social worker, play therapist (play lady), parents and other family members for play in the hospital or at home and communicate with all members.
3. Interact during play and help the child to express the feelings. Then interpret, analyze and handle the emotional and physical needs to provide necessary support and care.

4. Observe and record the child's behavior and the interaction patterns during playing.
5. Protect children if their play becomes too aggressive and guide them into less destructive types of play activities.
6. Encourage all children to participate in all planned play programs. Nurses may also have an opportunity to participate with the children during play.
7. Teach the parents and other family members about the importance of play for therapeutic value, recreational value and all round development of personality.

Nurse should serve as an advocate, a spokesman, a diagnostic observer, source of support, planner and teacher to promote play for the children at hospital and home.

Preparation of Child for Diagnostic Tests

Advancement of medical technology and laboratory science has a greater impact in the modern health care services. The clinical diagnosis is confirmed by laboratory investigations, X-ray, ultrasonography and other diagnostic techniques. Outcome of the management can also be evaluated by these procedures.

The children with the differences in physical and emotional functions from adult, require special physical and psychological preparations for the diagnostic procedures. The approaches towards children will differ than that of adults to remove fear and anxiety and to gain co-operation during these interventions.

The diagnostic procedures are done in a variety of settings including laboratories, outpatient department and inpatient settings. Regardless of the setting, infants and children of all ages and their parents should be prepared before any procedures are done. Verbal explanation cannot be understood by very young children, but they can understand the parent's or nurse's softly spoken words and the touch of comfort. Older children should have all procedures explained in ways they can understand. Nurses can fulfill their responsibilities through adequate explanation and increasing the trust of the parents and children.

The pediatric nurses should have specific knowledge about the diagnostic procedure and they should explore about the knowledge of parents and children before preparing them for any procedures.

For the *psychological preparation* of parents and children the following guidelines can assist the nurse:

- Emphasis on the positive outcome of the procedure, its importance and purposes.
- Timing of the preparation should be settled. The initial preparation for certain procedures can be done by the parents at home. In hospital, nurse can prepare the parents and child prior to the procedure. Preparation should be done, if possible, when the child is rested and alert.

- Verbal preparation to be done with the use of specific words to explain the procedure. Parents and child should understand the explanation rather than confusion. Explanation to be given according to the level of maturity and understanding and past experience with medical care and discomfort. Nonthreatening terminology is used to reduce anxiety. Information to be given about sensations during procedures, which is more important than that about where and how the procedures will be done. Anxiety-producing information should be given at the end of the preparation.
- Use of visual aids is important to make the verbal explanation more concrete. The nurse, parents and child can play out the procedure to be done using the materials like intravenous equipment, syringe, stethoscope, etc. through dramatic play. A doll can be used by the nurse to demonstrate the procedure.
- Role-playing of the procedure to be done in which the child will take an active part. For example, the diabetic child who requires insulin injections can role-play by giving an injection to a doll initially.
- Evaluation of the preparation can be done through the verbal explanations of parents and children or the use of teaching aids. The knowledge of parents and child concerning the procedure to be evaluated. The process may stimulate further questions that the nurse can then answer.

The *physical preparation* of the child vary from one procedure to others. The major aspects are positioning, privacy, asepsis, restraint, etc, should be done accordingly.

Collection of Specimens for Laboratory Examination

During hospitalization of children, the nurse may carry out or assist in certain diagnostic procedures, including collection of specimens of urine, stool, sputum, throat swab, blood and cerebrospinal fluid. These procedures help in diagnosis of various disease conditions and to determine the therapeutic effects of the treatment given.

Infants and young children may not be able to co-operate when specimens are collected. They may not be able to understand the instructions given by the nurse or handle the equipment to be used. Therefore, the nurse has to follow special approaches during collection of specimens with the help from parents or other health team members.

When specimens are collected from the particular child, they must be accurately labeled and accompanied by the fill up laboratory form when sent to the laboratory for immediate processing to find out the normal or abnormal findings and values.

Collection of Urine Specimens

Urine specimens for laboratory examinations can be collected as routine urine specimen, clean-catch specimen and catheterized specimen for culture. Children who are not toilet-trained pose the greatest problem to obtain urine specimen.

Routine urine specimen collection from older children, who can co-operate with the nurse or the mother is relatively easy, but is more difficult from infants. Pediatric urine collection bag is used for infants. The nurse should wash own hands thoroughly before the application of the urine collection bag. After the external genitalia of the child has been cleaned and thoroughly dried, the collection bag is attached to the perineum in the girls. For boys, the penis and scrotum are inserted into the opening of the bag. The infant or toddler is placed in semi-Fowler position and a diaper is placed in position to prevent the displacement of bag. The nurse must check the bag frequently to prevent the urine from leaking and to obtain a fresh specimen for laboratory testing. When the child voids, the bag is removed and the specimen sent to the laboratory.

Clean-catch urine specimen: It is examined for rough estimation of number of bacteria present. In infant and small child, this specimen is obtained in a sterile urine collector. To obtain the specimen, the child's genitalia to be cleaned with soap and water using cotton balls and then rinsed with an antiseptic solution. After the genitalia is thoroughly cleansed, the skin is rinsed with sterile water and dried. When the child has voided, the urine is emptied into a sterile container. To obtain clean-catch specimen from preschool or older child, a sterile container or sterile specimen bottle can be used. Parents may assist in collection of urine. Adequate explanation to be given to the parents.

Urine can be collected as midstream specimen, but it is difficult to obtain from small children. If able to co-operate, the child voids a small amount into an unsterile container and then voids into a sterile container. Twenty-four hours urine collection may be needed in some children.

Collection of Stool Specimens

A stool specimen is collected by using spatula or spoon to transfer a freshly passed stool to a clean covered specimen container. The specimen should not be contaminated by urine. If a stool specimen cannot be obtained, a rectal swab may be taken by gently inserting a swab as far into the rectum as a thermometer is placed and twisting when removing it. Stool specimens and rectal swabs must be sent to the laboratory promptly, especially when it is examined for ova, parasites and cysts.

Collection of Blood Specimens

Blood specimens may be collected by laboratory technicians, physician or nurses. Nurse's responsibility is to prepare sterile articles and collection tubes or containers. The preparation of child for co-operation is very important. The older children are able to co-operate after an explanation of the procedures. The infants and young children cannot understand a verbal explanation. So mummy restraint to be used to complete the procedure quickly. Usually femoral vein puncture or antecubital fossa venipuncture is done to collect the specimen. After the puncture, firm pressure should be exerted over the vein for 3 to 5 minutes to prevents leakage of blood into the subcutaneous tissues following the collection of blood samples.

Children of all ages may fear the taking of samples of their blood. Explanation and application of band-aid may assure the children. Strict asepsis should be followed during collection of blood.

Peripheral capillary blood samples are taken from children by ear-lobe stab or finger stick methods. Peripheral blood samples are taken from infants by a heel stick.

Avoid contamination of specimen during and after collection of blood. Send the specimen to laboratory with label and filled up form. Help the child to verbalize the feeling.

Collection of Throat Swab

Collection of throat swab is an uncomfortable procedure. A sterile swab is used to obtain for throat culture. During collection of throat swab, the nurse should not permit it to touch the lips or tongue on entering or being removed from the mouth. The swab should touch only the most inflamed areas of the throat and tonsils. A tongue blade may be used to depress the tongue, so that the swab can be taken easily. The swab is then placed in a sterile container (test tube) to prevent it from drying prior to examination. Outside of the container should be kept clean to protect persons handling them. Special instructions, like not to wash mouth in the morning, before collection of swab, to be explained. Parents should assist during collection of swab to hold the child and to immobilize the child's head, which should be slightly tilt backward to obtain throat swab. The specimen to be sent to the laboratory promptly.

Collection of Sputum

The sputum specimen from a child who is too young to cough productively is difficult to collect. A suction device called mucus trap is used to obtain such specimen from trachea or bronchi. Children who are old enough to cough deeply and productively may be instructed to do so to collect the sputum specimens. Sputum to be collected with adequate instruction and should not mix with saliva or material from the throat. It can be collected most easily early in the morning before the child has had an opportunity to cough and swallow what was produced overnight.

Administration of Medications

Administration of medication is the most important nursing responsibility. The need for accuracy in preparing and giving medications to children is greater than that of adult. Since the pediatric dose is often relatively small in comparison with the adult dose, a slight mistake in the amount of a administered drug represents a greater error.

Safety Measures in the Administration of Drugs

Each child has five 'rights' during administration of medication, which will prevent most drug errors. A 'sixth' right has been added to this listing because it also will provide for a measure of safety when parents give medication to their child. These rights include the following:

The right patient, the right drug, the right dose, the right route, the right time and the right of the parents and the child "to know" (or right information). Other rights during administration of drugs include right assessment, right evaluation, right documentation and right to refuse treatment.

The right of the parents and child to know indicates the right to ask and the right to receive an answer to their questions regarding prescribed drug, its action and side effects. The nurse or the doctor is responsible for sharing this information to use the drug safely.

Medication History

Before administering medications to a child, it is important to obtain medication history. Some information such as presence of drug allergies can be obtained during history taking at the time of admission. Details information regarding name of the drugs, the dose and schedule, the reason for taking the drugs and any adverse reactions should be recorded for those drugs taken in the past and those being taken recently. If the baby is on breastfed, information to be collected regarding any medications taken by the mothers. These history can help to evaluate the child's tolerance and effectiveness of the drugs.

Calculation of Drug Dosage

Although most medications are supplied by the pharmaceutical companies in a convenient form or strength for a standard adult dose and children dose, but often children dosages are calculated as fractions of the adult dose.

Dosages based on the child's body surface area, give the most accurate results. The formula for determining a child's dose of medication based on body surface area is as follows:

a. $\dfrac{\text{Child's body surface area}}{\text{Adult's body surface area}} \times$ Adult dose = Estimation of child's dose.

b. Body surface area of child $(m^2) \times$ dose/(m^2) of surface area = Estimation of child's dose.

- Manufacturer's recommendations of drug dose per kg of body weight is usually followed for the drug therapy of children

Approach to Parents and Child

Parents can help the nurse to follow useful approaches during administration of medication. They may even be responsible for giving medications to their children. Older children may be responsible for own medication, if they are capable.

Administering medications to young children present a challenge to pediatric nurse. They may not co-operate during the procedure because of previous uncomfortable experiences depending upon the level of emotional, physical and intellectual development.

The nurse should follow the following suggestions to gain co-operation from children during administration of drugs:

- Prepare the child honestly with trusting relation and explanation.
- Approach positively and confidently.
- Encourage the child to participate in taking drugs.
- Distract the child to focus attention away from the procedure.
- Accept the child's reaction to the procedure.
- Reinforce the child's efforts to control and praise for co-operation.

Routes of Administration of Medications

The most common routes of giving medications are oral and parenteral. Rectal administration and instillation of drops into nose, ear and eye are also practiced in children. Intrathecal administration and inunction may be indicated for some children.

Oral administration of drugs: Pills, tablets and capsules are given to the older children who are able to co-operate in swallowing these forms of drugs. Liquid medications (syrup) are given generally to children below the age of 5 to 6 years because of the danger of aspiration of solid forms of drugs.

Liquid medications may be measured and given in the prescribed amount using various devices. These include glass or plastic medicine cup, 5 ml teaspoon, medicine dropper and plastic syringe. Accuracy is the prime importance in the measuring and administration of medications.

Infants generally accept medications put into their mouths that can be readily swallowed. The medication should be given along the side of the tongue slowly to prevent choking. The child can be placed on lap or in a semisitting position to prevent aspiration.

Toddlers and preschool children usually resist or refuse to take oral medications. They need explanation for co-operation. Sometimes these children need to restraint by the nurse's hand or by the parent. The child's head is held firmly and medication is given slowly to prevent aspiration.

The older child may also refuse to take oral medication. The nurse should approach firmly and positively. Explanation for co-operation and support help the child to receive the medication.

Parenteral administration of drugs: Parenteral route of giving medications means administering medications not through alimentary canal but by injection through intramuscular, intravenous, subcutaneous, etc.

1. *Intramuscular (IM) administration:* Injection of any kind can hurt and be painful. Preparation for an intramuscular (IM) injection should be given just before it is done, so that children do not have time to build up their anxieties. The child's reaction to the injection depends upon level of the neurological maturity. The infants usually cry due to injection but older children try to get away and need restraining so that the injection can be given as safe and painless as possible.

   Selection of site of injection is very important. Intramuscular injection should be given at a site away from major blood vessels and nerves and with adequate muscle tissues to retain and absorb the injected medicine. The IM injection sites in older children and adolescents are the same as for adults, i.e. the posterior gluteal, ventrogluteal, deltoid and quadriceps femoris muscles (rectus femoris). The preferred sites for infants and small children are ventrogluteal, vastus lateralis and rectus femoris muscles (Figs 8.3A to D).

   General principles of IM injection to be followed with strict aseptic technique. When injecting less than 1 mL of medication, use a tuberculin syringe for accuracy. After medication is drawn from vial, draw up additional 0.2 to 0.3 mL of air into the syringe, thus clearing needle of medication and preventing medication seepage from the injection site. Needle to be inserted at 45 degree angle in a downward direction toward the knee, when given in rectus femoris muscle. For other site insert needle perpendicular to surface on which the child is lying. The amount of medication should be 1 or 2 mL. After injection, massage the site, unless contraindicated. The complication of fibrosis and contracture of the muscle can be diminished by massage, and range of motion exercises to disrupt and stretch immature scar tissue when multiple

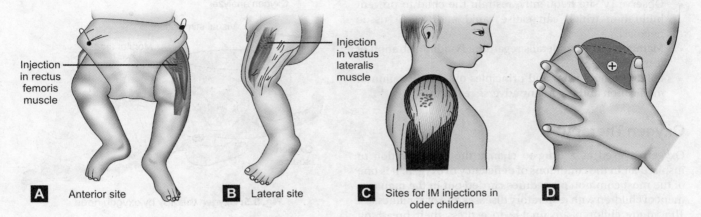

Figs 8.3A to D: Sites of intramuscular injection in children: (A) Rectus femoris; (B) Vastus lateralis; (C) Deltoid; (D) Ventrogluteal

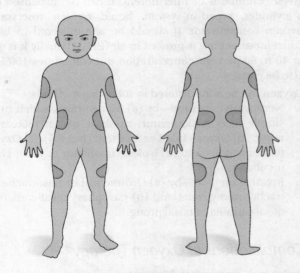

Fig. 8.4: Sites for insulin injection (SC)

injections are being administered. The drug is recorded along with the site of injection, so that injection sites can be rotated.

2. *Subcutaneous (SC) administration:* Certain drugs like insulin and heparin that are not irritating or available in heavy suspensions can be safely injected in small amounts subcutaneously. The sites, same as for IM injection can be used but additional areas of loose areolar tissue like anterior abdominal wall, interscapular or subscapular areas may also be utilized. A small syringe and needle are used and inserted in 45 degree angle holding the pinch of skin firmly between the thumb and index finger. The advantage of subcutaneous route include the presence of many sites for injection and rotation and unlikelihood of damage to vital nerves and blood vessels (Fig. 8.4).

3. *Intravenous (IV) administration:* Intravenous drugs are given more in pediatric practice. They are given to children who require a high serum concentration of a drug and to children who cannot absorb drugs from the gastrointestinal tract because of chronic diarrhea and other problems.

Several types of intravenous drug delivery systems are available. Three methods that can provide absolute control of drug delivery time are: (1) volume control set for single or intermittent administration of drug, (2) manual retrograde injection infusion for children whose fluids are restricted and (3) infusion pump system for continuous durg infusion. With these system only one drug is infused at a time and no flushing of intravenous system is required. Microdrip (60 drops makes 1 mL) is usually used for continuous infusion.

The nurse must be aware of the following aspects when giving drugs intravenously:

- The drug must be prepared for IV use.
- Strict aseptic precautions to be followed.
- Dilute IV medication and inject slowly as prescribed.
- Be knowledgeable regarding the used drugs in details.
- Intravenous drugs generally are not administered with blood or blood products.
- Only one antibiotic at a time should be given and should not be mixed with other drugs.
- Check the site of infusion for proper placement and signs of infiltration and any reactions.
- Heparin lock is used to provide a site for the intermittent administration of intravenous medications. Usually a blood vessel on the dorsum of the hand is used for the site of insertion. After insertion the heparin lock is flushed with a diluted solution of heparin (0.5 to 1.0 mL of a solution of 10 units of heparin per mL of physiologic saline solution). It is reflushed every 2 hours, especially after medication is given, to prevent clot formation.

- Observe IV site frequently, restrain the child to prevent infiltration which can cause rapid and severe tissue necrosis.
- Maintain record in details regarding IV administration of drugs.
- Follow general rules and principles of administration of medication and report any adverse reaction.

Oxygen Therapy

Oxygen is used as a drug to change the concentration of inspired air in the conditions of deficiency of oxygen. It is one of the most common procedures carried out in the management of children with respiratory diseases and other illnesses. The young children are unable to express their breathing discomfort. The pediatric nurse should have knowledge, good observation skill and ability for assessment of need for oxygen therapy.

Purpose of Oxygen Therapy

Oxygen is administered to achieve satisfactory level of PaO_2, range between 60 and 80 or 90 mm Hg. It is used as a temporary measures to relieve hypoxemia and hypoxia, but does not replace definite treatment of underlying cause of these conditions.

The general purposes of oxygen therapy are:
1. To correct hypoxemia and hypoxia.
2. To increase oxygen tension of blood plasma.
3. To restore the oxyhemoglobin in red blood cells.
4. To maintain the ability of body cells to carry on normal metabolic functions.

Assessment of Need for Oxygen Therapy

Oxygen administration is indicated in numbers of medical and surgical conditions. The need for oxygen is assessed by the followings:
1. Observing symptoms of respiratory distress and hypoxia i.e. inadequate breathing pattern, laboured respiration, dysrhythmias, cyanosis, change of activity like restlessness, lethargic and unresponsiveness, change in level of consciousness, hypothermia, etc.
2. Analysis of Arterial Blood Gases (ABGs) for PaO_2, $PaCO_2$, pH, HCO_3, etc.
3. Pulse oximetry.
4. Measuring of inspired O_2 concentration (FiO_2)

Methods of Oxygen Administration

It depends upon age and condition of the child, cause of hypoxia, required concentration of oxygen and ventilatory assistance, available facilities etc. Oxygen therapy can be

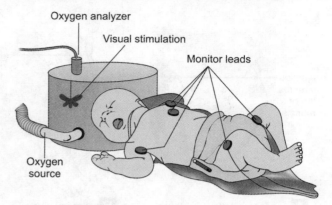

Fig. 8.5: Oxygen therapy by oxygen hood

given continuous or intermittent. It can be dispensed from a cylinder, piped-in-system, liquid oxygen reservoir or oxygen concentrator. It should be administered in higher concentration than is present in air (21%). Usually it is given in 40 to 60 percent concentration but sometimes 100% can also be given.

Oxygen can be administered by following methods:
1. Noninvasive method—by (a) oxygen mask which can be simple face mask, venturi mask or partial rebreathing mask, (b) Oxygen hood or face tent (Fig. 8.5). (c) Oxygent tent or canopy and (d) Isolette incubator or other closed incubator.
2. Invasive method—by (a) Orotracheal or nasotracheal or tracheostomy route and (b) nasopharyngeal catheter or nasal cannula or nasal prong.

Complications of Oxygen Therapy

Prolonged exposure to high concentrations of oxygen may result in constriction of cerebral blood vessels leading to irreversible brain damage and constriction of retinal blood vessels causing retinopathy of prematurity or retrolental fibroplasia. Pulmonary complications are pulmonary congestion, bronchiolar edema, bronchopulmonary dysplasia (in neonates), respiratory depression, necrotizing bronchiolitis, etc. Long-term complications due to oxygen toxicity are chronic pulmonary diseases, seizure disorders and epilepsy.

Safety Precautions during Administration of Oxygen

1. Oxygen acts as a drug—it must be prescribed and administered in specific dose in terms of rate, concentration and duration.
2. Humidifier and regulator must be used.
3. Oxygen should be warmed to room temperature.

4. It should be given at lowest concentration and for shortest period of time to achieve satisfactory level of SpO_2 or PaO_2. It is important to monitor PaO_2 that should not exceed 100 mm of Hg, as there is no clinical signs which indicate hyperoxia that result in oxygen toxicity.
5. Oxygen therapy to be discontinued gradually.
6. Precautions to be taken to prevent fire hazards.
7. General principles of oxygen administration to be followed. The child should be observed frequently. Recording of O_2 therapy to be maintained.

Care of Neonate in Incubator

Incubators are apparatus for maintaining optimal conditions of high risk preterm neonates. It is essential to provide an ideal microenvironment. The main functions of incubators are isolation, maintenance of thermoneutral ambient temperature, desired humidity and administration of oxygen. It is desirable to nurse extremely low birth weight stable babies (less than 1000 g) in the incubator. There should be easy access to the baby for all nursing procedures and easier observation of the baby from a distance. It should be easy to clean.

The incubator may be portable type for transport of sick babies or stationed in the nursery. It can be open box type or closed type. The closed type incubators (isolette) are used for intensive care and equipped with port holes for access to the infant. The servo-control system is ideal in isolette incubator. Skin sensor is affixed to the abdominal skin midway between umbilicus and xiphisternum and incubator is set for maintenance of desired skin temperature between 36.5°C and 37.5°C. Infant nursed under servo-mode should be watched to ensure that skin probe is in place. There should be in-built audio and visual alarms for set temperature, high body temperature, air flow, probe or sensor failure, etc.

Sterile water to be used in the humidity tank to prevent infection. As incubators are a potential source of infection, most centers are now using incubators without adding any water in the humidity chamber.

Expert nursing skill is essential for intensive care of the high risk neonates in the incubator. The incubator should be kept ready to receive the baby at any time. It should be checked for working condition with all its monitors functioning well. It is placed in a suitable place away from any heat source. Keep the incubator warm for use and decide the desirable temperature according to baby's weight and age. When the baby is placed in the incubator, suitable position to be done and the baby is kept naked for good observation. Sensor probe to be fixed on the abdomen by tape when the baby-mode incubator is used. It gives the reading of skin temperature. The heater inside the incubator warms the air to help to reach the set temperature of the baby. Be alert about the warnings given by monitors and take prompt action.

Close and constant observation to be done through transparent canopy. Provide gentle care and disturb the baby least. Use portholes to approach the baby, one side portholes for clean procedures, e.g. feeding, suctioning, injections, etc. and other side for dirty procedures like changing, cleaning, etc. Use gloves during procedures and special care to be taken to keep the portholes clean. Provide tactile stimulation to the baby at regular interval. Don't use the same incubator for more than seven days continuoulsy. Routine care of the baby should be provided with precautions of prevention of infection. Explanation to be given to the parent regarding indications and importance of incubator care, condition of the baby and possible outcome. Parents can be involved in baby care, whenever possible for routine activities.

After care of incubator is also important to prevent cross infection. All parts of the incubators to be disinfected and sterilized. All detachable parts should also be cleaned with antiseptic lotion. Formalin/formaldehyde may be used to sterilize the incubator. In general, infection-control measures to be followed when caring the baby in incubators.

When the baby is removed from an isolette or incubator, it is important that the infant should be dressed and wrapped with adequate clothing to conserve heat. A knitted cap should be used to prevent heat loss from the head. The parents should be informed about the routine care and warning signs for problems of the baby.

Techniques of Feeding

Maintenance of fluid and nutrition is vitally important for the sick child. An ill child can be given fluid and nutritional support to avoid the problems of severe depletion. These are given in several way, i.e. oral feeding, gavage feeding, gastrostomy feeding, intravenous and subcutaneous infusion and hyperalimentation. The choice of feeding method depends upon the age and condition of the child.

Oral Feeding

Feeding by mouth is preferable from physiologic stand point to other methods of feeding. Oral feeding utilize normal gastrointestinal metabolic processes and maintain intestinal mucosal integrity and function. Liquid, soft or solid feeding are given depending upon the child's condition.

Infants and young toddlers are encouraged to take adequate amounts of feeding at frequent intervals. Forced feeding to be discouraged because it may lead to vomiting. Diet planning to be done according to the cause of illness and to assist the child in maintaining or improving the level of growth and development already achieved before the illness.

Older children should offer feeding that they enjoy based on their likes and dislikes. Nurse can involve the children for planning of diet along with their parents and should keep record of fluid and food taken by the children.

Gavage Feeding

When the sick infant or child cannot take food by mouth, feeding can be given by gavage, i.e. administration of liquid nourishment through a stomach tube. It can be given intermittently or continuously.

The preterm baby who is unable to suck or swallow or who becomes fatigued with the effort of feeding should be fed by gavage. Infants or children having congenital anomalies of the throat or esophagus, difficulty in swallowing, respiratory distress or unconsciousness may be fed by gavage.

The gavage tube is passed into the stomach through the mouth or the nares. The tube may be inserted and removed at each feeding or it may be left securely in place for 24 to 72 hours depending upon the condition of the individual child or on the policy of the hospital; General principles for insertion of tube or gavage feeding to be followed. The following special considerations to be practiced:

- Positioning to be done on right-side or back with a folder towel places under shoulders to elevate the head slightly. The head of the bed in older child is elevated during feeding.
- Application of mummy restraint may be necessary to control the child's movements during tube insertion. Infants hand may be restrained using a soft restraint, to prevent grasp of gavage tube and it's removal.
- For gavage feeding of infant, sterile equipment to be used. Clean equipment may be used for older children.
- Feeding amount should be calculated.
- Sterile water or saline is used to lubricate the tube. Do not use oil because of the danger of aspiration into the lungs.
- For infants, tube is passed through the mouth. Small infants usually breaths through nose, so tube in the nostril can inhibit breathing. For older infants and children, pass the tube through more patent nostril.
- Feeding tube can be measured for correct length of insertion by two methods (a) measuring from the tip of the nose to the bottom of the ear lobe and then to the tip of the xiphoid process of the sternum and (b) measuring from the nose to the ear lobe and then to a point midway between the xiphoid process and umbilicus. For orogastric feeding tube from the tip of the nose to ear lobe and to midpoint between end of xiphoid process and umbilicus. For neonates, measure from the bridge of the nose to the lower tip of the ear lobe and then to the level of the stomach, to the midpoint between the xiphoid process and the umbilicus.
- Test the correct position of the tube in the stomach.
- The flow of feeding should be slow by gravity. Do not apply pressure. Elevate reservoir of feed (syringe barrel)

15 to 20 cm (6–8 inches) above the child's abdomen and in neonates 10 to 12 cm only.

- Feeding should be given about 5 mL per 5 to 10 minutes or 15 to 20 minutes total time.
- When feeding is completed the tube to be flushed with small amount of sterile water or air.
- If the catheter is to be left in place, it is capped or clamped to prevent entrance of air into the stomach and to prevent loss of feeding.
- Burp the child if possible after the feeding.
- Observe the child for any problem and place on right side for at least one hour.
- Record time of feeding, the type, amount of feed and response of the child to the feeding. Intake and output chart to be maintained.

Gastrostomy Feeding

If the sick child has an upper gastrointestinal tract anatomic abnormality or requires prolonged gavage feeding or has side effects from gavage feeding, then feeding can be given by gastrostomy or jejunostomy. Gastrostomy feeding is more preferable to jejunostomy feeding because digestion that normally occurs in the stomach is by-passed when jejunostomy is used.

A gastrostomy tube is inserted through the abdominal wall into the stomach while the child is under general anesthesia. The type of tube used may be a plain or a Foley's or any self-retaining catheter.

The procedure for feeding a child through a gastrostomy is similar to that of gavage feeding. The infant fed through a gastrostomy tube should be given the opportunity to satisfy the need for sucking. Care of the skin around the gastrostomy is very important to prevent irritation and infection. The area to be kept clean and covered with sterile dressing. The dressing must be changed and ointment to be used to aid in healing. After the wound heals, a dressing may not be necessary.

If the gastrostomy tube is a Foley's catheter, slight traction to be made to make certain that the balloon is at the gastrostomy opening. It must be secured in place, so that it does not move to pyloric sphincter and occlude it.

During feeding, elevate tube and reservoir to 10 to 12 cm (4 to 4¾ inches) above abdominal wall. Do not apply pressure to start flow of feed. Feed the child slowly taking 20 to 40 minutes. Avoid air entry during feeding and instill clear fluid when the feeding is completed. Place the child on right side or in Fowler's position after feeding. Record the procedure accurately.

When the child no longer needs the gastrostomy feeding, the tube is removed and the abdominal opening closes and contracts spontaneously or may need surgical closure.

Intravenous Infusion

Intravenous infusion of fluid is the most frequently used therapeutic measures in the care of children. The nurse has an important role and responsibility in monitoring this type of therapy. Although many of the principles used in administering parenteral fluids to adults are same and applicable in the care of children, there are some very important difference exist in the preparation of parents and child, calculation of flow rates, veins used for infusion, equipment and procedures and methods of protecting the child and the site of infusion.

Preparation of Parents and Child

Adequate explanation, showing another child who is having an intravenous infusion and restraint may be necessary to help them to co-operate with the procedure and to reduce their anxiety. Generally venipuncture is done in the treatment room and parents (one or both) can allow to support the child during the procedure. Older children should be instructed to use controlled breathing to control pain by inhale slowly and exhale through the mouth. The nurse should appreciate the child for co-operation and allow play materials to divert the feeling.

Calculation of Flow Rates

Nurse must calculate the flow rate to maintain desired amount of fluid intake. If a microdropper is used (60 drops makes 1 mL), the procedure is easy because the number of milliliters to be given per hour is the same as the number of drops per minute. If a microdropper is not used, the nurse can compute the flow rate by the following standard formula. In this formula, the drop factor, written as gtt (or drops) per mL (listed on the infusion set) depends on the type of infusion used. The formula is:

$$\frac{\text{Volume (capacity) of solution}}{\text{Time interval in minutes}} \times \text{drop factor} = \text{drops per minutes}$$

Veins Used for Intravenous Infusion

Several sites may be used for the injection of intravenous fluid. Scalp veins are preferred sites in the newborn and early infancy. Superficial scalp veins have no valves, they can be infused in either direction. For this procedure, an area of infant's scalp may have to be shaved carefully to visualize the site of venipuncture easily.

During infancy, the superficial veins of the hand, wrist, arm and foot may also be used for infusion. The sites used for giving IV infusion to older children are determined on the basis of accessibility. The child who is right handed would probably be happier if the infusion were given in the left arm.

Equipment and Procedure

All equipment should be sterile and scalp vein needles, IV set and IV solution and other required articles should be arranged accordingly. Restraint may be applied as appropriate and positioning to be done. Flow rate to be regulated as prescribed. Intravenous infusion pump may be used. The nurse must be familiar with the function of infusion pump and its use. Continuous monitoring of IV infusion is very important. Maintenance of intake and output chart should be done strictly. General principles of IV therapy to be followed as for adults.

Protecting the Child and the Site of Infusion

Protection of the site of infusion is important responsibility. Position of the part, limit the movement and secure the site with nonirritating tape, but do not obstruct the view of site. Parents and child should be explained about the problems of displacement of needle.

Another important responsibility of the nurse is to protect from infection and infiltration of fluid due to dislodgement of needle.

Infusion pump and tubing should be checked for running of fluid or any problems. If the infants and children are too ill to move their extremities or if their extremities are restrained, then passive range of motion exercises must be given periodically to promote comfort and ensure flexibility of muscles and joints. Older children should be provided with play activities as much as possible during the infusion.

Total Parenteral Nutrition or Hyperalimentation

Total parenteral nutrition (TPN) or intravenous alimentation is used to fulfill the total nutritional needs of those who cannot receive feedings by way of gastrointestinal tract. It is administered in small preterm infants, infants who have severe gastrointestinal anomalies and infants or children having intractable diarrhea or vomiting, extensive burns, inflammatory bowel disease or chronic bowel obstruction.

The usual intravenous solution contains electrolytes and sugar but no protein and fat, which are necessary for growth and maintenance of body tissue. The highly concentrated solution used in TPN contains hypertonic glucose, protein, electrolytes, vitamins, minerals and trace elements. Intralipid solution or emulsified fat that can be given intravenously can supply the required fatty acids. Iron can be administered by intramuscular injection or by transfusion.

This solution is given continuously by means of an infusion pump through a catheter places in the superior vena cava; which is reached by way of the external jugular, internal jugular or subclavian vein. Small peripheral veins cannot be used for this injection of the concentrated TPN.

Careful assessment of the infant or child having TPN is necessary because of danger of sepsis, fluid electrolyte imbalance, hyperglycemia, hypoglycemia and faulty rate of infusion. The prevention of infection is of paramount importance from the time of insertion of catheter. Special nursing care and accurate recording of intake and output, along with child's general condition are additional nursing responsibilities.

Procedures Related to Elimination

Constipation may be an indication of illness and the sick children many times become constipated during periods of hospitalization. They may become constipated because of inactivity, decreases muscle tone, inadequate hydration, dietary change or medications. Constipation is managed by adequate amount of fluid, diet, exercise, privacy, medications and enema. Some conditions may require the formation of ostomy for the purpose of elimination.

Enemas

Enemas are given to encourage the expulsion of feces and flatus, to soften stools, or to soothe mucous membranes. The reason for giving the enema determines the type of fluid to be used and the kind of enema to be given. The children should be explained and prepared adequately for the procedure. The procedure for giving enema to the child is similar with that for the adult but some alterations are necessitated by the anatomy and physiology of the child.

- The catheter size should be 10 to 12 french and should be inserted only 2 to 4 inches into the rectum depending upon the size of the child.
- Temperature of the solution should be 105°F or 40.5°C.
- An isotonic solution or physiologic saline is used. Tap water alone is not used because of the danger of a fluid shift and overload.
- The amount of fluid given depends on the size of the child. Infants are given 150 to 250 mL, young child 250 to 350 mL, older child 300 to 350 mL and adolescent 500 to 750 mL.
- The infant or young child is positioned by placing pillow under the head and back. The buttocks are places upon the bed pan, which has been covered with soft pad under the lower lumbar area. Pillows also can be arranged beneath the older child's back for comfort, when the bedpan is used.
- The enema can should not be held more than 18 inches above the level of the child's hips so that solution may run slowly by gravity and without pressure into the bowel. For infants and young children, 50 mL syringe barrel attached to a catheter may be used instead of enema can.
- Parents or nurse must hold the buttocks together to help the child retain the fluid, especially in infants and young

children. The older children need explanation for co-operation.
- The results of enema should be recorded carefully.
- For an oil retention enema, a funnel or syringe may be used. It is given with 100°F (37.7°C) temperature and 75 to 150 mL amount. Pressure over the anus to be given after retention enema so that it will not be immediately expelled. Peristalsis stimulation is avoided. A cleansing enema is given 30 to 45 minutes after the oil retention enema.
- Commercially prepared disposable pediatric enemas may be used only when specially prescribed. They can result in rapid, harsh action and can be dangerous when used on dehydrated children or on those who have megacolon.

Ostomies

The formation of an ostomy for the purpose of elimination is usually done in the infants and children having anorectal malformations and Hirschsprug's disease or congenital megacolon.

The surgical creation of a new opening on the surface of the body (abdominal wall) into the colon is a colostomy and into the ileum is an ileostomy. An ileal conduit is formed when the surgeon makes a short segment of small intestine into a conduit or pipeline for urine. The ureters are joined to one end of the intestinal conduit and the other end is made into a stoma on the skin surface.

The condition requiring an ostomy are mainly high anorectal malformations, intestinal atresia, Hirschsprung's disease, intestinal malrotation (volvulus), necrotizing enterocolitis, chronic ulcerative colitis, extensive injury or peritonitis following abdominal surgery.

Preparation of child and family: General principles of preparation for the procedure same as other surgery. Spot to be marked on the abdomen of child, preoperatively, where the ostomy will be done. Ostomy care to be taught to the parents and family members. Adequate explanation to be given about the indications of stoma, care of the stoma, use of colostomy bag, possible complications and necessary medical help.

Nursing management following surgery: Ostomy care can be given in two ways, i.e. without ostomy bag and with ostomy bag. During first one or two days following surgery, when the bag is not applied just after surgery, the stoma to be kept exposed to air and to be checked for bleeding. Care of the skin around the stoma is of vital importance. After the child has a liquid stool, the area is cleansed with soap and water and the skin is protected with aluminum paste or zinc oxide as prescribed by the doctor. A dressing made of squares of gauze or tissue paper with a hole cut in the middle to fit around the stoma, is placed over the protective substance.

The purpose of dressing is to absorb irritating drainage. It must be replaced after each liquid stool.

The stoma may be fitted with an ostomy bag in the operating room depending upon the type of ostomy and the surgeon's choice. During the first few days, postoperatively the child usually has a nasogastric tube, so there is little drainage from the stoma except for blood and mucus.

For infants, a small ostomy bag or a urine collection bag may be used to collect the liquid stool. Larger size bags are available for children and adolescents. To facilitate adherence of the bag and to protect the skin from irritation, a liquid skin barrier may be used which is applied only on healthy skin. The skin barrier (stomahesive) or other peristomal covering is available which is made of gelatin, pectin and other substances. It is available in powder, paste or wafer forms. The wafer form can be cut to fit the stoma, thus protecting the skin.

When an ostomy bag is used, soaps containing perfume and creams should not be used on the skin because they interfere with adhesion of the bag. Plain water is recommended to cleanse the area, as soap of any kind tends to further dry the skin.

If a sigmoid colostomy has been done on an infant, the stools are usually formed, so it is not necessary to use collecting device. Vaseline may be put on the skin around the stoma and a diaper can be applied.

Care of the colostomy and ileostomy in the infant and young child is based on the same principles and is essentially the same as that for an adult, with the following exceptions:

1. Colostomy irrigation is not part of management in small children. Irrigation is primarily for the purpose of regulating the colostomy to empty at regular intervals. Because children have bowel movements at more frequent intervals, this type of control is not feasible. Irrigation should be done only in preparation for diagnostic tests or surgery and occasionally for the treatment of constipation.
2. Observation of drainage for amount and characteristics is important to provide fluid replacement and prevent dehydration.
3. Prevention and treatment of skin excoriation around the stoma is primary concern. Ostomy bag to be checked every 2 hours for leakage and to be changed as soon as leakage is suspected.
4. Teach the parents about the importance of emptying the bag when it is 1/4 to 1/3 full and about the treatment of skin breakdown.
5. For older children with ostomies, "potty training" can be given for ostomy pouch emptying.
6. Care at home to be taught to the parents, family members and older children with the help from community health nurse. Important aspects of home care are:
   - Ostomy bag should be changed at least once a week or more frequently.
   - The child can take bath with the bag off, allowing for inspection of the stoma and the abdominal skin.
   - Encourage care of ostomy as part of normal activities of daily living.
   - Observe for signs of stomal complications which include ribbon like stool, diarrhea, failure of evacuation of stool or flatus, and bleeding.
   - Small frequent meals to be provided for the child with avoidance of foods that cause gas and diarrhea such as cabbage, spicy foods, beans, fruits, etc.
   - Measures to be taken to prevent infections (virus) and dehydration.
   - Encourage medical follow-up, good health and hygiene and supportive care from ostomy group.

Basic Care of Children Undergoing Surgery

The infant and children have different types of surgical problems than that of adults. Especially the congenital malformations are the important causes of surgical interventions in children. Another common surgical problem in children is acute abdomen. Success of surgery in pediatric population depends upon expert team approach with special attention on replacement of fluid loss, continuous monitoring of vital signs to detect complications, prevention of infections and emotional support.

Surgery can be planned or unplanned, i.e. elective or emergency. It is potentially stressful experience for children. They may not understand the reason for surgery and can think of an unjustifiable attack on their bodies. Potential threat for surgery to the children are physical harm, pain, injury, death, separation from parents, strange and unknown situation at operation room, fear of anesthesia and surgery, etc.

Preparation of children for surgery is an important aspect and should be based on child's age, developmental stage, level of personality and past experience. It should begins with preparation for admission to the hospital. In emergency surgical interventions, preparation should be done in modified ways but basic approach should be same. For day care surgery, which is usually a minor procedure, preparation should be done according to the type of operation.

Preoperative Nursing Management of Children

Preoperative nursing management for children include psychological preparation, physical preparation, protective measures and preoperative teaching. Details nursing history and physical assessment are done as for other pediatric admissions to the hospital. The nurse should give special attention to the history of other surgical interventions the child has had and the reactions of the child to those experiences. Necessary laboratory and radiological investigations should be performed as required.

Psychological Preparation

During preoperative period the nurse should develop trusting relationship with the child and parents. Parents must present during the stressful experience of the child. The nurse should assess the level of understanding and anxiety of the child and parents and their coping abilities. The following nursing interventions help to promote co-operation and reduce fear, anxiety and negative emotional reactions of the child and parents. These interventions include:

- Discuss about the type of surgery. Explain the information to the child and parents.
- Explain about the preoperative medication which can cause discomfort.
- Discuss about anesthesia and operating room set up and transportation to OT.
- Explain about the limitation of diet, nothing per mouth at least 4 to 6 hours prior to surgery or as directed by the anesthesiologist.
- Demonstrate the equipment to be used postoperatively such as oxygen mask. IV fluid set, urinary catheter, etc.
- Describe the postoperative discomfort and pain which may be relieved by medications.
- Explain about the recovery room care and set up.
- Demonstrate the procedures to prevent postoperative complications such as deep-breathing and coughing exercise.
- Do not remove favourite toys and other objects to prevent loss of security. Encourage child to play with cap, gown, mask and gloves with the dressed doll.
- Assure the child that the parent will be nearby and waiting for him or her.

Physical Preparation

- Monitor temperature, pulse, respiration, blood pressure, body weight, skin rash or any other abnormalities. Record the findings and report to the appropriate authority.
- Give nothing by mouth for the period prescribed prior to surgery or at least 4 to 6 hours before operation. Take the child away from the area where other children are taking food.
- Maintain good hydration, if needed IV fluid therapy to be administered as prescribed.
- Make certain that all other prescribed preoperative procedures have been completed such as collection of investigation report, anesthetic check up, signature in consent form, antiseptic dressing of operative area, bowel clearance, nasogastric tube insertion, hygienic measures (bathing, OT dressing), etc. Shaving of the operative area may not be necessary on children or may be done after they are anesthetized.
- Check for any loose teeth, secure the loose tooth and report.
- Remove nail polish and makeup if any.
- Eye glasses, hearing aids may be worn to the OT and then taken to the recovery room or can be given to the parent to prevent loss or damage.
- Ask the child to empty the bladder to prevent bladder incontinence or distension.
- Administer prescribed preoperative medications in time. Encourage the child to cry or scream for the injection or for the fear of operation.
- Transfer the child to the OT at the given time and handover to the OT nurse with all necessary things, records, reports and case sheet.

Protective Measures

- Obtain an informed written consent for anesthesia and surgical intervention as a legal protection.
- Check that all laboratory reports (blood, urine), X-ray and any other tests are included in the case sheet.
- Record complete information regarding premedication, preoperative procedures, child's emotional and physical state to protect from legal problems.
- Make sure that identification band for the child is attached securely to prevent faulty identification.
- Allow one familiar person to stay with the child to avoid fear of strange. The child should not be left alone to provide a sense of security and emotional protection. There is chance of fall or physical injury when premedication are given, so to protect from accidental injury the child should be attended by familiar one.
- Make sure that the child is send to the OT with all documents and necessary precautions.

Postoperative Nursing Management of Children

Nursing responsibilities in the postoperative management include meeting both physical and psychological needs of the child. Operation bed and necessary articles to be kept ready for receiving the child and to provide immediate post-anesthetic care in the recovery room or in the pediatric unit.

Immediate postoperative care

- Receive the child with details information about the operation performed and the case sheet recorded accurately.
- Check vital signs and give oxygen therapy, if needed.
- Maintain patent airway by placing the child on side or abdomen to allow secretions to drain and to prevent tongue from obstructing pharynx.
- Suction any secretions present.
- Restrain the child to prevent dislodging of IV channel, drainage tube and dressing.
- Monitor and record vital signs, blood pressure, bleeding, vomiting, dehydration, signs of shock, level of

consciousness, restlessness, skin color, cyanosis, pallor and other complications.

- Check the nasogastric tube (if any) and aspirate at the given interval and record the amount.
- Administer prescribed medications and record in the case sheet.
- Monitor IV infusion flow rate as directed.
- Check for any drainage tube and connect with the bottle or bag for continuous drainage.
- Give the child nothing per mouth till complete awake from anesthesia and begin feeding with sips of water when directed.
- Maintain intake and output chart accurately.
- Explain the parent about the treatment plan.
- Maintain warmth and cleanliness.

Care after recovery from anesthesia

- Continue to make frequent observations in regard to vital signs, behavior, hydration, urination, dressing, operative site, drainage, bowel sound, passage of flatus, crying, pain, or any signs of complications.
- Change the position frequently to minimize discomfort and complications.
- Administer prescribed medications with precautions and record the effects.
- Continue IV infusion, nasogastric aspiration and other drainage as required.
- Provide diet as prescribed. For major surgery, start oral feeding when bowel sound is audible, no vomiting present, no aspiration required and bowel movement established. First feeding is given usually with clear liquid, if tolerated advance slowly to full diet as per age. Note any vomiting or abdominal distension. Diet should contain high protein and vitamin 'c' to promote healing. High fluid intake should be encouraged.

- Maintain adequate rest periods and sleep. Allow early ambulation and self care as possible.
- Prevent infections by aseptic measures, appropriate wound care and change of dressing, breathing-coughing exercise, etc.
- Provide good general hygiene with special emphasis on mouth care, skin care, care of bladder and bowel.
- Follow preventive measures for postoperative complications like shock, hypoxia, hemorrhage, wound infections, abdominal distension, hypostatic pneumonia, atelectasis, retention of urine, thrombophlebitis, embolism, emotional stress, etc.
- Provide emotional support, reassurance, recreation and diversion.
- Plan for removal of stitches, if required, usually 5th to 7th day and prepare for discharge from hospital.
- Teach the parents regarding continuation of care at home, rest, diet, medications, special procedures and follow-up. Provide written instructions and arrange for referral to community health nurse whenever needed.

Nurse play vital role for improved care and better outcome of hospitalized child. In the care of sick child, pediatric nurses are responsible to maintain legal and ethical aspects. Negligence and malpractice are possible involving all areas of pediatric nursing practice. Intelligent and expert nursing care help to handle the problems related to child health care. Nursing personnel working in the hospitals or health care delivery system need to develop skill and competence to assess the problems of the sick child and to plan, implement and evaluate the care given to them. Nurses also need to anticipate the anxiety of the parents and to provide necessary support to the parents and family members. Family centered care, parental participation and more psychological approach should be emphasized during comprehensive care of the sick child.

Common Health Problems during Childhood

9

- Fever
- Excessive Cry
- Vomiting
- Diarrhea
- Constipation
- Abdominal Pain
- Abdominal Distension

- Allergies
- Poisoning
- Bites and Stings
- Foreign Bodies
- Multiple Injury
- Failure to Thrive
- Developmental Disorders

INTRODUCTION

Children are prone to various minor and major health problems. About 3/4th of the children are considered as unhealthy and surviving with impairment of physical and intellectual functions due to poor health status. Early detection and anticipation of the problems may prevent impairment, disability and fatal outcome. The common childhood problems found in health care settings or in community health units or at home, need immediate interventions. Nurses play vital role for the prevention and management of these conditions. Some of the common health problems during childhood period are discussed in this chapter.

FEVER

Fever or pyrexia is the elevation of body temperature above normal, i.e. 37°C or 98.4°F. It is very common health problem in children. It is a symptom related to various disease condition.

There is variations in increased body temperature. Pyrexia is classified as the followings:

- *Low pyrexia*—37.1°C to 38.4°C (99°F–101°F)
- *Moderate pyrexia*—38.4°C to 39.5°C (101°F–103°F)

- High pyrexia—39.5 to 40.6°C (103°F–105°F)
- *Hyper pyrexia*—Above 40.6°C (105°F).

Causes of Fever in Children

The heat regulating center in the hypothalamus is not well developed in the infants. So they cannot tolerate extreme heat or cold. Besides this, common causes of fever in infants and children are:

- Dehydration, excessive diuresis, hot environment and evening time of the day, excitement and exertion.
- Infections, e.g. ARI, malaria, meningitis, urinary infections, typhoid fever, measles, etc.
- Injury or disturbance of hypothalamus or brain.
- Side effects of drugs, toxins, vaccines, chemical substances, etc.
- Disease conditions like leukemia, systemic lupus erythematosus, tuberculosis, rheumatic fever, etc.

Clinical Manifestations Associated with Fever

The clinical features of particular cause of fever may be associated with the problem. But the features due to or related to fever include the followings:

- Hot dry skin, dehydration, flashed face.
- Thirsty, nausea, vomiting and loss of appetite.
- Headache, body ache, malaise, high colored scanty urine.
- Increased pulse rate and respiration rate.
- Chill, rigor, delirium, fainting attack or convulsions and other harmful effects may found on central nervous system due to prolonged hyperpyrexia.

Investigations

Detection of underlying cause of fever is very important to prevent harmful effects by early interventions. Thorough physical examination including details history of illness and related conditions help in clinical diagnosis. But various laboratory and radiological investigations are necessary to detect the exact cause and to implement the appropriate management. The following investigations may be planned:
- Urine for routine examination and culture-sensitivity test.
- Blood for total count, differential count, ESR, malarial parasite, Widal test, culture-sensitivity test, etc.
- CSF examination to detect CNS infections.
- Bone marrow examination.
- Throat swab culture to detect sore throat.
- Chest X-ray to exclude tuberculosis.

Management of a Child with Fever

Management of fever is initially symptomatic but the exact cause to be detected and management to be started in the earliest possible time. Antibiotic trial is not rational and may be harmful to the children.

Management depends upon the findings of history, physical examination and investigations. History should be collected regarding duration and pattern of fever, associated symptoms like convulsions, cough and cold, or recent vaccination. Detail physical examination should include head to foot examination, vital signs, blood pressure, neurological signs, examination of throat and all other systems.

Reduction of body temperature is the vital aspect of management. It can be done by giving tepid sponge, applying ice bag or fanning in cool airy environment with good ventilation. Administering antipyretic drugs, paracetamol 10 to 15 mg/kg of body weight, when body temperature is above 38.5°C or 101°F and repeating, if necessary.

Provision of rest and comfort to reduce metabolic rate and allowing more oral fluid to prevent dehydration are important supportive measures. Light, liquid and easily digestable high caloric diet to be planned according to child's condition. Maintenance of personal hygiene especially, special mouth care, care of skin and loose absorbent cotton clothing are essential. Arrangement of toys and other play materials help the child to cooperate and adjust with the illness.

Monitoring and recording of vital signs, condition of the child, therapeutic effects of the management should be done. Accurate technique to be followed for temperature measurement at same time and same method.

Early diagnosis of underlying cause and specific treatment of the condition should be initiated as soon as possible for better outcome.

EXCESSIVE CRY

Excessive cry can be defined as persistent crying of the child instead of fulfilling all biological needs and bodily comforts. When cry is present for a long period and beyond normal limit then it is termed as excessive cry, because to a particular extent cry is normal.

Cry is the only language which the neonates have. It is one of the first way to communicate with external environment for hunger, thirst, chill and need for mothering. Normal cry is lusty, frequent and encourage expansion of lungs.

Causes of Excessive Cry

There are various causes which makes the infant cry excessively. The causes can be divided into three groups.

Nonpathological Conditions

The common causes of excessive cry are mainly non-pathological. Mother or primary care giver or nurse should be good observer to find out the cause. These causes are hunger, thirst, wet nappy, chilling, high or low environmental temperature or excessive heat or cold, discomfort position, tight or over clothing, open safety pin, insect bites, over stimulation, sudden loud noise, etc.

Pathological Conditions

Serious causes of excessive cry are mainly related to pathological conditions. They include abdominal colic or distension, high fever, constipation, infections or inflammations (meningitis, otitis media, oral thrush), any accidental injury or surgical conditions.

Emotional Conditions

Emotional deprivation makes the child to cry excessively. Infants cry due to fear and helplessness when parents leave them or favorite toys are taken away.

The child can cry due to unanticipated events like change in food or routine activity, separation from parent, stranger approach, etc. Excessive cry can be found in anger and frustration due to lack of mothering, disturbed play, lack of sleep and inappropriate parent-child relationship.

Types of Cry

Quality of cry in infant is very important for assessing the problems and cerebral functions.

- Low, angry, lusty cry indicates normal infant.
- Persistent or continuous cry indicates hunger.
- Weak and whining cry indicates ill infant.
- High pitched, penitrating cry indicates cerebral irritation.
- Cat like screeching cry indicates chromosomal defect.

Management of Excessive Cry

- Assessment of cause and types of cry by close observation, physical examination and details history help in appropriate interventions.
- Nonpathological causes can be managed by the parents and family members by identifying the cause and removing it. Nurse should provide necessary guidance to detect the cause, whenever needed and when the child is brought to the health care setting for excessive cry.
- Emotional conditions need interventions by the nurses or professional persons to remove the cause of emotional deprivations. Parents usually need counseling and guidance on child rearing.
- Pathological conditions need to be diagnosed by necessary investigations and early interventions to be arranged. These children may require hospitalization, medications, surgical procedures and supportive measures to prevent complications. Nurse should assist and participate in the management by necessary assessment, planning, interventions and evaluation. Parental support and necessary explanation about the condition of the child are also important nursing responsibilities.

VOMITING

Vomiting is the most common symptom found during infancy and childhood. It is a reflex process governed by the vomiting center of the medulla oblongata. It can be defined as forceful expulsion of stomach content through the mouth. During vomiting, duodenum contracts in spasm, its' content reflux into the stomach and then through vigorous contractions of abdominal muscles, the stomach is emptied forcefully. Usually glottis and soft palate close the air passage to prevent aspiration of stomach content.

Occasional vomiting needs little attention. But frequent and persistent vomiting may be serious and requires further evaluation. It can lead to dehydration, electrolyte imbalance, metabolic alkalosis and aspiration of vomitus resulting asphyxia, pneumonia or atelectasis.

Vomiting can be accompanied by other features like excessive salivation, tachypnea, tachycardia, sweating, dilated pupil, pallor, etc.

Causes of Vomiting

Causes of vomiting can be grouped into nonorganic and organic causes.

Nonorganic Causes

The following nonorganic causes are found in various age groups:

Neonates: Swallowed amniotic fluid or blood, faulty feeding techniques, swallowed air due to erratic feeding, possetting and side effects of drugs.

Early infancy: Excessive cry, faulty feeding, overfeeding, rumination, introduction of soild, loneliness, etc.

Late infancy and childhood: Forced feeding, emotional disorders as attention seeking behavior in poor parent-child relationship, motion sickness, repetitive swinging movement, sudden excitement, fear, anxiety, unpleasant sight or odor and cyclic vomiting.

Organic Causes

Infections: Intrauterine infections, septicemia, meningitis, encephalitis, acute gastroenteritis, acute respiratory infections, pertussis, viral hepatitis, tonsilitis, otitis media, urinary tract infections, acute appendicitis, pancreatitis, necrotizing enterocolitis, etc.

Mechanical conditions: Congenital hypertropic pyloric stenosis, esophageal atresia, malrotation of gut, duodenal atresia, volvulus, intussusception, hiatus hernia, esophageal diverticulum, pylorospasm, gastroesophageal reflux, etc.

Neurological: Birth asphyxia, birth defect of central nervous system, birth injuries, intracranial SOL, hydrocephalus, intracranial hemorrhage, increased intracranial pressure, subdural hematoma, etc.

Metabolic: Diabetes mellitus, uremia, galactosemia, hypoglycemia, cholemia, hypercalcemia and inborn error of metabolism.

Toxic: Ingestion of irritant food or drug, food poisoning, allergic food intake, postnasal discharge or dripping.

Emotional: Anorexia nervosa, migraine, psychogenic habit vomiting, etc.

Assessment

The cause of vomiting is assessed by details history about the condition, complete physical examination and necessary investigations.

Thorough history to be collected about the vomiting episodes including duration, frequency and amount of vomiting, appearance of vomitus with or without presence of bile, blood, or fecal material, type and amount of oral intake and timing of vomiting in relation to oral feeding, etc. History of associated symptoms like fever, headache, earache, abdominal pain, weight loss, drowsiness, confusion, etc. should be excluded. History of exposure to any infected persons like diarrhea, mumps or any other infections are also essential.

A complete physical examination to be done including careful abdominal examination, auscultation of bowel sound and palpation for tenderness. Assessment of general condition, vital signs, blood pressure, urine output, hydration status, body weight are also important.

Laboratory and radiological investigations to be planned according to the probable cause of vomiting to confirm the diagnosis.

Treatment

No treatment is required for the children having vomiting due to nonorganic causes. Only sips of water to be given after vomiting. Parents need explanation and reassurance for the correct feeding technique and necessary modifications in child care practices.

The organic causes should be diagnosed early and medical or surgical management should be performed according to the particular condition and cause.

Nursing Interventions

- Continuous observation should be done to assess child's condition and recording of findings.
- Administration of IV fluid therapy to prevent fluid electrolyte imbalance and maintenance of intake and output chart.
- Administration of prescribed medications, especially antiemetics.
- Arrangement of planned investigations of blood, X-ray, ultrasonography of abdomen, scanning, etc.
- If not contraindicated, feeding should be given in small amount frequently with clear fluids, ice chips, milk, breastfeeding, diluted fruit juices, then gradually transfer to semisolid and solid food. High fat in diet to be avoided. Slight head-up position to be maintained during feeding.
- Care to be taken to prevent aspiration of vomitus by turning head to one side.
- General cleanliness and hygienic measures to be maintained. Especially after vomiting, neck folds, face, back of the ear to be cleaned. Mouthwash to be given.
- Involving parent in child care and providing emotional support to the parents.
- Following aseptic measures and universal precautions for prevention of cross infection.

- Participating in medical and surgical management.
- Teaching the parents about care during vomiting, feeding technique, hygienic measures, emotional care by love and affection, avoiding over protection, etc.

DIARRHEA

See the Chapter 16 related to gastrointestinal system.

CONSTIPATION

Constipation is a common problem found in children. It is infrequent passage of dry and hard stool often with difficulty and pain. The most common form of constipation is functional or nonorganic which is often familial. Chronic constipation is common but acute constipation may occur due to organic causes.

Causes of Constipation

The causes of constipation can be classified as follows:

Nonorganic Causes

Insufficient intake of food and starvation or under-nutrition, lack of fluid intake and dehydration, artificial feeding in infants, delayed introduction of solid food, lack of roughage in diet or low residue diet in older children, high protein and low carbohydrate ratio in diet, poor toilet training, unclean toilet, faulty bowel habit, lack of exercise, emotional disorders (like fear, anger) are usually found as nonorganic cause.

Organic Causes

Lack of muscle tone in chronic illness, malnutrition, rickets, intestinal parasitosis, cystic fibrosis, prolonged vomiting, hypertrophic pyloric stenosis, duodenal atresia, meconium ileus, intestinal obstruction, Hirschsprung's disease, anal fissure, anorectal malformation (stenosis, stricture), spinal cord lesions, cerebral palsy, cretinism, myotonic dystrophy, lead poisoning and adverse drug effect are the common organic causes.

The children with chronic constipation may have symptoms like abdominal discomfort, flatulence, anorexia, nausea, vomiting, headache, disturbed sleep, abdominal pain, rectal pain, etc. Other associated features may be found related to particular cause of constipation.

Management of constipation depends upon the specific cause. Diagnostic measures include details history of bowel pattern, through physical examination, laboratory tests (stool, urine, blood), radiological investigations (Barium enema) and abdominal ultrasonography. Organic causes are managed by medical or surgical interventions as needed for the particular condition.

The *management of nonorganic causes* includes the following interventions:

- Explanation and reassurance to the parents about the nature and cause of constipation.
- Increasing intake of fluid and water.
- Allowing balanced diet with high residual foods including roughage, more carbohydrate (adding sugar), leafy vegetables, fruits, etc.
- Encouraging the older child for regular bowel habit at a particular time every day and without hurry and distractions.
- Arranging suitable toilets and toilet seat.
- Improving hygienic measures and motivating the older child to solve own problem.
- If required, stool softener or mild laxative, or suppositories or enemas can be used. Suppository or medications should not be used frequently.
- If the condition worsen, medical help to be taken for detection of any organic cause and management.
- Informing the parents about the prevention of constipation by simple measures. Managing the nonorganic causes and appropriate toilet training are important aspect of prevention of constipation. Nurse should explain the preventive measures and answer the questions as asked by the parents and children.

ABDOMINAL PAIN

Abdominal pain is a common complaint and most children experience it at some time. Acute abdominal pain may be a serious problem requiring hospitalization and immediate interventions. Chronic and recurrent abdominal pain is common in school aged children which require thorough investigations and specific management.

Assessment of abdominal pain begins with collection of history regarding onset, duration, precipitating factors, location, severity, presence of other symptoms, etc. Abdominal examination in a relaxed and quiet approach helps to identify the cause which can be confirmed by other necessary investigations like examination of stool, urine and blood, X-ray abdomen, abdominal ultrasonography and endoscopy, etc.

Causes of Abdominal Pain

a. Acute abdominal pain are commonly caused by acute gastroenteritis, hepatitis, peritonitis, intestinal obstruction, appendicitis, necrotizing enterocolitis, pancreatitis, urinary tract infections, lower lobe pneumonia, abdominal trauma, etc.

b. Chronic and recurrent abdominal pain may be due to functional pain, milk allergy, chronic constipation, malabsorption, abdominal infections, dysentery, amebiasis, giardiasis, worm infestations, abdominal tuberculosis, irritable bowel syndrome, hydronephrosis, lead poisoning, abdominal epilepsy, Hirschsprung's disease, etc.

Abdominal pain may present with associated features like high grade fever, anorexia, nausea, vomiting, reduced activity level, jaundice-weight loss, abdominal mass, tenderness, distension, etc. Organic causes of abdominal pain may present with sudden onset of severe pain which may awakens the child from sleep, or as referred pain or localized pain in nonperiumbilical region. Inconsistent and nonspecific pain in periumbilical region indicates functional pain.

Management

Pain assessment is an important responsibility of nursing personnel. Exact cause of abdominal pain can be detected with good observation, history and physical examination.

Management of abdominal pain depends upon its nature and cause. Minor pain that resolve spontaneously does not require further attention. Persistent pain, which is severe enough to effect the activities, needs complete investigations.

Parents and older children should be explained and reassured about the nature of abdominal pain, possible management and prognosis. Psychogenic abdominal pain of the child requires relief of parental tension and conflict in the child. Development of trusting relationship with parents, child, and health care providers are essential.

Hospitalization may be required for symptomatic management of pain and treatment of particular cause. Acute abdominal pain may be due to surgical conditions and requires surgical intervention. Pain may be relieved by anticholinergic drugs. Oral intake of fluid and food may be allowed or restricted according to child's tolerance and associated features. Chronic abdominal pain may be treated at OPD or hospital admission may require to treat the exact cause.

ABDOMINAL DISTENSION

Abdominal distension is a common problem usually associated with intestinal obstruction and infections. It occurs when abdomen stretched out or inflated with air, gas and secretion and needs immediate attention.

Common causes of abdominal distension are acute gastroenteritis, intestinal obstruction, congenital malformation of GI tract, peritonitis, pneumonia, septicemia, electrolyte imbalance, etc.

Other associated features which may found with abdominal distension are abdominal pain, nausea, vomiting, absence of stool, respiratory distress, increased pulse rate, increased abdominal girth, loss of appetite, malaise, etc.

Management

Early detection of problem and prompt management of the condition help in prevention of complications. Assessment of the child's condition and detection of cause are the important aspects of management. Other measures include the followings:

- Gastric intubation to aspirate the GI secretions and to relief from distension. It also helps to reduce respiratory distress related to distension and to prevent possibility of aspiration of GI secretions to lungs.
- Administration of IV fluid to maintain fluid electrolyte balance. Maintenance of intake and output chart.
- Keeping the child in nothing per mouth till the distension is relieved.
- Monitoring vital signs and other problems and recording the findings.
- Protection from cross infection and maintenance of hygienic measures and elimination patterns.
- Explanation and reassurance to the parent and giving necessary instruction to participate in child care.
- Specific management of the cause by medical and surgical measures.

ALLERGIES

Allergy is an abnormal acquired immune response to a foreign substance. It is a state of changed reactivity in a host as a result of contact with an allergen. It is an adverse consequences resulting from the interaction of an allergen with humoral antibody and/or cellular immune response. Sensitization or an initial exposure to the allergen is required. Subsequent contact with the allergen result in a broad range of reactions.

Allergy is a problem of great importance in children. It is difficult to avoid allergy but early detection and prompt management are essential to prevent complications and recurrence.

The common allergens are various food items, drugs, animal hair, feathers, dust, pollens, insect bites, infections, cosmetics, oils, etc. These allergens are introduced by skin contact (e.g. cosmetics) or by inhalation (pollen)or by ingestion (food items) or injection (drugs).

The mechanism of allergy is not well understood, but the factors responsible for the condition include the followings:

a. *Hereditary predisposition:* Positive family history of allergy is found in about 60 percent of cases.
b. *Exposure to sensitizing factors:* Previous exposure of allergen is responsible for this immune response.
c. *Psychological factors:* Release of histamine in psychological disturbance may precipitate the allergic symptoms.

Asthma and eczema may develop due to emotional disturbances.

d. Infections are common allergens and allergic children are more liable to upper respiratory infections. Other conditions like acute nephritis, rheumatic fever, scabies, etc. have been associated with allergic reaction.
e. Drugs may produce allergic symptoms mainly antibiotics, aspirins, etc.

Types of Allergic Reactions

There are four types of allergic reactions:

1. *Type I (immediate):* It is rapid and immediate reactions of local or systemic anaphylaxis and mediated by IgE. The local response includes urticaria, asthma, angioedema and systemic reaction as life-threatening anaphylaxis. Allergen reaches the blood stream and triggering massive release of chemical mediators that produce laryngeal and pulmonary edema with severe bronchial obstruction and vasodilation which can cause shock due to increased vascular permeability.
2. *Type II (cytotoxic):* It is initiated by allergen as antigen-antibody reaction and mediated by IgG and IgM that causes cell damage. Transfusion reaction and drug reaction are type II allergic reaction which is produced due to lysis of blood cells and other cells.
3. *Type III (immune complex):* It occurs in sensitized people, when antibody (IgG and IgM) attached to antigen (allergen) creating a complex and damage the walls of blood vessels or the basement membrane. It causes local inflammation and massive complement activations. Serum sickness is a Type III reaction characterized by fever, joint pain, muscle pain, urticaria and lymphadenopathy. It develops in sensitized people who receive penicillin or sulfonamides or antitoxins.
4. *Type IV (cell-mediated):* This reaction is mediated by T-lymphocytes. Contact dermatitis is one of the type IV reaction. It occurs in many common allergens like rubber, leather, nickel, etc. Contact dermatitis is manifested by acute erythema, edema, itching and scaling. Delayed hypersensitivity reaction in skin test is another form of type IV reaction.

Clinical Manifestations

Local or systemic inflammatory response is manifested by redness, edema, heat, respiratory symptoms including wheezing, coughing sneezing and nasal congestion with increased blood eosinophil level.

The allergic diseases demonstrated in different type of reactions are as follows:

a. Type I allergic reactions are manifested as allergic rhinitis, asthma, acute urticaria, angioedema, atopic dermatitis and anaphylactic shock.

b. Type II allergic reactions are manifested as hemolysis in mismatched blood transfusion, hemolytic anemia, purpura, agranulocytosis due to drug hypersensitivity and some autoimmune diseases.

c. Type III allergic reactions are manifested as serum sickness, vasculitis, glomerulonephritis allergic alveolitis, rheumatic arthritis, SLE, farmer's lung and some other autoimmune diseases.

d. Type IV allergic reactions are found in contact dermatitis, homograft rejection, areas of necrosis, cessation in tuberculosis and some autoimmune diseases.

Management of Allergies

a. Management of allergic reactions includes avoidance of allergens after identification by careful history and skin test. Elimination of allergens and environmental control are the initial steps.

b. Drug therapy used for symptomatic relief of allergic manifestations and interruption of tissue damage as consequence of antigen-antibody reactions are very important. The used drugs are antihistamins, corticosteroids, adrenergics (epinephrine, salbutamol) and methylxanthines (theophylline) groups.

c. Immunotherapy or desensitization of allergens done by repeated injections of increasing amounts of allergic extract till the patient reaches an optimal tolerance level. This procedure is done in a well equipped health care facilities.

Nursing Interventions

In hospital and community, nurse can play an important role for the management of this condition by the following activities:

- Careful history taking to detect the allergens.
- Providing informations to the people and given health education about avoidance of common allergens, allergic reactions and its effects.
- Following preventive measures of allergic reactions like skin test for specific drugs, prevention of mismatched blood transfusion, etc.
- Keeping all emergency drugs ready in hands to manage life-threatening anaphylactic reactions promptly.
- Administering drug therapy and other management during hospitalization and providing routine need based care.
- Referring for desensitization therapy.
- Providing support to the child and parents including family members.

POISONING

Poisoning is one of the important accidental hazards among children. It may occur through ingestion, inhalation, injection or skin contact of poisonous substances. The children below five years of age are the common victim of this problem. It may occur as acute exposure of poisonous substance or may also occur due to chronic exposure of poisons.

Accidental poisoning in children is a serious challenge to the child health care due to its continuing morbidity and morality. Most cases of accidental poisoning are preventable. Nursing personnels are mostly responsible for the preventive measures to be taken at hospital and home. Health education is considered as the vaccine for prevention of accidental poisoning like other accidental hazards.

Common Poisoning Agents

Chemical products are swallowed commonly by the children which include kerosene, medicines, acids, insecticides, cosmetics, paints, bleach, etc. Poisonous seeds and plants are also ingested by the children due to their curious nature leading to poisoning. Bites and stings of animals and insects also cause poisoning. Carbon monoxide poisoning can happen when fires, stoves, heaters or ovens are used in rooms which do not have proper ventilation to let the gas out. Inhalation poisoning can also occur due to gas vapor, dust, fumes, spray, etc.

Nearly 75 percent of poisoning episodes are due to ingestion of nontoxic substance which requires reassurance to the children and parents. About 20 percent of poisoning episodes require urgent measures to remove the poison and approximately 5 percent of poisoning need intensive treatment.

Ecology of Poisoning

About 70 percent of all cases of accidental poisoning in children occur within third years of life. These children are active and try to explore unfamiliar objects by putting into their mouth and testing them. They have tendency to put objects into the mouth without knowing its consequences. Hyperactive male children are more prone to accidental poisoning. In adolescents, the intake of toxic agent may be a suicidal attempt.

Large families, small accommodation, careless storage of potentially poisonous household substances, easy availability of poisons, lack of time for supervision of children, lack of discipline and anticipatory guidance are the influencing factors of greater risk of poisonings.

Management of Poisoned Children

In minor poisoning, symptomatic and supportive treatment are usually not required but for moderate or severe poisoning, advanced symptomatic and supportive treatment are always necessary. Minor cases are having mild, transient and spontaneously resolving symptoms. Moderate cases are having pronounced and prolonged symptoms, whereas serious life-threatening symptoms are found in severe cases.

Antidotes are available for very few poisons and treatment is usually nonspecific and symptomatic and supportive.

Basic Principles of Management

a. Emergency stabilization measures.
b. Identification of poison.
c. Removal of poisonous substance and toxin.
d. Specific antidote therapy.
e. Promotion of excretion of toxin.
f. Supportive therapy.
g. Counseling to parents and children.

Steps of Management

1. Establish clear airway and provide ventilatory support, if the child is unconscious and having respiratory failure.
2. Place the child in semiprone position, if possible to minimize the risk of inhalation of gastric contents.
3. Assess the child's condition, level of consciousness, features of complications like metabolic acidosis, hypoglycemia, hyperkalemia, shock, renal failure, etc.
4. Identify the poison by careful history and find supporting evidence from the presenting features and physical signs.
5. Remove the unabsorbed poison by vomiting or gastric lavage. Vomiting is induced by (a) tickling the back of the pharynx by fingers or a spoon or (b) give salt water or warm water to drink or (c) give ipecac syrup. Induction of vomiting is contraindicated in corrosive or kerosene poisoning, unconscious child and child with absence of gag reflex. Precautions to be taken to prevent aspiration during vomiting.
   Gastric lavage is given with warm water or tap water and four or five washes to be given. It should be done promptly to remove the poison when vomiting does not occur quickly. Gastric lavage should not be performed in children with poor gag reflex or corrosive poisoning. In kerosene poisoning, lavage may be done very cautiously, when the child has consumed a large amount of kerosene and is brought quickly to the hospital, otherwise it is better to avoid stomach wash in case of ingestion of kerosene.
   Activated charcoal can be used as absorbent of the toxic agent in the GIT. For the comatosed patient with potentially serious overdose, gastric lavage is followed by administration of activated charcoal via an orogastric or nasogastric tube within 1 to 2 hours of ingestion. The dose should be at least 10 times of the dose of ingested toxic material.

Removal of poison may be needed from the skin and clothing in case of organophosphorus and related compounds which can prove as fatal as oral route absorption. All contaminated clothes to be removed and whole body including nail, skin folds, groin to be irrigated with water or saline as soon as possible after exposure and continue irrigating for at least 15 minutes. Eye contamination requires immediate local decontamination by copious irrigation with neutralizing solution (normal saline or water) for at least 30 minutes. Do not use acid or alkaline solution for eye irrigation.

Laxative and purgatives may be given in poisoning with substances which do not cause corrosive action on gastrointestinal mucosa. Increased motility of the gut may reduce absorption of poison.

6. Administer specific antidote according to the particular toxic agent. Specific antidote may be life saving but unfortunately they are not often available and are effective for less than 5 percent of poisoning cases. The commonly used antidotes are atropine for organophosphate, naloxone for opioid analgesics, neostigmine for anticholinergic poisonous seed (dhatura), pyridine-2-aldoxime-methiodide (PAM) for organophosphates, diazepam for chloroquine, flumazenil for benzodiazepines, etc.
7. Allow increased fluid intake to promote renal clearance by excretion of poison through the urine. Fluid diuresis by IV fluid therapy or diuretics like lasix or mannitol can be used to enhance the elimination of toxin. Hemodialysis or peritoneal dialysis can also be done to remove the poison in some cases. Hemoperfusion is more effective than hemodialysis in some selective poisoning but hemodialysis may be preferred for correction of acid-base and electrolyte imbalance simultaneously.
8. Provide supportive and symptomatic therapy. Oxygen, IV fluid and medications like anticonvulsive, antipyretics, analgesics, antibiotics may be needed. If the child is unconscious special care to be provided to prevent complications. Patent airway, removal of oropharyngeal secretions, position change, care of eyes, mouth and skin, care of bladder and bowel should be emphasized. Oral feeding to be allowed when condition permits. Continuous monitoring of child's condition and intake-output should be recorded for early detection of complications.
9. Keep all relevant documents and records accurately considering the medicolegal aspect.
10. Arrange for counseling of the parents and children and guide the parents for regular psychological follow-up. Teach the parents and family members about the prevention of accidental poisoning and need for parental supervision.

BITES AND STINGS

Bites and stings are one form of poisoning and common in infants and children. Animal bites and insects stings may lead to minor symptoms like pain and swelling to a life-threatening shock requiring immediate and urgent attention.

Common bites are dog bites and snake bites. Common stings are scorpian stings and stings by bees, ants, wasps, etc.

Dog Bites

Dog bite can result to a viral disease known as rabies or hydrophobia, especially due to bite of a rabid dog. There is possibility of contracting rabies from other animals (cat, monkey, horse, sheep, goat). Rabies in man is characterized by long incubation period, striking clinical presentation of hydrophobia and an almost invariably fatal outcome. Rabies in dogs takes two forms namely the furious and the dumb rabies. Once the dog manifests clinical signs of rabies, it generally dies within a week.

The virus-laden saliva (Lyssavirus type 1) of the infected animal comes in contact with the subcutaneous and muscular tissues of the host as a result of the bite, causing the picture of viral encephalitis. Transmission may occur through licks or aerosol or man to man (a case of a child biting its parents). The incubation period of rabies ranges between 20 and 90 days in 90 percent of cases, although it may vary from 10 days to over a year.

Clinical Manifestations

During the initial 1 to 4 days, the patient suffers from prodromal symptoms of fever, myalgia, headache, easy fatigability, sore throat and changes in mood. Paresthesias or fasciculations at the site of bite at this stage are highly suggestive of impending rabies. The prodromal stage is followed by widespread excitation and stimulation of all parts of nervous system. The patient is intolerant to noise, bright light or a cold draught of air. Aerophobia or fear of air may present. Examination may show increased reflexes and muscle spasms along with dilatation of the pupils and increased perspiration, salivation and lacrimation. Mental changes include fear of death, anger, irritability and depression. The symptoms are progressively aggravated and all attempts of swallowing liquid become unsuccessful. The characteristic symptom of hydrophobia may found even at the sight or sound of water due to spasm of muscles of deglutition. The patient may die abruptly during convulsions or may pass to the stage of paralysis and coma.

Diagnosis

The *diagnosis* of rabies can be made with the history of dog bite, the presence of paresthesias at the site of bite and hydrophobia. Confirmatory diagnosis of rabies can be made on postmortem as well as antemortem by a variety of tests. The eosinophilic cytoplasmic inclusions, the "Negri Bodies" are pathognomonic of rabies.

Management

Antirabies treatment consists of two important aspects, i.e. management of the wound and the rabies prophylaxis.

Management of the wound is the utmost importance. It is done by cleaning and washing the wound with soap and running water and then appling alcohol or tincture iodine or aqueous solution of iodine. Antirabies serum should be infiltrated around the wound, if the bite is less than 24 hours old. Tetanus toxoid should be given and antibiotics may be administered, if wound appears unhealthy. There is no need of cauterization or stitching or application of oil or turmeric over the wound.

Passive immunization with antirabies serum combined with local treatment of the wound and active immunization provides best-protection to the exposed individual. Rabies immunoglobulin should be given for all category III exposures (single or multiple transdermal bites or scratches and contamination of mucous membrane with saliva).

Active immunization by rabies vaccine can be provided even after exposure to the infection due to long incubation period of rabies. Presently available rabies vaccines are nervous tissue vaccines and tissue culture vaccines. The nervous tissue rabies vaccines are given by 7 or 14 daily doses subcutaneously depending upon the nature of exposure. The tissue culture vaccines are scheduled on days 0, 3, 7, 14 and 30 in intramuscular route for postexposure and on 0, 7, 28 days for pre-exposure rabies prophylaxis. Intramuscular injection should be given in anterolateral aspect of thigh and never use gluteal region. An additional 6th dose on the day 90 is considered optional for postexposure prophylaxis.

Immunization of the animals also helps in prevention of rabies. Treatment of rabies in man should be done at intensive care unit in the form of respiratory and cardiac support with strict isolation technique and intensive therapy. Rabies in humans almost inevitably ends in death, a few instances of recovery have been recorded.

Snake Bites

Snake bites continues to be an important public health problems in India and other countries. There are about 216 species of snakes identifiable in India, of which 52 species are known to be poisonous which are members of 3 families, i.e. Elapidae (cobra, krait), Viperidae (vipers) and Hydrophiidae (sea-snake). The venoms produced by the Elapidae and Hydrophidae are primarily neurotoxic. They act by blocking neuronal transmission at the neuromuscular junction causing death due to respiratory depression. The venoms produced by the vipers are primarily cytolytic causing cellular necrosis, vascular leak, hemolysis and coagulopathy leading to death due to hemorrhage, shock or renal failure.

Children under the age of 10 years account for 7 to 15 percent of all cases. Most bite occur in rural and semirural areas, usually in outdoors. Peak incidence occurs during the warm and humid months. Over two-third of the bites involve the lower limbs and about 40 percent over the feet alone.

Clinical Features

Clinical features depends upon the type of snakes and presented as local effects and systemic effects.

Elapids (cobra, krait) bites produce local pain followed by swelling within 2 to 3 hours and rapid necrosis sets in as wet gangrene. Systemic manifestations occur within 15 minutes to 10 hours after the bites, as neurotoxic and cardiotoxic features. Paralysis begins with ptosis and ophthalmoplegia followed by involvement of muscles of palate, jaws, tongue, larynx, neck, deglutition and respiratory. Cardiotoxic effects include tachycardia, hypotension and ECG changes. Hemolysis may also occur.

Vipers bites produce severe burning pain with dramatic appearance of edema, swelling, cellulitis, bullae and ecchymoses at the site of the bite. Continuous oozing or bleeding may occur. Local necrosis is slow in onset and resembles dry gangrene. Systemic manifestations may occur within 15 minutes or may be delayed by several hours and presented with bleeding from puncture sites, purpura, hematemesis, melena, epistaxis, hematuria, gum bleeding, intracranial hemorrhage, etc. Circulatory collapse, delirium and renal failure may occur.

First Aid Management

First aid management of snake bites includes reassurance, rest and moral support with immobilization of patient and bitten part in horizontal position. Manipulation of the bitten part, exertion and exercise must be avoided. Do not give alcoholic drinks or stimulants to the patient. Incision and suction of the wound is no longer recommended. A wide tourniquet or crepe bandage to be applied proximal to the bite site to occlude the lymphatics only, therefore it should not be too tight. It should be released and moved proximally as the advancing swelling augments the tightness of the bandage. The level of swelling should be marked. The patient should be transferred promptly for definitive medical treatment.

Hospital Management

Immediate *hospital management* should include management of shock, respiratory failure by mechanical ventilation and antivenom therapy. Neostigmine-atropine regimen can be effectively used in case of Elapids venom. Supportive care include fresh whole blood transfusion for blood loss, appropriate antibiotic therapy for secondary infection, wound care and hemodialysis in renal failure.

The overall mortality due to snake bite is about 10 percent. The major reason of poor outcome is the delay to reach to hospital for definitive treatment and nonavailability of antivenin in most hospitals. Awareness to be promoted to prevent snake bites and to avail medical facilities as early as possible, in case of snake bites.

Insects Stings

Insects stings are commonly found in rural and coastal areas. Scorpion stings are second only to snake bites as a cause of fatal envenomation. It occurs mainly in wet and summer months. The red scorpion is extremely dangerous. Insects stings also include bees, wasps, ants and beetles.

Scorpion stings may be fatal because scorpion venom is neurotoxic, cardiotoxic, hematotoxic and myotoxic and having wide range of local and systemic manifestations. The child may present following the scorpion stings with intense local pain, swelling and ecchymosis. Profuse perspiration, tachypnea, vomiting, hypersalivation, lacrimation, frequent passage of urine or stool are the most prominent features of autonomic storm. The child usually have convulsions, hemiplegia and other neurological deficits with shock, respiratory distress, acute renal failure, coagulopathy and cardiomyopathy.

Management

Management of scorpion stings should be done promptly as no first aid measures are of particular value. A tourniquet should be applied immediately with precautions. The wound should be washed with plain water and the part should be immobilized. Local anesthetics to be used (lignocaine) to reduce pain. Oxygen therapy, drugs and IV infusion to be started to manage shock. Symptomatic treatment to be given promptly with adrenergic blocking agent (prazosin), diuretic, bronchodilators and insulin which may be useful. The antivenom therapy and lytic cocktail regimen for scorpion stings are controversial. Tetanus prophylaxis should be given. Prevention of scorpion stings should be promoted.

Bees and wasps stings to be managed by local cooling, removal of visible sting, application of soothing lotion (calamine) or anesthetic cream, oral analgesic and antihistamine. Adrenaline may be needed in anaphylactic manifestations along with other supportive management. Ants stings may be managed by application of cold compresses, washing of sites with soap and water, applying local antiseptics, oral or topical antihistamines, oral corticosteroids and analgesics. Severe reactions necessitate immediate subcutaneous injection of 0.3 to 0.5 ml of 1:1000 solution of epinephrine and repeated at ten minute intervals, if necessary.

Nursing responsibility in relation to bites and stings are mainly promoting awareness about the prevention of this problem. Prompt management at hospitalization should be initiated to prevent complications and fatal outcome. Parental support and providing information about the probable outcome are important aspects of nursing liability.

FOREIGN BODIES

Children are fond of putting objects into various orifices either their own or others due to curiosity or innocence, during the oral phase of psychosocial development and thereafter. Objects inserted into the nose, ears, anus, vagina are usually easy to manage but foreign bodies in the mouth can be difficult and often life-threatening because they may track down into the respiratory tract or in the alimentary tract. Foreign bodies in the eyes may also create serious problem but in the soft tissue may be managed easily.

Foreign Bodies in the Respiratory Tract

Aspiration of foreign bodies into the respiratory tract is quite common in children. About 75 percent cases seeds, nuts and other vegetable matters are inhaled in the airways. Inert materials like glass bead, plastic piece (from toy, ball pen), stone, screw, etc. can also aspirate in respiratory passage. This problem is common in male toddlers. A definite history of foreign body inhalation is not always available. The child may present with acute airway obstruction.

The *clinical features* in the child with foreign body in the nose usually present with nasal obstruction, sneezing, discomfort and serosanguinous discharge. When the foreign body impacted in the larynx the child presents with sudden choking, aphonia and stridor or violent inspiratory efforts or even death, if impaction is complete. Foreign bodies in the trachea may present with spasmodic paroxysmal coughing, wheezing, hoarseness, hemoptysis, cyanosis and dyspnea. Foreign bodies in the bronchus may present with variable degree of tachypnea, cough, and wheezing. Prolonged impaction may lead to pneumonitis and bronchiectasis. Complications of long standing foreign bodies in the respiratory tract may present with repeated pneumonia, lung abscess, atelectasis and emphysema.

Diagnosis

The diagnosis of foreign body inhalation is best done by clinical features. Plain chest X-ray (including neck and diaphragm) usually helps to locate the foreign body, mainly the radiopaque materials. In very acute cases the child may have to be rushed to the operation theater for a diagnostic-cum therapeutic bronchoscopy.

Emergency Management

Emergency management of foreign body inhalation at home can be done with precautions by hanging the child upside down, thumping over the back, groping with fingers in the pharynx, backblows, chest thrusts, Heimlich maneuver, etc. In hospital, once the diagnosis is established or strongly suspected, bronchoscopy should be done as soon as possible. After bronchoscopy some children may need humidification, parenteral steroids, antibiotics and chest physiotherapy. Tracheotomy may be needed when large vegetable foreign body swells up and difficult to remove through larynx or in case of laryngeal obstruction. Thoracotomy and bronchotomy may be required in case of impacted long standing foreign bodies in the bronchus.

Foreign Bodies in the Alimentary Tract

Ingestion of foreign bodies is also common like inhalation. The majority of swallowed foreign bodies are spontaneously passed in the stool, some may require endoscopic or operative removal. The commonly ingested foreign bodies are coins, button cell, key, safety pin, rings, pencil sharper and sometime trichobezoar (bolus of hair) or cotton from cloths.

Initial features of foreign body ingestion may be same as foreign body inhalation but the coughing is not severe and there is minimal choking and gagging. This is usually followed by dysphagia, drooling of saliva and retrosternal or epigastric discomfort, if the foreign body gets impacted in the esophagus. When the foreign body passed beyond the esophagus, it remains asymptomatic and spontaneously removed in the stool within 4 to 5 days. Impaction of foreign body in the gastrointestinal tract may present with features of intestinal obstruction, peritonitis, etc.

To detect the impacted radiopaque foreign body, X-ray neck, chest or abdomen is helpful. Esophagoscopy and/or barium studies, ultrasonography may be needed to identify nonradiopaque substances.

When foreign body is impacted in the esophagus, it can be managed simply eating bulk of mashed potatoes or bananas which may help in forcing a foreign body down the esophagus into the stomach. Children with distressing symptoms with impacted foreign body should be referred for endoscopy. Smooth surface foreign bodies can be extracted by the Foley's

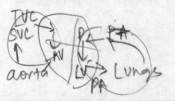

catheter from the esophagus. Some cases may need surgical removal. No need of use of purgatives when the foreign body passes down the stomach. Normal diet with roughage should be given with adequate amount of water. The child should be observed for any untoward symptoms. Passage of foreign body in the stool should be checked.

Foreign Bodies in the Eyes

Foreign bodies in the eyes is also common incident found in the children. Dust, sand, wood, glass particles, metal splinters, etc. may get enlodged into the eye, making injury of the cornea, conjunctiva, sclera and even the eye ball. The child may present with severe pain, lacrimation, foreign body sensation, photophobia, redness, itching and swelling. Severe infection may occur within hours in wood and plant foreign body.

The condition should be managed as emergency. Instruction to be given to avoid rubbing. If the foreign body is not embedded, it can be removed by corner of clean cloth or by blinking eyelids under water. The embedded foreign body should be removed through irrigation or cotton-tip applicator or magnet. Surgical removal may be needed in case of intraocular foreign body. Antibiotic therapy should be given to prevent infection. Aseptic eye care and follow-up are essential.

Preventive measures are important to reduce the incidence of foreign bodies. Children must be supervised and watched carefully by the caretakers. Harmful small articles and toys with detachable small parts should not be allowed to the child or to be kept out of their reach. A foreign body in any parts of the body should be managed immediately with special attention. Foreign bodies in the aerodigestive tract can be a life-threatening emergency requiring immediate management. It is, therefore, important that public awareness should be increased by health education about the different preventive approaches. Nurses are the key person to educate the people and make them aware about the prevention of these hazards.

MULTIPLE INJURY

Multiple injury is now commonly found in pediatric surgery unit which is difficult to manage and may have fatal outcome or multiple organ dysfuction or disability. Changing life style, increased number of road traffic accidents, sports or recreational injury, violence, etc. are the important causes of multiple injury in children. The child may be hospitalized with injury at different sites of the body. Head injury alongwith other bony injury of the limbs are very common. Intra-abdominal injury, chest injury, injury of the pelvic region may occur alone or in combination. Injury can occur in eyes or skin and superficial tissue. Commonly injuries are found as lacerating injury or blunt injury or penitrating injury. Sometimes superficial wounds or abrasions may or may not present along with internal injury.

The child may present with fractures and unconsciousness depending upon the severity of injury. Shock, hemorrhage, pain, convulsions, and respiratory distress may present which should be managed promptly.

Initial resuscitative management should emphasis on 'ABC' of resuscitation, i.e. airway clearance, breathing support and circulation maintenance. Establishment of patent airway and breathing support should be considered as prime important to save the life. Appropriate positioning, ventilatory support are essential with oxygen therapy. Maintenance of circulation may require for external cardiac massage, IV infusion and medications. Hemorrhage should be checked promptly. Analgesics to be administered to relieve pain. Patient should be assessed quickly for shock, level of consciousness, nature and extent of injury, and urine output. Indwelling catheterization to be done, whenever needed. Intake and output record to be maintained strictly. Continuous monitoring of patient's condition should be done and necessary measures to be taken for better outcome.

Specific treatment to be arranged for specific type of injury, when the patient's condition is stabilized. Necessary investigations to be done to detect the type of injury for appropriate management. Information to be given to the parents about the child's condition and encouraging them to participate in child care, as possible. Public awareness to be increased about preventive measures, traffic rules, protective devices, etc. to reduce the incidence of accidental injuries.

FAILURE TO THRIVE

Failure to thrive (FTT) is a common problem of children from poor socioeconomic group. This term was mentioned as early as 1915. Afterwards it was termed as 'Emotional deprivation' and as 'Maternal deprivation syndrome' by Bowlby, in 1969.

Failure to thrive can be defined as a chronic potentially life threatening disorder of infant and children who fail to gain weight and even lose weight. The children with FTT show failure of expected growth and noticeable lack of well-being. It indicates psychosomatic growth failure.

The physiologic concepts of FTT is based on inadequate parent-child relationship leading to disturbances of neuro-endocrine functions. The hyperactivity of adrenal cortex of the emotionally disturbed children may suppress the growth. Secretion of pituitary growth hormone may be inhibited due to abnormal sleep pattern and deprivation of food of the disturbed child.

Causes

Causes of failure to thrive can be grouped into three categories:

1. *Organic FTT:* It is usually associated with all serious pediatric illnesses like congenital heart diseases, malabsorption syndrome, intestinal parasitosis, tuberculosis, juvenile diabetes mellitus, cystic fibrosis, liver abscess, congenital pyloric stenosis, gastroesophageal reflux, etc.
2. *Nonorganic FTT:* It is a psychosocial problem due to disturbed parent child relationship leading to emotional deprivation, poverty, illiteracy, ignorance, faulty food habit and conflict in the family resulting social deprivation. All these lead to poor nutritional intake, feeding problems and failure of growth.
3. *Mixed FTT:* It is combined effect of both organic and nonorganic causes.

Management

Management of a child with FTT needs physical, social and emotional approach in home and hospital on immediate and long-term basis.

Initial assessment of child's physical and mental health status including the assessment of family condition and sociocultural influence are very important for the management of the child with FTT. Detailed collection of family history is the prime responsibility of the pediatric nurse. Thorough physical examination and laboratory investigations (stool, urine, blood) should be done to detect the organic cause. Growth chart also helps in diagnosis that should be followed, if maintained previously.

Hospitalization may be necessary to confirm the diagnosis and to treat the cause and complications.

Nursing Management

Nursing management should emphasize on supervision of optimum food intake, warm emotional care with love and affection from parent and family members with psychological stimulation to the child. Parental involvement in treatment plan and care is vital. Emotional support to the parents and necessary instructions are essential for improvement of parent-child relationship and resolution of emotional conflict of the child. Regular follow-up should be done for effective management. Referring may be planned, whenever needed, for social support and community assistance to improve socioeconomic status. Community health nurse should arrange regular home visit for follow-up and further assistance towards tender loving care of the child.

DEVELOPMENTAL DISORDERS

Developmental disorders are commonly found in children. There are several factors responsible for developmental problems which include poor socioeconomic status, genetic influence, prenatal and perinatal factors, environmental factors, hormones, nutritional deficiencies, chronic or repeated illness, lack of emotional stimulation, etc.

Developmental disorders are found as delayed development, failure to thrive, short stature, obesity, behavioral problems, maladjustment, poor school achievements, learning disabilities, hyperactive-attention deficit disorders, adolescent problems, antisocial behavior or juvenile delinquency, etc.

During periodic visits of the child to the primary health care workers, pediatric nurse or physician, the child should always be screened for behavioral development. A developmental problem should be suspected if the child is not able to perform the given tasks by the particular age or showing any behavioral disorders. It is possible to recognize severe developmental disorders early in infancy. Speech problems, hyperactivity and emotional disturbances are often not detected till the child is 3 to 4 years old. Learning disabilities are not picked up till the child starts schooling. The common development disorders are discussed below. The behavioral disorders are described in the next chapter (Chapter 10).

Short Stature

Short stature is the disorder of growth and development. It is termed when a child is having length or height below 3rd percentile for according to international standard and below 5th percentile according to ICMR standard and 3 SD (Standard deviations) of mean for age. The term dwarfism is no longer used for short stature. Disorders of growth are now-a-days referred as dysplasia. Short stature may either be proportionate or disproportionate.

The causes of short stature are mainly genetic heritance or familial, intrauterine growth retardation, malnutrition, malabsorption, chronic infections and infestations, endocrine disorders, (hypothyroidism, growth hormone deficiency, diabetes mellitus), emotional deprivation, constitutional delay in growth, rickets, caries spine, achondroplasia, chondrodysplasia, mucopolysaccharidosis, etc.

Short stature can be primary and secondary. Primary short stature is due to poor skeletal growth in genetic or prenatal causes. The skeletal age is unaffected. Secondary short stature is manifested as delayed height gain and impairment of bone age.

Detection of causes of short stature should be done with details history, clinical examination, routine laboratory investigations, hormonal assay, genetic study and estimation of bone age. Bone age or epiphyseal development is less than chronological age in cases of constitutional delay in puberty, markedly delay in hypothyroidism and hypopituitarism. It is moderately delayed in malnutrition and chronic illnesses. Bone age is in advance of the height age in children with genetic short stature, chondrodystrophies, trisomy 21, Turner syndrome, intrauterine infections and storage disorders.

Treatment of the specific cause by early detection, parental support and reassurance are important aspects of management. Prevention of emotional deprivation and nutritional deficiency conditions are essential. Parents need necessary information about the problem.

Obesity

Obesity is not a common problem in Indian child, where nutritional deficiencies are mostly found. But changes in lifestyle and child rearing practices are contributing towards this problem. Adolescents of affluent family are more prone to develop obesity. Hormonal changes, erroneous eating habits (chocolates, sweets, candies, snacks, ice cream), lack of outdoor play, excessive television watching, overprotective parenting and genetic predisposition are the important precipitating factors.

Obese children have low self-esteem and emotional problems leading to isolation, excessive appetite and more food intake causing further obesity. There is no difference in energy expenditure between obese and nonobese adolescents. Individuals with truncal obesity are more prone to cardiovascular disease and diabetes.

Weight reduction program is planned as dietary regulation with reduced calorie intake and increased physical exercise. Emotional problems to be handled carefully. Weight should be reduced gradually not abruptly. The child needs constant encouragement and supervision for the reduction of weight.

Adolescent Problems

Adolescence is the period of transition from childhood to maturity with rapid physical, intellectual, emotional and social growth. Remarkable changes in puberty occur by gaining of 50 percent of adult weight and 25 percent of adult height. In boys, dominant muscular development and in girls fat deposition are the characteristic changes along with other external physical changes. Emotional development includes formation of identity, self-concept and social relationship with peers and outgroups rather than family members. Development of heterosexual relationship, sexual maturation, romantic attraction to opposite sex and sex-role identity are important tasks of this group. Autonomy from parents, morality and career choice are accomplished during adolescence.

The special needs of adolescents include independence, status or worth, satisfaction of philosophy of life, appropriate orientation about sex and sexuality, guidance for selection of vocation or career, morality, etc. They also need affection, encouragement, appreciation and trust along with other emotional and physical demands.

The areas of stress in adolescents are related to body image, sexuality conflict, scholastic pressure, competitive situations, relationship with parents, siblings and peers, financial problems, career planning, decision-making about present and future roles, ideological conflicts, etc. They may feel sometimes confused, insecured, anxious, disoriented, isolated, worried, rigid and less happy. Their emotion fluctuate and subject to turbulent and unpredictable behavior. They are extremely sensitive to feeling and behavior. They are struggling for independence and consider friends extremely important.

Due to inadequate fulfillment of needs and deprivation in various aspects, adolescents are vulnerable to different problems, which requires special consideration.

Classification

Adolescent problems can be grouped into three categories, i.e. physical, sexual and psychological.

Physical problems of adolescents:
a. *Nutritional problems:* Under nutrition, obesity, anemia, puberty goiter, anorexia nervosa and bulimia.
b. *Infections:* Reproductive tract infections (RTIs) or sexually transmitted diseases (STDs), urinary tract infections, pelvic inflammatory diseases, tuberculosis, fungal infections, etc.
c. *Menstrual problems:* Amenorrhea, dysmenorrhea, menorrhagia, metrorrhagia, DUB, premenstrual syndrome, precocious puberty, pelvic mass, imperforate hymen, hematocolpos, etc.
d. *Disorders of breasts:* Breast asymmetry, breast hypoplasia, breast mass, abnormal nipples, galactorrhea or nipple discharge, fibro cystic disease in girls and gynecomastia in boys.
e. *Penoscrotal problems:* Penile hypoplasia, abnormal shape, size and curvature of penis, erectile or ejaculatory dysfunctions, genital warts, balanitis, balanoposthitis, hydrocele, ectopic testes, etc.
f. *Skin problems:* Acne, hirsuitism and fungus infections.
g. *Musculoskeletal problems:* Kyphosis, scoliosis.
h. *Miscellaneous:* Accidents proneness, delayed speech, hearing problems, visual problems (myopia), sleep disorders (hypersomnia, insomnia, narcolepsy), diabetes mellitus, excessive tallness, hypertension, endocrine dysfunctions, etc.

Sexual problems of adolescents: Precocious sexuality, sexual experimentation, premarital sex, unsafe sex, sexually transmitted diseases including HIV/AIDS, teenage pregnancy, unsafe abortion, early marriage, promiscuous sex, homosexuality, sexual abuse as sexual assault, rape, incest and excessive masturbation.

Psychological problems of adolescents:

a. *Emotional problems:* Anxiety, hypersensitivity, impulsiveness, moodiness, immaturity, withdrawal, maladjustment, frustration, etc.

b. *Motivational problems:* Lack of ambition, low aspiration level, feelings of frustration, negative attitude, lack of interests.

c. *Moral problems:* Feeling of guilt, confused ideas of right and wrong, delinquencies, violence, school truency, substance abuse, etc.

d. *Mental health problems:* Anxiety disorders, phobias, obsessive behavior, hypochondriasis, depression, suicide, acute psychosis, etc.

Maintenance of Adolescent Health

Health care providers are responsible to promote adolescent health through various approaches. Adolescents' needs to be fulfilled adequately in health and illness. Parents, family members, teachers and community leaders should be involved and encouraged to participate in the maintenance of adolescent health.

Maintenance of adolescent health includes the provision of adequate rest, sleep, balanced diet, good health habits and hygiene, healthy physical and emotional environment, education, recreation and diversion. They also need emotional support and adequate explanation about changes of puberty and personality, body image and present turmoil during adolescents. They should provide informations about future plan of life and sex education to prevent sexual calamities. They need safety, security and protection with independence and discipline. They should provide counseling and guidance whenever needed in social, moral and intellectual conflicts.

Adolescence mental hygiene should be promoted by the following approaches:

- Accept adolescent as unique individual.
- Respect their ideas, likes, dislikes, wishes and privacy.
- Involve in different activities and avoid criticism about no-win topics.
- Provide opportunity for choosing options and allow increasing independence within limitation of safety and well-being.
- Clarify house rules and consequences for breaking them and make the communication clear.
- Provide unconditional love and avoid comparisons with siblings and peers.
- Try to share adolescents feeling of joy and sorrow and to help them control emotions.
- Be available to answer questions, give informations and provide companionship.
- Explain the physiological basis of change of the body, sexual maturity and sex role.
- Provide sex education and instruct about sex hygiene.
- Allow learning by doing and assist in selection of career goals and preparation of adult role.
- Guide to develop philosophy of life and to satisfy it.
- Encourage in wise decision making and to be a well adjusted mature adult.

Behavioral Disorders in Children

10

- Behavioral Problems of Infancy
- Behavioral Problems of Childhood
- Behavioral Problems of Adolescence
- Nursing Responsibilities in Behavioral Disorders of Children

INTRODUCTION

Infancy and childhood are of paramount importance in determining and patterning the future behavior and character of the children. Childhood is the period of dependency. Gradually, children learn to adjust in the environment. But when, there is any complexity around them they cannot adjust with that circumstances. Then they become unable to behave in the socially acceptable way and behavioral problems develop with them.

Normal children are healthy, happy and well adjusted. This adjustment is developed by providing basic emotional needs along with physical and physiological needs for their mental well-being. The emotional needs are considered as emotional food for healthy behavior. The children are dependent on their parents, so parents are responsible for fulfilment of the emotional needs.

Every child should have tender loving care and sense of security about protection from parent and family members. They should have opportunity for development of independence, trust, confidence and self-respect. There should be adequate social and emotional interaction with discipline. The child should get scope for self-expression and recreation. Parents should be aware about achievements of their children and express acceptance of positive attitude within the social norms.

These all needs required to be satisfied to ensure optimum behavioral development. Sometimes children show a wide variety of behaviors which create problems to the parents, family members and society. Most of the problems are minor and do not have any permanent disturbances but produce anxiety to the parents. Major behavioral problems are the significant deviations from socially accepted normal behavior. These problems are mainly due to failure in adjustment to external environment and presence of internal conflict. Behavioral problems alway require special attention.

Causes of Behavioral Disorders

Behavioral disorders are caused by multiple factors. No single event is responsible for this condition. The important contributing factors are:

Faulty Parental Attitude

Overprotection, dominance, unrealistic expectation, over-criticism, unhealthy comparison, underdiscipline or over discipline, parental rejection, disturbed parent-child inter-action, broken family (death, divorce), etc. are responsible factors for development of behavioral problems.

Inadequate Family Environment

Poor economical status, cultural pattern, family habits, child rearing practices, superstition, parent's mood and job satisfaction, parental illiteracy, inappropriate relationship among family members, etc. influence on child's behavior and may cause behavioral disorders.

Mentally and Physically Sick or Handicapped Conditions

Children with sickness and disability may have behavioral problems. Chronic illness and prolonged hospitalization can lead to this problem.

Influence of Social Relationship

Maladjustment at home and school, disturbed relationship with neighbors, school teachers, schoolmates and playmates, favoritism, punishment, etc. may predispose behavioral problems.

Influence of Mass Media

Television, radio, periodicals and high-tech communication systems affect the school children and adolescence leading to conflict and tension which may cause behavioral disorder.

Influence of Social Change

Social unrest, violence, unemployment, change in value-orientation, group interaction and hostility, frustration, economic insecurity, etc. affect older children along with their parents and family members resulting abnormal behavior.

Common Behavioral Problems in Children

a. *Feeding problems*—Food fad, food refusal, overeating, vomiting, impaired appetite, pica, anorexia nervosa.
b. *Habit disorders*—Thumb sucking (finger sucking), nail biting, enuresis, encopresis, tics, breath holding spell, bruxism (teeth-grinding), rolling and head banging, trichotilomania.
c. *Speech problems*—Unclear speech, delayed speech, dyslalia, stammering or stuttering.
d. *Sleep problems*—Sleep walking (somnambulism), sleep talking (somnoloquy), night terrors, nightmares, insomnia, hypersomnia, narcolepsy, cataplexy.
e. *Educational difficulties*—School phobia, truancy, repeated failure, school absentism, hyperactive attention deficit disorders.
f. *Adjustment problems*—Disobedience, misconduct, temper tantrum.
g. *Emotional problems*—Negativism, jealousy, shyness, fear, anger, anxiety, timidity.
h. *Antisocial problems*—Delinquency, destructive attitudes, kleptomania (compulsive stealing), substance abuse, drug addicts.
i. *Sexual problems*—Masturbation, precocious sexuality, homosexuality, hypersexuality, incest, sexual assault, etc.

These behavioral problems may found to all children, but some problems are specific to particular age group. For example temper tantrum and breath-holding spell are common in toddlers. Thumb-sucking and nail biting are common in preschoolers. Enuresis and speech problems are common in school children and delinquency and drug abuse are common is adolescents. Details of these problems are discussed as problems of specific age group.

BEHAVIORAL PROBLEMS OF INFANCY

Manifestations of behavioral problems during infancy are found as resistance to feeding or impaired appetite, abdominal colic, stranger anxiety, resistance to parental interference to explore environment and vomiting as attention seeking behavior in disturbed parent-child relationship.

Resistance to Feeding or Impaired Appetite

During infancy feeding problems often develop at the time of weaning. Infant may refuse new foods due to dislike of taste or due to separation anxiety from mother. It may be due to forced feeding by the mother or may be due to indigestion of new food and abdominal colic. The infant may have painful ulcer in the mouth or sore throat causing difficulty in swallowing. There may be nasal congestion or any other pathological cause which need to be excluded.

Mothers usually become frustrated and anxious with this situation, so they need reassurance and guidance in rescheduling the feeding time and change of food items. Problems like mouth ulcer, sore throat, nasal congestion or any other conditions to be treated accordingly. Mother should be encouraged to provide tender loving care to her infant and to avoid separation.

Abdominal Colic

Abdominal colic is an important cause of crying in the children. Some infants may cry continuously for variable periods. This problem usually starts within the first week after birth, reaches a peak by the age of 4 to 6 weeks and improves after 3 to 4 months. The infants may cry loudly with clenched fists and flexed legs.

The cause of this colic is not clearly understood. It occurs commonly in overactive infants who are overstimulated by parents. It can be due to hunger, or improper feeding technique or physiological immaturity of the intestine or cow's milk allergy or aerophagy. Excessive carbohydrate in food may lead to intestinal fermentation and accumulation of gas which may cause abdominal distension and pain.

Abdominal colic of the baby increases anxiety and tension of the mother. She required explanation and help for solving the problem. Baby should be placed in upright position and burping can be done to remove swallowed air. Psychological bonding with infant to be improved. Presence of any organic cause to be excluded and necessary management to be arranged. Antispasmodic drugs may be administered to relief the colic. Frequent small amount feeding and modification of feeding technique are very important.

Stranger Anxiety (Separation Anxiety)

Mother is significant person during infancy for satisfaction of needs, feeling of comfort, pleasure and security. The infant does not belief any other persons except mother, because they have trust relationship with mothers only. In absence of mother, if any new person approaches, the child will start crying due to feeling of insecurity, fear and anxiety. This crying may upset the parent, but it is an indication that parent have done a great job in the emotional development of the infant by deep mother-child or parent-child bondage. Separation anxiety is a vital steps of emotional development and may continue up to 13 to 15 months of age. This anxiety usually reduced when the strangers gradually approach from distance in a familiar place specially in presence of the mother or father. In absence of parents, loving concern of the stranger is very important.

BEHAVIORAL PROBLEMS OF CHILDHOOD

Common behavioral problems of childhood are temper tantrum, breath-holding spell, thumb sucking, nail biting, enuresis, encopresis, pica, tics, speech problems, sleep disorders, school phobia, attention deficit disorders, etc. Details of these problems are discussed below.

Temper Tantrums

Temper tantrum is a sudden outburst or violent display of anger, frustration and bad temper as physical aggression or resistance such as rigid body, biting, kicking, throwing objects, hitting, crying, rolling on floor, screaming loudly, banging limbs, etc.

Temper tantrum occurs in maladjusted children. The activity is directed towards the environment not to any person or anything. It is normal in toddler, may continues to preschool period and become more severe indicating the low frustration tolerance. It is found usually in boys, single child and pampered child.

Temper tantrum occurs when the child cannot integrate the internal impulses and the demand of reality. The child become frustrated and reacts in the only ways he/she knows i.e. by violent bodily activity and crying, using great deal of muscular activity and striking out against environment. When no substitute solution is available temper tantrum result.

If temper tantrum continues, the child needs professional help from child guidance clinic. Parent should be made aware about the beginning of temper tantrum and when the child loses control. Parent should provide alternate activity at that time. Nobody should make fun and tease the child about the unacceptable behavior. Parent should explain the child, that the angry feeling is normal but controlling anger is an important aspect of growing up. The child should be protected from self-injury or from doing injury to others. Physical restraint usually increase frustration and block the outlet of anger. Frustration can be reduced by calm and loving approach. Overindulgence should be avoided. After the temper tantrum is over the child's face and hands should be washed and play materials to be provided for diversion. The child's tension can be released by vigorous exercise and physical activities. Parents must be firm and consistent in behavior.

Breath-holding Spell

Breath holding spell may occur in children between 6 months to 5 years of age. It is observed in response to frustration or anger during disciplinary conflict. The child is found with violent crying, hyperventilation and sudden cessation of breathing on expiration, cyanosis and rigidity. Loss of consciousness, twitching and tonic-clonic movements may also be found. The child may become limp and look pallor and lifeless. Heart rates become slow. There may be spasm of laryngeal muscles. This attack last for one or two minutes, then glottis relaxed and breathing resumed with no residual effects.

Parents and family members become very anxious with the attack. Attempt to prevent the spells is usually not successful. Parents need assurance about the harmless effects of the attack and should be tolerant, calm and kind. Identification and correction of precipitating factors (emotional, environmental) are essential approach. Over protective nature of parents may increase unreasonable demand of the child. The child can use secondary gain as advantages. Punishment is not appropriate and may cause another episodes. Repeated attacks of the spells need to be evaluated with careful history, physical examination and necessary investigations to exclude convulsive disorders or any other problems.

Thumb Sucking

Thumb sucking or finger sucking is a habit disorder due to feeling of insecurity and tension reducing activities. It may develop due to inadequate oral satisfaction during early infancy as a result of poor breastfeeding. In older children, this habit may develop when they are tired, bored, frustrated or at bed and want to sleep, but feel lonely.

If thumb sucking continues beyond 4 years of age then complications may arise as malocclusion and malalignment of teeth, difficulty in mastication and swallowing. It may cause deformity of thumb, facial distortion and speech difficulties with consonants (D and T) and GI tract infections.

If the child develops thumb sucking at the age of 7 or 8 years, it indicates a sign of stress.

Parents and family members need support and to be adviced not to become irritable, anxious and tense. Praising and encouraging child for breaking the habit are very useful. Distraction during bored time or engaging the thumb or finger for other activity to be practiced to keep the hand busy. The child should not be scolded for the habit. Consultation with dentist and speech therapist may be required to correct the complications. Hygienic measures to be followed and infections to be treated promptly.

Nail Biting

Nail biting is bad oral habit especially in school age children beyond 4 years of age (5–7 years). It is a sign of tension and self-punishment to cope with the hostile feeling towards parents. It may occur as imitating the parent who is also a nail biter. It is caused by feeling of insecurity, conflict and hostility. It may be due to pressurised study at school or home or due to watching frightening violent scenes. It may continue up to adolescence. The child may bite all 10 finger nails or any specific one. The bite may include the cuticle or skin margins of nail bed or surrounding tissue.

The cause for nail biting to be identified by the parents with the help of clinical psychologist and steps to be taken to remove the habit. The child should be praised for well kept hand by breaking the habit to maintain self-confidence. The child's hand to be kept busy with creative activities or play. Punishment to be avoided. Parents need reassurance and assistance to accept the situation and to help the child to overcome the problem.

Enuresis or Bed Wetting

Enuresis is the repetitive involuntary passage of urine at inappropriate place especially at bed, during night time, beyond the age of 4 to 5 years. It is found in 3 to 10 percent school children. The most frequent causes are small bladder capacity, improper toilet training and deep sleep with inability to receive the signals from distended bladder to empty it. The emotional factors responsible for enuresis are hostile or dependent parent—child relationship, dominant parent, punishment, sibling rivalry, emotional deprivation due to insecurity and parental death. The other factors include the child with emotional conflict and tension, desires to gain care and attention of parents as in infancy. Environmental factors like dark passage to toilet or cold or fear of toilets or

toilet at distance from bedroom may cause bed wetting at night. The associated organic causes may present, e.g. spina bifida, neurogenic bladder, juvenile diabetes mellitus, seizure disorders, etc. and need to be excluded.

Enuresis may be primary or secondary in type. Primary or persistent enuresis is characterized by delayed maturation of neurological control of urinary bladder, when the child never achieved normal bladder control usually due to organic cause. In secondary or regressive enuresis the normal bladder control is developed for several months after which the child again starts bed wetting at night usually due to regressive behavior like illness and hospitalization or due to any emotional deprivations.

Management of enuresis depends upon the specific cause. Assessment of exact cause is very essential by thorough history, clinical examination and necessary investigations. The organic causes are managed with specific treatment. Nonorganic causes to be managed primarily with emotional support to the child and parents along with environmental modification. The child needs reassurance, restriction of fluid after dinner, voiding before bed time and arising the child to void, once or twice, three to four hours later. Interruption of sleep before the expected time of bed wetting is essential. The child should be fully waken up by the parent and made aware of passing of urine at night. The child can assume responsibility for changing the bed cloths. Parents should not be worried about the problem.

Parents should encourage and reward the child for dry nights. Punishment and criticism may lead to embarrassment and frustration of the child. Bladder stretching during daytime to be done to increase holding time of urine, using positive reinforcement and delaying voiding for some time. Drug therapy with tricyclic antidepressant (Imipramine) are useful. Condition therapy by using electric alarm bell mattress is a effective and safest method, when the child wakes up as soon as the bed is wet. Supportive psychotherapy is important for child and parent. Changes of home environment to remove the environmental causes are essential.

Encopresis

Encopresis is the passage of feces into inappropriate places after the age of 5 years, when the bowel control is normally achieved. It is a more serious form of emotional disturbances due to unconscious anger, stress and anxiety. It can be primary or secondary encopresis like bed wetting. Associated problems are chronic constipation, parental overconcern, over aggressive toilet training, toilet fear, attention deficit disorders, poor school attendance and learning difficulties may be found with encopresis.

Assessment of this condition includes history of bowel training, use of toilets and associated problems. The child needs help in establishment of regular bowel habit, bowel training, dietary intake of roughage and intake of adequate fluid. Parental support, reassurance and help from psychologist for counseling of child and parents may be essential in persistent problems.

Geophagia or Pica

Pica is a habit disorder of eating nonedible substances such as clay, paints, chalk, pencil, plaster from wall, earth, scalp hair, etc. It is normal up to the age of two years. If it persists after two years of age, it may be due to parental neglect, poor attention of caregiver, inadequate love and affection, etc.

It is common in poor socioeconomic family and in malnourished and mentally subnormal children.

Children with pica may have associated problems of intestinal parasitosis, lead poisoning, vitamins and minerals deficiency. These children may have problems like trichotillomania (pulling out of scalp hair and swallow) and trichobezoar (a big palpable lump in the upper abdomen due to collection of swallowed hair).

Management of this problem is done with psychotherapy of the child and parents. Associated problems should be treated with specific management.

Tics or Habit Spasm

Tics are sudden abnormal involuntary movements. It is repetitive, purposeless, rapid stereotype movements of striated muscles, mainly of the face and neck. Tics occur most often in school children for discharge of tension in maladjusted emotionally disturbed child. It is outlet of suppressed anger and worry for the control of aggression.

Tics can be motor or vocal tics. Motor tics can be found as eye blinking, grimacing, shrugging shoulder, tongue protrusion, facial gesture, etc. Vocal tics are found as throat clearing, coughing, barking, sniffing, etc.

A special type of chronic tics is found as 'Gilles de la Tourette's Syndrome', characterized by multiple motor tics and vocal tics. It seems to be a genetic disorder with onset at around 11 years of age. It requires for special management with behavior therapy, counselling and drug therapy with heloperidol group of drug.

Parental reassurance and counseling of the child and parents usually useful to manage the simple motor or vocal tics.

Speech Problems

Speech disorders are common in childhood. These can be found as disturbances of voice (pitch disorder), articulation (baby talk) and fluency. Speech problems can be associated with organic causes like hearing defect, cleft lip and cleft palate, cerebral palsy, dental malocclusions, facial and bulbar paralysis, etc. The emotional deprivations are also very significant cause of speech disturbances. The common speech problems related to emotional disorders are stuttering or stammering, cluttering, delayed speech, dyslalia, etc.

Stuttering or Stammering

Stuttering or stammering is a fluency disorders begins between the age of 3 to 5 years probably due to inability to adjust with environment and emotional stress. It is characterized by interruptions in the flow of speech, hesitations, spasmodic repetitions and prolongation of sounds specially of initial consonants. It is commonly found in boys with fear, anxiety and timid personality. These children are usually rigid and have positive family history of language and speech difficulty.

Management of stuttering includes behavior modification and relaxation therapy to resolve the conflict and emotional stress, thus to improve self-confidence in the child. Parents need counseling to rationalize their expectations of child's achievement according to the potentiality. The child should be reassured and helped in breath control exercise and speech therapy. Criticism for speech problem and pressure for normal speech make the child more handicapped. These children are not mentally retarded, they may have normal or high IQ level. So they need encouragement and guidance. Stammer suppressors, psychotherapy and drug therapy may be needed for some children.

Cluttering

Cluttering is characterized by unclear and hurried speech in which words tumble over each other. There are awkward movements of hands, feet and body. These children have erratic and poorly organized personality and behavior pattern. They need psychotherapy.

Delayed Speech

Delayed speech beyond 3 to 3.5 years can be considered as organic causes like mental retardation, infantile autism, hearing defects or severe emotional problems. The exact cause must be excluded for necessary interventions.

Dyslalia

Dyslalia is the most common disorder of difficulty in articulation. It can be caused by abnormalities of teeth, jaw or palate or due to emotional deprivation. Treatment of the structural abnormalities and speech therapy should be done adequately. In absence of structural problems, the responsible emotional disorders or factors should be ruled out. The child need counseling. The parents should be informed about the modification of family environment and correction of deprivation.

Sleep Disorders

Sleep disorders are common in children with anxiety, tension and overactivity. These problems are present with or without physical symptoms of behavioral disorders. Disturbances of sleep usually occur in deep sleep, i.e. stage 3 or 4 of NREM (nonrapid eye movement) sleep. The common sleep problems are difficulty to fall asleep, night mares, night terrors, sleep walking (somnambulism), sleep talking (somniloquism), bruxism (teeth grinding), etc.

In *night mares*, the child awakens from a frightening bad dream and is conscious of surroundings. In *night terrors*, the child awakens during sleep, sits up with screaming and terrified to recognize the surrounding and after sometimes sleeps again.

In all these problems, the child should have light diet in dinner and pleasant stories or scene at bed time. No exciting games and pictures and frightening stories (ghost, murder, accidents) should not be allowed at night. Parents should allow relax comfortable bed and emotionally healthy environment to the child. In case of sleep walking, door and windows to be kept closed and dangerous objects to be removed. In advanced and prolonged problems consultation with doctors and psychologists is essential for specific drug therapy and psychotherapy.

School Phobia or School Refusal

School phobia is persistent and abnormal fear of going to school. It is common in all social group. It is an emotional disorder of the children who are afraid to leave the parents, especially mother, and prefer to remain at home and refuse to go to school absolutely. It is a symptom of crisis situation of developmental stages and 'cry for help', which needs special attention.

The contributing factors of school phobia are anxiety about maternal separation, overindulgent, over protective and dominant mother, disinterested father, intellectual disability of the students and uncongenial school environment like teasing by other students, poor teacher-student relationship, unhygienic environment, fear of examination, etc.

The child may complain of recurrent physical complains like abdominal pain, headaches, which subside, if the child is allowed to remain at home.

The problem can be managed by habit formation for regular school attendance, play session and other recreational activities at school, improvement of school environment and assessment of health status of the child to detect any health problems for necessary interventions. The most important aspect to manage this problem is family counseling to resolve the anxiety related to maternal separation.

Attention Deficit Disorders

Attention deficit disorders (ADD) are learning disabilities can be related to CNS dysfunction or due to presence of psychoeducational determinants. It is usually associated with hyperactivity and known as hyperactive attention deficit disorders. These children are lagging behind in intellectual and learning abilities with alteration of behavior patterns.

The cause of this problem is not understood clearly, but predisposing factors can be prematurity or low birth weight, brain damage due to infections or injury and interaction between genetic and psychosocial factors. Impulsive children with poor attention span, hyperactivity and more demanding attitude are more likely to show poor learning abilities.

The manifestations may be combinations of reading and arithmetic disability, impaired memory, poor language and speech development, inappropriate understanding of spoken words, etc. The child is usually overactive, aggressive, excitable, impulsive and inattentive. They may be easily frustrated, irritated and show temper tantrums. Social relationship and adjustment are poorly developed.

Management is done by team approach including pediatrician, psychologist, psychiatrist, pediatric nurse specialist, school health nurse, teachers, social workers and parents. The approaches of management include behavior modification, counseling and guidance of parents and appropriate training and education of the child. Drug therapy can help to improve the CNS dysfunction or other associated problems.

BEHAVIORAL PROBLEMS OF ADOLESCENCE

Common behavioral disorders of adolescence are excessive masturbation, delinquency, antisocial behavior, substance abuse, anorexia nervosa, etc. These problems need special attention and necessary interventions.

Masturbation

Masturbation or genital stimulation by handling the genitals gives pleasure to the children. The infants and toddlers do this out of pure curiosity. The older children masturbate due to anxiety or sexual feelings. Boys during teen years mostly engage with this practice. Girls may do it to a lesser degree, though the number of these practice is increasing in recent years. Boys may masturbate in front of friends but girls are more private. Children may play with each other's genitals or a child may play alone with own.

Adolescents experience sexual excitement and erection of penis or clitoris followed by relief during masturbation.

It contributes in developing sense of mastery over sexual impulses and help the adolescents to capacitate and prepare for heterosexual relations.

Parents should be informed, that masturbation is normal response during prepubescent and pubescent stage and has a role in physical and emotional development. It provides a variety of sexual experiences. It helps in tension release and development of sexual fantasies and future sexual behavior.

If parents told about harmful effects of masturbation, when the child experiences pleasure out of it, then there will be conflict in the child, which can be associated with guilt feeling and shame. This conflict may be expressed as physical symptoms like severe weakness, fatigue, aches and pains and later as neuroses with feeling of unworthiness and maladjustment.

In case of excessive masturbation, the child needs special attention, facilities for recreation and diversion, sex education and counseling. Parents should be explained to provide love, affection and attention to the older children with specific concern about their feelings. Punishment and threat can exaggerate the practice. Excessive masturbation can cause sexual maladjustment in future.

Juvenile Delinquency

Juvenile delinquency means indulgence in an offence by a child in the form of premeditated, purposeful, unlawful activities done habitually and repeatedly. Usually these children belongs to broken family or emotionally disturbed family with overcrowded unhealthy environment and having financial or legal problems.

The factors contributing to the problem are mainly (a) rapid urbanization and industrialization, (b) social change and changing lifestyle, (c) influence of mass media, (d) change in moral standards and value systems (e) lack of educational opportunities and recreational facilities, (f) poor economy, (g) unsatisfactory conditions at schools and colleges, (h) unhealthy student-teacher relationship and (i) lack of discipline.

The juvenile delinquent behavior includes lying, theft, burglary, truancy from school, run away from home, habitual disobedience, fights, ungovernable behavior, mixing with antisocial gang, cruelty to animals, destructive attitude, murder, sexual assault, etc. In a broad sense, delinquency is not merely juvenile crime, it includes all deviations from normal youthful behavior and antisocial activities.

These rebellious antisocial behavior is the protest and response to the constant frustration, maladjustment, low self-esteem, lack of love and affection and emotional conflict. It is more common in boys. It is found in the children with aggressive, dishonest, addictive, unethical, rigid and disciplinarian parents. Children and adolescent may involve in delinquent activities in a gang, as the part of gang activities, just to prove their adventure and brave nature.

Prevention

Prevention of juvenile delinquency is possible by elimination of contributing factors. The problem of delinquent behaviors is now increasing in India and other countries. Preventive measures to be emphasized by healthy family and school environment. Healthy parent-child relationship, tender loving care in the family, fulfilment of basic needs, educational opportunities, facilities for sports, exercise and recreation, healthy teacher taught relationship, etc. are important aspects of prevention.

Delinquent child needs sympathetic attitude with necessary guidance and counseling for modification of behavior. The child should be referred to child guidance clinic for necessary help. A team approach is necessary in management of this condition including social workers, psychologists, psychiatrists, pediatricians, community health nurse, school teachers, family members and parents. Modification of social environment and rehabilitation of the delinquent child should be promoted.

Substance Abuse

Substance abuse or drug abuse is an threatening social problem of school going and adolescence age group. It is periodic or chronic intoxication by repeated intake of habit forming agents. It is persistent or sporadic use of drugs or any substance inconsistent with or unrelated to acceptable medical and social patterns within a given culture.

The abused agents are mainly tobacco, alcohol, sleeping pill, tranquillizers, mood elevators, stimulants, opiates, LSD, cocaine, heroin and cannabis (*bhang, ganja, charas*).

The children with this behavioral disorders are having frustration, emotional conflicts and disturbed family and school relationship. They are victims of gang activities, wrong adventure, poor parental guidance and lack of recreation and education. They may involve in various antisocial activities like stealing, shoplifting and even begging. The substance abuse is commonly found in boarding public school.

Preventive Measures

Preventive measures of substance abuse include the followings:
- Provision of adequate facilities for recreation and entertainment, especially in the hostels.
- Proper channelization of energies of the adolescents into constructive activities.

- Inculcation of the dangers of drug abuse among students, their teachers and family members.
- Provision of mental health program and periodical psychiatric guidance facilities in schools.
- Strict implementation of drug control measures.

The ill effects of substance abuse to be informed to the public through individual or group health education or by mass media communication to create public awareness. Parents, teachers and family members are also responsible to provide emotional support to the older children to prevent frustration, conflict, confusion and mental tension. They should identify the addicts and arrange for deaddiction, wherever necessary. The addicted children need psychotherapy, deaddiction services and rehabilitation.

Anorexia Nervosa

Anorexia nervosa is a eating disorder occurs most often in adolescent girls. The problem is found as refusal of food to maintain normal body weight by reducing food intake, especially fats and carbohydrates. The affected adolescent girls practices vigorous exercise for weight reduction or induce vomiting by stimulating gag reflex to remain slim. It is a marked disturbance of body image. The adolescent thinks that they are fat even though they are under weight. Anorexia means loss of appetite, but in this condition the affected individual experience true hunger though they have absolute control over their appetite.

There is no specific organic cause of anorexia nervosa. The affected adolescent may have associated conditions like disease of liver, kidney, heart or diabetes. Parents of the affected adolescent may be anorectic and having conflict in relationship with the child or overprotective which lead to development of immaturity, isolation and excessive dependence.

The affected individual is characterized by undernutrition, marked weight loss, bizarre food intake patterns, dryness of skin, hypothermia, hypotension, bradycardia, amenorrhea, constipation, etc.

Management of the condition include psychotherapy, antidepressant drugs, behavior modification and nutritional rehabilitation. Parental counseling for modification of parent child relationship is essential. Hospitalization may be needed in complicated cases.

NURSING RESPONSIBILITIES IN BEHAVIORAL DISORDERS OF CHILDREN

Nurses play a vital role for prevention, early identification and management of behavioral disorders in children. Nurses themselves, need to have up to date knowledge and skill related to these problems. They can help the children, their parents and family in different aspects.

Nursing Responsibilities

Nursing responsibilities can be summarized as follows:

- Assessment of specific problem of the child by appropriate history and detection of the responsible factors.
- Informing the parents and making them aware about the causes of behavioral problems of the particular child.
- Assisting the parents, teachers and family members for necessary modification of environment at home, school and community.
- Encouraging the child for behavior modification, as needed.
- Promoting healthy emotional development of the child by adequate physical, psychological and social support.
- Creating awareness about psychosocial disturbances which may lead to behavioral problems during developmental stages.
- Providing counseling services for children and their parents to solve the problems, whenever necessary and for tender loving care of the children.
- Participating in the management of the problem child, as a member of health team along with pediatrician, psychologist and social worker. Organizing child guidance clinic.
- Referring the children with behavioral problems for necessary management and support to better health care facilities, child guidance clinic, social welfare services and support agencies.

Congenital Anomalies

11

- Concepts of Congenital Anomalies
- Etiology of Congenital Anomalies
- Diagnostic Approaches
- Common Congenital Anomalies

- Prevention of Congenital Anomalies
- Genetic Counseling
- Nursing Responsibilities Towards Congenital Anomalies

CONCEPTS OF CONGENITAL ANOMALIES

Congenital abnormalities are those defects and diseases which are substantially determined before or during birth and recognizable in early life. Some disorders are detected at birth, e.g. cleft lip and cleft palate. Some are obvious in early life like congenital dislocation of hip which is detected until walking commence and some may become apparent until much later in life, e.g. patent ductus arteriosus, which is diagnosed usually in school age or even later. Some disorders may remain unrecognized. Some defects are classified as major which may require surgical interventions, either as emergency or as elective. Some are classified as minor that have no functional implications, like skin tags in front of the ear.

Congenital malformations may be regarded as one form of reproductive failure. The favorable environmental and genetic factors result in normal reproduction and the unfavorable factors lead to sterility, abortion, stillbirth, preterm births or neonatal death. Congenital anomalies represent a relative reproductive success when compared to sterility or abortion. Prevention of congenital defects must be achieved by special attention to environmental factors rather than by attempting to improve heredity towards successful reproductive outcome.

Definitions

The terms congenital anomaly and congenital malformation are used interchangeably, but they are different in meaning.

A WHO document described the terms, the congenital anomaly being used to include all biochemical, structural and functional disorders present at birth and the congenital malformation should be confined to structural defects only, present at birth. The birth defects or congenital defects may be inherited genetically or acquired during gestation or inflicted during parturition.

Incidence

The global incidence of congenital disorders is estimated about 30 to 70 per 1000 live birth (1989). Approximately half of these infants have fatal outcome or lifelong chronic diseases. Actual numbers vary widely between countries. The most common congenital defects are congenital heart diseases and central nervous system malformations.

In India, the incidence of congenital defects is about 2.5 to 4 percent among children. It is considered as third most frequent cause of perinatal mortality in India. Congenital anomalies are also considered as one of the important cause of physical and mental handicapped conditions among survivors. Most common type of birth defect is CNS abnormalities, approximately 22 percent of all defects. In northern part of India, neural tube defects are most common, whereas in the rest of India, musculoskeletal disorders are commonly found.

Risk Factors

Some factors are considered to be significantly associated with incidence of congenital anomalies.

- Advanced maternal age, e.g. elderly mother has risk of birth of baby with Down's syndrome or other congenital anomalies.
- Consanguinity, i.e. baby born out of consanguineous marriages (among blood relations), e.g. marriage with first cousin or uncle-niece, are at risk of congenital defects like mental retardation.
- Maternal malnutrition especially folic acid deficiency can lead to CNS defects and iodine deficiency can lead to mental retardation or other congenital anomalies.

ETIOLOGY OF CONGENITAL ANOMALIES

The causes of most of the congenital anomalies are not fully understood. Majority of the causes are unknown or due to complex interaction between genetic and environmental factors and is considered as multifactorial. Approximately 65 percent cases may be due to multifactorial, whereas about 25 percent cases are due to genetic factors and about 10 percent cases are due to environmental factors. Genetic disorders again can be classified as (a) chromosomal abnormalities, (b) unifactorial (single gene or Mendelian) diseases and (c) multifactorial disorders.

Genes are the units of heredity. They contain hereditary information encoded in their chemical structure for transmission from generation to generation. They affect development and functions of the individual, both normal and abnormal. It is said, that we inherit about 50,000 genes from the father and 50,000 from the mother. Allele, one of two or more alternative forms of a gene at corresponding sites (loci) on homologous chromosomes, determine alternative characters in inheritance.

Since genes are contained in the chromosomes. Genes also occur in pairs. If the genes comprising a pair are alike (DD), the individual is described as homozygous for that gene, and if it is different (Dd), the individual is described as heterozygous.

A gene is said to be dominant when it manifests its effect both in the heterozygous and the homozygous state. A gene is said to be recessive when it manifests, its effect only in the homozygous state. Genes are usually stable, but sometimes normal genes may be converted into abnormal ones, this change is called mutation. Mutation is a regular phenomenon in nature. The natural mutation rate is increased by exposure to mutagens such as ultraviolet rays, radiation or chemical carcinogens.

Genetic Factors

Congenital anomalies are inherited through the genes in the ovum or sperm. The anomalies may be related to chromosomal abnormalities, single gene disorders or polygenic inheritance. Single gene disorders may be either autosomal or X-linked inheritance, which may be dominant or recessive traits. There are about 3000 known genetic disorders.

Chromosomal Abnormalities

Chromosomal abnormalities occur either in the form of numerical or structural alterations and found time to time in human beings. They arise in various ways, i.e. non-disjunction, translocation, deletion, duplication, inversion, isochromosomes and mosaicism. The most common chromosomal abnormality related to autosomes is Down's syndrome or Trisomy 21.

Single Gene Disorders

Single gene disorders are found as autosomal dominant inheritance, autosomal recessive inheritance and X-linked inheritance. The principal characteristics of the autosomal and X-linked inherited disorders are as follows:

Autosomal-dominant traits: In this condition, every affected child has at least one affected parent (except mutations). An affected individual needs only be heterozygous for the given allele. Male and female offspring are equally affected (50:50). There is a risk of 50 percent involvement of each sibling of an affected individual, if the parent is affected. There are affected individuals in several generations. Examples of autosomal dominant inherited diseases are—achondroplasia, hereditary spherocytosis, osteogenesis imperfecta, Marfan syndrome, Huntington chorea, polydactyly, polycystic kidney, retinoblastoma, etc.

Autosomal-recessive traits: In this disease, each parent of an affected individual must carry at least one mutant allele (normal parents are carriers). Every affected individual is homozygous for the given allele. Individuals possessing a single mutant allele do not show the trait. Either sex may be affected and there is a 25 percent risk of involvement of the siblings of an affected individual. The disease tends to be rare but more severe than dominantly inherited traits. Examples of autosomal recessive inherited diseases are—albinism, cystic fibrosis, galactosemia, microcephaly, sickle cell anemia, Tay-Sachs disease, thalassemia, phenylketonuria, Hirschsprung disease, etc.

X-linked inheritance or sex-linked inheritance: X-linked disorders are inherited abnormalities in which the abnormal genes are carried on the sex (X) chromosomes. The known two types are, X-linked recessive and X-linked dominant. The Y-chromosome is known to carry only one genetic trait, i.e. hairy ears. Therefore, all of the known sex-chromosome disorders involve one of the X-chromosomes.

The *principal characteristics* of X-linked traits are as follows:

i. *X-linked recessive traits:* In this disorders, affected individuals are nearly always male. The mother is usually a carrier and she transmits the disease to 50 percent of her sons. One half of carrier mothers' daughters will be carriers. Affected males transmit their mutant allele to each of their daughters and none of their sons. The uninvolved sons do not transmit the disease. Examples of X-linked recessive diseases are color blindness, hemophilia A and B, glucose-6 phosphate dehydrogenase deficiency, hydrocephalus, Duchenne type of muscular dystrophy, etc.

ii. *X-linked dominant traits:* In this conditions, the hemizygous male will exhibit the full disease. All the daughters and none of the sons of affected males are affected. The homozygous female will have severe disease and all of her children will be affected. The heterozygous female will have a milder form of the disease and there is a 50 percent chance that her children will be affected. The best examples of this type of inheritance are orofaciodigital syndrome type-I, hereditary hematuria, incontinentia pigmenti, etc. This inheritance is rarely found.

Polygenic or Multifactorial Inheritance

Each individual carries a variable number of genes which, if combined in a certain way, but as yet unknown way with a mate's gene, can cause physical defects in offspring. A polygenically determined abnormality is the result of a combination of these multiple genes, that is no one specific gene is totally responsible for the defect. The intrauterine and postnatal environment can be influential in this form of inheritance, and may be responsible for the polygenetic disorder. Multifactorial inheritance is a combination of polygenic and environmental factors.

Some examples of multifactorial inheritance are pyloric stenosis, cleft lip and/or palate, isolated heart disease, anencephaly, meningomyelocele, diabetes, idiopathic epilepsy, asthma, schizophrenia, mental retardation, colon cancer, coronary artery disease, etc.

If the parents are unaffected, the recurrence risk of the specific defect is usually given in the range of 3 to 5 percent. If one parent is affected the risk is more. The more siblings affected, the higher the risk or recurrence in future offspring, even as high as 11 to 21 percent.

Environmental Factors

Various environmental factors are responsible for occurrence of congenital anomalies. Teratogenic agents of the environment adversely affect the normal cellular development of the embryo or fetus causing birth defects. The common environmental factors are:

- Intrauterine infections especially by STORCH (Syphilis, Toxoplasmosis, Rubella, Cytomegalovirus and Herpes Virus).

- Drugs intake by the mother during pregnancy like steroid hormones, stilbestrol, anticonvulsants, folate antagonists, cocaine, lithium, thalidomide, etc.
- X-ray exposure during pregnancy.
- Maternal diseases like diabetes, cardiac failure, malnutrition, folic acid deficiency, iodine deficiency disorders, endocrine abnormalities, etc.
- Abnormal intauterine environment like bicornuate uterus, septed uterus, polyhydromnios, oligohydromnios, fetal hypoxia, etc.
- Maternal addiction with alcohol, tobacco or smoking (active or passive).
- Environmental pollution, especially air pollution.

Effects of the teratogens depend upon the severity of exposure, the gestational age of fetus at the time of exposure and the maternal and fetal immune response to the teratogenic agents. The fetus is potentially susceptible to some teratogenic effect even after the completion of organogenesis. The ultimate effect may be death, malformations, growth retardation of fetus or functional disorders.

DIAGNOSTIC APPROACHES

An accurate and early diagnosis is of primary importance. It depends upon the available facilities for diagnostic tests. It is now possible to identify the healthy carriers of a number of genetic disorder like hemophilia, thalassemia, inborn errors of metabolism, etc. There are thousands of known genetic diseases and hundreds of established patterns of malformation syndromes, so it may be difficult to diagnose all conditions accurately. But various prenatal and postnatal investigations help to detect the congenital abnormalities for necessary care and management.

Prenatal Diagnosis

Advanced medical technology helps in the detection of congenital anomalies in intrauterine period by the following diagnostic measures:

- Amniocentasis in early pregnancy, about 14 to 16 weeks, helps in prenatal diagnosis of chromosomal abnormalities (Down's syndrome) and many inborn errors of metabolism (Tay-Sachs disease, galactosemia).
- Chorionic villus sampling for cytogenetic study to detect chromosomal aberration especially in advanced maternal age.
- Estimation of maternal serum alpha-fetoprotein and chorionic gonadotropin to screen out neural tube defect and trisomy.
- Ultrasonography for fetal profile.
- Fetoscopy with special fetoscope or endoscope.
- Amniography with radio-opaque dye to diagnose soft tissue abnormalities.

- Fetal blood sampling and skin scraping test, protein assay and DNA diagnosis.
- Radiography.
- Antenatal screening of maternal diseases, metabolic and endocrinal functions by regular examination, laboratory investigations and details family history.

Prenatal diagnosis of congenital anomalies helps the parents to decide for the medical termination of pregnancy or to allow the birth of a malformed baby or some time for intrauterine corrective surgical interventions.

Postnatal Diagnosis

Postnatal diagnosis is easy by various approaches. Details maternal and family history along with thorough physical examination of the newborn baby help in diagnosis. There are numbers of screening tests for early diagnosis of genetic abnormalities like sex chromosome abnormalities, congenital dislocation of hip, PKU, congenital hypothyroidism, sickle cell disease, cystic fibrosis, Duchenne muscular dystrophy, congenital adrenal hyperplasia, G6PD deficiency, etc.

Biochemical assay, cytogenetic study, blood test, hormonal assay, radiography, ultrasonography, etc. are useful to detect different anomalies for early management.

COMMON CONGENITAL ANOMALIES

There are thousands of known congenital anomalies affecting various system of the body. Most common problems are related to central nervous system. Lists of known and common congenital anomalies of different systems are given below. The details of these problems are discussed in the respective chapters (Figs 11.1 to 11.9).

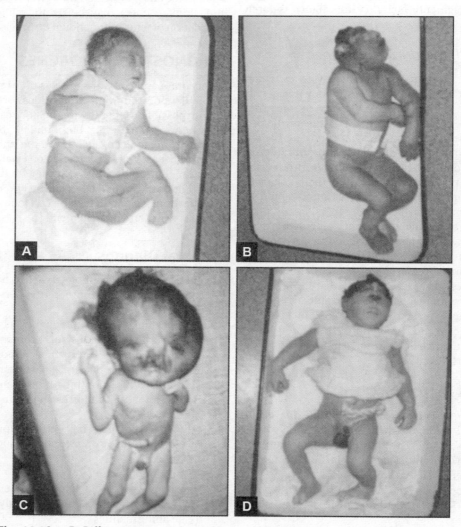

Figs 11.1A to D: Different congenital anomalies in still birth baby *(For color version, see Plate 3)*

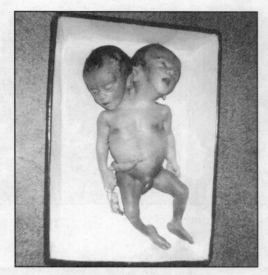

Fig. 11.2: Double headed monster
(For color version, see Plate 4)

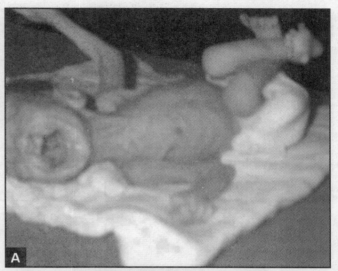

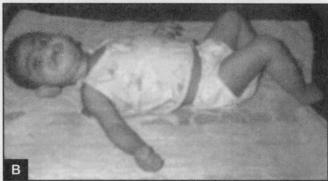

Figs 11.4A and B: Cleft lip and cleft palate
(For color version, see Plate 4)

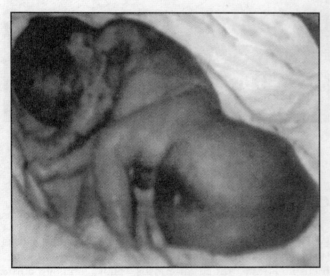

Fig. 11.3: Sacrococcygeal teratoma
(For color version, see Plate 4)

Central Nervous System Defects

Congenital anomalies of central nervous system include—Anencephaly, spina bifida occulta, spina bifida cystica (meningocele, meningomyelocele, meningoencephalocele, encephalocele), hydrocephalus, microcephaly (microencephaly), macrocephaly, syringomyelia, tethered spinal cord, diastematomyelia, porencephaly, schizencephaly, agenesis of cranial nerves, etc.

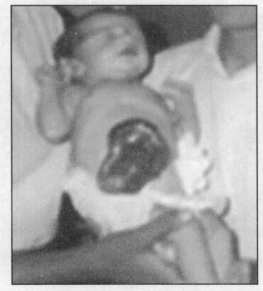

Fig. 11.5: Gastroschisis *(For color version, see Plate 4)*

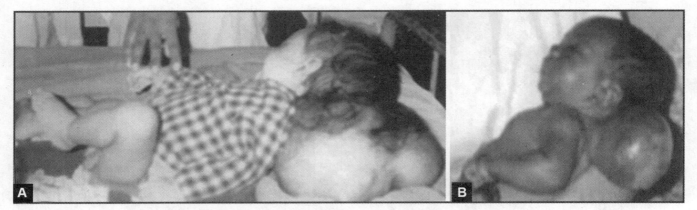

Figs 11.6A and B: Meningoencephalocele *(For color version, see Plate 5)*

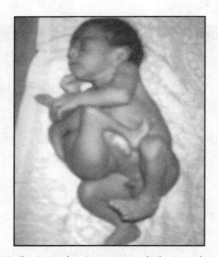

Fig. 11.7: Conjoined twin, one twin baby is without head
(For color version, see Plate 5)

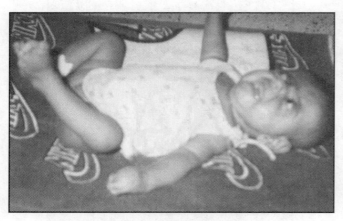

Fig. 11.8: Multiple congenital anomalies
(For color version, see Plate 5)

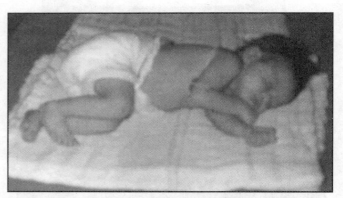

Fig. 11.9: A neonate with congenital obstructive jaundice
(For color version, see Plate 5)

Congenital Heart Diseases

Congenital heart diseases include ventricular septal defect (VSD), atrial septal defect (ASD), patent ductus arteriosus (PDA), coarctation of aorta, transposition of great vessels, tricuspid atresia, truncus arteriosus, Fallot's tetralogy, aortic stenosis, pulmonic stenosis, aortic or pulmonary artery dilatation, mitral or aortic regurgitation, Ebstein's anomaly, dextrocardia, etc.

Gastrointestinal System Abnormalities

The congenital abnormalities of gastrointestinal system include: Tracheoesophageal fistula, esophageal atresia, congenital pyloric stenosis, duodenal atresia, meconium ileus, malrotation of gut, congenital megacolon (Hirschsprung disease), anorectal malformations, exomphalos, umbilical hernia, diaphragmatic hernia, femoral hernia, congenital intestinal obstruction, gastroschisis, etc.

Respiratory System Abnormalities

The congenital anomalies of respiratory system include; choanal atresia, tracheoesophageal fistula, congenital atelectasis, pulmonary agenesis, congenital stridor, congenital cyanosis, etc.

Abnormalities of Genitourinary System

Renal agenesis, congenital hydronephrosis, congenital polycystic kidney, horse-shoe kidney, posterior urethral valves (PUV), hypospedias, epispedias, ectopia vasicae, congenital phimosis, congenital hydrocele, undescended testis, congenital inguinal hernia, ambiguous genitalia, malformations of reproductive organs, etc.

Musculoskeletal Abnormalities

Club foot, (talipes), congenital dislocation of hip, osteogenesis imperfecta, polydactyl, webbed fingers and toes (synductyl), amelia, phocomelia, congenital scoliosis, Marfan syndrome, mucopolysaccharidoses (Hurler syndrome, Hunter syndrome), muscular dystrophies, etc.

Blood Disorders

Thalassemia, hemophilia, sickle cell anemia, congenital spherocytosis.

Metabolic Disorders

Cystic fibrosis, phenylketonuria (PKU), G-6PD deficiency, porphyria, congenital lactose intolerance, glycogen storage diseases, mucopolysaccharidoses, Tay-Sachs disease, Gaucher disesase, Wilson's disease, galactosemia, inborn errors of metabolism, etc.

Endocrinal Abnormalities

Congenital hypopituitarism (dwarfism), congenital hypothyroidism (cretinism), congenital adrenogenital hyperplasia, congenital goiter, diabetes mellitus.

Chromosomal Abnormalities

Down's syndrome (Trisomy 21), Patau's syndrome (Trisomy-13), Edward's syndrome (Trisomy-18), Turner syndrome (XO), Klinefelter's syndrome (XXY, XXXY), Cri du chat syndrome (cat like cry of infant).

Miscellaneous

Many congenital malformation do not fit into particular categories of either matabolic or chromosomal disorders or to a specific system. They may found as a single defect or as syndrome, which include cleft lip and/or palate, congenital cataract, congenital glaucoma, retinoblastoma, color blindness, congenital deafness, deaf and dumb, mental retardation, microagnatha, albinism, hemangioma, pseudohermophroditism, situs inversus, Prader-Willi syndrome, Apert syndrome, congenital biliary atresia etc.

PREVENTION OF CONGENITAL ANOMALIES

Prevention of congenital anomalies can be possible by health promotional measures, specific protection, early diagnosis and specific management. Prevention of these abnormalities is more approachable than the curative management. According to Penrose (1961), major advances in the prevention of malformations must be achieved by attention to environmental factors rather than by attempting to improve heredity. Environmental modification is more within reach than genetic control.

Preventive Measures

The preventive measures should include the following aspects:
- Genetic counseling is the true preventive measure of congenital anomalies.
- Reducing and discouraging consanguineous marriages. When blood relatives marry each other there is an increased risk in the offspring of traits controlled by recessive genes and those determined by polygenes.
- Avoiding late marriage of females and avoidance of pregnancy beyond the age of 35 years.
- Promotion of health of girl child and prepregnant health status of the females by prevention of malnutrition, anemia, folic acid deficiency, iodine deficiency, etc.
- Encouraging the immunization of all girl child by MMR (Mumps, Measles, Rubella).
- Increasing attention to the protection of individuals and whole communities against mutagens such as X-ray and other ionizing radiations and also for chemical mutagens (drugs, alcohol).
- Immunization by anti-D immunoglobulin to the 'Rh-negative' mothers after abortion or first child birth to prevent Rh-hemolytic disease of the newborn which is a genetically determined immunological disorder.
- Elimination of active and passive smoking of tobacco by mothers.
- Avoidance of drug intake without consulting physician in the first trimester of pregnancy.
- Prevention of intrauterine infections and promotion of sexual hygiene along with general hygienic measures.
- Efficient antenatal care especially removal of teratogens, periconceptional supplementation of folic acid, prevention of maternal malnutrition by adequate diet, prenatal diagnosis of suspected genetic disorders and

maternal diseases, appropriate treatment of maternal diseases and infections, prevention of fetal hypoxia, etc.
- Promotion of therapeutic abortion of abnormal fetus and fetus with gross congenital anomalies, after prenatal diagnosis.
- Discouraging reproduction after birth of a baby with congenital anomalies, without genetic counseling. The risk of malformations in subsequent pregnancies is increased by 10 times.
- Increasing public awareness about the risk factors and etiological factors of congenital anomalies and their preventive measures.
- Promotion of detection of genetic carriers, e.g. both partners should arrange to test for thalassemia carrier before marriage.
- Reducing the frequency of hereditary disease and disability in the community to as low as possible by *negative eugenics*. The persons who are suffering from serious hereditary disease are debarred from producing children or sterilized, there should be no serious objection to marriage. *Positive eugenics* can be promoted to improve the genetic composition of the population by encouraging the carriers of desirable genotypes to assume the burden of parenthood.

GENETIC COUNSELING

The most immediate and practical service that genetics can render in medicine and surgery is genetic counseling. It is a problem-solving approach or communication process in relation to genetic disorders or congenital anomalies in the family. This process helps in providing appropriate informations and advice about the course of action in relation to occurrence or risk of occurrence or recurrence of genetic problems in a family. It is nondirective information to the individual or family who discuss the importance to their own situations. It may be prospective or retrospective.

Prospective genetic counseling allows for the true prevention of disease. This approach aims at preventing or reducing heterozygous marriage by screening procedures and explaining the risk of affected children (thalassemia, sickle cell anemia).

Retrospective genetic counseling is mostly done at present, after a hereditary disorder has already occurred within the family. The methods which could be suggested under retrospective genetic counseling are (a) contraception (b) termination of pregnancy and (c) sterilization depending upon the attitudes and cultural environment of the couples involved.

Reasons for Seeking Genetic Counseling

- A child has been born with a diagnosed congenital defect or a group of malformations.

- A medical problem has affected more than one member of the family and suspected to be genetic.
- A family has one or more mentally retarded children or having delayed physical and mental developmental milestones.
- Exposure of some environmental agents (teratogen, mutagen).
- Closely related couples want to know their risk of having a child with a birth defect.
- When one person wants to marry, but known about hereditary problem in one or both family.
- A genetic disorder is detected during prenatal diagnosis.

The informations received by the families during genetic counseling can affect the parents and normal siblings' decision about having future children and also about the care of the affected child throughout the life. The informations help the individual or families about the present and future possible genetic disorders and the various options available for safeguarding from recurrence of such a disorder or minimizing its adverse effects.

For effective genetic counseling the following prerequisites to be satisfied:
- Obtain accurate prenatal, natal and postnatal history along with medical history of the disorder and family history.
- Prepare a pedigree chart or family tree.
- Detailed recording of clinical examination of the affected child.
- Confirmation of the diagnosis by relevant investigations.
- Information regarding support groups for the benefit of the family and available management facilities and follow-up.
- Awareness about the emotional reactions of the parents and their acceptance of the malformed child.

Genetic counseling can be done by group of specialist including physicians, geneticists, psychologists, biochemists, cytologists, pediatric nurse specialist and social worker. Counseling can be done to the individual parent or to the family according to the nature of problem. It can be provided in as little as one session and as many sessions as the counselor and family feel they need to understand the complexities and emotional response of the disorders. It is important after a single counseling session to emphasize for follow-up meeting whenever any problem or questions arise.

NURSING RESPONSIBILITIES TOWARDS CONGENITAL ANOMALIES

As a member of the team, the nurse has the responsibility of being liaison among the family, referring physician or agency and the medical-genetics team. The nurse is usually the first person with whom the family has contact. The nurse can help the family by assuring them and explaining about importance of accurate diagnosis for appropriate management. Nursing personnel can provide following interventions for the management of the affected child.

- Collection of details history, especially history of prenatal, natal and postnatal period along with history of family illness.
- Preparation of pedigree chart by interview and home visit.
- Identification of present problems, its nature and severity, for necessary interventions.
- Participation in diagnostic investigations, treatment, follow-up and research project.
- Provide necessary information to the parents and family members.

- Motivate the family members for genetic counseling and referring to the genetic clinic.
- Participating in genetic counseling proccess with special training, personal experience, knowledge and competency.
- Provide emotional support and answer questions asked by the counselee.
- Guide the family for rehabilitation of the child and for available social and economical support through social welfare agencies.
- Promote public awareness about the prevention of congenital anomalies by individual or group health education or by mass media information.

Nutritional Deficiency Disorders

12

- Ecology of Malnutrition
- Assessment of Nutritional Problems
- Protein-energy Malnutrition
- Vitamins and their Deficiency Disorders
- Minerals and their Deficiency Disorders
- Community Nutrition Programs

INTRODUCTION

Nutritional deficiency disorders are major public health problem in India and other developing countries. They affect vast majority numbers of population and responsible for approximately 55 percent of childhood death. They are important factors behind childhood illness like ARI, diarrhea, perinatal insult, etc. They considered as leading killers and significant cause of childhood mortality and morbidity. They contribute towards various physical and mental handicapped conditions in later life. Though the frequency of nutritional deficiency disorders is difficult to estimate, the condition is still threatening, especially in our pediatric population.

In India, there are about 60 million malnourished children and every month about one lack children die due to effects of malnutrition. About 2.5 million children of our country are threatened by blindness in early childhood (1–5 years) because of lack of vitamin 'A' and about 12000 to 14000 go blind every year because of this deficiency which is eminently curable. About 75 to 80 percent of the hospitalized children suffer from some degree or type of malnutrition. Approximately 25 percent pediatric beds are occupied by patients whose major problem is malnutrition or in whom malnutrition is indirectly responsible for hospitalization.

On a global scale, the five principal nutritional deficiency diseases that are being accorded the highest priority action are kwashiorkor, marasmus, xerophthalmia, nutritional anemias and endemic goiter. These diseases represent the tip of the iceberg of malnutrition, a much larger population are affected by hidden malnutrition which is not easy to diagnose.

The effects of malnutrition on the community are both direct and indirect. The direct effects are the occurrence of frank and subclinical nutritional deficiency diseases such as kwashiorkor, marasmus, vitamin and mineral deficiency disorders. The indirect effects are a high morbidity and mortality among young children, retardation of physical and mental growth and development, lowered vitality of the people leading to lowered productivity, permanent disability and reduced life expectancy.

Definition of Malnutrition

Malnutrition has been defined as a "pathological state resulting from a relative or absolute deficiency or excess of one or more essential nutrients." It comprises four forms—Undernutrition, overnutrition, imbalance and the specific deficiency. Protein-energy malnutrition, vitamin deficiency disorders and mineral deficiency diseases are important nutritional problems in our country.

ECOLOGY OF MALNUTRITION

Malnutrition is a man-made disease of human society. The ecology of malnutrition is complex with numbers of influencing factors like disease conditions, infections, socio-economic status, cultural practices and available health and other services.

Infections and Disease Conditions

Infectious diseases are important responsible factors for malnutrition in children. Malnutrition predisposes to infection and infection to malnutrition, it is a vicious circle. ARI, diarrhea, intestinal parasitosis, measles, whooping caugh, tuberculosis, malaria, all contribute to malnutrition directly or indirectly. Deliberate restriction of food during illness, loss of appetite, increased catabolism during fever and poor absorption in intestinal parasitosis are leading cause of malnutrition.

Poor Socioeconomic Status

Poor economical status and social structure are the important factors for the development of malnutrition. Nutritional deficiency conditions are by-product of bad-economy, insufficient education, ignorance, lack of knowledge regarding food values, inadequate sanitary environment, large family size, disturbed family (broken family, alcoholism), closely spaced families with repeated pregnancies, working mothers, infants with low birth weight and prematurity, etc. These factors bear most directly on the quality of life and are significant determinants of malnutrition, primarily by dietary deficiency.

Population explosion, natural disaster (like flood, earthquakes, draughts), unequal distribution of available food, scarcity of food at the family level in accordance with physiological needs, increased expenditure for clothing and entertainment rather than food, etc. are also contributing towards malnutrition.

Cultural Influences

Deficiency of food materials is not the only cause of malnutrition. Many deep-rooted beliefs, customs, practices, superstition, food taboos, ignorance about food value, food habits and attitudes, religious belief, food fads, cooking practices, etc. have powerful influence to cause malnutrition.

Faulty child rearing practices and care of antenatal mothers influence the nutritional status of the infants and children. Inadequate diet in antenatal period and maternal malnutrition lead to low birth weight, prematurity, neonatal infections etc. which pose a bad start for the infants causing high mortality or poor growth of the survivors. Failure of lactation, inadequate breastfeeding, increasing numbers of working mothers, delayed weaning, adoption of bottle feeding by premature curtailment of breastfeeding, feeding with commercially produced foods with diluted formula, starvation during diarrhea and other illnesses are very significant contributing practices leading to malnutrition.

Inadequate Health and Other Services

Malnutrition is the outcome of several factors. Health sector with the help of other sectors and adequate resources can combat the problems of malnutrition by different approaches. But inadequacy of resources in relation to the extent of problem makes it unmanageable. It seems that 50 percent of the nutritional problems can be solved by nutrition education only, but it is still a weak component of health services. Nutritional assessment, nutritional supplementation and nutritional rehabilitation are not sufficiently provided for the vulnerable population, especially for the children of rural, tribal and backward areas.

ASSESSMENT OF NUTRITIONAL PROBLEMS

Assessment of nutritional status of the malnourished children is more easy than that of borderline (mild or moderate) or subclinical nutritional disturbances of the children. The assessment of nutritional status of an individual involves various techniques.

- Assessment of dietary intake by details history of dietary patterns, specific food consumed and its amount, quality and adequacy in relation of nutrient value.
- Anthropometric examination of the child including weight, length/height, mid-upper arm circumference, skin fold thickness, are valuable indicators of nutritional status. In young children, head circumference and chest circumference are also measured to assess patterns of growth and development and deviations from average size.
- Clinical examination of the child to assess deficiency signs and associated problems. Thorough head to foot examination is done to detect the classical signs of various deficiency states.
- Assessment of associated problems like tuberculosis, malabsorption syndrome, any infections or infestations should be made to find out the probable cause of nutritional deficiency.
- Laboratory investigations to be done to exclude the underlying cause including routine examination of stool, urine, blood, and X-ray. Estimation of hemoglobin, serum proteins, enzymes, blood levels of nutrients like vitamins, iron, amino acid, etc. to be done whenever indicated.
- Assessment of ecological factors, morbidity and mortality patterns in the community help to detect the nutritional status of the particular community, as these situations influence the nutritional status of an individual.

PROTEIN-ENERGY MALNUTRITION

Protein-energy malnutrition (PEM) has been identified as a major public health and nutrition problem in India. It can be defined as a group of clinical conditions that may result from varying degree of protein deficiency and energy (calorie) inadequacy. Previously, it was known as protein calorie malnutrition (PCM) (Figs 12.1A to D).

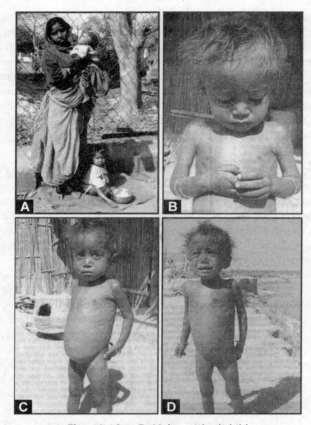

Figs 12.1A to D: Malnourished child

The incidence of PEM in India in preschool children is about 1 to 2 percent. The great majority of cases of PEM, nearly 80 percent are the mild and moderate cases which frequently go unrecognized. This problem exists in all states. Nutritional marasmus is more common in occurrence than kwashiorkor.

PEM is primarily due to an inadequate intake of food (food gap), both in quantity and quality. Infections, especially ARI, diarrhea, measles and worm infestations lead to the condition which increase in requirements for calories, proteins and other nutrients, while decreasing their absorption and utilization and considered as important cause of PEM. There are numerous other contributory factors for the causation of PEM (as discussed in ecological factors of malnutrition). The first indicator of PEM is under weight for age which is easy to detect by growth chart maintenance. These charts indicate at a glance whether the child is gaining or losing weight.

Classification of Protein-energy Malnutrition

The PEM is a broad range of condition ranging from growth failure to overt kwashiorkor or marasmus. It may be classified according to severity or level of deficiency. Classifications are done based on achievement of expected weight or height according to given age.

There are several classifications of PEM; known as syndromal classification, Gomez classification, Welcome or International Classification, Classification by Indian Academy of Pediatrics (IAP), Jelliffe Classification, MC Laren Classification, Waterlow Classification, Arnold Classification, WHO Classification, Gopalan Classification, etc. Some of the Classifications are as follows:

Syndromal Classification

- Kwashiorkor
- Nutritional marasmus
- Prekwashiorkor
- Nutritional dwarfing.

Classification by Indian Academy of Pediatrics

- When the child is having weight more than 80 percent of expected weight for age, considered as normal. The grade of malnutrition is described as follows:
- Grade I — between 71 and 80 percent of expected weight for the age.
- Grade II — between 61 and 70 percent of expected weight for that age.
- Grade III — between 51 and 60 percent of expected weight for that age.
- Grade IV — 50 percent or less of weight expected for that age.

In case of demonstrable edema in the child, the letter 'K' is placed in front of the evaluated grade.

Gomez Classification

According to this classification, PEM is graded with reference to the weight for age as percentage of the expected weight (Harvard Standard). It is an international classification that takes a weight of more than 90 percent of expected for that age (50th percentile) as normal. The grade of malnutrition are as follows:

- Grade I — Weight between 75 and 90 percent of expected for the age.
- Grade II — Weight between 61 and 75 percent of expected for the age.
- Grade III — Weight less than or equal to 60 percent of expected for the age.

WHO Classification

WHO recommends three term, i.e. stunting, under weight and wasting, for assessing the magnitude of malnutrition in under five children.

Stunting is defined as a child below 2 standard deviation (SD) score from the median height for age of NCHS reference population (–3 SD for severe stunting).

Under weight is defined as a child below 2 SD from the median weight for age of NCHS reference population (–3 SD for severe under weight).

Wasting is defined as a child below 2 SD from median weight for height of NCHS reference population (–3 SD for severe wasting).

National Center for Health Statistics (NCHS), USA, is the most popular international standards (WHO, 1993).

Clinical Features of PEM

Clinical features of PEM depend upon severity and duration of nutritional inadequacy, age of the child, relative lack of different foods and presence or absence of associated infections. Kwashiorkor and nutritional marasmus are two extreme forms of PEM. These extreme forms account for a small proportion of cases of PEM, whereas a much larger number of children suffer from mild to moderate nutritional deficiency.

When the dietary intake is inadequate for a short period, the body adjusts its metabolism to compensate for the deficiency to some extent. If deficit of food persists for a longer period, the malnourished children conserve energy by reducing physical activity. Moderately malnourished children appear more slow and less energetic. If the nutrition deficit continues longer, growth of the child is affected. As the nutritional deficiency exaggerates with infections, the child may become marasmic or may develop kwashiorkor.

Kwashiorkor

Kwashiorkor was first described by Dr. Cicely Williams in 1933, but the particular term "Kwashiorkor" was introduced in 1935, according to local name for the disease in Ghana. The term was said to mean "red boy" due to characteristic pigmentary changes.

This nutritional deficiency condition is mainly found in preschool children but may occur in any age. The childhood infections like ARI, diarrhea, measles, etc. may precipitate the disease. Dietary history reveals deficient intake of both protein and calories but protein lack is more predominant.

The *presenting features* can be divided into two groups, i.e. essential and nonessential features.

Essential features of kwashiorkor
- Marked growth retardation with low weight and low height gain.
- Muscle wasting with retention of some subcutaneous fat.
- Psychomotor changes characterized by mental apathy with listless, inertness, lack of interest about the surrounding, lethargy, dullness and loss of appetite.

- Pitting edema, especially over the pretibial region, due to hypoalbuminemia, and increased capillary permeability with damage cell membrane.

These essential features are to be considered as the minimal diagnostic criteria for kwashiorkor.

Nonessential features of kwashiorkor: These features are variable and may or may not be present in the children.
- *Hair changes:* Hair changes are found as light colored hair or reddish brown color hair which becomes thin, dry, coarse, silky with easy pluckability. The affected child may have alopecia with alternate band of light and dark color hair as 'flag sign' which indicates period of inadequate, adequate and inadequate nutrition over a prolonged period.
- *Skin changes:* It is found initially with erythema and hyperpigmented skin patches but later found as desquamated and hypopigmented patch with the appearance like old paint flaking off the surface of the wood (flaky-paint dermatosis). The child may also have crazy-pavement dermatosis, mosaic dermatosis, reticular pigmentation, pyodermas, scabies and indolent sores and ulcers over the exposed parts or limbs.
- *Superadded infections:* These children usually suffer from repeated infections of GI tract with diarrhea, vomiting, anorexia and dehydration. Respiratory infections (ARI, tubeculosis), skin infections and septicemia, are common and difficult to manage in these patients.

Other usual associated features in these children are manifestations of minerals and vitamin deficiencies, hepatomegaly, intestinal parasitosis, metabolic disorders, malabsorption syndrome with stunted growth.

Nutritional Marasmus

Nutritional marasmus is also termed as infantile atrophy or athrepsia. It is common in infants and may found in toddlers and even in later life. Dietary history reveals both proteins and calories inadequacy in diet in the recent past with predominant lack of calories. The child looks like old person with wizened and shrivelled face due to loss of buccal pad of fat. Initially the child is irritable, hungry and craves for food, but in later stages may become miserable, apathetic and refusal to take anything orally.

The clinical features are subdivided into essential and nonessential features.

Essential features of nutritional marasmus
- Marked growth retardation with less than 60 percent of expected weight for age and subnormal height/length.
- Gross wasting of muscle and subcutaneous tissue.
- Marked stunting and absence of edema.

Nonessential features of nutritional marasmus
- Hair changes usually not present or may be hypopigmented.

- Skin looks dry, scaly with prominent loose folds and having reduced mid-upper arm circumference.
- Superadded infections are common. Skin infections and diarrhea with vomiting and abdominal distention usually occur.
- Liver usually shrunk and the child is having craving for food and hunger.
- Psychomotor changes usually present with irritability, apathy and miserable appearance.
- Features of mineral deficiencies (anemia) and vitamin deficiencies are usually found.

Grading of nutritional marasmus is done depending upon the areas of loss of fat. Grade I is considered when there is loss of fat from axilla, grade II for loss of fat from abdominal wall and gluteal region, grade III for loss of fat from chest and back and grade IV for loss of buccal pad of fat.

Marasmic Kwashiorkor

It is condition where the child manifested both the features of marasmus and kwashiorkor. The presence of edema is essential for the diagnosis and other features of kwashiorkor may or may not be present.

Prekwashiorkor

It is a condition when the child is having features of kwashiorkor without edema. If the early management is initiated by early diagnosis of the condition, the child may be protected from full-blown kwashiorkor.

Nutritional Dwarfing

It is condition when the child is having significant low weight and height for the age without any overt features of kwashiorkor or marasmus. It is usually seen when the PEM continue over a number of years.

Management of PEM

Management of PEM is carried out mainly by nutritional rehabilitation. It can be done at home or in nutritional rehabilitation center (NRC) or in health center or hospital, depending upon the severity of the condition. The child with severe PEM need hospitalization for initial treatment of the associated life-threatening problems, correction of metabolic abnormalities and beginning of intensive feeding with follow-up.

Domiciliary Management

Children with mild to moderate malnutrition without any infections and complications can be managed at home.

Parent should be made aware about the dietary management and other care, with necessary instructions, health education, nutritional counseling and demonstration. It is necessary to be sure that child will be managed by parent appropriately with improved intake of recommended diet, by less expensive locally available foods. Community health nurse or Anganwadi worker should supervise and provide necessary guidance by regular home visit. Follow-up visit to be made for medical supervision, evaluation of weight gain and improvement of nutritional status.

Management in Nutritional Rehabilitation Center

Management of PEM is planned at nutritional rehabilitation center (NRC), in day care NRC or residential NRC according to the available facilities, when home management is not ensured adequately. Government institutions or NGOs can provide this rehabilitation services to the malnourished children.

Management at Hospital

Hospitalization may be needed in advanced cases of PEM with infections and other complications. Children weighing less than 60 percent for age with edema, severe dehydration, severe diarrhea, hypothermia, shock, infections, jaundice, bleeding, persistent loss of appetite and age less than one year should be admitted and managed in the hospital. Children having severe wasting or edematous undernutrition also need hospitalization.

Prompt efficient management is required to save the life and irreversible handicapped conditions. Severe malnutrition usually carries about 20 percent mortality. The initial management in the hospital should be done with treatment of complications and metabolic abnormalities along with correction of specific deficiencies and intensive feeding.

Feeding should be started as early as possible. If oral feeding is not possible, nasogastric tube feeding to be given. Frequent small amount feeding according to child's tolerance to be provided initially with milk-based diet, then semisolid food items are given orally. The diet should provide and contain high protein and high calorie. To begin with a daily intake of 80 to 100 kcal/kg/day for maintenance requirement, which need to be gradually increased to 150 kcal/kg/day of energy and 2 to 3 g/kg/day of proteins. Total amount of fluid intake should be within 100 to 125 mL/kg/day. Higher intake of protein is not necessary, it is safer to obtain 10 to 15 percent of calories from dietary protein. Fat should be supplemented to make the food energy dense. Minerals and trace elements to be supplemented but iron and vitamin 'B' complex are not useful in initial therapy.

During initial management of one week, a child with kwashiorkor will lose weight and a marasmic child gains little or nothing because the tissue gains are masked by excess body water loss. Intensive feeding helps to recover lost weight. Emotional and physical stimulation and preparation for discharge along with training of mother for home care are essential aspects. Recovery may take place in 6 to 8 weeks.

Discharge from hospital is planned when the child has achieved a weight about 85 to 90 percent of the normal weight for height and complications are treated effectively. Mother should be provided with necessary information regarding continuation of nutritional support at home along with regular medical check-up to prevent relapse and to promote adequate growth and development. Necessary hygienic measures, immunization coverage and other routine care of the children to be emphasized to the parents.

Complications and Prognosis of PEM

PEM has acute and long-term complications which influence the outcome. The acute complications are systemic or local infections, severe dehydration, shock, dyselectrolytemia, hypoglycemia, hypothermia, CCF, bleeding disorders, hepatic dysfunction, sudden infant death syndrome (SIDS), convulsions etc.

The long-term complications include cachexia, growth retardation, mental subnormality, visual and learning disabilities.

Prognosis depends upon good hospital and domiciliary care. Acute complications may lead to poor prognosis and fatal outcome.

Preventive Management of PEM

There is no simple solution of the problem of PEM. Prevention of PEM needs various approaches from all levels. Nutrition education is the high priority to prevent this problem. Other preventive measures include the followings:

Health Promotion

- Improvement of health of prepregnant state, pregnant mother and lactating women towards healthy mother for healthy child.
- Promotion of exclusive breastfeeding up to 4 to 6 months of age to prepare firm base of child health and promotes nutritional status.
- Appropriate weaning practices and necessary nutritional supplementations.
- Improvement of family dietary habit with locally available, low cost food items for balanced diets.
- Nutrition education and nutrition counseling to promote correct feeding practices, food habits, food hygiene,

safe water, environmental sanitation and to eliminate misconceptions regarding food and feedings.
- Improvement of home economics, earnings, income generating activities, adequate dietary budget and diet planning for family members.
- Birth spacing and regulating family size.
- Promotion of educational status especially women literacy to improve the family health.
- Provision of nutritional supplementation from ICDS centers and schools (Mid-day meal).
- Maintenance of healthy family environment, congenial for physical, social and psychological development of children.

Specific Protection

- Provision of balanced diet with adequate proteins and energy for all children according to the age
- Immunization against vaccine preventable diseases
- Promotion and maintenance of hygienic measures (hand-washing, food hygiene)
- Food fortification to enrich the food items.

Early Diagnosis and Treatment

- Periodic health check-up of all children for health supervision and maintenance of 'growth chart'.
- Detection of growth lag or growth failure as early as possible.
- Early diagnosis and management of infections, worm infestations and common childhood illnesses (ARI, diarrhea, measles, malaria).
- Promotion of early rehydration therapy in the child having diarrhea, without restriction of feeding.
- Implementation of supplementary feeding programs and services.

Rehabilitation

- Nutritional rehabilitation services
- Hospital management of advanced PEM cases
- Follow-up care.

Nursing Responsibilities for the Management of PEM

Nursing personnel can provide both preventive, curative and rehabilitative services to the children with PEM at home and hospital. The nursing responsibilities include the followings:
- Assessment of nutritional status of the children with collection of appropriate dietary history, including history of breastfeeding, weaning, food habits, balanced

diet, socioeconomic status, presence of illness, etc. Physical examination and anthropometric assessment also important to detect the nutritional deficiency states.

- Assisting in diagnostic investigations whenever necessary.
- Maintenance of growth chart by regular health check-up at home, clinic or health centers for early detection of growth failure.
- Participating in the hospital management in complications and life-threatening situations related to PEM and other related illnesses.
- Implementing nutritional rehabilitation activities.
- Encouraging the parents for home care and follow-up at regular interval.
- Nutrition education, demonstration and counseling according to identified problems of particular child. Informing about breastfeeding, weaning, balanced diet, food hygiene, personal hygiene (handwashing), appropriate feeding practices and food habits, cultural taboos, irrational belief, quality of common foods, food values, food preservations etc.
- Promoting preventive measures for individual, family and community to overcome the problem of PEM.
- Co-operating with other team members and acting with different sectors for the implementation of various nutritional services (e.g. working with Anganwadi workers).
- Maintaining records and reports related to nutritional assessment of individual or community.
- Assisting in implementation of national nutritional programs for prevention of various malnutrition.
- Participating in nutritional research project and assisting in modification of nutritional behaviors by creating awareness in individual, family and community towards appropriate nutritional practices for better nutritional status.

VITAMINS AND THEIR DEFICIENCY DISORDERS

Vitamins are organic compounds, considered as essential nutrients, required by the body in very small amounts. Vitamins do not provide energy but help the body to use other nutrients. Since the body is generally unable to synthesize vitamins, they must be provided from external sources, i.e. from diet, for maintenance of normal health. The balanced diet supplies the vitamins required for an individual.

Vitamins are divided into two categories:

1. Fat soluble vitamins: Vitamins A, D, E, and K
2. Water soluble vitamins: Vitamins B-complex and Vitamin C.

Each vitamin has specific functions to perform and deficiency of particular vitamin may result to specific deficiency disorders. Vitamin deficiency may occur as such or in combination with other nutritional disorders like PEM.

Vitamin 'A' Deficiencies

Vitamin 'A' (Retinol and beta carotene) is indispensable for normal vision. It helps to form retinal pigments, rhodopsin and iodopsin, for vision in dimlight. It is essential for normal functions of glandular and epithelial tissue of skin, eye, digestive, respiratory, urinary and reproductive systems. It promotes bone and teeth development. It acts as anti-infective and antioxidant agent. It reduces the risk of lung, breast, oral and bladder cancers. The recommended daily allowances for infant 300 to 400 micrograms and adolescents 750 micrograms.

The *sources* of vitamin 'A' are both animal foods (retinol) and plant foods (carotenes). The food items rich in retinol are liver, egg yolk, butter, cheese, ghee, whole milk, fish, meat and fish liver oils. The plant foods are the cheapest sources of vitamin 'A' include grean leafy vegetables (spinach, drumstick leaves, amaranth), cereals and pulses, green and yellow fruits and vegetables (like ripe-mango, orange, papaya, pumpkin), roots (carrots), fortified foods like vanaspati, margarine, milk, etc.

Vitamin 'A' deficiency (VAD) is a systemic disease with major effects on eye. This deficiency is usually associated with malnutrition, chronic diarrhea, malabsorption syndrome, cystic fibrosis of pancreas, hepatic insufficiency, measles and prematurity.

Subclinical cases of vitamin 'A' deficiency is manifested as infections of respiratory and/or urinary or GI tract. Earliest manifestations of ocular problems are defective dark adaptation as night blindness due to inefficient formation of rhodopsin. Clinically first sign is conjunctival xerosis as dry and wrinkled conjunctiva. Conjunctival xerosis leads to formation of Bitot's spots. These are triangular pearly white or yellowish foamy spots on bulbar conjunctiva on either side of cornea. Afterwards corneal xerosis and ulceration may manifest. In advanced stages, keratomalacia, as softening necrosis, and ulceration of cornea may develop. Keratomalacia is irreversible and one of the major cause of blindness in Indian population.

According to WHO (1976), syndrome of xerophthalmia is classified as primary signs and secondary signs in 6 to 36 months old children.

Primary signs	*Secondary signs*
X1A - Conjunctival xerosis	XN - Night blindness
X IB - Bitot's spots	XF - Xerophthalmic fundus
X2 - Corneal xerosis	XS - Corneal scars.
X3A - Corneal ulceration	
X3B - Keratomalacia.	

Extraocular manifestations of vitamin 'A' deficiency include phrynoderma or toad skin, hyperkeratosis, dry scaly skin, hypertrophy or atrophy of tongue, growth retardation, susceptibility to various infections (respiratory, urinary, intestinal), renal stone, interference with reproductive functions and may rarely to hydrocephalus.

Treatment of vitamin 'A' deficiency to be done immediately on diagnosis by oral vitamin 'A' administration in a different dose depending upon the age. Parenteral water soluble vitamin 'A' is recommended in case of impaired oral intake, persistent vomiting and severe malabsorption. Local treatment in case of corneal ulcer should be done to prevent secondary infections.

Excess of vitamin 'A' can lead to acute manifestations of toxic effects including nausea, vomiting, dizziness, increased intra-cranial tension and papilledema. This syndrome is known as pseudotumor cerebri. Chronic intoxication of vitamin 'A' can cause anorexia, dry itchy skin, skin disquamation, sleep disorders, painful extremities, sparse hair, enlargement of liver and spleen, hypoplastic anemia, teratogenicity, etc.

Prevention of vitamin 'A' deficiency includes the following approaches:

- Administration of vitamin 'A' oil supplementation—one dose of one lakh units along with measles vaccination at 9 months of age followed by eight more doses of 2 lakhs units every 6 months interval (18, 24, 30, 36, 42, 48, 54 and 60 months) up to 5 years of age.
- Improvement of dietary intake of vitamin 'A' with recommended daily allowances for particular age with vitamin 'A' containing food items.
- Reduction, early detection and management of childhood illnesses like PEM, ARI, diarrhea, measles, worm infestations, etc.
- Early detection of signs and symptoms of vitamin 'A' deficiency diseases for prompt therapeutic interventions.
- Creating awareness about preventive measures by health education and nutrition demonstration against 'VAD'.

Vitamin 'D' Deficiencies

The nutritionally important forms of vitamin 'D' are vitamin D_2 or calciferol and vitamin D_3 or cholecalciferol. Vitamin 'D' stimulates normal mineralization of bones and teeth and promotes intestinal absorption of calcium and phosphorus. It enhances tubular reabsorption of phosphate and calcium. It also contributes towards normal growth and development of children.

Important Sources

The important sources of vitamin 'D' are sunlight and animal foods. Ultraviolet rays of sunlight acts on 7 dehydrocholesterol, which is present under the skin to synthesize vitamin D_3. Foods of animal origin are only sources of vitamin 'D' in diet which include liver, egg yolk, butter, cheese, fish, fish liver oil and milk. Recommended daily allowances for infants is 5.0 micrograms (200 IU) and for children 5 to 10 micrograms (200–400 IU).

Deficiency of vitamin 'D' leads to rickets, bony deformity, growth retardation and muscular hypotonia in children and osteomalacia in adult women.

Despite such a lot of sunshine, the incidence of rickets due to vitamin 'D' deficiency continues to be high in India and other developing countries. It may be due to poor dietary intake of vitamin 'D' and also due to poor exposure to sunlight. Disturbed metabolism, poor synthesis of vitamin 'D' from the skin, malabsorption state, diarrheal diseases and excessive phylate with low calcium and low phosphate containing diet may also be other causes of rickets in malnourished children.

Rickets

Clinical manifestations of vitamin 'D' deficiency is mainly found as rickets. It is usually developed in children between 6 months to 2 years of age. It is a disease of growing bones. In ricket, the process of proliferation, degeneration and calcification of bones are incomplete. The condition may occur in older children with malabsorption or other systemic disorders.

Initially the clinical features of rickets are vague with irritability, restlessness and sweating over the head especially during sleep.

The early sign of rickets is craniotabes, which develops due to softening and thinning of skull bones, mainly occipital and posterior parietal bones, which felt like ping-pong ball, if compressed by thumb. Other features include large size head, delayed closure of fontanels, frontal and parietal bossing and box-shaped head with flat vertex. The bony deformities of chest include prominent costochondral junctions (rachitic rosary), pigeon chest deformity, horizontal depression of lower border of chest (Harrison's groove) and violin shaped deformity of chest (pectus excavatum). The spinal deformities include scoliosis, kyphosis or lordosis. The child usually has deformities of limbs like knock-knee (genu valgum), bowlegs (genu varum), broadening of wrists and ankles. Other features are coxavera, flat feet, delayed eruption of teeth, protuberent abdomen due to marked hypotonia of abdominal muscles (pot-belly), visceroptosis, growth failure and neonatal cataract. Rickets due to vitamin 'D' deficiency should be differentiated from renal or celiac rickets.

Diagnosis of rickets is based on the clinical features, biochemical findings and X-ray findings (especially of wrist). Specific *treatment* consists of administering a single massive dose of vitamin 'D' orally or intramuscularly. Gross orthopedic deformity needs surgical correction (osteotomy). Associated problems like malabsorption, steatorrhea, if present, should be treated. Diet should have adequate amount of vitamin 'D' from animal foods. The child should be encouraged to play outside for longer period for exposure to sunlight. Poor response to adequate vitamin 'D' therapy indicates refractory or resistant type of rickets due to primary hypophosphatemia (X-linked vitamin-'D' resistant rickets), or vitamin 'D' dependent rickets.

Overdose of vitamin 'D' for a long period results in toxic symptoms such as hypotonia, anorexia, nausea, abdominal cramps, diarrhea or constipation, irritability, polydipsia, pallor, drowsiness and failure to thrive. Calciuria may occur due to hypercalcemia. Calcification of soft tissue (heart, renal tubules, blood vessels, bronchi, stomach), cardiac arrhythmias and renal failure may also occur in hypervitaminosis 'D'.

Prevention of Vitamin 'D' Deficiency

Prevention of vitamin 'D' deficiency can be done by the following measures:

- Health education and promotion of awareness about the causes and prevention of vitamin 'D' deficiency diseases.
- Exposure of the child to sunlight, avoidance of overclothing and provision of proper housing.
- Improvement of dietary habit to include foods of animal origin rich in vitamin 'D'.
- Regular health supervision of children to detect the features of vitamin 'D' deficiency conditions and early interventions for prevention and treatment.
- Adequate treatment of childhood diseases like malabsorption states, diarrheal diseases, etc. which interferes with poor synthesis of vitamin 'D'.
- Congenital rickets though rare can be prevented by preventing osteomalacia of mothers.
- Promotion of supply of milk with vitamin 'D' fortification.

Vitamin 'E' (Tocopherol) Deficiency

Alpha-tocopherol is biologically most potent among other fat soluble compounds of tocopherols and tocotrienols. Functions of vitamin 'E' is less understood. It helps in cell maturation and maintenance of stability of biological membranes. It minimizes oxidation of carotene and linoleic acid in the intestine. It acts as an antioxidant and used as a free radical scavenger. It has antineoplastic effects.

Sources of vitamin 'E' include vegetable oils, sunflower oil, soyabean, wheat, germs, leafy vegetables, egg yolk, etc. Nuts and polyunsaturated vegetables oils are rich sources. Seeds, whole wheat grains are good sources.

Deficiency of vitamin 'E' in mothers may lead to prematurity. In preterm babies, vitamin 'E' deficiency may cause hemolytic anemia, skin changes, jaundice, edema, retinopathy of prematurity, intraventricular hemorrhage, bronchopulmonary dysplasia, etc. Children with vitamin 'E' deficiency usually suffer from malabsorption states, cholestatic disease, ataxia, muscle weakness, dysarthria, muscular dystrophy and growth impairment. Reproductive functions impaired in later life due to this deficiency.

Preventive measures include dietary improvement of mother and child and creating awareness about the functions of vitamin 'E' and its deficiency conditions.

Vitamin 'K' Deficiency

Vitamin 'K' is found mainly in two major natural forms, vitamin K_1 and K_2. Therapeutically water soluble analogues of vitamin 'K' acts to stimulate the production and/or the release of certain coagulation factors (II, VII, IX and X) in the liver.

Vitamin K_1 is available mainly in fresh green leafy vegatable (especially dark green), soyabeans, tomato, fruits, liver, egg yolk and milk. Cow's milk is richer sources of vitamin 'K' than human milk. Vitamin K_2 is synthesized by the intestinal bacteria flora.

Deficiency

Deficiency of vitamin 'K' leads to prolonged blood clotting time due to decreased prothrombin level. The condition is manifested in newborn as bleeding from GI tract, intracranial hemorrhage, bleeding from umbilical stump and other hemorrhagic diseases. In infant, this condition may be related to inadequate colonization of intestinal bacterial flora, chronic diarrhea, malabsorption syndrome, worm infestations, biliary tract obstruction and prolonged use of oral broad spectrum antibiotics.

Prevention

Prevention of coagulation defects due to hypo-prothrombinemia in the newborns can be done by administration of vitamin K-1 mg in intramuscular route. Prophylactic use of vitamin 'K' to every infant immediately after birth remains controversial. Excessive administration of vitamin 'K' may cause hemolytic anemia, hyperbilirubinemia and kernicterus especially in preterm and G6PD deficient infants. In older infant, early weaning and intake of food containing vitamin 'K' can prevent this problem.

Vitamin 'B' Complex Deficiencies

Vitamin 'B' is a water soluble compound. Vitamin 'B' complex group includes B_1, B_2, B_5, B_6, B_{12} and folic acid. Other vitamins of 'B' complex group, whose functions and nutritive value are not fully understood, are pantothenic acid, para-amino benzoic acid, biotin, carnitine, inositol, choline, etc.

Thiamine or Vitamin B_1 Deficiency

Vitamin B_1 or thiamine is essential co-enzyme for utilization and metabolism of carbohydrate and proteins. In thiamine deficiency, there is accumulation of pyruvic and lactic acids in the tissues and body fluids. Vitamin B_1 has vital role in the nutrition of heart and peripheral nerves. It is required for the synthesis of acetylcholine and its' deficiency results in impaired nerve conduction.

Vitamin B_1 is available in all natural foods, i.e. whole grain cereals, wheat, gram, pulses, oilseeds and nuts especially groundnuts. Meat, fish, eggs, vegetables and fruits contains smaller amount of thiamine. During process of milling, thiamine is lost from rice. Further losses take place during washing and cooking of rice.

Deficiency of thiamine occurs due to poor dietary intake of vitamin B_1 containing food, malabsorption states and prolonged illness. The deficiency condition is mainly beri-beri. Wernicke-Korsakoff syndrome and subacute necrotizing encephalopathy may also occur due the deficiency vita-min B_1.

Beriberi may occur as dry beriberi, wet beriberi, infantile beriberi and the meningitic form.

Dry beriberi or chronic neurologic involvement is characterized by anorexia, indigestion, weight loss, weakness, diarrhea, constipation, edema, drowsiness, apathy, ataxia, peripherial neuritis, nystagmus, hoarseness, vocal cord paralysis and diminished deep tendon reflexes.

Wet beriberi or acute cardiac involvememt is characterized by congestive cardiac failure with dyspnea, cyanosis, tachycardia, edema and hepatomegaly.

Infantile beriberi may found between 2 to 4 months of age of breast-fed baby of a thiamine deficient mother with peripheral neuropathy.

Meningitis form of beriberi is manifested with convulsion, dilated pupils, bulging anterior fontanel and coma.

In order to prevent thiamine deficiency, health education should be given on balanced diet and thiamine rich foods (parboiled and undermilled rice). Adequate antenatal diet, treatment of prolonged illness and improvement of socioeconomic status help to prevent thiamine deficiency. Prophylactic use of vitamin B_1 to the children with persistent vomiting or prolonged gastric aspiration and those who go on long fasts, prevents the deficiency state.

Riboflavin or Vitamin B_2 Deficiency

Vitamin B_2 is a co-enzyme in metabolism of protein, fatty acid and carbohydrate. It helps in cellular oxidation.

Rich sources of vitamin B_2 in natural foods are milk, egg, liver, green leafy vagetables, etc. Meat and fish contain small amounts. Cereals and pulses are relatively poor sources but germination increases the riboflavin content in them.

Deficiency of riboflavin is manifested as angular stomatitis, cheilosis, (fissuring of lips), magenta tongue, glossitis, nasolabial seborrhea, seborrheic dermatitis, dysquamation, etc. It may cause keratitis, watering of eyes, photophobia, blurring of vision, burning and itching of eyes. Peripheral neuropathy, hyperesthesia, pain sensation, growth failure and delayed tissue repair may be found as other manifestations.

This deficiency occurs due to restricted protein intakes and malabsorption of protein. It may also occur in neonates under phototherapy (due to photo-degradation) and following administration of certain drugs. It may be associated with vitamin B_1 deficiency.

Prevention of vitamin B_2 deficiency can be done by promoting intake of riboflavin containing food and preventing faulty absorption.

Niacin or Vitamin B_5 Deficiency

Niacin or Nicotinic acid is essential for carbohydrate, fat and protein metabolism. It helps in the normal functions of skin, gastrointestinal, nervous and hemopoietic system. Tryptophan, an essential amino acid acts as the precursor of vitamin B_5.

Sources of vitamin B_5 are the natural foods like milk, liver, cheese, cereals, pulses, ground nuts, fish, etc.

Deficiency of niacin results in pellagra. It is characterized by three 'Ds'—diarrhea, dermatitis and dementia. Other features include glossitis, stomatitis, dysphagia, nausea, vomiting, loss of appetite, anemia and mental changes like depression, irritability and delirium. Dementia is encountered much less in children than adults. Dermatitis is found in exposed skin as pigmented scaly cracked area on neck (casal necklace), back of hands, lower legs and face (cheeks). Pellagra is found in malnutrition and in jower and maize eater. It may occur in chronic diarrhea, malabsorption and anorexic states.

Preventive measures of niacin deficiency include promotion of well-balanced diet containing leguminous food and animal protein along with avoidance of only maize and jower eating. Pellagra is the disease of poverty. Improvement of socio-economic status and agricultural development will help to overcome the problem. Health education to be given, to create awareness about the preventive measures, to the family members and school children, because pellagra usually occurs in school-going age.

Pyridoxine or Vitamin B_6 Deficiency

Pyridoxine helps in metabolism of carbohydrate, proteins and fatty acid. It is essential for normal functions of brain and nervous system. It has also a role in blood formation and maturation of polymorphonuclear cells.

Sources of vitamin B_6 are natural foods like liver, egg, meat, wheat germ, soyabeans, peas, pulses, cereals, etc. Small amount of pyridoxine is available in milk and vegetables.

Deficiency of pyridoxine is manifested as convulsions, peripheral neuritis, irritability, microcytic hypochromic anemia (not responding to iron therapy,) as seborrheic dermatitis around nose and eyes, gastrointestinal upset as loss of appetite, abdominal discomfort and diarrhea. This deficiency is rare in children, especially of nutritional origin, but can occur in association with INH therapy in tuberculosis.

Prevention of pyridoxine deficiency is possible by simple balanced diet as it is widely distributed in natural foods. Vitamin B_6 supplementation is necessary in prolonged INH therapy and in use of other drugs like hydralazine, penicillamine, etc. Relative deficiency can occur when protein intake is increased. So balanced diet with adequate amount of protein and vitamin B_6 containing food to be provided in the child's diet.

Cyanocobalamin or Vitamin B_{12} Deficiency

Vitamin B_{12} co-operates with folate for the synthesis of DNA. Separately it is essential for the synthesis of fatty acid in myelin. It may have some role in carbohydrate and fat metabolism, growth of lactobacilli in intestine and for maturation of RBCs. Intrinsic factor of stomach is required for its absorption from ileum.

Sources of vitamin B_{12} are only the animal foods such as liver, meat, egg, milk, fish, cheese, etc. It is not available in vegetable foods. It is synthesized in the colon by the bacteria.

Deficiency of vitamin B_{12} is associated with juvenile pernicious anemia, a megaloblastic anemia due to lack of intrinsic factors in the stomach and achlorhydria. Gastrectomy, surgical removal of ileum, intestinal tuberculosis, long-term therapy with PAS or neomycin and malabsorption state may also result to vitamin B_{12} deficiency. It can be found in the child of vegetarian mother and in the child who is strictly vegetarian.

Other vitamin B_{12} deficiency conditions are demyelinating lesions of spinal cord with numbness and tingling sensation of fingers and toes.

Preventive measures include adequate amount of animal food in daily balanced diet and early detection of features of deficiency condition for necessary treatment. Vitamin B_{12} supplementation to be done in the conditions, when there is risk for deficiency state.

Folic Acid or Folates or Folacin Deficiency

Folic acid or folate is required for normal development of blood cells in the marrow and in the production of purines and pyrimidines which is essential for the synthesis of DNA.

Sources of folic acid are leafy vegetables, cereals, fruits, milk, egg, liver, meat and dairy products. Overcooking and heat destroy folic acid in foods.

Deficiency of folic acid results in megaloblastic anemia, weakness, anorexia, glossitis, cheilosis, gastrointestinal upset as diarrhea, abdominal distention and flatulence. Folic acid deficiency may found separately or associated with vitamin B_{12}, iron and protein deficiency. Treatment of folic acid deficiency is done with 1 to 2 mg folic acid orally.

Prevention of folic acid deficiency is possible by proper cooking process and avoiding dietary insufficiency of folic acid. Adequate treatment of chronic liver disease, malabsorption syndrome, recurrent diarrhea and worm infestations should be done promptly.

Vitamin 'C' or Ascorbic Acid Deficiency

Vitamin 'C' is a water soluble vitamin and most sensitive to heat. It is required for formation of collagen and intracellular matrix in teeth, bones and capillaries. It helps in tissue oxidation, maturation of RBCs, absorption of iron and metabolism of tyrosine and phenylalanine. It stimulates phagocytic activity of WBC and production of antibody. It seems that vitamin 'C' helps in prevention of common cold and protection against infections.

Sources of vitamin 'C' are mainly amla, guava and other fresh fruits like tomato, orange, lemon. It is also available in green leafy vegetables, peas, beans, etc. Small amount of vitamin 'C' is present is roots, tubers, fresh meat and fish.

Deficiency of vitamin 'C' causes scurvy with features of swollen and bleeding gum, subcutaneous bruising, bleeding under the skins or in joints, delayed wound healing and anemia. Other manifestations of vitamin 'C' deficiency are weakness, irritability, apprehensive look, tenderness and pain over the extrimities with frog-like position giving impression of pseudoparalysis which occur due to subperiosteal hemorrhage. Scorbutic rosary may result from posterior displacement of the sternum and prominent costochondral junction. Hemorrhage in the internal organ may occur as hematuria, malena, orbital or conjunctival bleeding.

Prevention of vitamin 'C' deficiency can be done by providing vitamin 'C' containing fresh food items and encouraging breastfeed. Vitamin 'C' supplementation should be given to the artificially-fed babies. Adequate treatment to be done for gastrointestinal disturbances.

Management consists of giving a loading dose of 500 mg of vitamin 'C' followed by daily dose of 100 to 200 mg for several weeks orally. Improvement after treatment can be assessed by X-ray study within two weeks. It may takes months to disappear the subperiosteal hemorrhages.

MINERALS AND THEIR DEFICIENCY DISORDERS

Minerals are nutritionally significant for human being. They are essential for growth, repair and regulation of body functions. Major essential minerals are calcium, phosphorus, sodium, potassium and magnesium. Trace elements required by the body are iron, iodine, fluorine, zinc, copper, cobalt, chromium, manganese, molybdenum, selenium, nickel, tin, silicon and vanadium. There are some trace minerals with no known function which include lead, mercury, boron, aluminium, etc.

Calcium

Calcium is an important mineral element of the body, mainly utilized in formation of bones and teeth. It is also involved in blood coagulation, cardiac function, nerve conduction, muscle contraction and metabolism of enzymes and hormones. It also plays an important role in the transformation of light to electrical impulses in the retina and to relay electrical and chemical messages to the cells. Calcium metabolism is regulated by calcitonin, vitamin 'D' and parathyroid hormone.

Sources

Sources of calcium are mostly milk and milk products, egg and fish. The cheapest sources are green leafy vegetables, cereals, and millets (ragi). Rice is deficient of calcium. Calcium absorption is aided by vitamin 'D', vitamin 'C' and lactose and hindered by excess dietary intake of oxalic acid, phytic acid, fat, fibers and phosphate.

Deficiency

Deficiency of calcium may produce rickets and hypocalcemic tetany with muscle cramps, numbness, tingling sensation of limbs etc. It may also result in growth retardation, dental caries, osteoporosis, osteomalacia, insomnia, skin problems, joint pain and palpitation.

Prevention

Prevention of calcium deficiency to be done by increased dietary intake of calcium containing food, promoting calcium absorption by avoiding excess dietary intake of phytic acid, (cereals), increasing dietary protein intake and treating chronic diarrhea.

Hypercalcemia may occur in hyperparathyroidism, hypervitaminosis 'D', multiple myeloma and bone neoplasms. Severe and progressive hypercalcemia is characterized by anorexia, vomiting, constipation, hypotonia, mental retardation, cardiac anomalies, hypertension, etc.

Phosphorus

Phosphorus plays a vital role in metabolism of proteins, fat and carbohydrates. It is essential for formation of bones and teeth, synthesis of phospholipids and regulation of acid-base equilibrium.

Significant dietary sources are milk, meat, fish, egg yolk, cereals and pulses. Phosphorus is widely available in foodstuffs, so its deficiency occurs rarely.

Deficiency of phosphorus may lead rickets in growing children. Hyper-phosphatemia results in renal failure.

Sodium

Sodium is an important electrolyte, present in all body fluids. It is essential for maintenance of osmotic pressure, irritablity of muscle and nerves for acid-base balance. It is available in common salt, drinking water, vegetables, milk, egg, meat, etc.

Deficiency

Deficiency of sodium results in hyponatremia due to excess loss through secretion, vomiting, gastric aspiration, diarrhea, diuresis, etc. The clinical features of low sodium are dehydration, weakness, lassitude, dizziness, nausea, anorexia, hypotension, syncope and convulsions.

Hypernatremia and sodium retention may result in excessive sodium intake with high protein diet and characterized by edema (peripheral and pulmonary) and CNS symptoms like dullness, convulsions and coma.

Potassium

Potassium is an important element for muscular contraction, conduction of nerve impulses, cell membrane permeability and enzyme action. It is essential for maintenance of osmotic pressure, fluid electrolyte balance and integrity of cardiac muscle exitability, conduction and rhythm.

All foods contain potassium and mostly available in meats, milk, cereals, vegetables, legumes, dried fruits and fruit juices.

Deficiency

Deficiency does not occur in normal healthy child. *Hypokalemia* develop in starvation, malnutrition, gastroenteritis, steroids and diuretics therapy. It may also found in excessive vomiting, gastric aspiration, loss of gastrointestinal secretion, in various disease condition and in fluid therapy with potassium-free solution. Hypokalemia is manifested as tachycardia, ECG changes, marked muscle weakness, hypotonia, abdominal distention and drowsiness.

Hyperkalemia

Hyperkalemia results from increased extracellular potassium, most often due to renal failure and excess potassium therapy. The clinical features of this condition are mainly muscle weakness, abdominal distention, restlessness, diarrhea, abnormal cardiac rythm, cardiac arrest and ventricular fibrillation.

Magnesium

Magnesium is present in all body cells. It is essential for formation of bones and teeth, enzymatic actions, carbohydrate metabolism, synthesis of fatty acids and proteins. It helps in the metabolism of calcium and potassium. It requires for cardiac function and effects on myoneural junctions.

Sources of magnesium are bananas, milk, cereals, nuts, meats and green leafy vegetables. *Deficiency* condition is usually associated with PEM, malabsorption syndrome, chronic renal failure, diarrhea, persistent vomiting, gastric aspirations and hypocalcemia. The clinical features of *hypomagnesemia* are CNS symptoms like irritability, convulsions, areflexia or hyperreflexia, ataxia, muscular weakness and tetany.

Hypermagnesemia may occur in diminished urinary excretion and manifested as muscular weakness, low BP, sedation, extreme thirst and even respiratory muscle paralysis.

Iron

Iron has great significance as nutritional element. It is an important mineral in the formation of hemoglobin and myoglobin. It helps in the development and function of brain, regulation of body temperature, muscular activity and catecholamine metabolism. It is essential for production of antibodies enzymes and cytochromes. The most important function of iron is oxygen transport and cell respiration.

There are two forms of iron, heme-iron and nonheme iron. Best sources of heme-iron are liver, meat, egg and fish which also promote the absorption of nonheme iron present in plant foods. Sources of nonheme iron are vegetable in origin, e.g. grean leafy vegetables (spinach, drumstick leaves, coriander leaves), legumes, nuts, cereals, oilseeds, jaggery, dried fruits, etc. Foods which inhibit iron absorption are milk, egg, tea and excess fiber. But vitamin 'C' containing food items promote iron absorption.

Deficiency of iron leads to nutritional anemia of microcytic hypochromic nature. Other conditions which may arise due to iron deficiency are impaired cell mediated immunity, susceptibility to infection, increasing morbidity and mortality due to related complications.

Excess of iron and deposition of abnormal iron pigment (hemosiderin) in the tissue may occur in iron poisoning, excessive breakdown of RBCs in hemolytic anemia and repeated blood transfustion (as in thalassemia).

Prevention of iron deficiency requires for iron rich dietary intake by child and mother, treatment of chronic blood loss and worm infestations alongwith promotion of iron absorption by changing diet habit.

Iodine

Iodine is a significant micronutrient essential for synthesis of thyroid hormones—thyroxin (T_4) and triiodothyronine (T_3). It is also required in small amount for growth and development.

Important *sources* of iodine are seafoods, (seafish, seasalt) and vegetable grown in soil rich in iodine. Smaller amount is available from milk, meat and cereals. Fresh water is very poor source of iodine. Some foods interfere with iodine utilization by thyroid glands and termed as 'goitrogens'. The vegetables like cabbage and cauliflower may contain goitrogen.

Iodine deficiency disorders (IDD) include goiter, hypothyroidism, cretinism, dwarfism, deaf-mutism, subnormal intelligence, impaired physical and mental growth and delayed motor milestones.

Prevention of IDD includes improvement of dietary intake of iodine containing food in balanced diet, compulsory use of iodised salt and creating awareness about the use and preservation of iodised salt.

Fluorine

Fluorine is essential for normal mineralization of bone and formation of tooth enamel. The main source of fluorine is drinking water. It is also available in trace amount from foods like seafish, cheese and tea. Inadequate fluorine intake leads to dental caries. Excess fluorine in diet results in toxic effects and produce a clinical syndrome called fluorosis. It is found as dental flurosis and skeletal flurosis. Manifestations of the condition are mottling of teeth, dental destruction, exostoses with myelopathy, peripheral neuropathy and formation of new bone. Excess intake of fluorine may lead to crippling skeletal deformity of spine and joints and genu valgum.

Zinc

Zinc is a trace element and essential component of many enzymes. It helps in the synthesis of nucleic acid, proteins, lipids and carbohydrates. It is required for a synthesis of insulin in pancreas and for the development of cell immunity. It is also needed for vitamin 'A' metabolism by promoting mobilization from the liver. It promotes wound healing process.

Zinc is available from vegetable and animal foods like meat, milk, fish, cheeze, nuts, whole wheat, etc. Zinc deficiency leads to growth failure, delayed wound healing, liver disease, hypogonadism, anorexia, alopecia and behavior changes. Balanced diet provides normal requirement for the prevention of the deficiency states. Growing children, antenatal and lactating mother require more amount of zinc.

Copper

Copper is required for connective tissue formation, iron metabolism, myelin production, melanin synthesis, cell respiration and energy utilization. It is present in various enzymes.

Dietary sources of copper are seafood, meats, legumes, nuts, milk, sugar, cereals etc. *Deficiency* of copper results in anemia, neutropenia, hypopigmentation of hair and skin, osteoporosis, fracture and defective immune system. Genetic defects of copper metabolism may give rise to Wilson's disease and Menke's kinky hair syndrome. Wilson's disease may present as hepatic dysfunction and neurological involvement. *Hypocupremia* occurs in patient with nephrosis. *Hypercupremia* may be found in excessive intake of copper which may result from eating food prepared in copper made cooking vessels or may be associated with several acute and chronic infections, leukemia, severe anemia, hyperthyrodism etc.

Other minerals are also responsible for various healths problems in human beings. Recently, it is found that *cobalt deficiency* and cobalt-iodine ratio in the soil may produce goiter, because cobalt may interact with iodine and affect its utilization. *Selenium deficiency* may be associated with PEM and selenium administration to children with kwashiorkor resulted in significant weight gain. Selenium deficiency in combination with vitamin 'E' deficiency reduces antibody production. Excess absorption of *molybdenum* has been shown to develop bony deformities and deficiency of molybdenum, is associated with mouth and esophageal cancer, dental caries and Keshan disease.

COMMUNITY NUTRITION PROGRAMS

The Government of India have initiated several large-scale supplementary feeding programs and programs aimed at overcoming sepecific deficiency diseases through various Ministries to combat malnutrition. The *National Nutritional programs* include the followings:

- Vitamin 'A' prophylaxis program as one of the components of the National program for control of blindness.
- National program for the prevention of nutritional anemia (consisting distribution of iron and folic acid tablets).
- Iodine—Deficiency disorders control program (as a part of National goiter control program to supply iodised salt).
- Integrated Child Development Services Scheme (ICDS) for supplementary nutrition.
- Balwadi nutrition program for food supplementation.
- Mid-day meal program (also known as School Lunch Program) for school children.
- Special nutrition program in urban slums, tribal areas, and backward rural areas for nutrition benefit of children below 6 years, pregnant and nursing mothers.
- Applied nutrition program with the assistance of UNICEF, WHO and FAO to improve the nutritional status of the mothers as well as the infants and children especially by health education on nutrition.

Improvement of nutritional status of the people can be achieved by nutritional programs which may be initiated at national, community and individual level. Family level preventive measures to be encouraged by health education. Community levels measures include early detection of malnutrition, growth chart maintenance, integrated health package, nutrition education, family planning, promotion of educational status and appropriate technological approaches.

Fluids, Electrolytes and Acid-base Disturbances

13

- Body Fluids
- Electrolyte Composition of Body Fluids
- Acid-base Balance
- Fluid Imbalance

- Electrolyte Imbalance
- Acid-base Imbalance
- Clinical Conditions Requiring Fluid Therapy
- Monitoring of Fluid and Electrolyte Imbalance

BODY FLUIDS

Stable internal environment is maintained by the balance of body water and electrolytes. Disturbances in the fluid and electrolyte balance is very common problem usually found in association with several disease conditions. Growing children are more susceptible to disturbances of fluid and electrolyte balance during their illnesses. Correction of imbalance and maintenance of fluid and electrolyte balance are the prime importance for the management of any disease conditions.

Water is the largest component of human body. Total body water (TBW) in full-term neonates is approximately 75 to 80 percent of body weight and gradually reduces to 60 percent by one to two years of age.

Total body water consists of two major compartments, i.e. intracellular fluid (ICF) and extracellular fluid (ECF) and the two minor compartments, i.e. transcellular fluid (TCF) and slowly exchangeable fluid (SEF) compartments. Intracellular fluid volume represents 35 to 40 percent of body weight and is the sum-total of fluids from the cells in different locations. Extracellular fluid volume represents 20 to 25 percent of body weight and consists of plasma water and interstitial water. Transcellular fluid volume represents about 2 percent of body weight, its most important components being gastrointestinal secretions, urine in kidney and lower urinary tract, CSF, aqueous humor and synovial, pleural and peritoneal fluids. Slowly exchangeable fluid volume represents 8 to 10 percent of body weight and is contained in bones, dense connective tissues and cartilages.

Table 13.1 Distribution of total body water

Fluid compartments	Infants	Older children
• Intracellular fluid (ICF)	40%	35–40%
• Extracellular fluid (ECF)	35–40%	20–25%
- Interstitial	–	15%
- Transvascular (plasma)	–	5%
- Transcellular	–	1–3%
• Total body water	75–80%	60%

Distribution of total body water as percent of body weight is shown in Table 13.1.

Regulation of body water is controlled by its intake and excretion. Water intake is stimulated by thirst. Thirst is regulated by the center in the midhypothalamus and also by the volume of body water. It is inter-related with anti-diuretic hormone (ADH) and activated when ECF water deficit is about 2 percent. It remains the major early defense mechanism against hypertonicity and dehydration.

Kidney regulates the water balance and osmolality of body fluids by controlling the excretion of solutes and free water under the influence of ADH and natriureteric peptides. Natriureteric peptides are body's defense against volume expansion. Osmolality is the number of osmotically active particles per 1000 g of water in solution mOsm/kg. The number of dissolved particles in a solution determines osmolality, i.e. tonicity of body fluids.

Antidiuretic hormone secretion is regulated by intracellular and plasma osmolality and by the volume of ECF. Hypovolemia is more potent stimulus of ADH secretion than hyperosmolality. Fall in plasma and resultant reduction in renal perfusion triggers the release of aldosterone from adrenal cortex. Aldosterone causes active transport of sodium at the distal tubular level, so that sodium and water is retained in the extracellular space, thereby regulating the ECF volume.

Situations in which ADH secretion is high include, hypertonicity of ECF due to administration of IV hypertonic saline solution, fall in plasma or ECF volume, drugs like phenobarbitone, epinephrine, histamine, analgesics and emotional stress.

Situations in which ADH secretion is inappropriately high in relation to osmolality of blood include, meningitis, encephalitis, GB syndrome, CNS tumors, head injury, subarachnoid hemorrhage, perinatal asphyxia, tuberculosis, pneumonias and some malignancies.

Antidiuretic hormone secretion is inhibited when excessive water is administered resulting dilution of the body fluids and hypotonicity. The ADH act primarily by increasing the permeability of the renal collecting ducts to water.

ELECTROLYTE COMPOSITION OF BODY FLUIDS

Body fluid is not only water. It contains electrolytes, which have the capability of conducting an electric current in solution. These substances may be charged positively and called cations or charged negatively and termed as anions.

The important cations are sodium, potassium, calcium and magnesium. Important anions are chloride, bicarbonate, sulfate, organic acids and protein acids. Sodium and chloride are the principal electrolytes in the ECF, while potassium and phosphates are the principal electrolytes in the ICF. Concentration of electrolytes of body fluids is shown in Table 13.2.

The ECF and ICF compartments are normally in osmotic equilibrium except for transient changes. A change in the osmolality of either compartment from the normal, leads to rapid movement of water across the highly permeable cell membrane to achieve an equilibration of osmolality. Normally, water flows from a region of low osmolality to that of high osmolality. Since sodium chloride is the principal osmotic agent in ECF, regulation of body water depends on regulation of sodium. The kidney is the main organ involved in regulation of water and sodium balance. The main role in regulation of this balance is of ADH, aldosterone and thirst mechanism. Both renal and extrarenal mechanisms play role in regulation of potassium balance which include aldosterone production and promotion of potassium movement into the cells by alkalosis and insulin.

Table 13.2 Electrolyte composition of body fluids

Electrolytes	ICF	ECF	Interstitial fluid
Cations (mEq/L)			
• Na^+	9.0	140.0	147.0
• K^+	158.0	4.5	4.0
• Ca^{++}	3.0	5.0	2.5
• Mg^{++}	30.0	2.0	1.0
Anions (mEq/L)			
• Cl^-	4.0	103.0	114.0
• HCO^-_3	10.0	25.0	30.0
• Proteins	65.0	15.0	0
• Phosphates	95.0	2.0	2.0
• Organic acids	4.0	6.0	7.5
• Sulfates	22.0	–	1.0

ACID-BASE BALANCE

Acid-base balance is an essential part of fluid-electrolyte management.

An *acid* is a chemical substance that dissociates in solution, releasing hydrogen ions (a proton donor). An acidic solution has a pH below 7.0.

A *base* is a substance that combines with acids to form salts. It dissociates to give hydroxide ions in aqueous solutions. Its molecule or ion can combine with a proton (hydrogen ion) as hydrogen ion acceptor.

A *buffer* is a substance that reduces the change in free hydrogen ion concentration of a solution when an acid or base is added.

The concentration of hydrogen ions determines the acidity of body fluids. When the concentration of hydrogen ion is higher, the fluid is acidic. If the concentration of these ions is less, the fluid is basic or alkaline. In a neutral solution, the number of H and OH ions is equal. The hydrogen ion concentration is dependent on the ratio of pCO_2 and bicarbonate.

The term pH is used to indicate acidity, alkalinity and neutrality. Higher pH indicates alkalinity and lower pH denotes acidity. A neutral solution has a pH of 7. Blood pH is 7.4 ± 0.05 which means it is slightly alkaline.

Regulation of body pH is maintained by the following mechanisms.

Chemical Buffer System of the Body

A buffer is a substance that can absorb or donate H^+ ion and thereby mitigate changes in pH. The four important chemical buffer systems in the body include, bicarbonate-carbonic acid buffer, phosphate buffers, hemoglobin buffer and protein buffers. Bicarbonate-carbonic acid buffer is the most important system that converts strong acids to a weak carbonic acid.

Respiratory Regulatory Mechanism

This mechanism provides support to the bicarbonate carbonic acid buffer system by eliminating excess CO_2 through rapid breathing.

Renal Mechanisms

It helps in the elimination of excess acids and bases by reabsorption of bicarbonate in the proximal tubules and excretion of H^+ ions as phosphate buffer salts and ammonium ions.

With these mechanisms the acidity and alkalinity of body fluids are kept in a state of equilibrium, so that the pH of arterial blood is maintained at about 7.35 to 7.45. Disturbances in acid-base balance can occur due to primary respiratory or metabolic events with resultant increase or decrease in body acid or base. If the acid-base imbalance is predominantly metabolic in nature, changes in pH, HCO_3, pCO_2 occur in the some direction (all are reduced or increased and the main alteration is in HCO_3). If the imbalance is predominantly respiratory in origin, changes in HCO_3^- and arterial pCO_2 are opposite to changes in pH and main alteration is in pCO_2. The most serious acid-base disturbances are of mixed type when both respiratory and metabolic disorders result in pH changes in the same direction. The acid-base status of an individual is determined by measuring pH, pCO_2, Hb concentration and other indices of blood gas analysis for effective interventions.

FLUID IMBALANCE

Fluid imbalance may occur when the normal physiological requirements of fluids is not maintained to replace obligatory urinary and insensible losses and the water required for metabolic activity. The requirement of fluids depends upon body weight, body surface area, metabolic rate and age of the individual. Disease conditions which affect water loss from the body or the total caloric expenditure require modification in the maintenance of water requirement. Modifications of fluid requirement may also be necessary to prevent fluid imbalance in renal diseases, respiratory, gastrointestinal and cardiovascular problems and even in excessive sweating. Neonates and infants need special attention for the prevention of fluid imbalance, because

they are more prone to develop this problem due to several reasons peculiar for this age.

The fluid imbalance is found as dehydration and over-hydration or water intoxication.

Dehydration

Dehydration is the most common fluid imbalance due to excessive loss of body water. It is a clinical state that results from fluid deprivation or from fall in total quantity of electrolytes. It is more common in infant and children. The important causes of dehydration in children is diarrhea and vomiting. It may also occur in diabetes insipidus, hyperglycemia and renal losses.

Dehydration can be hypotonic, isotonic or hypertonic. The most common type is isotonic dehydration with proportionate loss of water and solutes from ECF. The ICF volume remains intact as there is no redistribution of fluid.

In hypotonic dehydration, the depletion of solutes in ECF is much more than the water losses. Hypotonicity of ECF leads to shift of water from ECF to ICF causing further contraction of ECF and shock.

In hypertonic dehydration, excess loss of water proportionate to the solutes causing movement of water from the cells in the ECF leading to intracellular dehydration.

Assessment of Dehydration

The successful management of dehydration in infants and children can be possible by accurate assessment of degree of dehydration and initiation of rehydration therapy according to the child's condition.

Clinical history and physical examination are the major aspects of assessment of hydration status. Details history should include the amount of urine output, vomitus and diarrheal losses. Physical examination should be done to exclude the signs of dehydration which include dryness of mucous membrane (mouth, tongue, eyes), absence of tears, sunken eyes, presence of thirst, restlessness and irritability, lethargy or unconsciousness and cold extremities. Skin turgor and capillary filling time to be assessed which, considered as reliable marker of dehydration. Pulse rate, respiration rate and blood pressure should be checked and interpreted in relation to the child's age. Signs of shock and CNS signs should be detected for early interventions.

Laboratory investigations are essential for further assessment of fluid and electrolyte deficits and to guide the subsequent therapy in severely dehydrated patients. These are not essential for starting the management. The most helpful investigations are serum electrolytes, blood urea and creatinine, acid-base status, plasma osmolality, hematocrit values and urine specific gravity.

Management of Dehydration

(Dehydration to be managed promptly after accurate assessment of hydration status. In severe dehydration and shock rapid expansion of intravascular volume is required to maintain vital functions) This is achieved by rapid intravenous infusion of 100 to 120 mL/kg of isotonic, iso-osmotic solution (Ringer's lactate) or normal saline or plasma. The goal is to achieve normal urine output, correction of potassium deficit and acidosis and to enable the patient to return to oral rehydration as early as possible.

(Correction of total fluid deficit by rehydration therapy is very important aspect of management by intravenous fluid or oral rehydration therapy (ORT)) Total correction of fluid and electrolyte deficit can be achieved safely and rapidly through ORT in most of cases with dehydration. (In patients with severe dehydration, once the intravascular volume deficit has been corrected and urine flow is established, rest of the deficit can be corrected by ORT) (In diarrheal dehydration, rapid ORT is superior to conventional slow or rapid intravenous rehydration therapy)

Intravenous rehydration is recommended if there is severe dehydration or if there is persistent vomiting, paralytic ileus or child is unconscious or too sick to drink ORS.

(There should be provision of maintenance fluids and electrolytes balance and replacement of ongoing losses and to monitor the child's hydration status for effective outcome of therapy.) Mother should be involved during rehydration therapy, especially in ORT. (Hydration should be reassessed at regular interval to determine whether rehydration therapy is essential furthermore or not) (Maintenance of intake and output record is vital responsibility of nursing personnel during rehydration therapy)

Over Hydration or Water Intoxication

Acute water intoxication may occur due to inattentive or unintentional excessive infusion of salt free or poor salt glucose solution or due to plain water enema. Hyponatremia is usually present with the condition. The child may present with distended neck veins, pulmonary crepitations or wheeze and dependent edema. The child may have convulsions and shock due to cerebral edema resulting from sudden water overload and ECF dilution.

Water restriction and diuretics (furosemide) are effective management of the condition. In severe cases peritoneal dialysis with hypertonic glucose could be useful.

ELECTROLYTE IMBALANCE

Common electrolyte disturbances or dyselectrolytemias in sick children include hyponatremia, hypernatremia, hypo-

kalemia, hyperkalemia, hypocalcemia and hypomagnesemia. Most common are hypo- or hypernatremia and hypo- or hyperkalemia.

Hyponatremia

Hyponatremia is termed when serum sodium level is less than 130 mEq/L. It occurs due to water retention, sodium loss or both.

Hyponatremia is commonly found in hospitalized children with acute diarrhea, pneumonia, meningitis, sepsis, heart failure, hepatic failure and renal diseases.

Etiology of Hyponatremia

- Primary sodium deficit with sodium depletion resulting in (a) renal sodium losses in prematurity, chronic diuretic therapy, osmotic diuresis in diabetes mellitus, renal tubular acidosis, adrenal insufficiency with mineralocorticoid deficiency, etc. (b) extrarenal sodium losses due to vomiting, diarrhea, nasogastric drainage, burns, cystic fibrosis and excessive sweating (c) nutritional deficits in water intoxication, poor sodium concentration in IV fluid, paracentesis, CSF drainage and burns.
- Primary water excess with water gain due to excess IV fluids, tap water enema, hypothyroidism, syndrome of inappropriate ADH secretion, glucocorticoid deficiency and psychogenic polydipsia.
- Abnormal retention of sodium and water in nephrotic syndrome, cirrhosis of liver, CCF, renal failure.

Clinical Manifestations

The hyponatremia is presented with restlessness, confusion, convulsions, hypotension, heart failure and unconsciousness. The patient may be asymptomatic. The features depend upon the severity of the condition. Usually the patients with sodium level between 120 and 130 mEq/L are asymptomatic.

Management

Symptomatic hyponatremia is managed by administering 3 percent solution of sodium chloride (saline), 10 mL/kg body weight at the rate of 1 mL per minute intravenously to correct the sodium deficit. Thereafter, calculated extra sodium should be administered slowly in 24 to 48 hours. Fluid restriction may be required in some cases (SIADH, renal failure) to safeguard against pulmonary edema and CCF. Furosemide may be administered along with 3 percent saline if CNS symptoms are associated with the condition. Fluid should not be restricted in hyponatremia accompanying hypoproteinemia. Rapid correction of sodium deficit, in both symptomatic and asymptomatic hyponatremia, should be avoided to prevent pontine myelinosis.

Hypernatremia

Hypernatremia is termed when serum sodium is more than 150 mEq/L. It results from deficit of water with respects to sodium stores due to water loss in diarrhea, vomiting, diuresis and burns or excessive sodium intake. It can be associated with any state of hydration, i.e. dehydration, overhydration or normal hydration status.

Etiology of Hypernatremia

- Excessive sodium gain in faulty preparation of ORS formula, accidental substitution of sodium chloride for glucose in infant formula feeding, excessive sodium bicarbonate during resuscitation, IV administration of hypertonic saline, hypernatremic enema, high sodium content in breast milk and salt poisoning.
- Excessive water loss or deficit in diabetes mellitus, more loss of water than solute loss in AGE, poor water intake, inadequate breastfeeding, increased insensible loss of water especially in prematurity, fever, and hyperventilation.

Clinical Manifestations

The clinical features of hypernatremia include irritability, confusion, twitching, seizures, tough and doughy skin and subcutaneous tissue, intracranial hemorrhages and coma. Metabolic acidosis with deep rapid breathing is usually present. Hypotenison and dehydration may also be found. The condition can be complicated with permanent neuromotor sequelae.

Management

Hypernatremia should be treated promptly with rapid intravenous infusion of Ringer lactate or saline to correct hypovolemia. Underlying cause to be ruled out to manage the condition with specific treatment. It may be essential to control GI fluid losses and fever, withholding diuretics, treatment of hypokalemia or hypercalcemia or correction of faulty ORS therapy.

If the child is conscious, ORS or free water and breast-feed should be given orally. Child's condition to be monitored frequently. CNS symptoms like convulsions need anticonvulsive and mannitol therapy. Peritoneal dialysis is indicated if the serum sodium level is 180 mEq/L or more. In patients with hypernatremia that has developed over a period of hours, rapid correction (1 mEq/L/hour) is safe and improves prognosis. Maintenance fluid requirements in hypernatremia to be reduced by 25 percent to prevent complications.

Hypokalemia

Hypokalemia is termed when serum potassium level is less than 3.5 mEq/L. The most common causes are AGE, septicemia, diuretic therapy and hepatic failure especially in malnourished child. It may develop due to reduced potassium intake, high renal losses and extrarenal losses.

Etiology of Hypokalemia

- Reduced potassium intake in PEM.
- High renal losses of potassium in diuretic therapy, renal tubular defect, acid-base imbalance (alkalosis, diabetic ketoacidosis) and endocrinopathies (thyrotoxicosis, cushing syndrome, primary aldosteronism).
- High extrarenal losses of potassium in diarrhea, vomiting, frequent enemas, biliary drainage, profuse sweating, etc.
- Decrease in muscle mass in myopathies.
- Familial hypokalemic periodic paralysis.

Clinical Manifestations

Hypokalemia affects the bioelectric processes including muscle contraction, nerve conduction and myocardial pacing.

The *clinical features* of this condition include weakness of skeletal muscle, hypotonia, diminished reflexes, abdominal distention, poor peristaltic movement, paralytic ileus, respiratory distress and paralysis. Cardiac problems in this condition include various arrhythmias, ECG changes and cardiac arrest. Prolonged hypokalemia decreases the capacity of kidney to concentrate urine leading to hypokalemic nephropathy and polyuria.

Management

Management of hypokalemia consists of slow administration of potassium over 24 to 28 hours and treatment of underlying cause. Oral administration is safer than IV route, especially in massive urinary losses. In life-threatening hypokalemia with ECG abnormalities rapid correction is recommended. Potassium infusion should be given using infusion pump at the rate of 0.3 to 0.35 mEq/kg/hour till the ECG becomes normal. Infusion rate should not exceed 0.6 mEq/kg/hour. Infused fluid should not contain more than 40 mEq/L of potassium. Higher rates and concentrations may cause cardiac depression. Potassium should be administered only when urinary flow is established. Monitoring of child's condition, especially the urinary output, cardiac features and fluid intake are important nursing responsibility. Intake-output chart and rate of infusion pump should be recorded accurately.

Hyperkalemia

Hyperkalemia is termed when serum potassium level is more than 5.5 mEq/L. The causes of hyperkalemia are the followings:

- Excessive intake of potassium mainly through IV infusion.
- Impaired excretion of potassium in acute or chronic renal failure, Addison's disease, hypoaldosteronism, potassium-sparing diuretics, etc.
- Shifting or release of potassium from tissues into ECF in case of acidosis, hemorrhage, burns, hemolysis, sepsis, tissue necrosis, insulin deficiency, crush injuries, etc.
- Drug therapy with digoxin toxicity and succinylcholine.

Clinical Manifestations

Mild hyperkalemia is usually asymptomatic. When severe, the effects are mainly found on cardiac and skeletal muscles. The features include muscular weakness, paresthesias, shock, bradycardia or cardiac arrhythmias and ECG changes. The condition may be complicated with heart block, ventricular fibrillation, flaccid paralysis and tetany.

Management

Mild hyperkalemia (5.5–6 mEq/L) is managed by stopping the potassium intake and offending drugs. Moderate hyperkalemia (6–8 mEq/L) is managed with glucose-insulin infusion and/or sodium bicarbonate infusion and additional supportive measures along with discontinuation of potassium intake.

Severe hyperkalemia (more than 8 mEq/L) should be managed with IV calcium gluconate for reversing the electrophysiological abnormality effectively. Sodium-bicarbonate, glucose-insulin therapy and other additional supportive measures to be provided considering the condition as a medical emergency. Continuous ECG monitoring is must in case of acute hyperkalemia. Intravenous or nebulized salbutamol therapy may be needed in some cases. Dialysis may be required in refractory cases or in cardiac arrhythmias. Sodium polystyrene sulfonate, a potassium binding ion exchange resin, can be administered orally or per rectum 4 to 6 hourly, 1 g/kg in 10 percent dextrose, especially for the long-term management of hyperkalemia. Continuous monitoring of child's condition and supportive nursing measure promotes better prognosis.

ACID-BASE IMBALANCE

Acid-base imbalance is found as acidosis or alkalosis. They can be metabolic or respiratory in origin. *Acidosis* is actual or relative increase in the acidity of blood due to an accumulation of acids or an excessive loss of bicarbonate. The hydrogen ion concentration of the fluid is increased lowering the pH. It may occur commonly due to diabetic ketoacidosis, impaired kidney functions, pulmonary insufficiency, drowning, etc. *Alkalosis* is a pathological condition due to accumulation of base in or loss of acid from the body. It may be found along with hypokalemia, metaboic disorders and respiratory problems.

Metabolic Acidosis

Metabolic acidosis means accumulation of acid and the metabolic acidemia indicates actual lowering of blood pH because of elevation of hydrogen ion concentration above normal. The accumulation of acid may be managed normally by the buffer mechanism or the compensatory respiratory mechanism. Metabolic acidosis occurs due to increase in acids other than carbonic acid. It results from either excessive production or decreased excretion of H^+ ions or excessive loss of bicarbonates from the body. It may found with increased anion gap or without an increase in anion gap.

Anion gap is defined as the difference between measured cations (Na^+ and K^+) and measured anions (Cl^- and HCO_3^-). It occurs due to accumulation of anionic substances (acids).

Etiology of Metabolic Acidosis

- Metabolic acidosis with increased anion gap. It occurs due to overproduction of endogenous acids in diabetic ketoacidosis, or in case of under excretion of fixed acids in advanced renal failure or in ingestion of excess exogenous acids by salicylates and alcohol.
- Metabolic acidosis without an increase in anion gap (hyperchloremia). It results from loss of bicarbonate in severe diarrhea or from the kidney in renal tubular acidosis, nephrotoxic drugs, etc.

Clinical Manifestations

The clinical features of mild metabolic acidosis are nausea, vomiting, headache and abdominal pain. In chronic acidosis, the child may have anorexia, lethargy and fatigue. When pH is below 7.2, there is deep and rapid respiration (Kussmaul breathing) with features of peripheral vasodilatation. The child becomes drowsy, confused and stuporous. Cardiac dysarrhythmias, muscle weakness and flaccidity may also present. Severe metabolic acidosis, may lead to vascular collapse, shock, myocardial depression, increased pulmonary vascular resistance, hyperkalemia and depressed cerebral and cellular metabolism.

Management

The child should be assessed to detect the severity of the problem. Detail history and physical examination should include assessment of urine output, fluid intake, dietary habits, recent fasting, presence of associated problems (like diabetes mellitus, renal diseases, liver dysfunction, etc.) and intake of medicine like aspirin and alcohol. Investigations should be done for ABG analysis and serum potassium level.

Correction of acidosis is usually not recommended in mild and moderate cases. Treatment of underlying condition improves acidosis.

Severe acidosis requires urgent management with sodium bicarbonate and IV fluid. Sodium bicarbonate is the safest and most effective alkalinizing agent. One-half of the calculated amount of sodium bicarbonate may be administered immediately and another half in 12 to 24 hours as a slow infusion. Sodium bicarbonate must be diluted with at least equal volume of distilled water. In cardiorespiratory problems O_2 therapy and mechanical ventilation may be needed. Potassium is essential to prevent hypokalemia and calcium gluconate should be administered separately to prevent tetany. Sodium overload may occur while correcting acidosis with sodium bicarbonate. Other alkalinizing agents such as THAM (trihydroxymethyl-aminomethane) can be used where sodium bicarbonate administration is considered hazardous. The THAM rapidly increases pH of body fluids and tissues including CNS and transiently lower pCO_2. Severe acidosis with renal failure or hyperosmolar state is best managed by dialysis.

Supportive nursing measures should include frequent oral hygiene, change of position, safe environment with minimal stimulation and continuous monitoring of the condition.

Respiratory Acidosis

Respiratory acidosis develops due to retention of CO_2 in pulmonary insufficiency. It occurs as a result of decreased elimination of CO_2 from the body due to poor ventilation which leads to accumulation of carbon dioxide in the body and generation of carbonic acid. Acute respiratory acidosis is characterized by a primary rise in pCO_2, above 45 mm Hg which remains at this high value for no longer than 6 to 12 hours. Sustained elevation of pCO_2 beyond 12 hours is termed as chronic respiratory acidosis.

Etiology or Respiratory Acidosis

- *Acute respiratory acidosis:* It may develop in the following conditions:
  - Airway obstruction due to birth asphyxia, bronchial asthma, foreign body inhalation, laryngeal edema and aspiration.
  - Lung diseases like RDS in newborn, pneumonia, peumothorax, pulmonary edema, pulmonary embolism, etc.

  - Neuromuscular diseases like GB syndrome and polio-myelitis.
  - Brainstem lesion with central depression.
  - Overdose of opium and sedatives.
- *Chronic respiratory acidosis:* It may develop in asthma, cystic fibrosis, bronchiectasis, interstitial fibrosis, kypho-scoliosis, paralysis of respiratory muscles, asphyxiating thoracic dystrophy, etc.

Clinical Manifestations

Clinical features of respiratory acidosis depends upon degree of hypercapnia. The child usually presents with headache, irritability, restlessness or depression due to increased intracranial pressure. There is alternation of consciousness varying from drowsiness to deep coma. Muscular tremors, flushing of skin or perspiration, tachycardia and hypotension may present. Shock and ventricular fibrillation may develop.

Management

Management of the condition should emphasis on treatment of underlying cause and improvement of alveolar gas exchange by assisted ventilation. Oxygen therapy with high flow rates may help to remove excess CO_2. Tight fitting mask or head box may cause dangerous elevation of pCO_2. Sodium bicarbonate may be administered as life-saving measures, if there is hyperkalemia or ventricular fibrillation and should be given after establishment of ventilation. Intravenous fluid should be administered to maintain hydration and fluid balance. Child's condition should be monitored to detect the anoxic damage due to condition.

Metabolic Alkalosis

Metabolic alkalosis occurs due to loss of H^+ ions or an excess of bicarbonate ions in the body associated with hypoventilation and compensatory increase in pCO_2 with high pH. It is classified into two types, i.e. chloride responsive and chloride resistant, on the basis of urinary chloride levels. In chloride responsive variety urinary chlorides are less than 10 mEq/L and in resistant type it is usually more than 10 mEq/L.

Etiology

Metabolic alkalosis usually develops in persistent vomiting in hypertropic pyloric stenosis, or in prolonged gastric aspiration as a result of loss of chloride and body fluids. Prolonged diuretic therapy and excess intake of alkali can cause metabolic alkalosis. Hypokalemia can lead to this condition due to shift of hydrogen ions into the cells in order to conserve potassium. Other causes of this problem are hyperaldosteronism, Cushing's syndrome and Bartter's syndrome which can lead to chloride resistant alkalosis.

Clinical Manifestations

The patient with metabolic alkalosis may present with hypoventilation, apathy, confusion, drowiness, convulsions and coma. The child may develop tetany, laryngospasm and cardiac arrhythmias due to hypocalcemia and hypokalemia. The child usually have signs and symptoms of underlying cause with pH above 7.55.

Management

Management depends upon type of the metabolic alkalosis. In chloride responsive cases, management is done with saline and potassium chloride. In chloride resistant type, mild cases respond to sodium chloride restriction, spironolactone therapy and potassium supplements. Severe cases should be managed with HCl (through central venous line) or with HCl producing substances such as ammonium chloride in intravenous route. Underlying cause should be diagnosed and appropriate management to be done.

Respiratory Alkalosis

Respiratory alkalosis occurs when there is a fall in arterial pCO_2. It usually develops due to hyperventilation in case of assisted ventilation and in psychogenic or neurogenic hyperventilation (hysteria). It may develop in CNS disorders (severe hypoxia, trauma, infections, tumor,) CCF, hepatic insufficiency and septicemia.

Clinical manifestations of the condition include numbness, tingling, paresthesis and light headedness. Features of tetany may present in severe cases. Unconsciousness may develop due to vasospasm of cerebral vessels in case of hypercapnia.

Management of the condition is done by treatment of underlying cause. Sodium bicarbonate therapy is not indicated.

Mixed Acid-base Disorders

Mixed acid-base disorders are conditions where more than one primary acid-base disturbance occurs. The common four types of mixed acid-base disorders are:

1. Respiratory acidosis and metabolic acidosis.
2. Respiratory and metabolic alkalosis.
3. Respiratory alkalosis and metabolic acidosis.
4. Respiratory acidosis and metabolic alkalosis.

Mixed acid-base disorders are suspected when the compensatory response falls outside the expected range.

CLINICAL CONDITIONS REQUIRING FLUID THERAPY

Parenteral fluid therapy may be required in a wide variety of clinical situations to provide normal or adjusted maintenance

Table 13.3 Daily maintenance requirements of fluids and electrolytes

Requirements	By body weight	By surface area
Water		
• Up to 10 kg	• 100 mL/kg	
• 11–20 kg	• 1000 mL + 50 mL/kg for extra weight above 10 kg	• 150 mL/m² (range 1200–1800 mL)
• > 20 kg	• 1500 mL + 20 mL/kg for extra weight	
Sodium	3–4 mEq/kg/day	40–60 mEq/m²
Potassium	2–3 mEq/kg/day	30–40 mEq/m²
Chloride	3–4 mEq/kg/day	

fluid needs or to replace abnormal deficits. Modification of maintenance water requirement may be required in certain clinical conditions because of changes in metabolic rate.

- Maintenance fluid therapy with deficit replacement and replenishment of concurrent fluid losses
  - Continuous gastrointestinal fluid losses in vomiting, diarrhea, nasogastric tube aspiration, colostomy, etc.
  - Burn injury
  - Diabetic ketoacidosis.
  - Pyloric stenosis
  - Salicylate intoxication.
- Maintenance fluid therapy
  - Unconscious or sick child who is unable to take oral fluid.
- Adjusted maintenance fluid therapy
  - Postoperative patient
  - Oliguria or anuria
  - Raised intracranial pressure
  - Cardiac failure.
  - Edema.
  - SIADH (Syndrome of inappropriate secretion of ADH)

Daily maintenance requirements of fluids and electrolytes on the basis of body weight and surface area are shown in Table 13.3.

MONITORING OF FLUID AND ELECTROLYTE IMBALANCE

Fluids and electrolytes should be administered according to the guidelines for specific condition. During parenteral fluid therapy, clinical and biochemical indicators of water and electrolyte status should be monitored closely to make necessary adjustments to maintain homeostasis in an individual child. During intravenous infusion in early resuscitation phase (0–2 hours), pulse rate, blood pressure, capillary refill time and sensorium should be monitored continuously. Urine output to be measured everyone hourly. Subsequently recording of intake and output, body weight and detection of renal compensatory mechanisms or consequences due to fluid excess or deficit are the most important concerns. Clinical parameters should be reviewed at least 8 hourly and laboratory tests should be done daily to adjust intake of water and electrolytes accordingly. Body weight should be recorded daily. Clinical monitoring is considered as sufficient to detect early fluid imbalance.

The important parameters for clinical monitoring include body temperature, pulse, respiration, blood pressure, chest sound, skin turgor, condition of mucous membrane, level of consciousness, capillary refill time, body weight, urine output (1–3 mL/kg/ hour), urine specific gravity, and intake-output record.

Laboratory investigations may be done for urine osmolality, plasma osmolality, serum sodium, serum potassium, blood urea, serum creatinine, ABG analysis, etc.

Monitoring of fluid electrolyte imbalance is vital during fluid therapy to detect the disturbances of the delicate balance. The goal of fluid and electrolyte therapy should be achieved to maintain normal volume and tonicity of body fluids necessary for supply of nutrition at the cellular level.

14

Common Communicable Diseases in Children

- Common Viral Infections
- Common Bacterial Infections
- Common Parasitosis in Children

INTRODUCTION

Communicable diseases continue to be a major health problem in India, especially among children. A communicable disease is an illness caused by an infectious agent or toxic product and is transmitted by direct or indirect contact between the reservoir host and the susceptible individual. The transmission can occur from man to man, animal to animal or from the environment (through air, dust, soil, water, food, etc.) to man or animal. Infectious disease is the disease caused by growth of pathogenic microorganisms in the body. It is not necessarily contagious. Contagious diseases are transmitted through contact (e.g. STD, leprosy and scabies).

Nurses assume responsibility for assessing the potential conditions for children to develop these disease and promoting awareness to prevent them. They are also responsible for assisting to identify specific communicable diseases, providing care in the hospital or home and educating family members for home care.

COMMON VIRAL INFECTIONS

Common viral infections among children are measles, chickenpox, viral hepatitis, influenza, mumps, poliomyelitis, HIV/AIDS, dengue syndrome, etc. Other less common viral infections include, German measles, herpes simplex infection, herpes zoster, GB syndrome, infective mononucleosis, cytomegalic inclusion disease, etc.

Measles

Measles is a highly infectious disease of childhood caused by measles virus. It is characterized by fever, catarrhal symptoms of the upper respiratory tract followed by typical rash. In our country, it is a major cause of ill health and morbidity. It is a significant contributor to childhood mortality, especially in the malnourished children below the age of 3 years.

Measles is endemic in all parts of the world and it tends to occur in epidemics.

Epidemiology

The causative agent of measles is the specific measles virus, a RNA virus of the genus morbillivirus, of paramyxoviridae family. Human body is the only reservoir of this infection. The only source of infection is a case of measles. Infective materials are secretions of nose, throat and respiratory tract of the infected patient. The period of communicability is approximately 4 days before and 5 days after the appearance of rash. One attack of infection gives life-long immunity.

Mode of transmission is mainly by droplet infections and droplet nuclei. Portal of entry is the respiratory tract and sometimes through conjunctiva. It can spread directly by air borne route or by indirect contact with fomites. Incubation period is 10 to 15 days.

Measles usually occurs in the children between the age of one year and 5 years. Infants are protected by maternal antibodies up to 6 months of age. It is rare in infants of 6 to 12 months. Before 6 months it is uncommon. It may found around 6 months in mild form. Sometimes it may occur in older children. The disease is found in very severe form in malnourished children.

Measles usually occurs in winter and spring months but may found in all seasons. It is common in poor community and related to social belief as "Curse of the goddess". Parents prefer to visit temple rather than consulting doctor and usually provide neglected care and negligible foods.

Pathological Changes

Pathological changes are related to the invasion of virus in the respiratory epithelium which results in local multiplication and viremia. The infection spreads to reticuloendothelial system and causes secondary viremia which produces systemic symptoms. Superficial blood vessels of skin and mucous membrane are affected and formed inclusion bodies. This multinucleated giant cell can be demonstrated in both epidermis and oral epithelium.

Clinical Manifestations

Clinical features of measles are manifested in three stages, i.e. prodromal or pre-eruptive stage, eruptive stage and convalescent or post-measles stage.

Prodromal (catarrhal) or pre-eruptive stage usually starts after 10 days of infection and lasts 3 to 5 days. This stage is manifested with fever, malaise, coryza, sneezing, nasal discharge, brassy cough, redness of eyes, lacrimation and often photophobia. Lymphadenopathy may also present. Vomiting and diarrhea may present is some children. The important characteristics of this stage is appearance of Koplik's spots, grayish or bluish-white spots, fine tiny grain like papules on a faint red base, smaller than head of a pin. These spots appear before the appearance of rash. They are found on the buccal mucosa opposite the first and second lower molars. The spots usually disappear a day after the rash appears. Practically the spots are observed in only a small number of cases.

Eruptive stage is characterized by a typical irregular dusky-red macular or maculopapular rash which found behind the ears and face first, usually 3 to 5 days after the onset of the disease. Then it spreads to neck, trunk, limbs, palms and soles in next 3 to 4 days. Fever usually rise again or regress gradually within 3 days. Anorexia, malaise and cervical lymphadenopathy may present. Fever and rash usually disappear in 4 to 5 days in the same order of appearance. There is fine shedding of superficial skin of face, trunk and limbs, leaving brownish discoloration which may persist for 2 months or more.

Convalescent or post-measles stage is the period of disappearance of constitutional symptoms, fever and rash. But usually the child remains sick for number of days and lost weight. There may be gradual deterioration into chronic illness due to bacterial or viral infections, nutritional and metabolic disturbances or other complications.

Investigations

Usually clinical features help in diagnosis, no investigations needed. But serological tests, viral isolation, ELISA test to detect the presence of measles antibody and routine blood examination can be done.

Complications

Complications of measles are potentially dangerous and fatal than the disease. The common complications are:

1. *Respiratory tract infections,* as bronchopneumonia, laryngitis, laryngotracheobronchitis, bronchiolitis, activation of primary tuberculosis, otitis media and mastoiditis. These are most common complications causing long-term problems.
2. *Neurological complications:* These include encephalitis, febrile convulsions, sub-acute sclerosing panencephalitis, GB syndrome, cerebral thrombophlebitis, brain abscess, hemiplegia, retrobulbar neuritis, mental retardation, etc. CNS infections are most serious complications and may be fatal.
3. *Gastrointestinal complications:* These include persistent diarrhea, appendicitis, stomatitis, enteritis, cancrum oris (noma), etc.
4. *Other complications* are myocarditis, acute glomerulonephritis, DIC and bleeding diathesis, keratitis and corneal ulcer secondary to vitamin 'A' deficiency, malnutrition, etc.

Management

There is no specific management for measles. The symptomatic management is done with antipyretic, antihistaminics/antipruritics, cough sedatives, vasoconstrictor nasal drops and vitamin 'A' supplementations. Antibiotics may be given in superadded bacterial infections. The use of antiviral drugs, gammaglobulins and steroids are doubtful.

Good nursing care and supportive measures promote the outcome. They include isolation, rest, calm and quiet environment, dimlight, good nourishing diet, adequate amount of fluid, oral hygiene, general cleanliness, meticulous skin care and daily bath, tepid sponge to reduce fever, clearing nasal and mouth secretions, eye care and careful observation for features of complications. Early detection and management of complications should be done promptly to prevent poor prognosis.

Preventive Measures

Active immunization with live attenuated measles vaccine is administered 0.5 mL subcutaneously in single dose at 9 to 12 months of age. A booster dose of measles vaccine is now recommended at the age of 16 to 24 months. It provides protection to the susceptible children for the life time. MMR vaccine can be administered for protection against measles along with mumps and rubella.

Passive immunization with gamma globulin can be administered intramuscularly 0.25 mL/kg for infants and 0.5 mL/kg for the children more than one year. It provides short-term immunity.

Isolation of the infected child and appropriate disposal of infected materials are necessary to prevent spread of infection to others.

Prognosis

Prognosis of a well-nourished child with measles is usually good. Measles is self-limiting disease unless it is complicated. Approximately 90 percent of death may occur in severe respiratory and neurological complications. The survivors of post-measles encephalopathy may have neurological deficits as long-term sequelae.

Poliomyelitis

Poliomyelitis is an acute viral disease caused by the RNA enterovirus, called as poliovirus. It has three serotypes, i.e. type-1 (Burnhide), type-2 (Lansing) and type-3 (Leon). Type-1 is the most common and type-2 is the least common cause of paralytic poliomyelitis. Type-1 causes large epidemics, type-2 is found as small outbreaks and type-3 as small epidemics. At present number of poliomyelitis cases is reduced because of intensified 'pulse polio' immunization program to eradicate the disease from our country.

Epidemiology

Man is the only reservoir and natural host of the virus. Mild and subclinical infections play dominant role in the spread of infection. The infectious materials are feces and oropharyngeal secretions of an infected persons. The cases are most infectious in the period 7 to 10 days before and after onset of symptoms. The virus is excreted in the stool for 2 to 3 weeks, sometimes for 3 to 4 months. The poliovirus can live in water for 4 months and in stool for 6 months in a cold environment.

Mode of transmission is mainly the feco-oral route, directly through contaminated fingers and indirectly through contaminated water, milk, foods, flies and articles of daily use. Infection can spreads through droplets in the acute phase of disease when the viruses present in the throat and oropharyngeal secretions. Incubation period is usually 7 to 14 days, but may range from 3 to 35 days.

Poliomyelitis is commonly found in infancy (approximately 50%) and childhood. The most vulnerable age is between 6 months and 3 years. Maternal antibody can protect the infant for first few months of life. Male children are more affected than female. Predisposing factors are intramuscular injection, trauma, operative procedures (e.g. tooth extraction, tonsillectomy), strenuous exercises, etc.

Poliomyelitis is more likely to occur during rainy season. The environmental sources of infections are contaminated water, food, finger and flies. Overcrowding place, poor sanitation, lack of hygienic practices, urban slum and villages facilitate the exposure of infection.

Pathology

Poliomyelitis is primarily an infection of the human alimentary tract, but the virus may infect the central nervous system and produces inflammation of gray matter of the spinal cord. The virus multiplies in the intestine and spreads to the surrounding lymph nodes and reticuloendothelial structures. The viremia may develop for a short period. Proliferation of the virus and invasion of the nerve structure occur when the virus particles are not neutralize by the antibody. Virus primarily invades the anterior horn cells of spinal cord, bulbar nuclei, vermis and nuclei of the roof of the cerebellum. Viruses usually reach the nervous system through blood stream and possibly through olfactory neural pathway. Poliovirus selectively damages motor and autonomic nervous system. The areas which are not usually affected include the white matter of the spinal cord, cerebellar hemispheres and nonmotor part of the cerebral cortex. Neurological damage may be mild and transient or severe and extensive.

Clinical Types of Poliomyelitis

The infections with poliovirus may present as the following clinical types:

- Asymptomatic poliomyelitis (silent or inapparent) or subclinical infections
- Abortive poliomyelitis or minor illness
- Nonparalytic poliomyelitis
- Paralytic poliomyelitis including four subtypes, i.e. spinal, bulbar, bulbospinal and encephalitic.

Clinical Manifestations

1. *Asymptomatic poliomyelitis:* Approximately in 90 to 95 percent of the susceptible persons, infected with the virus and the infection is asymptomatic. They are subclinical cases and considered as silent or inapparent.

2. *Abortive poliomyelitis:* The illness aborts in 4 to 8 percent of cases. It is usually mild and self-limiting illness. Due to viremia it may manifest as fever, sore throat, headaches, nausea, vomiting, anorexia and abdominal pain. Neurological features are usually not present.

3. *Nonparalytic poliomyelitis:* It occurs about in one percent of all infections. The virus enters the nervous system without destroying the cells. This condition may present as febrile illness due to viremia. The additional presenting features are meningeal irritation as neck rigidity, headache, backache, pain in legs, neck pain, nausea and vomiting. No paralysis occur in these cases and the patient remains conscious. The neck and back stiffness can be demonstrated by the kiss-the-knee test, tripod signs and head drops signs.

   Kiss-the-knee test consists in directing the child to sit up and kiss own knees. The test is positive, if he fails to do so without bending the knee. This occurs due to neck rigidity.

   Tripod signs is elicited by asking to child to sit up. The test is positive, if he assumes a tripod position while doing so.

   Head drop sign is tested by placing the hand under the patient's shoulder and the trunk is raised. The test is positive, when head lags behind limply.

   Recovery of nonparalytic cases is rapid. The disease usually lasts 2 to 10 days. The disease is synonymous with aseptic meningitis.

4. *Paralytic poliomyelitis:* It occurs in less than one percent of all infections. The virus invades CNS and result varying degree of paralysis. The most important feature is acute asymmetrical flaccid paralysis (AFP). History of fever along with acute flaccid paralysis is suggestive of poliomyelitis. The clinical features of paralytic type depend upon the site of involvement. It can be found in four subgroups, i.e. spinal form, bulbar form, bulbospinal form and encephalitic form.

   a. *Spinal form* of paralytic poliomyelitis may involve the extremities, neck, abdomen, diaphragm and intercostal muscles. Paralysis of spinal muscles may occur suddenly and manifested with fever, constitutional symptoms, muscle pain, hyperesthesia, tremors, diminished deep tendon reflexes and asymmetrical flaccid paralysis of the muscles. Flaccid paralysis commonly occurs in the lower limbs than upper limbs and large muscles are more affected than small muscles. Maximum paralysis occurs on 2nd or 3rd day of illness and usually descending type. The child may have frog-like position and phantom hernia may develop during crying due to weakness of the abdominal wall. Bladder and bowel involvements are common and lead to urinary retention and constipation. The child may present with respiratory difficulty due to involvement of diaphragm and intercostal muscles. There is no sensory loss in the affected part.

   b. *Bulbar poliomyelitis* is less common form but most severe due to involvement of vital medullary centers and paralysis of muscles innervated by cranial nerves. The clinical features include dysphagia, nasal speech, dyspnea and facial paralysis. Paralysis of vagus nerve causes the weakness of soft palate, pharynx and vocal cords. So, nasal speech and hoarseness of voice develop. Breathing and swallowing become difficult. Regurgitation of fluid and aspiration of secretions may cause atelectasis and pneumonia. Due to involvement of respiratory center, there is shallow, irregular breathing with diminished oxygen saturation. Damage of vasomotor center may occur and found as rapid, weak thready pulse and rise in blood pressure. The skin becomes dusky red and mottled. The patient become restless, confused and unconscious. Bulbar polio may or may not be associated with paralysis of spinal muscles.

   c. *Bulbospinal poliomyelitis* is manifested with combined features of both bulbar form and spinal form. It is found in about 25 percent cases of paralytic polio.

   d. *Encephalitic form* of poliomyelitis is less common. The patient is found with irritability, tremors, drowsiness, convulsions and unconsciousness. Paralysis may be upper motor neuron type.

Diagnosis

Poliomyelitis cases are diagnosed primarily by history and physical examination. The characteristic clinical features along with asymmetrical acute flaccid paralysis are useful to detect the case. Lumber puncture can help to diagnose the condition, but is best to avoid, because it may cause development of paralysis. CSF study helps to exclude the possibility of bacterial meningitis and shows a moderate increase in cells and an inconsistent elevation of protein. Poliovirus may be isolated from the CSF, urine and oropharyngeal secretions. Stool examination for 3 consecutive days may demonstrate the presence of poliovirus. Polio antibody can be detected in serum during convalescence period.

Management

No specific treatment is available for poliomyelitis. The prompt symptomatic and supportive management help in good prognosis. Good nursing care plays vital role for recovery and better outcome.

Hospitalization is necessary for all paralytic polio cases. Strict bed rest preferably on hard bed with minimum and gentle handling of the affected part are very essential. Positioning of the patient to be done to keep the airway patent and head to be turned to one side for gravity drainage of oropharyngeal secretions. Suctioning to be done whenever necessary to clear the air passage. Neutral position of the limbs to be maintained by little flexion of knees, straight hips, shoulder abducted at right angles and affected feet at right angles to the legs with support by sand bags or foot boards. Overstretching of the paralyzed limbs should be avoided.

Analgesics may be administered to relief pain. Hot moist pack or dry heat with infrared lamp or hot tub bath may be useful to reduce pain of the affected part.

Antihypertensive drugs may be needed in some cases. Mild sedative tranquilizer may be given in spinal paralysis to relief anxiety.

In case of respiratory failure, the patient should be managed in ICU with assisted ventilation in the mechanical ventilator. Continuous monitoring of patient's condition with pulse oxymetry should be performed. Tracheostomy may be necessary in constriction of hypopharynx and paralysis of vocal cords. Special care should be taken in case of tracheostomy.

Maintenance of fluid-electrolyte balances are very important in acute phase of illness. Later, appropriate nutritious diet to be provided. Continuous bladder drainage may be necessary to manage the retention of urine. Constipation should be managed, if present. Hygienic care should include special mouth care, skin care and eye care.

When muscle pain and spasm is relieved, then full range passive physiotherapy should be provided to prevent deformities and promote muscle power. Physiotherapy is performed with tolerance for 10 minutes, 2 to 3 times per day. Active physiotherapy should be started when condition permits. Parental involvement in the care of the child is very essential. Emotional support to the child, parents and family members help to reduce their anxiety and promote better coping and cooperation.

Rehabilitation of the paralyzed child should be planned according to the degree of involvement. Corrective splints brace or other orthotic devices may be necessary for the handicapped child. Surgical correction of the deformities may be done in later stages.

Complications

a. *Pulmonary complications:* Most important pulmonary complication is respiratory distress. It is a serious life threatening problem and develops due to one or more of the factors, i.e. paralysis of diaphragm and intercostal muscles, obstruction of upper respiratory passage, involvement of medullary respiratory center or vagus nerve and local lung conditions like pneumonia, atelectasis, pulmonary edema, etc. Respiratory failure may also develop.

b. *Cardiovascular problems:* Heart failure, myocarditis, hypertension and cardiac arrest.
c. *Gastrointestinal problems:* GI bleeding, perforation, fecal impaction.
d. *Urinary problems:* Transient paralysis of bladder, urinary tract infection and renal stone.
e. *Postpolio residual paralysis (PPRP) and bony deformities.*

Prognosis

About 5 to 10 percent cases of polio may be complicated with respiratory paralysis. It is not always fatal and many patients may survive with prompt management. Prognosis is generally worse in sudden onset with high fever and in older children. Mortality rate is about 5 to 7 percent and mostly due to respiratory failure. Among survivors, signs of recovery are found in the first few weeks, then recovery slows down during the next 6 months. Recovery may continue slowly up to 2 years. Postpolio residual paralysis may found among survivors of paralytic polio along with bony deformities. Prognosis varies from complete recovery to complete paralysis.

Preventive Measures

Active immunization with oral polio vaccine (OPV) is the important preventive measures. Trivalent OPV-2 drops is administered orally in 3 doses at one month intervals from 6 weeks of age onwards. In institutional delivery; 'O' dose OPV is given at birth. A booster dose of OPV is given at 16 to 24 months of age.

Global eradication of poliomyelitis is a great concern. Considering polio is an eradicable disease because man is the only host, there are no carriers, no animal reservoir, safe effective vaccine is available and the immunity is the life-long. India also accepted the eradication program as 'pulse polio immunization'. The strategy for eradication is four pronged: (a) high routine immunization coverage with OPV, (b) supplementary immunization in the form of National Immunization Day (NID) or Pulse Polio Immunization Program, (c) effective surveillance system, and (d) final stage consisting of mopping up by door to door immunization campaigns.

AFP surveillance is also important to detect where and how wild polio virus is circulating or to verify when it has been eradicated. Every case of AFP, in any child under 15 years, is to be reported. Stool examination is done for 3 samples for virus isolation and follow-up is made at 60 days of illness to check for residual paralysis.

Other preventive measures include avoiding of provocative factors during epidemics like intramuscular injections (even DPT), over exhaustion, chilling and operative procedures (tooth extraction). Children should be kept away from overcrowding places and swimming pools. Promotion of personal hygiene (especially hand washing), use of latrine, and avoidance of open-field defecation, promotion of environmental sanitation, safe water and food hygiene are also important measures for the prevention of poliomyelitis.

Viral Hepatitis

Viral hepatitis is the infection of the liver caused by different viruses. Previously hepatitis 'A' virus and hepatitis 'B' virus were only known as causative agents of viral hepatitis, but at present at least 5 specific viruses are well-recognized, i.e. hepatitis A, hepatitis B, hepatitis C, hepatitis D and hepatitis E virus. Hepatitis A, C, D, E, viruses are RNA virus and hepatitis 'B' is a DNA virus.

Newer hepatitis viruses, whose exact role in human disease is yet to be fully ascertained, include hepatitis F and hepatitis G virus and GB agent (GB virus A, GB virus B). There are several nonhepatotropic virus like cytomegalovirus (CMV), Epstein-Barr virus (EBV), varicella-zoster, herpes simplex, mumps virus, HIV, adenovirus and ECHO virus also can cause hepatitis.

Hepatitis 'A'

It is an acute infectious disease caused by hepatitis 'A' virus (HAV). It was previously known as infective hepatitis. The disease is manifested as nonspecific symptoms such as fever, chills, headache, fatigue, generalized weakness, aches and pains followed by anorexia, nausea, vomiting, dark urine and jaundice. The disease is benign in nature with complete recovery within several weeks.

The exact incidence of the disease is difficult to estimate due to occurrence of subclinical and asymptomatic cases. The condition is reported as endemic, sporadic and epidemics.

Epidemiology

The hepatitis 'A' virus is an enterovirus of the picornaviridae family. It multiplies only in hepatocytes. Virus is fairly resistant to heat and chemicals and can survive more than 10 weeks in well water. It can withstand heating to 60°C for one hour and is not affected by chlorine in the doses usually used for chlorination. The reservoir of infection is the human case only. There is no evidence of chronic carrier state. Period of infectivity is maximum between 2 weeks before and one week after the onset of jaundice. Infective materials are mainly infected stool, blood, serum. Other body fluids can also be infective during the brief stage of viremia. The virus is excreted in stool and urine.

Mode of transmission is mainly feco-oral route directly from person to person by contaminated hands and utensils or indirectly by the way of contaminated water, food and milk or by the flies. Hepatitis 'A' can also be transmitted by parenteral route by blood and blood products or by contaminated needle during the stage of viremia. Sexual transmission may also occur by oral or anal contact. Incubation period is 15 to 45 days with an average of 25 to 30 days. This may vary according to the dose of ingestion of virus.

Hepatitis 'A' infection is more common in children than adults. Clinical severity increases with age. One attack gives prolonged immunity and may last for life. Second attack may only found in about 5 percent of cases.

The favorable environments of HAV infection are rainy season with heavy rainfall, poor sanitation, over-crowding areas, poor personal hygiene mainly inadequate hand washing practices, improper cooking, poor food hygiene and unsafe water supply. Water borne and food borne epidemics are found.

Pathology

There is damage of liver cells in centrilobular region. Damage of hepatocytes is mediated by a cell-mediated immune response. Circulating antibodies help in limiting the dissemination of infection.

Clinical Manifestations

The infection may remain asymptomatic or can be seen as acute or subacute clinical hepatitis. Onset is usually acute with prodromal phase of illness for one to two weeks. The child may present with moderate fever, severe malaise, nausea, anorexia, vomiting, headache, and upper abdominal pain. When prodromal phase is over, the patient passes dark urine and clay color stool. Jaundice appears as yellowish discoloration of sclera and skin which may present for one to 4 weeks. Liver and spleen may be palpable. The condition may be complicated with fulminant hepatitis (rare) and hepatic failure. Relapse may occur.

Investigations

History of illness and clinical examination of the patient help to diagnose the condition. Laboratory investigations may be done to assess bilirubin level, SGOT, SGPT, ESR and anti-HAV antibody. HBs Ag test can be done to be sure that the infection is not by hepatitis 'B' virus.

Management

There is no specific treatment of acute hepatitis. Complete bed rest should be continued till the transaminase level is high. Carbohydrate rich food with glucose and adequate protein should be allowed in diet. Fat should be restricted. Frequently small amount of feeds to be given according to patient's tolerance. Adequate amount of fluid should be given. Vitamin supplementation can be given as supportive measures. Intravenous glucose may be needed in severe vomiting.

Preventive Measures

Hepatitis 'A' can be prevented by promoting safe water, improving food hygiene, personal hygiene and environmental sanitation. The best means of reducing the spread of infection are the simple measures of personal and community hygiene like hand washing before eating and after toileting, sanitary disposal of excreta to prevent contamination of water, food, milk and provision of safe water by appropriate water treatment and purification.

Disinfection of stool and fomites of the infected persons is important control measures. Passive immunization can be provided by anti-HAV gamma globulin to the close contacts of a case of hepatitis 'A', the efficacy lasts for six months.

Active immunization against hepatitis 'A' can also be provided by several available inactivated or live attenuated vaccines. But only four inactivated hepatitis 'A' vaccines are currently available internationally. All four vaccines are similar in terms of efficacy and side effects. The dose of vaccine, vaccination schedule, age for which the vaccine is licensed, varies from manufacturer to manufacturer.

Hepatitis 'B'

Hepatitis 'B' is an acute systemic infection with major pathology in the liver caused by hepatitis 'B' virus (HBV). It was previously known as serum hepatitis. It is a global problem and a major public health problem in India.

Epidemiology

Hepatitis 'B' virus is a DNA virus, originally known as 'Dane Particle'. It replicates in the liver cells. HBV has three distinct antigens, a surface antigen also known as 'Australia antigen' (HBs Ag), a core antigen (HBc Ag) and an 'e' antigen (HBe Ag). They stimulate the production of corresponding antibodies. These antibodies and their antigens constitute very useful markers of HBV infections.

Mode of transmission is mainly the parenteral route. Hepatitis 'B' is essentially a blood-borne infection. It is transmitted by infected blood and blood products transfusion, dialysis, contaminated syringes and needles, skin pricks, handling of infected blood, accidental inoculation of infected blood during immunization, dental procedures, tattooing, ear or nose piercing, ritual circumcision, acupuncture, etc. Occasionally percutaneous inoculations may occur accidentally by sharing shaving razor blade and tooth brush.

Perinatal vertical transmission may occur from HBV carrier mother to their babies during third trimester or at the time of delivery or in early puerperal period. Horizontal transmission from child to child also may occur. Physical contact between children with skin diseases like impetigo, scabies, cut injury, sharing same bed or contact during play are the major routes or spread of HBV in children.

Other routes of transmission are sexual contact. Infected insect bites (mosquito, bed bugs) is also suspected as route of transmission by blood sucking.

Incubation period is 45 to 180 days, lower doses of virus result longer incubation period. The median incubation period is lower than 100 days.

Man is the only reservoir of infection which can be spread either from carriers or from cases. Infective materials are contaminated blood (main source of infection) and body secretions (saliva, vaginal secretions, semen) of infected persons. Period of communicability is usually several months to years (in chronic carriers). About 10 percent patients become carriers. HBV infection may occur during early childhood and in perinatal period. High-risk groups of HBV infections among children are recipients of blood and blood product transfusion, infants of HBV carrier mothers and homosexual or IV drug users (adolescent group).

Clinical Manifestations

Clinical features of hepatitis 'B' are similar to those of the other types of viral hepatitis. The onset is insidious. Nausea and vomiting are uncommon and anorexia is mild. The illness may be asymptomatic with minimal liver damage and carrier state. It may be found as acute or chronic hepatitis. Acute hepatitis 'B' is presented as hepatitis 'A'. Jaundice may present or absent. Fulminant hepatitis and complications are more common. Extrahepatic manifestations are characteristics in hepatitis 'B' infection. Those include serum sickness like syndrome (rash, arthralgia, urticaria), purpura, polyarthritis nodosa, glomerulonephritis, severe aplastic anemia, pleural effusion, myocarditis and pericarditis.

Chronic hepatitis 'B' is presented in two forms, i.e. chronic persistent hepatitis and chronic active hepatitis. Chronic persistent hepatitis (about 70%) manifested without clinical jaundice and general condition remains good. This condition is benign in nature with elevated transaminases and recovers completely. Chronic active hepatitis (about 30%) manifested with chronic jaundice, increased hepatic enzyme level and may be complicated with cirrhosis of liver and hepatic failure.

Fulminant hepatitis and subfulminant viral hepatitis may occur secondary to hepatitis 'B' and presented as hepatic failure, within 2 weeks, of jaundice and encephalopathy from 2 weeks to 3 months after the onset of jaundice. Chronic carriers can be complicated as hepatocellular carcinoma.

Investigations

History of illness, physical examination and laboratory tests for WBC count, SGPT, alkaline phosphatase, HBsAg, antibody to HBc Ag, etc. help to diagnose the condition.

Management

No special treatment is required for acute hepatitis 'B'. Bed rest and general supportive measures are important. No specific dietary restriction needed except in hepatic failure. Chronic persistent hepatitis needs no specific treatment. Chronic active hepatitis can be managed with alpha-interferon, adenine arabinoside and acyclovir.

Fulminant hepatitis should be treated with antibiotics (neomycin or ampicillin) for gut sterilization and protein-free diet, rich in carbohydrate. Lactulose is administered by nasogastric drip to inhibit colonic organism to form ammonia. Intravenous 10 percent glucose is given. Exchange blood transfusion and plasmapheresis may be helpful to manage the crisis of hepatic failure.

Preventive Measures

Active immunization is provided by administering hepatitis 'B' (HB) vaccine. The dose of HB vaccine in the child below 10 years is 10 microgram in 0.5 mL intramuscular for recombinant vaccine. Second dose is given after one month of first dose and third dose after 6 months. Older children need doubled dose. Hepatitis 'B' vaccine should be given to the recipient of blood and blood product transfusion and to all children. Passive immunization can be provided by hyperimmune hepatitis 'B' immunoglobulin (HBIg) in postexposure conditions like accidental needle prick, mucocutaneous exposure of infected blood and neonates of HBs Ag positive mothers. The recommended dose is 0.06 mL/kg intramuscular within 24 hours of exposure.

Neonates of HBsAg positive carrier mothers should receive HBIg and HB vaccine IM at separate site within 12 to 24 hours of birth followed by 2nd and 3rd dose of vaccine at one month and 6 months of age. HB vaccine can be administered to them within 7 days of birth for first dose.

Other preventive measures include universal precautions for prevention of spread of infection, appropriate sterilization technique and increasing public awareness about the mode of transmission. Promotion of HB vaccination, screening of blood donors, avoidance of commercial blood donation and precaution of carriers to prevent spread of infection.

Other Viral Hepatitis

Hepatitis 'C' virus also termed as post-transfusion, non-A, non-B virus. It is transmitted by transfusion of blood and blood product or by parenteral, sexual or vertical route or by household contact. Majority of the infected hepatitis 'C' individual remain asymptomatic. Clinically this condition cannot be differentiated from other viral hepatitis. Incubation period varies from 2 to 24 weeks with an average of 7 to 9 weeks. Symptomatic cases are found as chronic hepatitis with jaundice which can lead to cirrhosis of liver or liver cancer. Interferon is the only drug found effective in treatment of HCV. Use of interferon is expensive and may have serious side effects. Relapse may occur. Prevention of transmission of HCV is most important aspect of management which include health education to inform general public and health care workers about the risk of transmitting infection with the use of unsterile equipment and infected blood and blood products.

Hepatitis 'D' virus or delta hepatitis is transmitted as hepatitis 'B' virus. Chronic asymptomatic carriers of HBV are at risk of developing delta hepatitis and subsequent chronic liver disease and cirrhosis. Its incubation period is about 2 to 8 weeks and usually presented as fulminant hepatitis.

Hepatitis 'E' virus is transmitted by feco-oral route through contaminated drinking water. It was found as epidemic in Delhi in 1955 to 1956. It is also found as sporadic and endemic cases in developing countries. Incubation period is 2 to 9 weeks and presented as self-limiting acute viral hepatitis. The clinical features are same of hepatitis 'A'. The condition can be complicated as fulminant hepatitis. There is no specific treatment, only supportive care should be provided. No vaccine available and passive immunization is not effective. The preventive measures include safe drinking water, appropriate sewage disposal and improvement of general hygienic practices.

Chickenpox (Varicella)

Chickenpox is an acute and highly communicable disease caused by varicella-zoster (V-Z) virus. It is characterized by sudden onset of low grade fever, mild constitutional symptoms and vesicular rash, appearing on the first day of illness. It is found as both epidemic and endemic form throughout the world.

Epidemiology

The causative agent of chickenpox is V-Z virus, a DNA virus and also called as "human (alpha) herpes virus-3". The source of infection is usually a case of chickenpox. Man is the only reservoir. The virus found in oropharyngeal secretions, lesions of skin and mucosa. The virus can also be found in the vesicular fluid during the first 3 days of illness. The scabs are not infective. The period of infectivity is mainly 1 to 2 days before and 4 to 5 days after the appearance of rash. The virus usually tends to die out before pustular stage and absent in crusts. The disease is highly communicable and secondary attack rate of chickenpox is very high. It is approximately 90 percent in household contacts.

Mode of transmission is by droplet infection and by droplet nuclei. Majority patients are infected by direct face to face personal contact. Portal of entry is the respiratory tract. Infections usually do not spread through fomites, because the virus is extremely labile. The virus can transmit through placental barrier and can infect the fetus. So infection during pregnancy presents risk for fetus and neonates and may cause limb atrophy, skin scaring, microcephaly, neurological and ocular anomalies. Incubation period is usually 14 to 16 days with a range from 7 to 21 days.

There is no age limit for this illness, though majority of the cases are young children of 5 to 10 years of age. One attack gives durable immunity. Second attacks of chickenpox are rare. Neonates are usually protected by maternal antibodies for first few months. But may be affected in absence of maternal antibodies.

Chickenpox shows some seasonal variation and found during first 6 months of the year. Transmission is more favorable in overcrowding areas. About 90 percent of the nonimmune inmates of the same house are affected.

Pathology

Pathological changes are limited to skin and respiratory tract. The skin lesions found as macules which quickly develop into papules and vesicles with scab and crust formation. The vesicles are formed in prickle cell layer of skin. Degeneration of cells in the vesicles result in multinucleated giant cells containing intranuclear inclusions. The inclusion bodies and foci of necrosis may be present in esophagus, pancreas, liver, adrenal gland and genitourinary tract. Varicella may cause disseminated interstitial pneumonia, encephalitis, perivascular demyelination. The V-Z virus may remain latent and can cause herpes-zoster in later life. The virus has a potential for oncogenicity.

Clinical Manifestations

The clinical presentation of chickenpox may vary from a mild illness with only a few scattered lesions to a severe febrile illness with widespread skin lesions. Inapparent infections may occur in approximately 5 percent of susceptible children.

The clinical course of chickenpox can be divided into two stages, i.e. pre-eruptive and eruptive stage.

The *pre-eruptive* or prodromal phase presents with sudden onset of mild to moderate fever, back pain, shivering and malaise for a short period (about 24 hours). This stage may be overlooked in some cases.

The *eruptive stage* manifests with rash which can be first sign. It appears usually on the day, the fever starts. The eruptions pass through the stages, i.e. macule, papule, vesicle, pastule and crusts or scabs.

The distribution of rash is symmetrical and first appears on the trunk and scalp; then on the face, arms and legs. The trunk is covered profusely, whereas extremities and face are having scanty rash. Mucosal surface including buccal, pharyngeal and conjunctiva are generally involved. Axilla may be affected but palms and soles are usually not involved. The rash progresses rapidly through the different stages and all stages of rash may be seen at the same time in the same area. This characteristics feature of rash in chickenpox termed as pleomorphism. Rash appears in 2 to 4 crops and temperature rises with each fresh crop of rash. The superficial, pleomorphic and centripetal distribution of rash are found. The vesicles look like dew-drops and superficial, which easily ruptured and surrounded by an area of inflammation. They are not umbilicated and may form crusts without being pastules. Scabbing begins after 4 to 7 days of the appearance of rash. Itching may be severe in pastular stage. Rarely the rash may become hemorrhagic and the disease becomes severe in patients with immunosuppressive therapy (steroid).

Complications

In most cases, chickenpox is mild and self-limiting. The mortality rate is less than one percent in uncomplicated cases. Though rare, the following complications may be found. They include superadded skin infection (cellulitis, abscess), septicemia, bronchopneumonia, encephalitis and neurological problems, like cerebellar ataxia, optic neuritis, facial nerve palsy, etc. Other complications include suppurative arthritis, osteomyelitis, myocarditis, hepatitis, glomerulonephritis, appendicitis, myositis, thrombocytopenia, purpura fulminans, Reye's syndrome and herpes zoster.

Diagnosis

Chickenpox is usually diagnosed by clinical manifestations. It should be differentiated from other skin lesions like impetigo, herpes urticaria, etc. It is differentiated from smallpox, which is already eradicated. Laboratory investigations are difficult. Virus isolation, antibody test can be done.

Management

There is no specific treatment. Symptomatic and supportive management are essential.

Antipruritic drugs and mild sedation may be needed to relief from itching. Antiviral, acyclovir, can be given orally to healthy children above 12 years to reduce the severity of illness and duration. Antipyretics should be given to treat fever but aspirin should be avoided to prevent Reye's syndrome. Antibiotics may be required in secondary skin infections. Steroid is contraindicated.

Supportive nursing measures should be provided with application of local calamine lotion or potassium permanganate lotion and sponge bath with antiseptic lotion. Nail to be cut short. Oral hygiene to be maintained by special mouth care with nonirritating mouthwash and saline gargle. Soft tooth brush should be used to prevent mucosal injury.

Maintenance of general cleanliness is very essential to prevent secondary infections. Rest, restriction of movement and isolation for 6 days after appearance of rash are important measures to prevent spread of infection. Disinfection of articles contaminated with nasal and throat secretions is also helpful and essential as control measures.

Prognosis

Chickenpox is usually a self-limiting disease with good prognosis. In case of serious complications like encephalitis especially in immunocompromised children the prognosis may be worse.

Preventive Measures

A live attenuated chickenpox vaccine is now available for active immunity which is effective in more than 80 percent of exposed individuals. This vaccine should be administered within 3 days of exposure to a case of Chickenpox.

Passive immunity can be provided by Varicella-Zoster Immunoglobulin (VZIg) which is equally effective and indicated in the children with leukemia, steroid therapy, susceptible pregnant women and neonates whose mothers develop chickenpox 2 days before and 5 days after delivery.

Mumps (Epidemic Parotitis)

Mumps is an acute infectious desease caused by a specific virus affecting the glandular and nervous tissues. Clinical presentations are nonsuppurative enlargement and tenderness of one or both the parotid glands. Other organs may also be affected. Constitutional symptoms vary and may be silent. Majority of the cases (85%) belongs to pediatric age group. Morbidity rate is usually high but mortality rate is very negligible.

Epidemiology

Mumps is found worldwide in endemic form. The causative agent is myxovirus parotitis, a RNA virus. The source of infection is both clinical and subclinical cases. The subclinical cases are about 30 to 40 percent of all cases. Virus can be found in the saliva or from the surface of Stenson's duct. It has been also found in blood, urine, human milk and in CSF. The period of communicability is usually 4 to 6 days before the onset of clinical symptoms with salivary gland swelling and a week or more thereafter. When the swelling of the gland is subsided, the case should not be considering as infectious. Secondary attack rate is about 86 percent.

Mode of transmission is mainly droplet infection and direct contact with infected person. Saliva, fomites and air-borne droplets spread the disease. Incubation period is generally 18 days with a range from 2 to 4 weeks.

Mumps usually affects the children of 5 to 15 years of age group, but no age is exempted with no previous immunity. The disease is less severe in children than adult. One attack of clinical or subclinical infection gives life-long immunity. Man is the only reservoir of infection and no carrier state exists.

Mumps can occur throughout the year, but the peak incidence is in winter and spring. Overcrowding may lead to epidemics.

Pathology

The virus enters through the nose or mouth. It proliferates in the parotid glands and the respiratory mucosa and produce viremia. The virus is localized in the salivary glands (mainly the parotids) and CNS and brings about the clinical symptoms. The mumps virus can also affect testes, pancreas, ovaries and prostate.

Clinical Manifestations

Mumps is manifested as generalized viral infection. Approximately one-third cases are asymptomatic. The initial features are fever, headache, nausea, malaise, anorexia and sore throat. Earaches and pain behind the ear on chewing and swallowing are diagnostic features found usually within 24 hours of onset. Tender edematous swelling of the parotid glands is found within 1 to 3 days. The enlargement of gland displaced the ear lobe upwards and outwards. The submaxillary and sublingual glands may also be involved later. The disease usually begins unilaterally but in 75 percent cases it affects both sides within 48 to 72 hours. Tenderness and pain usually subside within 3 days and swelling disappear within 10 days.

Half of the cases may have asymptomatic CNS involvement. Neurological manifestations may be noticed as aseptic meningitis, encephalitis, auditory nerve damage, GB syndrome, facial palsy, facial neuritis, transverse myelitis and cerebellar ataxia.

Complications

In mumps, complications are common but usually not serious. The most common complication is orchitis-epididymitis which cause severe pain, swelling with tenderness and result in testicular atrophy and sterility. Oophoritis may occur in female adolescents. Mumps in the first trimester of pregnancy may lead to fetal mortality or LBW baby.

Meningoencephalitis is another serious complication which found in about 10 percent of the cases and can be fatal. CNS involvement may lead to various long-term neurological complications.

Other complications of mumps include as pancreatitis, hepatitis, nephritis, myocarditis, pericarditis, thyroditis, mastoiditis, nerve deafness, arthritis, ITP, ocular paresis, facial palsy, hydrocephalus, etc. Diabetes may develop in some children following mumps.

Diagnosis

The diagnosis of mumps is made by clinical examination for tender swelling of the parotid glands along with history of exposure of the infection. On examination of mouth, swelling of the glands is evident. The opening of parotid gland (Stensen's duct), opposite to second upper molar, is found puffy and red.

Laboratory investigations may be needed in CNS involvement and for clinical diagnosis. Complement fixation test, CSF study, blood count and virus isolation can be done. The condition should be differentiated from other problems of parotid glands.

Management

There is no specific treatment for mumps. The symptomatic management includes antipyretics and analgesic to treat fever and pain. Steroids may be administered to relief pain and swelling in case of orchitis. Bed rest and local support to be provided for the child with orchitis. Warm saline mouth wash and liquid diet is needed in difficulty of chewing. The child should be kept isolated. Early detection of complications and prompt management to be done to prevent long-term sequelae.

Preventive Measures

Active immunization is recommended as combined MMR vaccine (Mumps, Measles, Rubella) or rubella-mumps vaccine. Live attenuated vaccine is now available for the prevention of mumps. Use of mumps vaccine is controversial.

Passive immunization by gammaglobulin can be given after exposure but its protective effect has not been established.

The control of mumps is difficult because the disease becomes infectious before the diagnosis in made. Long variable incubation period and occurrence of subclinical cases also make the control of transmission more difficult.

Isolation of the affected child, disinfection of infected articles and surveillance of contacts are needed as control measures of the condition.

Dengue Syndrome

The dengue syndrome is one of the most important emerging disease in the tropical and subtropical regions affecting urban and periurban areas. It can occur in epidemics and endemics.

Dengue syndrome is arthropod borne viral disease caused by dengue virus (arbovirus). This infection may be found as asymptomatic cases. Symptomatic cases can be presented as: (a) 'classical' dengue fever (DF), (b) dengue hemorrhagic fever (DHF) and (c) dengue shock syndrome (DSS).

The geographic distribution and number of cases increased greatly in last 30 years. There was a pandemic of dengue in 1998, which was reported from 56 countries. Over the past 10 to 15 years, dengue has become a leading cause of hospital admission and death among children next to diarrhea and ARI, in the south-east Asian region. About 95 percent of dengue death occur in children below 15 years.

In India, dengue is widely prevalent as endemics and sometimes as epidemics. All four serotypes (1–4) of dengue virus are found as causative agents. There was a outbreak of dengue in 1996 in Delhi. In 2001, outbreak has been reported in Rajasthan, Tamil Nadu, Karnataka, Gujarat, Delhi and Haryana. In 2005, there is an outbreak of dengue in Kolkata and other districts of West Bengal.

Epidemiology

The etiological agent of the dengue syndrome is dengue virus, of the family Flaviradae, having four distinct antigenically related serotypes (1, 2, 3, 4). The reservoir of infection is both man and mosquito. The transmission occurs in cycle, man-mosquito-man. Aedes aegypti mosquito is the main vector. Other species *A. albopictus, A. polynesiensis* and *A. scutellaris* are also responsible for dengue outbreak. All ages and both sexes are susceptible and children are having milder disease. The disease is widely prevalent in cities with high population density.

Mode of transmission is through bite of the female Aedes mosquito. This mosquito lives indoor and breeds in stored water. It bites the patient at daytime during viremia and sucks the infected blood. The virus multiplies in the salivary glands of the mosquito. After 3 to 14 days, the infection transmitted to other person by the bites of infected mosquito. Movement of the infected persons from one place to other spread the infection more, rather than that of the vector. The incubation period is about 3 to 15 days with an average of 5 to 7 days.

Clinical Manifestations

Dengue syndrome is clinically presented in three forms. The classical benign form is termed as dengue fever. The more serious forms are called dengue hemorrhagic fever and dengue shock syndrome, according to the presence of clinical features. Two main pathophysiological changes occur in DHF/DSS. They are: (a) increased vascular permeability that gives rise to loss of plasma from the vascular compartment leading to hemoconcentration, low pulse pressure and other signs of shock and (b) disorder in the hemostasis involving thrombocytopenia, vascular changes and coagulopathy.

Dengue Fever

Clinical features of dengue fever include sudden onset of moderate to high fever, bradycardia, chills, intense headache, muscle and joint pain with restriction of movement. Retro-orbital pain on movement of eye or eye pressure and photophobia may develop within 24 hours. Other common features are extreme weakness, anorexia, vomiting, consti-pation, bad taste, sore throat, chest pain and abdominal discomfort. Flushing of face is often present. Skin rash may appear in upper limbs and trunk within 3 to 4 days after the onset of fever. Fever is biphasic usually subsides by lysis with profuse sweating. The condition may be complicated with convulsions, tonsillitis, pharyngitis, rhinitis, diarrhea, lymphadenopathy and hepatosplenomegaly. The child generally recovers within 7 days.

Dengue Hemorrhagic Fever

It is manifested with acute onset of high continuous fever, epigastric discomfort, abdominal pain, tenderness at right costal margin with palpable liver. Moderate to severe thrombocytopenia, hemoconcentration and polyserositis developed. Petechiae, purpura and ecchymosis are present on extremities, axillae, face and palate. There is easy bruisability and petechiae are also seen on skin and the mucosa. Prolonged bleeding occurs at needle prick and venipuncture site. The patient may be complicated with circulatory failure and shock or may recover spontaneously. Febrile convulsions may occur particularly in infants. Epistaxis, gum bleeding, hematemesis and/or malena may present. The tourniquet (Hess) test usually becomes positive.

Dengue Shock Syndrome

Dengue shock usually found after 2 to 7 days of fever. The patient presents with cold congested blotchy skin, rapid and weak pulse, lethargy, restless and acute abdominal pain before the onset of shock. Hypotension and reduced pulse pressure are found. Fatal outcome may occur if not treated adequately, otherwise complete recovery occurs within 2 to 3 days with prompt management of shock. Good prognosis is indicated by good appetite and adequate urine output.

Complications

Dengue hemorrhagic fever or shock syndrome may be complicated with intracranial bleeding, encephalopathy, con-vulsions, renal failure, hemolytic uremic syndrome, hepatic failure, and iatrogenic problems like sepsis, pulmonary edema, overhydration and electrolyte imbalance.

Diagnosis

History of illness and clinical features of dengue fever should be supported by a positive tourniquet (Hess) test. The diagnostic investigations include blood examination, stool examination for occult blood, virus isolation, IgM antibody estimation, etc.

Blood examination shows raised hematocrit (20% above baseline), thrombocytopenia, leukopenia, lymphocytosis, prolonged prothrombin and partial thromboplastin time. Other common findings are hyponatremia, raised SGPT level and hypoproteinemia.

Management

There is no specific treatment for dengue fever. Symptomatic management should be done with bed rest, hydrotherapy and antipyretics (paracetamol) for high fever. Analgesics for pain may be used, but salicylates (aspirin) should be avoided, because it may precipitate bleeding tendency and metabolic acidosis. Oral fluid intake with ORS or fruit juice are preferred to plain water. Maintenance of fluid and electrolyte balance and adequate nutrition are important. Monitoring of vital signs (TPR, BP), intake and output chart are very essential. Blood transfusion may be needed in severe hemorrhagic manifestations. Management of shock and other complications should be done promptly with IV fluid therapy and other supportive measures.

Patient should be discharged when body temperature becomes normal, for at least 24 hours, urine passed normally, improved appetite, no respiratory distress and stable hematocrit and platelet count.

Prognosis

Dengue fever is self-limiting and benign in nature. Full recovery is possible with appropriate management. In DHF, mortality is about 40 to 50 percent, but intensive care may reduce the mortality to as low as 2 percent.

Preventive Measures

Vector control by prevention of mosquito breeding in stored water and killing larva are important measures for prevention of dengue syndrome. Personal protective measures (mosquito net) should also be promoted along with effective treatment of infected persons. Isolation of the patient during first few days of illness under bed-nets is essential measures. There is no satisfactory vaccine against the disease.

HIV/AIDS in Children

Children are innocent victim of HIV/AIDS. HIV or human immunodeficiency virus infection leads to AIDS, i.e. acquired immunodeficiency syndrome. It is fatal illness and a pandemic disease with large number of infected children throughout the world. Approximately 0.8 million children, below 15 years of age are infected as estimated by WHO, at the end of 2001. Pediatric AIDS in developing countries comprises 15 to 20 percent of all cases against only 2 percent of the West.

Global HIV/AIDS epidemic:
- Number of children under 15 years living with HIV in 2006 is 2.3 million (approx.).
- AIDS death in 2006 among children under 15 years is about 380, 000.

In India, HIV/AIDS is presenting as epidemic. There is epidemic shifts from the highest risk group (commercial sex workers, drug users) to bridge population (clients of sex worker, STD patients, and partners of drug users) and then to general population. The trends indicate that HIV infection is spreading in two ways, from urban to rural areas and form individual practising high risk behavior to the general population. Data from antenatal clinics indicate rising of HIV prevalence among women which in turn contribute to increasing HIV infection in children.

Epidemiology

HIV is a protein capsulated RNA virus of retrovirus family, having two serotypes HIV1 and HIV2. It can mutate rapidly and developing new strains continually. HIV1 is more pathogenic then HIV2. Mode of transmission and clinical manifestations are same in two types. The virus can be easily inactivated by heat (56°C for 30 minute) or 0.2 percent sodium hypochlorite or one percent glutaraldehyde. It is relatively resistant to ionizing radiation and U-V light. The reservoir of infection is the case or carriers. Once an individual is infected, the virus remains in the body for life-long. Since the incubation period may be the years, the symptomless carriers can infect other people for long times.

The source of infections is the infected blood, semen and CSF. Lower concentrations have been detected in breast milk, saliva, tears, urine and cervical and vaginal secretions. The virus has also been identified in brain tissue, lymph nodes, bone marrow and skin. The most important sources are blood and semen.

Mode of transmission is mainly by sexual route in adult. Parent to child transmission is major concern in pediatric HIV/AIDS which include vertical transmission (90%) from infected mother to fetus or from infected mother to child. Transmission may occur in uterus (30–35%), during delivery (60–65%) and also through breastfeeding (1–3%). Children may get infection other than perinatal transmission through blood and blood product transfusion, organ transplantation, contaminated needle prick, use of contaminated instruments during surgical procedures or any skin piercing instruments during ear piercing, tattooing, acupuncture and circumcision. Sexual transmission may occur in sexually active adolescents. Horizontal transmission accounts for only 10 to 15 percent cases of HIV/AIDS in children. Total perinatal transmission is about 2.56 percent in India, in 2002, among reported HIV cases. HIV is not transmitted by food, water, mosquito bites, or casual contact like social kissing, hand shaking, hugging, sharing feeding articles, using public toilets, etc.

Neonates born to mothers with risk factors can be infected with HIV/AIDS. Risk factors of pediatric HIV/AIDS include— mother using IV drugs, indulging in promiscus sexual behavior and having heterosexual or bisexual sex partners. History of blood and blood products transfusion in case of thalassemia and hemophilia also considered as important risk factors of children for HIV infection.

Incubation period of HIV infection is uncertain. It may vary from few months to 6 years or more to develop AIDS from HIV infection. It depends upon lifestyle of the infected person and supportive care of the infected child. Natural history of HIV infection is not yet completely understood.

Pathogenesis

HIV infection is primarily the immune system disorder with depletion of CD4+ helper 'T' lymphocytes. HIV selectively infects the T helper cells apart from several other cells in the immune system, i.e. B cells, microphages and nerve cells. When the virus multiplicates, the infected T helper cells are destroyed. Depletion of CD4+ lymphocytes in blood and lymph nodes are the important characteristic of AIDS. There is reversal of helper/suppressor T cell ratio which tends to persist. As the disease progress, the functional abnormalities of T cells may result as abnormal response of lymphocytes to antigens, mitogens and allogeneic cells and failure to produce normal amount of interleukin-2, interferon and other lymphokines. T cell defect leads to defect in B cell activity resulting polyclonal hypergammaglobulinemia (raised IgA, IgG and IgM) leads to failure to form antibody to antigens. There is disturbance of complement and phagocytic activity along with widespread lymphoid infiltration.

Initially, after one to three weeks of infection there is viremia and decline of CD4+ cells. A long asymptomatic period may found due to decline in viremia as a result of vigorous cellular and humoral response of the immune system. But in long-term, there is steady decline in the number of CD4+ cells. Opportunistic infections usually occur when CD4+ cell count fall below approximately 200 to 400/mL. Death may occur due to infections, neoplasm and cachexia.

Clinical Manifestations

At birth, HIV infected infants are generally asymptomatic. After that clinical features may appear in two forms, i.e. rapid progressive (80%) and slow progressive (20%). In rapid progressive disease, the onset of symptoms set in from 3 to 4 months of age and in slow progression the child may present clinical features as late as 8 years.

Clinical features depend upon pre-existing immuno-deficiency conditions like prematurity or viral immuno-suppression or presence of other infections. The infected children may be asymptomatic or mildly symptomatic or moderately or severely symptomatic.

The infants born to mothers with risk factors/HIV infected may present with low birth weight, failure to thrive, microcephaly, hepatosplenomegaly, lymphadenopathy and *Pneumocystic carinii* pneumonia. Recurrent otitis media, chronic sinopulmonary infection, oral thrush, chronic diarrhea, chronic parotid swelling, unexplained anemia, thrombocytopenia and recurrent infection may develop. Cardiac or kidney disease may also found. Kaposi's sarcoma is uncommon in childhood AIDS.

Transfusion associated AIDS in children may present with *Pneumocystic carinii* pneumonia, Kaposi's sarcoma, chronic lymphadenopathy with recurrent pyrexia, night sweats, weight loss, chronic diarrhea, hepatosplenomegaly and other viral infections (E-B virus, hepatitis 'B' virus). Adolescents above 12 years of age present with same clinical features as adults.

WHO criteria for diagnosis of pediatric AIDS in developing countries, such as India are as follows:

Major Criteria

- Weight loss or abnormally slow growth
- Chronic diarrhea for over one month
- Prolonged or intermittent pyrexia for over one month.

Minor Criteria

- Generalized lymphadenopathy
- Oropharyngeal candidiasis
- Recurrent common bacterial infections
- Persistent cough for over one month
- Generalized dermatitis
- Confirmed HIV infection in the mother.

Note: The existence of 2 major and 2 minor criteria in the absence of other known causes of immunodeficiency is diagnostic of AIDS.

Clinical Staging

WHO clinical staging system for HIV infection and related disease in children:

- Stage 1 – Asymptomatic
  - Persistent generalized lymphadenopathy
- Stage 2 – Unexplained chronic diarrhea
  - Severe persistent or chronic candidiasis outside the neonatal period
  - Weight loss or failure to thrive
  - Persistent fever
  - Recurrent severe bacterial infections
- Stage 3 – AIDS defining opportunistic infections
  - Severe failure to thrive
  - Progressive encephalopathy
  - Malignancy
  - Recurrent septicemia or meningitis

Complications

There are numbers of complications in HIV/AIDS disease. These complications include recurrent infections, opportunistic infections, acute and chronic ENT infections, hearing loss, tooth and gum diseases, drug related toxicities, failure to thrive, developmental delay, malabsorption and wasting. Chronic atopic dermatitis and other skin reactions, cardiomyopathy, nephropathy, neuropathy, neutropenia, anemia, thrombocytopenia and psychological crisis.

Laboratory Investigations

The following investigations can be done to confirm the diagnosis for a suspected case of AIDS:

- ELISA test (Enzyme-linked immunosorbent assay test) is done for screening test for anti-HIV IgG detection.
- Western blot test is performed as confirmatory test.
- CD4 count—Use of CD4 count to assess HIV associated immunosuppression are not free from problem, because normal CD4 count is higher in infants and children and they have opportunistic infections at higher levels of CD4 count.
- T cell ratio and T cell growth factors.
- HIV culture and HIV antigen test.
- HIV specific PCR (polymerase chain reaction) to detect viral nucleic acid.
- TLC, DLC, platelet count.
- Quantitative measurement of immunoglobulin levels and circulating immunocomplex testing.

Maternal antibodies transmitted to fetus or child remain at significant level until 18 months. So IgG antibody tests are not reliable indicators of infection status to a child before 18 months of age.

Management

There is no curative treatment of HIV/AIDS. No vaccine is available for prevention of the condition. Preventive measures are the important aspect of management. Children should be protected from contacting the HIV infection from the adult.

If the child becomes infected, early diagnosis and prompt management should be initiated for the associated problems and opportunistic infections. Improvement of general health and promotion of living standard help in prolongation of life of the infected child.

Specific supportive management should be provided for the clinical problems of HIV/AIDS. Nutritional support and management of diarrhea, fever, cough, pain, etc. should be arranged as complaints for or by the patient. Tuberculosis, pneumonia, candiasis, Kaposi's sarcoma, herpes zoster, etc. should be managed accordingly. Family counseling and social support are important aspect of supportive management.

The specific therapy with antiretroviral drugs is indicated when the child have signs of immunodepression or HIV associated symptoms. The drugs which can be used for the children are zidovudine, didanosine, zalcitabine, stavudine and lamivudine as nucleoside analogs. Other drugs like protease inhibitors (ritanavir, indinavir, saquinavir, nelfinavir) and non-nucleoside reverse transcriptase inhibitors (nevirapine, delavirdine) can also be used as antiretroviral combination therapy. These drugs suppress the HIV infection but do not cure the disease. They are useful for prolongation of life in severely infected patients.

Nursing Interventions

Nursing management should be planned according to the nursing diagnosis to overcome the associated problems. Adequate history of illness, physical examination, analysis of relevant records and reports and assessment of psychological status are essential for identification of problems. The important nursing diagnoses related to HIV infected patient are as follows:

- Risk for infections related to immunodeficiency state.
- Altered nutrition related to anorexia, pain abdomen and malabsorption.
- Altered oral mucosa related to stomatitis, or candidiasis.
- Diarrhea and dehydration related to enteric pathogens and infections.
- Altered body temperature, more than normal, due to HIV infection and secondary infections.
- Pain related to advanced HIV diseases.
- Altered growth and development related to HIV infections and CNS involvement.
- Ineffective family coping related to chronic fatal illness of the child.
- Fear and anxiety related to diagnostic and treatment procedures.
- Knowledge deficit regarding transmission of HIV infection, care at home and available social support.

Implementation of nursing care should include preventing infections, maintaining adequate nutrition, improving integrity of oral mucosa, minimizing the effects of diarrhea and preventing dehydration, assessing general conditions and vital signs, controlling fever, promoting growth and development, reducing fear and anxiety, improving coping abilities, informing and educating about care of the child at home and prevention of transmission.

Prevention of HIV/AIDS

Preventive measures are best attempt to control the global problem of HIV/AIDS. Until a vaccine or more effective curative treatment of the disease becomes available, the best means of preventive measure is health education. It helps the community people to make life-shaving choices and avoidance of risk behaviors, thus to protect the children, the innocent victims from the fatal disease.

Four basic approaches to the control of HIV/AIDS include: (a) prevention by health education to make life-saving choices and avoiding blood-borne HIV transmission, (b) antiretroviral treatment with combination therapy or postexposure prophylaxis, (c) specific prophylaxis for HIV manifestations, e.g. isoniazid for tuberculosis and (d) primary health care approaches with integrated care in MCH, FP and health education.

Parent to child transmission can be prevented by avoiding indiscriminate sexual practices of adults and use of condom. Meticulous screening of blood and blood products, avoidance of commercial blood donation, promotion of voluntary blood donors, screening before organ transplant will help to prevent blood route transmission. Other preventive measures include sterilization of syringe and needle for injections or immunization, maintenance of aseptic techniques during delivery and in surgical or dental interventions, precautions for exposure to body fluids, motivation to avoid IV drug abuse, and unsafe sex among adolescents, creating awareness among traditional practitioners (barbar, tattoo maker, quacks) about avoidance of spread of HIV infection, promoting community awareness about transmission of HIV infection by unsafe practices, i.e. ear piercing, circumcision, etc.

Vertical transmission can be prevented by zidovudine prophylaxis to the infected pregnant women and to the infants till 6 weeks of life, born to the infected mother.

Postexposure prophylactic (PEP) treatment can be given with antiretroviral drugs (AZT monotherapy) for 4 weeks within hours following accidental exposure to the virus by needle stick injury.

HIV positive women should be informed and explained about the possibilities of the infection of the future offspring. Acceptance of pregnancy and its continuation should be judged by the couple according to their own decision.

Immunization of HIV Positive Children

Routine pediatric immunization must be given to HIV infected infants and children with some modifications. Oral polio vaccine (OPV) and BCG should be omitted, in symptomatic HIV positive children. Hepatitis 'B', inactivated polio vaccine and MMR can be administered to them. Children with asymptomatic HIV infection should receive BCG vaccine with other vaccines except OPV. These immunization will provide specific prophylaxis from associated complication of HIV infection.

COMMON BACTERIAL INFECTIONS

Common bacterial infections in children include tuberculosis, typhoid fever, tetanus, diphtheria, whooping cough and leprosy. Other childhood communicable diseases include hemophilus influenzae 'B' (HiB) disease, meningococcal infections, helicobacter pylori infections, toxic shock syndrome, STDs/RTIs, congenital syphilis and nosocomial infections. These communicable diseases are preventable by vaccination and by some preventive measures. Awareness about the preventive aspects is important approach to control these diseases. Nursing personnel are responsible for hospitalized and home-based care of these conditions and prevention of the diseases by various controlling measures.

Diphtheria

Diphtheria is an acute infectious bacterial disease caused by toxigenic strains of *Corynebacterium diphtheriae*. The disease is characterized by inflammation of epithelial surface, formation of a membrane in the upper respiratory tract and presence of severe toxemia due to the effect of powerful exotoxin.

Diphtheria is found as an endemic disease in India, but a rare condition found in developed countries. The incidence of the disease is declining due to increased coverage of childhood immunization with DPT vaccine.

Epidemiology

The causative agent of diphtheria is a gram positive, non-motile bacteria named as *Corynebacterium diphtheriae*. It has no invasive power but produces powerful exotoxin. The bacilli may survive for short period in dust and fomites. It can be killed by heat and chemical agent. The source of infection may be a case or a carrier. Cases can be found as subclinical or as frank clinical. Carriers are common source of infection (95%). Infective materials are nasopharyngeal secretions, discharge of skin lesions, contaminated fomites and infected dust. Period of infectivity may vary from 14 to 28 days from the onset of disease but carriers are infective for longer period.

Mode of transmission is mainly droplets infection. The disease can be transmitted directly from skin lesions or through contaminated objects (utensils, care articles, toys, etc.). Portal of entry is mainly respiratory tract. Other routes of entry are cuts, wounds, ulcers, and occasionally through eye, genitalia, middle ear, etc. Incubation period is 2 to 6 days.

Diphtheria affects mainly the children of one to five years of age. It can be found even in preschool and school children. Infants of the immune mothers are protected for few weeks or months of life. The disease occurs in all seasons but found more in winter or in autumn.

Pathology

The diphtheria bacilli proliferate and liberate powerful exotoxin which causes local and systemic lesions. The exotoxin causes necrosis of the epithelial cells and liberates serous and fibrinous material to form a grayish-white pseudo-membrane. The surrounding tissue becomes inflamed and edematous.

The exotoxin mainly affects the heart, kidney and central nervous system. Myocardial fibers degenerate and disturbance of conduction system developed. Toxic damage of CNS leads to polyneuritis. Inflammation of renal interstitial tissue occurs due to degeneration of renal tubular cells.

Clinical Manifestations

The clinical features depend upon the site of lesion, location of membrane, its extent and age of the patient. Diphtheria can occur on different location, i.e. faucial, laryngeal, nasal and cutaneous.

The onset of the disease is acute with fever (usually 39°C), malaise, headache, anorexia, delirium, drowsiness and toxic appearance.

Faucial or pharyngotonsillar diphtheria is the most common type in children. The clinical features of this condition include sore throat, difficulty in swallowing, muffled voice, low grade fever, prostration, tachycardia, redness and swelling with localized exudate over fauces. The important feature is formation of whitish-gray membrane adherent to the underlying mucosa over tonsils, anterior pillar, uvula and pharynx. Attempt to remove the membrane results bleeding, the maneuver should be avoided to prevent greater liberation of the damaging exotoxin. In severe cases, cervical lymphadenopathy and edema of submandibular area may be found giving a characteristic 'bullnecked' appearance.

Laryngeal diphtheria is most serious type but less common form. It is manifested with hoarseness of voice, aphonia, croup, brasy or barking cough, restlessness, prostration, dyspnea, chest retraction, cyanosis, cervical lymphadenopathy and edema of neck ("Bull neck"). The membrane is formed over the larynx or may be the extension of the membrane of the throat (faucial diphtheria) lower down into the larynx. The membrane may cause respiratory obstruction and respiratory failure as it may extend below to tracheal or bronchial tree.

Nasal diphtheria is uncommon but the important source of spread of infection to others. It is mildest type and may extend to pharynx. It is usually localized to the septum or turbinates of the nose. It is presented with serosanguineous discharge from the nose and excoriation of upper lip with minimum toxic features.

Other sites of diphtheria may be skin, ears, eyes and genitalia. Skin diphtheria is found as chronic tender ulcer surrounded by erythema and covered with a membrane.

Complications

Various complications may occur in case of diphtheria. They are mainly myocarditis, paralysis (pharyngeal, palatal, ocular or general) bronchopneumonia, nephritis, polyneuritis, hepatitis, vasomotor disturbances like hypotension and cardiac failure.

Diagnosis

History of illness, physical examination to exclude clinical features, throat examination and throat swab smear to detect diphtheria bacilli help to confirm the diagnosis. Culture on Loeffler medium demonstrates the growth of gram positive pleomorphic bacilli and results are available within 8 hours. Fluorescent antibody technique is of great value for quick diagnosis.

Management

The specific management of diphtheria is done by prompt initiation of treatment with antidiphtheritic serum (ADS), an antitoxin to neutralize the circulatory exotoxin. It is administered IM or IV after skin test. The dose of ADS depends upon the type of diphtheria, extent of membrane and degree of toxemia. ADS may be given as repeat dose for better improvement. Desensitization is needed in case of sensitivity to ADS. Close observation of the patient is very important to detect the untoward reactions and complications.

Antibiotic therapy, preferably penicillin or erythromycin, should be administered for 2 weeks to eradicate the bacilli and to stop production of diphtheria toxin. Only after three negative culture the patient should be considered as free of bacteria and cured. Carriers also need effective treatment to prevent spread of infection.

Supportive measures include isolation of infected child, bed rest for 2 to 3 weeks, easily digestible diet with high calorie, drug therapy with antipyretics and sedative. In case of seriously ill patient, IV fluid, oxygen therapy, nasogastric tube feeding may be needed for maintenance of fluid electrolyte and nutritional requirements. Frequent removal of oropharyngeal or nasal secretion is essential. Tracheostomy may be required in respiratory obstruction. Mechanical ventilation may be needed in case of respiratory failure. Cardiac complications should be detected early by close monitoring and necessary management should be initiated promptly.

During recovery phase, if schick test is positive, diphtheria toxoid should be given since not all patients develop adequate immunity after the disease.

Prognosis

Prognosis depends upon type of illness, initiation of specific therapy and available treatment facilities. If left untreated about 50 percent cases may die. With effective treatment by specific therapy only 4 to 5 percent cases may die due to various complications, like respiratory obstruction, respiratory paralysis, myocarditis and circulatory collapse. Among survivor permanent cardiac damage and paralytic sequelae may found.

Preventive Measures

The most reliable preventive method of diphtheria is active immunization by DPT and DT to all children by universal coverage. Isolation of cases, disinfection of contaminated articles and chemoprophylaxis of all household contacts and carriers are important preventive measures to control the disease. All close contacts need to have Schick test and throat swab culture before administering chemoprophylaxis. Passive immunization with ADS may be given to the carriers with negative Schick test and positive culture with unknown immunization status.

Whooping Cough (Pertussis)

Whooping cough is a highly communicable acute bacterial infections of the respiratory tract. It is a lethal disease manifested as an insidious onset of mild fever with irritating cough which gradually becomes paroxysmal with the characteristic inspiratory whoop. The clinical spectrum of the disease varies from severe illness to atypical and mild illness without 'whoop'. About 50 percent of total cases are found among preschooler. A single attack gives life-long immunity in majority of cases. It is also called at 'hundred days cough'.

Whooping cough occurs in all countries of the world as epidemic or endemic form. At present, there is marked decline of number of cases of this disease due to increased immunization coverage with DPT vaccine.

Epidemiology

The causative agent of whooping cough is 'Bordetella pertussis', a nonmotile rodshaped gram-negative bacillus. Other microorganisms which may cause pertussis like mild illness are *Bordetella parapertussis, Bordetella bronchiseptica, Hemophilus hemolyticus* and adenovirus (type 1, 2, 3 and 5).

Bordetella pertussis infects only man. The source of infection is a case of pertussis. Chronic carrier state does not exist. Infective materials are nasopharyngeal and bronchial secretions and contaminated objects. Infective period may be from a week after exposure to infection to about 3 weeks after the onset of the paroxysmal stage. The disease is most infectious in the catarrhal stage.

Mode of transmission is mainly droplet infection and direct contact. Children get infections from other children and playmates during coughing, sneezing and talking which sprayed the bacilli in air. Fomites spread the organism less, unless freshly contaminated. Incubation period of the disease is about 7 to 14 days but not more than 3 weeks.

Whooping cough is mainly the disease of the infants and preschool children. Highest incidence is found among the children below 5 years age and highest mortality is found in infants below 6 months, especially in undernourished children with other respiratory infections. The disease is more common in female child.

Pertussis may occur throughout the years but more cases are found in winter and spring. Overcrowding place, poor environmental sanitation and lower social living are the influencing factors of the disease.

Pathology

The causative agent of whooping cough liberates a number of antigens and toxins which result in pathological changes of respiratory tract from nasopharynx to bronchioles. They produce inflammatory reaction of the mucosa and secretions (phlegm), which is responsible for most of the clinical manifestations. Attachment of the pathogens to the respiratory epithelium, local epithelial damage, diminished phagocytic function and disrupts mucociliary clearance are the mechanism of pathological changes. The systemic manifestations are produced by the pretussis toxin. Cerebral damage results due to respiratory obstruction and apnea.

Clinical Manifestations

The clinical manifestations of whooping cough are found in three stages, i.e. first catarrhal stage, approximately 2 weeks duration, second paroxysmal stage about 2 to 4 weeks duration and third convalescent stage about 2 weeks duration.

Catarrhal stage: Onset of the disease is usually insidious with symptoms of rhinitis, sneezing, lacrimation, fever and irritating cough. Initially, cough is usually disturbing at night and later both in night and day time.

Paroxysmal or spasmodic stage: In this stage there is rapid paroxysmal, explosive and repeated series of cough in expiration followed by a sudden deep violent inspiration with crowing sound or whoop. The whoop sound is produced due to rushing of air through half open glottis during inspiration. Sometime whoop may be present with or without cyanosis and apnea. Paroxysms may occur in every hour or more frequently. It may be followed by vomiting. The patient looks suffocated with congested red face, anxious look, sweating, congestion of neck and scalp veins, confused and restless. The patient usually coughs up thick tenacious mucous. The condition is complicated with periorbital edema, subconjunctival hemorrhage, ulcer of frenulum of the tongue (due to repeated thrusting of tongue over the teeth), exhaustion, dehydration and convulsions.

The paroxysms of cough are precipitated by eating, sneezing, drinking and cold air.

Convalescent stage: During this stage severity of paroxysm decreases and the interval between paroxysm increases. Patients' general condition and appetite improve. Habit pattern of cough may persist for weeks or months. This stage may be prolonged due to pulmonary and other complications.

Complications

Complications of pertussis includes the followings:
a. *Respiratory complications:* Atelectasis, bronchopneu-monia, bronchiectasis, emphysema, peneumothorax, pneumomediastinum, flaring up of pulmonary tuber-culosis and hemoptysis.
b. *Neurological complications:* Encephalopathy, intra-cranial hemorrhage, persistent seizures, hemiplegia, paraplegia, ataxia, aphasia, blindness, deafness, mental subnormality, etc.
c. *Miscellaneous:* Alkalosis due to persistent vomiting, epistaxis, subconjunctival hemorrhage, rectal prolapse, hernia (umbilical and inguinal), otitis media, frenular ulcer, growth failure and malnutrition.

Investigations

Clinical diagnosis of whooping cough is easy during second stage of illness. Laboratory investigations are needed for isolation of organism and detection of toxins. Nasopharyngeal swab culture or cough plate method is used for isolation of causative organism. ELISA test is done to measure antibody to antigen and pertussis toxin. Blood examination shows remarkable high absolute lymphocytosis, extremely low ESR and WBC count is initially low but afterwards rises far beyond normal (20–50 thousand per cm). Chest X-ray helps to detect perihilar infiltration, atelectasis or emphysema.

Management

The patient with severe illness should be hospitalized and need bed rest, antibiotic therapy, symptomatic treatment and supportive care.

Antibiotics should be started by early diagnosis in the catarrhal stage to prevent severity and spread of infection. The drug of choice is erythromycin 40 to 50 mg/kg/day in 4 divided doses for 2 weeks orally. Other antibiotics like roxithromycin, azithromycin and clarithromycin for 5 to 7 days also give good results.

In case of severe paroxysmal cough, bronchodilator (salbutamol, albuterol) should be administered by nebulization, otherwise 0.3 to 0.5 mg of salbutamol per kg/day in three divided doses may be given.

Betamethasone (0.75 mg/kg/day) may be useful in severe coughing paroxysms. Pertussis immunoglobulin may be helpful in the first week of disease to reduce whoop.

Complications of pertussis should be detected as early as possible and prompt specific management should be initiated.

Supportive nursing care is significant aspect of management. It includes isolation of the patient, liberal use of oxygen to prevent hypoxia and cerebral anoxia, removal of secretions, positioning to relieve respiratory discomfort, maintenance of fluid and electrolyte balance to prevent alkalosis and dehydration. Other measures include appropriate dietary intake by small frequent well-tolerated food, minimal gentle handling during care, avoidance of precipitating factors of cough, close and continuous observation and recording for complications and child's condition. Administrations of prescribed medications, emotional support to parents and child, hygienic measures, parental involvement in child care and related health teaching to the parents are important aspects of nursing care.

Prognosis

Prognosis depends upon age of the child and presence of complications. Most of the deaths occur below the age of one year. Mortality rate is higher in malnourished children and with the presence of ARI. The associated complications obviously influence the immediate outcome and sequelae. The high morbidity and mortality is related to nature of complications.

Preventive Measures

Active immunization is the best measure for prevention of pertussis. DPT should be administered with 3 doses from 6 weeks of age at one month interval. A booster dose is given after one year of 3rd dose or at 16 to 24 months of age.

Pertussis vaccine should not be given to a child with history of convulsion associated with progressive neurological manifestations. Encephalopathy may develop following pertussis vaccine.

Other preventive measures are isolation of infected case, disinfection of secretions and contaminated articles and chemoprophylaxis of contact cases.

Tetanus

Tetanus is an acute infectious bacterial disease caused by *C. tetani* and characterized by muscular stiffness and painful paroxysmal spasms of the voluntary muscles caused by the powerful neurotoxin of the causative organism. The mortality rate of this disease tends to be very high.

Tetanus is one of the leading cause of neonatal death. Neonatal tetanus considered as a killer disease second only to measles among the six-killer vaccine preventable diseases.

Tetanus is found all over the world. In India, tetanus is an endemic infection. The important factors contributing to the incidence of the disease are lack of hand washing and unhygienic delivery practices, delivery by untrained persons, traditional birth customs and lack of interest in immunization among antenatal mothers. Inadequate medical care facilities with lack of primary health care services are important factors contributing to neonatal tetanus.

The incidence of tetanus is highest among agriculture-based community in rural areas and in livestock raising areas. It is common at periods of life when an individual is more exposed to trauma (childhood, adolescent). The number of neonatal tetanus is declining mainly due to significant increase in immunization coverage of pregnant women with tetanus toxoid. Childhood tetanus is also reducing with the improvement of coverage of DPT/DT/TT vaccines.

Epidemiology

The causative agent of tetanus is *Clostridium tetani*, a gram-positive, anaerobic, spore bearing organism. The spores are highly resistant to injurious agent, boiling, phenol, cresol, etc. The spores are best destroyed by steam under pressure at 120°C for 20 minutes or by gamma radiation or ethelene oxide (EO) sterilization. *C. tetani* germinates under anaerobic conditions and produces a potent exotoxin (tetanospasmin) having lethal toxicity. The natural habitat of the organism is mainly the soil and dust. The bacilli are found in the intestine of cattles, horses, goats and sheep which are excreted in their feces. The organism not transmitted from person to person.

The mode of transmission is mainly contamination of wound with tetanus spores. The injuries and accidents which can lead to tetanus are pin prick, skin abrasion, puncture wounds, burns, animal bites, insect stings, human bites, unsterile surgery, intrauterine fetal death, bowel surgery, dental interventions, infections, chronic skin ulcers, compound fractures, unsterile cutting of umbilical cord, gangrenous limbs, eye infections and otitis media. Incubation period is 6 to 10 days. It may range from one day to several months.

Tetanus is a disease of the active age group. Children are prone to all kinds of trauma and are at risk of occurring the disease. It is more common in new born due to non-aseptic delivery condition, specially due to cutting of cord with unclean instruments or when the umbilical cord is dressed with soil, ashes, cow dung, etc. Male children are more sensitive to tetanus toxin than females. Tetanus is an important environmental health problem.

Pathology

The spores of *C. tetani* invade the human host through an injury. Under anaerobic conditions, the spores transform into vegetative forms and multiply and elaborate the exotoxin. The exotoxin reaches the CNS through the lymphocytes in the circulation or through the absorption at the myoneural junctions. All parts of the nervous system are affected. The toxin acts on the motor end plates in muscles, motor nuclei in the nervous system, spinal cord, the brain and sympathetic system. Its principal action is to block the inhibition of spinal reflexes. Pathological changes are noted mainly in the striated muscles including diaphragm and intercostal muscles.

Types of Tetanus

Based on related causes tetanus can be grouped as traumatic, otogenic, neonatal, puerperal and idiopathic (without definite history of an injury, which may be due to microscopic trauma). Clinical types are localized, generalized and cephalic.

Clinical Manifestations

Localized tetanus is manifested with pain, constant rigidity and muscle spasm in the region of injury. It may be associated with otitis media. This condition may recover fully within a few weeks or may progress to generalized tetanus.

Generalized tetanus is the most common type. The onset of this condition is usually sudden with rapid progression of muscle spasm and cramps. The initial feature is the 'lock jaw' or trismus due to stiffness of the masseters which make the difficulty in opening mouth. It is followed by generalized muscle spasms, precipitated by external stimuli like touch, loud sounds, bright light, etc. Other features are difficulty in swallowing, restlessness, irritability, headache, neck rigidity, spasms of facial muscles (risus sardonicus), spasms and rigidity of muscles of back and neck make the body arch backward like a bow (opisthotonic position) and constant

spasm of the muscles of the extremities and abdomen. Other presentations include convulsion, tetanic spasm with clenching of jaws and hands, spasm of laryngeal muscles with respiratory distress, cyanosis and over exhaustion. Initially there is constipation and retention of urine due to spasm but afterwards fecal and urinary incontinence may found. Vertebral fracture and spinal cord compression may occur due to severe muscle spasm. Hypertension, excessive sweating, tachycardia and arrhythmias are observed due to sympathetic nerve involvement. The patient remains conscious all the time.

Cephalic tetanus is rare variety and manifested as paralysis of one or more of the cranial nerves (usually 7th) with gradual spastic manifestations of whole body. In majority of the cases complete recovery occur.

Neonatal tetanus develops due to unhygienic delivery or contamination of umbilical stump. Manifestations unually occur between 2 days and 2 weeks of age. The neonate presents with unexplained crying, refusal of feeds and apathy. On forceful feeding, reflex spasm of masseters and pharyngeal muscles leads to trismus (lock Jaw), dysphagia and choking. It is followed by spasms of limbs, generalized rigidity and opisthotonos. Reflex laryngeal spasm may lead to apnea and cyanosis. Continued spasm may cause to pyrexia, tachypnea, tachycardia, acidosis and dehydration. Superadded infections are common.

Complications

a. *Respiratory complications:* Aspiration pneumonia, atelectasis, pneumothorax, mediastinal emphysema.
b. *Cardiovasuclar complications:* Hypertension or hypotension, arrhythmia, myocarditits.
c. *Miscellaneous:* Injury of tongue or oral mucosa, intramuscular hematoma and vertebral fracture during tetanic convulsions, fluid and electrolyte imbalance, malnutrition.

Diagnosis

History of illness and clinical manifestations are sufficiently diagnostic. Laboratory investigations can be done to detect the causative organism from the discharge of the wound or from the ear or from necrotic tissue.

Management

The specific management should aims at neutralization of the toxin and removal of the *Cl.tetani*.

1. Human tetanus immunoglobulin 500 to 3000 IU should be given intramuscular immediate on admission to hospital. It is safest and most effective treatment without any complications. Antitetanic Serum (ATS) can be administered after skin test with 30,000 to 1,00,000 IU, IM or IV. 2.

Antibiotic is administered and penicillin is the choice. Cephalosporin also can be used. Antipyretics is given to treat fever. Sedative and muscle relaxant is given with diazepam or phenobarbitone every 2 to 4 hours with calculated dose to control spasms. IV fluid therapy and oxygen therapy are essential. Mechanical ventilation may be needed in respiratory paralysis. Tracheostomy may be required in persistent laryngeal spasm.

Supportive measures with special nursing care to be provided. The patient should be placed in isolation in a separate quite room with complete rest and close observation. Minimum disturbance and gentle handling to be maintained. Suctioning of oropharyngeal secretions, comfortable positioning, oxygen therapy, IV fluid therapy, hygienic measures and constant monitoring with recording of vital signs are important essential measures. Initially oral feeding should be avoided and nasogastric tube feeding should be given. Administration of medications should be done following specific precautions (e.g. skin test for penicillin). Care of wound or injury or umbilical stump or ear discharge need special attention. Special care to be taken for tracheostomy and for mechanical ventilation. Pyridoxine therapy may give gratifying results in neonatal tetatus with conventional regimen.

Prognosis

Prognosis is worse in the onset of symptoms within first week of life and presence of high fever, tachycardia and apnea with laryngeal spasm. The mortality rate is as high as 50 to 75 percent. Survivors usually do not have any neurological complications except in prolonged apnea which may complicate with cerebral palsy, paralysis, mental retardation and behavioral problems. The mortality rates can be reduced by excellent nursing care and prompt management facilities.

Preventive Measures

Active immunization of pregnant women with tetanus toxoid and infants and children with DPT, DT, TT are the best definite method of prevention.

In case of an injury with open wound, both active immunization with T. Toxoid and passive immunization with tetanus immunoglobin should be given. Antitetanic serum (ATS) is not usually used as prophylactic purpose. Thorough wound cleaning with antiseptic lotion is also very important measures.

Increasing awareness about the clean and aseptic delivery, safe care of umbilical cord and improvement of immunization status of mothers and children are significant preventive measures to reduce neonatal and childhood tetanus.

Tuberculosis

In developing countries like India, tuberculosis is a common pediatric problem and an important killer of children. India accounts for nearly one third of global burden of tuberculosis. The incidence of tuberculosis is markedly increasing due to increasing number of HIV/AIDS. Another problem associated with this condition is increasing number of multidrug resistant new patients.

Tuberculosis is a specific infectious chronic disease caused by 'Mycobacterium tuberculosis'. The disease primarily affects the lungs causing pulmonary tuberculosis. It can also affect meninges, intestine, bones, joints, lymph glands, skin and other tissues of the body.

Epidemiology

Mycobacterium tuberculosis is acid fast bacilli which rapidly inactivated by sunlight and UV light. In recent years, a number of atypical mycobacteria have been isolated i.e. M. Kansasii, M. scrofulaceum, M. intercellulare and M. fortuitum. All these are mainly saprophytic having different characteristics. Disease attributed to them have resembled pulmonary tuberculosis and chronic cervical lymphadenitis.

The most common source of infection is a human case, who is untreated or not fully treated. The bacilli are discharged in the sputum for years in a case of pulmonary tuberculosis. The bovine source of infection is infected unboiled milk. Bovine tuberculosis is not a problem in this country due to practice of boiling milk before intake. The patients are infective as long as they remain untreated. Effective antimicrobial treatment reduces the infectivity by 90 percent within 48 hours.

Mode of transmission is mainly droplet infection and droplet nuclei during coughing and sneezing in sputum positive patient of pulmonary tuberculosis. Nasopharyngeal secretions also may transmit infection. Infected spits of sputum of careless open cases of TB dries up and remains in the dust and air which may be important source of infection through inhalation. Extrapulmonary tuberculosis and sputum negative cases contribute in minimal transmission of infection. Transplacental transmission may occur causing congenital tuberculosis.

Incubation period may be weeks, months and years. It depends upon host parasite relationship, closeness of contact, extent of disease and sputum positivity of the source cases. Average incubation period is 3 to 8 weeks.

There is sharp rise in incidence of tuberculosis from infancy to adolescent in the developing countries, though tuberculosis affects all ages. In India from an average of one percent in the "under-5 age group", the infection index climbs to above 30 percent at the age of 15 years. The risk factors of tubercular infection are inherited susceptibility, intercurrent infections like measles, pertussis and malnutrition.

Tuberculosis is a social disease. There are so many social factors which contribute to the occurrence and spread of this disease. These factors are poor housing, poor ventilation, overcrowding, air pollution, less sunshine, population explosion, undernutrition, poor quality life style, lack of education and health awareness, large families, early marriages and poor economy.

Pathology

The child is infected from an open case of tuberculosis. The common mode of entry of tubercle bacilli is inhalation. Occasionally the organism may enter by ingestion and rarely through abraded skin. Majority (95%) of the primary tuberculosis occur in the lungs. The tubercle bacilli reach the finest bronchioles and alveoli where they are taken up by phagocytes. Bacilli multiply and set up a pathological lesion 'tubercle', a central area of caseation and necrosis surrounded by a ring of small round of lymphocytes. A number of such tubercle may merge to form the primary focus, also described as Ghon focus. The primary focus may be found in any portion of the lungs, but is often found sub-pleurally in the lower part of upper lobe of right lung. The infection spreads to the regional lymph nodes through the involved lymphatics. The regional glands become enlarged and caseous and may be associated with pleural reaction to form primary complex. The Ghon focus usually shows slow healing with calcification and fibrosis. The primary complex may be reactivated, following reinfection especially at the time of puberty.

The primary infection afterwards may spread through the lymphatics and the blood stream and carried in different parts of the body, i.e. meninges, peritoneum, bone, joints, kidney, spleen, liver, lymph glands, etc. Tuberculous meningitis and miliary tuberculosis are more likely to occur. Local spread may cause pleural effusion, atelectasis, obstructive emphysema and endobronchial segmental tuberculosis.

Congenital tuberculosis may occur from transplacental transmission or the fetus inhaling bacilli from liquor amnii as a result of the tuberculosis focus in the placenta. This condition is characterized by enlargement and caseation of the glands at pecta hepatis and disseminated tubercles throughout the liver. This comprises the primary complex and formation of tubercles. Scatterly through the lungs, spleen, brain, meninges and other viscera.

Clinical Manifestations

Clinical features usually vary with insidious onset and depend upon the site of infections. The most common site is intrathoracic infections (40%) and CNS tuberculosis (approximately 30%).

In intrathoracic tuberculosis, primary focus may be asymptomatic, especially in infants and young children. The condition may be symptomatic after the attack of whooping cough or measles. In older children, the features are manifested with vague symptoms like malaise, fatigue, anorexia, weight loss, failure to thrive, low grade fever, tachycardia, night sweats and pallor. Large size primary complex may stimulate pneumonia and the child is presented with high fever, cough, dyspnea and cyanosis. Splenic involvement may occur in some children. Hilar lymphadenitis is an important feature of primary complex. It is usually impossible to detect this lymphadenitis by clinical examination. Approximately 95 percent of primary complex heals uneventfully and remaining becomes progressive primary disease. The bacilli may spread to the surrounding and may produce massive lymphadenopathy and bronchial involvement.

The adenitis are found as enlargement of glands with fever, weight loss, cough and anorexia. Hilar, paratracheal, mediastinal, cervical and mesenteric glands are involved.

Tracheal and endobronchial spread of infection results in tracheal obstruction with stridor, cyanosis and bronchial narrowing with persistent wheezing, dyspnea and paroxysmal cough. Obstructive emphysema, pleural effusion, tuberculous bronchiectasis and caseous bronchopneumonia may also develop in progressive disease.

Segmental lesion are commonly found due to bronchial compression by the enlarged caseating glands which may perforate into the bronchus. The clinical picture thus varies from minimal signs and symptoms to severe constitutional disturbances. Previously this segmental collapse was also termed as epituberculosis. The patient may have hectic temperature, dry cough and wheezing which may complicate to bronchiectasis.

Miliary tuberculosis in children may occur within a year of the primary infection. It is the result of hematogenous dissemination and is characterized by extensive miliary mottling of lungs and involvement of spleen, liver and other tissues. It may be found as pulmonary type or septicemic type or meningitic type.

Chronic pulmonary tuberculosis is infrequent in younger children and may found in girls above seven years. The commonest site of isolated lesion of this type is the apex of the lungs.

Extrathoracic tuberculosis is mainly found in CNS (meninges), abdomen (intestine, peritoneum), bone, joints, lymph glands, skin and genitourinary tract. Tuberculosis may occur in any part of the body (pericardium, ears, eyes) where the disease has a high prevalence.

Diagnosis of Tuberculosis

Tuberculosis should be suspected in the children with growth failure, malnutrition, pyrexia with unknown origin (PUO), prolonged cough, recurrent chest infection, painless enlargement of lymph gland, asthma, pleural effusion and in pneumonia not responding to antibiotic therapy and unsatisfactory recovery from measles or pertussis or typhoid.

The diagnosis of tuberculosis is done based on history of illness with special emphasis on history of exposure to infection in family or in neighbors. Clinical examination, radiology and laboratory investigations help to confirm the diagnosis.

The laboratory investigations should include isolation of AFB by bacteriological examination, histopathology, immunodiagnosis and other supportive investigations.

The effective confirmatory investigation is the bacteriological isolation of the AFB. Sputum examination or laryngeal swab or peritoneal fluid in abdominal TB and CSF study in CNS involvement are very useful to confirm the diagnosis.

Histological study of the biopsy material or FNAC from affected part are helpful method for confirmation of the disease.

Immunodiagnosis of antitubercular antibody and antigen by the radioimmunoassay can be performed as an accurate and specific method.

Tuberculin test (Mantoux test) is done by intradermal injection of 0.1 mL (5–10 TU) of standard dilution of tuberculin (PPD or OT) into the anterior aspect of the left forearm to raise a wheal of about 6 to 8 mm in diameter. Reading of the reaction is noted after 48 to 72 hours. The induration of 10 mm or more is generally considered as positive. Below 5 mm induration indicates negative reaction.

BCG test is performed by intradermal injection with BCG vaccine in the left deltoid region. An induration of more than 5 to 6 mm after 3 days of injection is accepted as positive reaction.

Blood examination for ESR shows elevation during active phase of the disease, though the test has no diagnostic value.

Radiology is an important diagnostic approach of childhood tuberculosis. X-ray and CT scan of the affected part help in diagnosis of tuberculosis.

Management

The specific management is done with antitubercular drugs. The bactericidal drugs are streptomycin, isoniazid, rifampicin, pyrazinamide and ethionamide. The bacteriostatic drugs are ethambutal, para amino salicylic acid (PAS), thiacetazone, kanamycin, cycloserine, viomycin, capreomycin, etc.

Majority of the cases can be successfully treated with effective and minimum toxic drugs like isoniazid, rifampicin, ethambutol, streptomycin and pyrazinamide. These drugs are considered as first line of drugs. The second line of drugs used in drug resistant cases and in toxicity of first line drugs. They include cycloserine, kanamycin, PAS, ethionamide, capreomycin. Other drugs which can be used for resistant cases are quinolones, amikacin, ampicillin, ciprofloxacin.

The patients with pulmonary and extrapulmonary tuberculosis are now treated with short course chemotherapy regimen for 6 months or 9 months duration or more whenever necessary, in intensive phase and continuation phase treatment schedule. DOTS (Directly observed therapy short-term) is now practiced in India, under Revised National Tuberculosis control program. WHO recommended anti-tubercular treatment regimens have also produced cure rates approaching 100 percent when drug-taking has been fully supervised. WHO has recommended 6 months regimen, 8 months regimen and 12 months regimen depending upon the child's condition for the treatment of childhood tuberculosis.

Drug resistant cases should be managed on the basis of type of resistance which can be primary, natural, acquired, initial or multidrug type of resistance. Relapse cases and defaulter cases need special attention for management.

Baby born to the mother with tuberculosis, diagnosed in 3rd trimester or during delivery should be considered as special condition. Breastfeeding must be continued. BCG vaccination should be given at birth. Chest X-ray to be done to detect the lung condition and drug therapy to be started depending upon the findings.

Steroid (prednisolone) can be used as anti-inflammatory agent in the treatment of tuberculosis. The indications are TB meningitis, miliary tuberculosis, renal tuberculosis, precardial or pleural effusion, endobronchial tuberculosis or segmental lesion and in extremely ill patients or terminally ill children. It is administered with the dose of 1 to 2 mg/kg/day during first 6 weeks of infection and can be continued for 1 to 3 months.

Surgical interventions may be needed though number of surgery has greatly reduced. The common indications for surgical interventions are pleural effusion, bronchiectasis, cavity formation, ascites, cold abscess, pott's spine, CNS tuberculosis with hydrocephalus, GI bleeding and for diagnostic approaches (biopsy, bronchoscopy).

Supportive nursing measures should include general nursing care and drug compliance. All drugs should be administered in a single daily dose on an empty stomach. The drugs are safe if used in the recommended dosage schedule. Supervised drug therapy is essential in home based management. Hepatotoxicity may be found in malnourished children or in disseminated disease. Avoidance of defaulter, assessment of any adverse effects and complications are very important. Good diet with balanced intake of protein and vitamins are essential. Fresh air, sunshine, hygienic measures, necessary rest and ambulation should be promoted. Follow-up at regular interval even by home visit and involvement of family members in continued care are essential part of management.

Prognosis

Prognosis of tuberculosis depends upon age, duration of infection, type of disease, site of infection, nutritional status, living condition, socioeconomic status, intercurrent infections resistance to drugs, early diagnosis, continuation of treatment and facilities available.

Prognosis is worse in miliary tuberculosis, TB meningitis, chronic pulmonary tuberculosis, TB with malnutrition and drug resistant cases.

Adequate treatment facilities with anti-tubercular drugs and improvement of BCG vaccination help to bring the declining trends of mortality and morbidity pattern with increased life span of tuberculosis patient.

Preventive Measures

The most important preventive measure is active immunization by BCG vaccination. Improvement of immunization coverage and creating awareness about the preventive measures are best approach for prevention of tuberculosis. Promotion of health status of the vulnerable children should be achieved by health education.

Early detection of tuberculosis patients with prompt and adequate treatment help to prevent spread of infection. Completion of treatment schedule, prevention of defaulter cases, identification and treatment of relapse cases are important aspect of prevention of the disease.

Chemoprophylaxis should be given to high risk infants and children especially in household contact, BCG adenitis and baby born to mother with tuberculosis.

Sources of infection need adequate treatment after tracing them out. Familial and extra familial contacts should be find out from the school teacher, food venders, domestic servants and visitors.

Health education is the most important aspect of prevention of tuberculosis. The information and explanation should include mode of transmission, early symptoms, treatment facilities, regularity of treatment, home care, methods of coughing and sneezing, disposal of sputum, prophylaxis of contact and BCG vaccination. Health education should also include hygienic living with good housing, improved environmental sanitation, better living condition, well ventilation, avoidance of dampness, overcrowding and indiscriminate spitting, prevention of malnutrition, promotion of balanced diet, intake of boiled milk, family support, acceptance of family based treatment of tuberculosis patient and rehabilitation of them.

Typhoid Fever (Enteric Fever)

Typhoid fever is an acute bacterial systemic infection caused by *Salmonella typhi*. The illness is characterized by prolonged typical continuous fever for 3 to 4 weeks with prostration, relative bradycardia and involvement of spleen and lymph nodes. The term enteric fever indicates both typhoid and paratyphoid fever. This condition may found as epidemics, endemics and sporadics. In India, typhoid fever occurs in endemics. It is found all over the world where water supplies and sanitation are sub-standard. The disease is uncommon in developed countries.

Epidemiology

The causative agent of typhoid fever is *S. typhi* (90%). *S. typhi* has three main antigens (O, H, Vi). It can be readily killed by drying, pasteurization and common disinfectants. Man is the only reservoir of infection in the form of cases and carriers. The case may be mild, missed or severe. A case or carrier is infectious as long as bacilli are found in stools and urine. The carriers may be temporary (incubatory or convalescent) or may be chronic. Convalescent carriers excrete the bacilli for 6 to 8 weeks. A chronic carrier excretes bacilli for more than a year or several years after the clinical attack. In most chronic carrier, organisms persist in gallbladder or biliary tract. Carrier state is more common in under-five children. Fecal carriers are often found than urinary carriers. Primary sources of infection are stool and urine. Secondary sources of infection are contaminated water, food, fingers or hands and flies.

Mode of transmission is mainly feco-oral route or urine-oral routes. Infection takes place directly through soiled hands contaminated with stool or urine of infected patients or carriers. Indirect transmission occurs by the ingestion of contaminated water, food, milk or through flies. Vegetables grown in the sewage firm and washed in contaminated water promote the transmission. Typhoid bacilli may survive for about 7 days in water, one month in ice or ice cream and 70 days in soil irrigated with sewage under moist or cold condition. Food provides shelter to the bacilli, where they can multiply or survive for sometimes. The bacilli grow rapidly in milk without changing the taste and appearance.

Incubation period is usually 10 to 14 days with a range of 3 days to 3 weeks depending upon the dose of bacilli ingested. It is shortest in food-borne and longest in water-borne.

The incidence of typhoid fever is highest in 5 to 19 years of age group. More cases are found among males, but carriers are more in females. The disease is found throughout the year but more in summer and rainy season with increased number of flies. Pollution of drinking water supply, open field defecation and urination, poor food hygiene and personal hygiene, health ignorance, illiteracy and poor socio-economic conditions are important contributing factors.

Pathology

Mode of entry of typhoid bacilli is oral route. The organisms proliferates in the lymphoid tissue of intestines mainly in the ileum. The payer's patches become swollen and necrosed with ulceration which may lead to hemorrhage or perforation. The bacilli enter the blood stream through the intestinal lymphoid tissue and infect the liver with focal necrosis. Infection leads to enlargement and congestion of spleen. Mesenteric glands and lymph glands also become enlarged. Destruction of bacilli in the reticuloendothelial cells promotes release of endotoxin which causes toxemia and involvement of vital organs. The bacilli grow readily in the bile and may cause infection of the gall-bladder with chronic carrier state. Bacteremia may result to bronchial inflammation, osteomyelitis, meningitis, skin lesions, myocarditis and muscle degeneration.

Clinical Manifestations

The clinical presentations of typhoid fever in children may found suddenly, though classically the onset of the disease is gradual. The child usually present with rapid rise of temperature, extreme malaise, loss of appetite, headache, vomiting, coated tongue, abdominal pain and distension. When toxemia is severe the child may have apathy, cloudiness of consciousness and delirium. Bradycardia is not common in children. Diarrhea is usually found than constipation. Abdomen feels doughy, spleen is palpable one or two cm below costal margin and liver may also be palpable.

Typhoid rash as macular red rose spots may appear on about 6th day of illness. Rash may be visible on the trunk or may not be visible on pigmented skin especially in Indian children.

Sometimes the child may present with clinical features of bacillary dysentry, respiratory infection or meningitis along with typhoid fever.

Typhoid fever of infant and early childhood may present with fever, convulsion and anemia due to secondary blood loss or hemolysis from autoantibodies.

Neonatal typhoid may occur from vertical transmission. Neonates usually present with vomiting, abdominal distention, diarrhea, and fever with variable intensity, about 72 hours after birth. Other features may include convulsions, jaundice, loss of appetite, weight loss and enlargement of liver.

Complications

a. *Abdominal:* Intestinal perforation, GI bleeding, hepatitis, cholecystitis, peritonitis, gastroenteritis, urinary tract infection, liver abscess, fatty liver, pancreatitis.

b. *Neurological:* Encephalopathy, meningitis, hemiplegia, transverse myelitis, G.B. syndrome, cranial nerve involvement, psychiatric problems like depression, schizophrenia.

c. *Hematologic:* Hemolytic anemia, bone marrow depression.

d. *Cardiovascular:* Toxic myocarditis, pericarditis, endocarditis, venous thrombosis.

e. *Respiratory:* Pneumonia, bronchitis, empyema, pulmonary infarction, pleurisy.

f. *Miscellaneous:* Parotitis, bed sores, otitis media, tonsillitis, alopecia, chronic osteomyelitis, supportive arthritis, superficial abscesses.

Diagnosis

Clinical manifestations are useful for diagnosis of typhoid fever. The following laboratory investigations may be done to support the diagnosis.

- Routine blood examination—shows normal or low WBC count. Eosinophils may be low or completely absent.
- Blood culture in first week of illness shows *S. typhi* in about 75 percent of patients.
- Widal test is positive, 60 percent in 2nd week and 80 percent in third week.
- Bone marrow culture is highly sensitive (90%) for diagnosis of typhoid fever.
- Stool and urine cultures may show *S. typhi* after 2 weeks of illness and in suspected chronic carriers.
- Rapid serodiagnostic procedures like counter immunoelectrophoresis, ELISA test and coagglutination test are the simple modern specific diagnostic measures.

Management

Specific antimicrobial therapy for the treatment of typhoid fever in children is chloramphenical 50 to 100 mg/kg/day in 4 divided dose for 10 to 14 days. Other drugs which can be used are ampicillin, amoxicillin, cotrimoxazole, etc. The drug therapy with chloramphenical is associated with high relapse rate, drug resistance, bone marrow toxicity, high rate of chronic carrier, etc.

The newer cephalosporins including ceftriaxone, cefoperazone are the drug of choice (50 to 100 mg/kg/day) in single or two divided doses IV for 5 to 10 days.

Corticosteroid is given to the children with severe toxic state, prolonged illness, altered mental function and shock. Dexamethasone 3 mg/kg first dose followed by 1 mg/kg 6 hourly for another 8 doses is administered.

Symptomatic management with antipyretics, hydrotherapy and maintenance of fluid and electrolyte balance by IV fluid therapy are essential. Blood transfusion may be needed in intestinal perforation or hemorrhage. Nutritious diet to be provided. Early detection of complications and prompt management promote better prognosis.

Surgical management may be required in intestinal perforation and gallbladder infection in chronic carriers.

Supportive nursing care is important for better prognosis. Bed rest, skin care, good orodental hygiene and frequent mouth care with antiseptic mouth wash, adequate fluid intake or IV fluid therapy, administration of prescribed medications, tepid sponge to treat fever and continuous monitoring of patient's condition are important aspects of nursing measures. Isolation of patient and care of bladder and bowel are essential. Prevention of constipation or care during diarrhea, prevention of urinary retention, observation for frank or occult blood in stool and careful disposal of stool and urine are important. Diet should be planned with adequate calories, protein, iron and vitamins by liquid or semisolid food. Assessment and recording of vital signs and drug effects or any features of complications should be emphasized. Parental involvement in child care and necessary instructions to parents for continuing care at hospital and home are essential.

Prognosis

Prognosis of typhoid fever is generally good with adequate treatment. High morbidity and mortality is associated with malnutrition, age of the child (infancy), antibiotic resistant strain of organisms and presence of complications like perforation, severe bleeding, meningitis and endocarditis. In India, the mortality rate is about 1 percent and in untreated cases it is more than 10 percent. Relapse may occur in about 10 to 20 percent cases. Multiple relapse may occur in a single patient. Relapse usually occurs within 6 weeks of previous attack.

Preventive Measures

Control of case and carrier of the disease with improvement of sanitation and immunization are important. Isolation of patient, hygienic disposal of stool and urine of infected person, disinfection of contaminated articles, adequate hand washing practices, immunization of susceptible children and contact cases are important preventive measures. Health education is the most significant method of controlling this disease by increasing awareness about safe water, food hygiene, food handling, hand washing, kitchen hygiene, personal hygiene, sanitary sewage disposal, control of flies, hazards of contaminated food and water and mode of transmission of the disease, etc.

Active protection can be provided by use of typhoid vaccine. Three types of vaccines are available, i.e. whole cell vaccine, vi-vaccine and oral vaccine.

Whole cell vaccine is given with two doses of SC injection with 0.5 mL for the children more than 10 years of age and 0.25 mL for young children. It has 70 percent efficacy and side effects of fever, malaise, local pain and swelling.

Vi-vaccine is given as a single dose with 0.5 mL SC or IM. It has 70 to 80 percent efficacy for five years. Dose may be repeated after 5 years. No side effects observed for this vaccine. It is not given to children below 2 years of age.

Oral vaccine (typhoral) is available as a capsule and recommended for children older than 6 years on three alternate day (one capsule each on day 1, 3 and 5). Efficacy is 70 to 80 percent with 3 to 5 years immunity.

Leprosy (Hansen's Disease)

Leprosy is a chronic infectious disease caused by *Mycobacterium leprae*. It affects peripheral nerves, skin, muscles, eyes, bones, testes and internal organ.

Leprosy is not particularly a disease of children as was once believed, but in endemic areas, the disease is acquired commonly during infancy and childhood. The youngest case seen in South India was an infant of 2.5 months. Incidence rates generally rise to a peak between 10 and 20 years of age and then fall. However the presence of leprosy in child population is of considerable epidemiological importance. A high prevalence of infection among children means the disease is active and spreading in the community. Leprosy is widely prevalent in India (3.8/10,000) with high prevalence rate (above 7/10,000) in Jharkhand, Bihar, Chhattisgarh, Orissa and above 3/10,000 in Delhi, Uttar Pradesh, Tamil Nadu, Andhra Pradesh and Maharashtra.

Epidemiology

The causative agent of leprosy is a acid fast bacilli—*Mycobacterium leprae*. The most important source of infection is multibacillary cases. The inapparent infections are also common source of infection. The major portal of exit is the discharge from nasal mucosa during sneezing or blowing. The bacilli can also exit through ulcerated or broken skin of positive cases or through hair follicles of intact skins. Among household contact of lepromatous cases, 4 to 12 percent is expected to show signs of leprosy within 5 years.

Modes of transmission are mainly droplet infection and contact transmission. Contact transmission may occur between infectious patient and healthy but susceptible person, by direct skin to skin contact or indirect contact with contaminated soil and fomites (contaminated clothes and linen). Bacilli may also be transmitted via breast milk from lepromatous mother or by insect vectors or by tattooing needles.

Incubation period is 3 to 5 years or more for lepromatous cases. The tuberculoid leprosy is having shorter incubation period.

There is least sex difference in children below 15 years of age, males are more affected. The disease is more common in rural areas with more humidity and in overcrowding place. Lack of ventilation within households close contact, poor personal hygiene and presence of infectious cases are the risk factors for transmission of the infection. Leprosy is a social disease. The psychosocial factors like fear, guilt, social stigma, wrong belief about incurability, hiding the disease and delay or refusal of treatment, poverty, illiteracy are important factors related to the disease and its transmission.

Classification

There are various classification of leprosy. The Indian classification includes five types. It is clinicobacterial classification done by Indian Leprosy Association (1981), also known as Hindu Kusht Nivaran Sangh. The *five types* are as follows:

a. *Indeterminate type:* These are early cases with one or two vague hypopigmented macules and definite sensory impairment. These lesions are smear negative.
b. *Tuberculoid type:* These cases are manifested with one or two well defined lesions which may be flat or raised, hypopigmented, erythematous and are anesthetic. These lesions are also smear negative.
c. *Borderline type:* These cases are found with four or more lesions, which may be flat or raised, well or ill defined, hypopigmented, erythematous and with sensory impairment or loss. These lessons are bacteriologically may or may not be positive. It can degenerate from boderline tuberculoid to borderline lepromatous, if left untreated.
d. *Lepromatous type:* These cases are presented with diffuse infiltration or numerous flat or raised, poorly defined, shiny, smooth, symmetrically distributed lesions. These lesions are smear positive.
e. *Pure neuritic type:* These cases are having nerve involvemet without any skin lesion. These lesions are smear negative.

Following introduction of multidrug therapy the leprosy cases now are classified as major two types:

1. *Paucibacillary leprosy:* It accounts for about 60 percent of total leprosy patients. It includes smear negative, indeterminate, tuberculoid, borderline tuberculoid and pure neuritic type. It can be found as single lesion or 2 to 5 lesions.
2. *Multibacillary leprosy:* It includes smear positive cases, lepromatous type and borderline lepromatous cases. It has more than 5 lesions.

Clinical Manifestations

The major clinical features of leprosy are hypopigmented patches, partial or total loss of cutaneous sensation in the affected areas, presence of thickened nerves and presence of leprosy bacilli in the nasal smear or skin. In advanced cases, presence of nodules or lumps in the skin of face or ears, planter ulcer, loss of fingers and toes, nasal depression, loss of eye brows, glove and stocking anesthesia of hands and feets, contracture of medial two fingers from ulnar involvement, foot drop, claw toes and other deformities are found.

Allergic lepra reactions, particularly while on treatment with sulfone drugs, constitute a characteristic feature. It may be acute or sub acute inflammation resulting in bouts of acute exacerbation. Existing lesions in skin and mucous membranes become more thickened and erythematous. Fresh lesions may appear and intensity of lesions may increase. Reaction can be type I (reversal reaction) or type II (erythema nodsum leprosum—ENL). High fever, arthralgia, adenopathy, iridocyclitis, orchitis and erythema nodosum, the so called Arthus phenomenon, are prominent among the various lepra reaction.

Diagnosis

History of illness, family history of leprosy cases, history of contact, presence of clinical features and related complaints, any treatment taken are important diagnostic aspects. Physical examination to be done thoroughly to detect skin lesions, thickened nerves, presence of nodules or macules and testing for loss of sensation or any other complaints.

Bacteriological examination of skin smear, nasal smear or nasal blows or nasal scraping are important diagnostic approaches. A punch biopsy from the edge of the skin or nasal lesion confirm the clinical diagnosis.

Other investigations include histamine test, foot pad culture, immunological tests for detection of CMI or humoral response including lepromin test, lymphocyte transformation test (LTT), leukocyte migration inhibition test (LMIT), FLA-ABS test (Fluorescent leprosy antibody absorption test), monoclonal antibody test, ELISA test and radio immune assay.

Management

Multidrug therapy (MDT) is recommended and scheduled for the treatment of Paucibacillary (PB) and Multibacillary (MB) leprosy cases with dapsone, rifampicin, clofazimine, ethionamide, protionamide, quinolones (ofloxacin), minocycline and clarithromycin.

For multibacillary cases combination of rifampicin, dapsone and clofazimine are recommended for 12 months. Paucibacillary cases should receive combined therapy with dapsone and rifampicin for 6 months. Single lesion PB leprosy cases is treated with single dose of a combination of rifampicin, ofloxacin and minocycline. The treatment duration varies according to the type of disease. Treatment should be continued till all signs of disease activity have subsided.

Type I reaction is treated with prednisolone 1 mg/kg for 12 weeks. *Mild type II reaction* can be treated with aspirin and *severe type II* is managed by prednisolone therapy.

Rehabilitation of leprosy patient with correction of deformities are integral part of management.

Supportive nursing care is very important both in hospitalized and home based care. These include isolation of infected cases, good hygienic care, balanced diet, care of affected hands and feet, prevention of injury, promotion of use of shoe, aseptic care of any wound, emotional support, involvement of family members, follow-up and health education.

Prognosis

Childhood leprosy is self healing. Adequate treatment should be given to prevent complications and promote healing. Prognosis is usually good with prompt initiation of treatment by early diagnosis. The long-term complications are neural involvement, reactive episodes and deformities of face, hands and feet.

Preventive Measures

Isolation of infectious cases, adequate treatment of affected individual by MDT, chemoprophylaxis of the contact person with dapsone, immunoprophylaxis by BCG vaccine and screening (individual or mass) of susceptible population (school children, household contacts) are important preventive measures. Adequate treatment of infectious patient with MDT is most significant measure because it can turned the patient to noninfectious with dapsone therapy for 90 days or with rifampicin for 3 weeks. Local (nasal) application of rifampicin (drops or spray) may destroy all bacilli within 8 days.

Health education is important for increasing public awareness about the nature of illness, mode of transmission and factors promoting the illness. Information to be given about importance of early diagnosis and initiation of treatment of compliance of drug regimen. Home based care and follow-up at regular interval are essential aspect of prevention.

Hospital Acquired Infections (Nosocomial Infections)

Hospital acquired infections (HAI) are those infections which developed within the hospital or produced by cross infections from one patient to another, from doctors, nurses, visitors, attendants or other hospital staff during hospital stay.

HAI is localized or systemic conditions that results from adverse reactions to the presence of infectious agents which was not present at the time of hospital admission. Highest incidence of this infection is found in neonatal intensive care units (NICU) or other ICU.

Causes of HAI in Children

- Hospital delivery without aseptic technique.
- Congenital or intrauterine infections from mothers.
- Intravenous procedures.
- Neonatal resuscitation, assisted ventilation and any respiratory procedures like suctioning, endotracheal intubation, etc.
- Nonjudicious use of broad spectrum antibiotics.
- Delayed initiation of oral feeding and artificial feeding.
- Surgical interventions and inappropriate wound management.
- Invasive procedures, care in PICU/NICU and use of unsterile articles.
- Inadequate isolation technique of infected patients and malpractice related to barrier nursing.
- Infections among hospital staff.
- Poor hospital environment laden with microorganisms i.e. hospital dust, linen, bed cloths, furniture, etc.

Risk Factors

The responsible factors of hospital acquired infections are immunocompromised children, long hospital stay, lack of hand washing practices, preterm or LBW baby, serious illness, corticosteroid therapy, use of indwelling catheter, care in ICU, etc.

Mode of Transmission

There are different routes of transmission of HAI. The common routes of spread of cross infection are:

- *Contact spread:* There are two routes of contact transmission, i.e. direct or indirect routes. Organisms may spread directly from contaminated hands of doctors and nurses to the susceptible host or from other patients by physical contact. Indirect contact may occur through feeding articles, syringe and needles, suction equipment, venous or arterial catheters, renal dialysers, contaminated linen, bed pans, sputum cups etc.
- *Vehicle spread:* Contaminated inanimate vehicle serves as the vector for transmission of infectious agent to different individuals, e.g. contaminated food and water, blood and its products, IV fluids, etc.
- *Vector-borne spread:* Both external and internal vectors can spread infections. External vectors are flies which transmits diseases like *Shigella* and *Salmonella*. Internal vectors are mosquitoes which are responsible for biological transmission.
- *Air-borne spread:* Droplets released during coughing and sneezing by the infected persons and hospital dusts are important route of dissemination of infections from the source to the victim.

Common HAI

- *Respiratory tract infections:* About 15 to 20 percent of all HAI are LRTI, pneumonia, pulmonary tuberculosis, *Pneumocystis-cariniipneumonia, Chlamydia,* etc.
- *Urinary tract infection* caused by simple or indwelling catheterization.
- *Surgical wound infections* due to inadequate sterilization method, improper wound dressing and hospital dust.
- *Miscellaneous:* IV therapy associated infection, gastroenteritis, oral thrush, umbilical sepsis, pyoderma, eye infections, etc.

Prevention and Control Measures of HAI

- Emphasis on hand washing practices.
- Practice of strict aseptic technique in invasive procedures.
- Improvement of sterilization and disinfection practices and procedures.
- Appropriate care of instruments, catheters, syringe, needle, dressing, etc.
- Maintenance of general cleanliness of the unit including floor, toilets, wash basins, furniture and all other articles and equipment used for patient care.
- Adequate bed spacing and preventing overcrowding.
- Wearing of gown, cap, mask and changing of shoes in ICUs. Avoidance of hanging mask around the neck.
- Wet mopping and damp dusting and no brooming. Vacuum cleaning should be emphasized.
- Screening of source of infection among hospital staff at regular interval, especially the susceptible persons.
- Adequate management of waste disposal—stool, urine, blood, infected body fluids, dressing, etc.
- Isolation of infectious patient, e.g. smear positive pulmonary tuberculosis, infected neonates and children with communicable diseases.
- Provision of barrier nursing, separate cubicle or glass pane partition for infectious patients.
- Special care of resuscitation equipment and intensive care units.
- Carbolization and disinfection of cot, bed linen and other used articles of patients after death or discharge.
- Improvement of hygienic measures of patients.
- Health education for increasing awareness and to provide information to the public about the sources and mode of transmission of common HAI.
- Compliance and adherence to the infection control practices and in service educational program for hospital staff about the HAI preventive measures.
- Each hospital should have infection control committee to formulate policies, supervise and ensure the practices of infection control measures, along with safe disposal of hospital waste. (See Appendix XXVIII for waste disposal).

COMMON PARASITOSIS IN CHILDREN

Childhood parasitosis is commonly found as intestinal parasitic infestations with giardiasis, amebiasis, worm infestations and cryptosporidiosis. Other parasitic diseases like malaria, filaria, kala-azar, hydatid disease also affect the children. These conditions are preventable by various means. Early detection and prompt management of these conditions prevent complications and promote child health.

Malaria

Malaria is a protozoal disease caused by arthropod borne infection with malarial parasite (plasmodium), which is transmitted by infected female anopheline mosquito.

Malaria is found in about 100 countries in the world. Urban and periurban areas with unfavorable ecological changes, civil unrest and population movement with large number of unprotected, nonimmune and physically weakened refugees contribute a lot to new malaria outbreaks. Large numbers of children under the age of 5 years are killed by the disease mainly from cerebral malaria and anemia. It is commonly found in rural areas with restricted access to adequate treatment. Malaria control was emphasized through "Roll back Malaria initiative", launched in 1998 by WHO, UNICEF, UNDP and World Bank with special emphasis on children.

In India, number of malaria cases was dropped down from 6.74 million cases in 1976 to 2 million cases in the year 2000, with the implementation of modified plan of operation. Malaria has been a serious problem in North Eastern states of India due to topography and climatic conditions. The responsible constraints and problems for slow progress of malaria control is mainly related to forests (forested hills, forest fringe areas), mobile tribal population, limited health infrastructure, nonavailability of drugs in village level and irrigated dry areas or desert areas. In urban and periurban areas, malaria situation is influenced by poor sanitation and poor group living in slum and unplanned settlements.

Epidemiology

Malaria is caused by four distinct species of the malaria parasite (*P. vivax, P. falciparum, P. malariae* and *P. ovale*). In India, *P. vivax* causes 70 percent of all infections, 25 to 30 percent due to *P. falciparum*, about 1 percent due to *P. malariae* and *P. ovale* is rarely found.

The life cycle of malaria parasite under goes the human cycle (asexual cycle) and mosquito cycle (sexual cycle). Man is the intermediate host and mosquito the definitive host.

The asexual cycle or schizogony starts when an infected mosquito bites an individual and injects sporozoites. In the human cycle the parasite passes through hepatic phase and erythrocytic phase. Sexual forms (i.e. male and female gametocytes) of the parasite develop in human host, which are infective to mosquito.

The sexual cycle or sporogony starts when gametocytes are ingested by the mosquito during feeding on an infected person. The gametocyte continues further development in the mosquito to develop into an oocyst. Sporozoites liberate from mature oocyst and migrate to the salivary glands of the mosquito. The mosquito becomes infective to man when these sporozoites are ready to be released in the blood of the human host following the mosquito bite.

Reservoir of infection can be a patient who can also be a carrier of several plasmodial species at the same time. Children are more likely to be gametocyte carriers than adults, and better reservoir than adults.

Mode of transmission is mainly vector transmission by female anopheline mosquito. Direct transmission may occur accidentally by hypodermic, IM or IV injections or blood transfusion. Anyone having malaria should not be accepted as blood donor until three years afterwards. Congenital malaria rarely may occur to the newborn from an infected mother.

Incubation period varies depending upon the types of parasite. It is 12 days (9–14 days) for *P. falciparum*, 14 days (8–17 days) for *P. vivax*, 17 days (16–18 days) for *P. ovale* and 28 days (18–40 days) for quartan or *P. malariae*.

Period of communicability extents as long as mature, viable gametocytes exist in the circulating blood of the infected individual in sufficient number to infect vector mosquitoes. It is usual for *P. vivax* and *P. ovale* to relapse more than 3 years after patient's first attack. Relapse of *P. falciparum* usually not found after 1 to 2 years of first attack. *P. malariae* infection causes prolonged low level asymptomatic parasitemia and may persist ever for 40 years or more.

Malaria affects all ages. Infant and young children are considered as high risk group in some areas. Newborns have some resistance to *P. falciparum* due to presence of fetal hemoglobin, in first few months of life. Outdoor life and wearing of less clothing with more exposed body parts are the risk factors of getting infection. Poor housing with ill-ventilated and inadequate lighted rooms are considered as resting place for this mosquitoes. Population mobility, wandering tribal, agriculture based rural areas, human habits like sleeping outdoors, refusal of insecticide spraying inside house, avoidance of use of personal protection by using mosquito nets and collection of stagnant water, pools, ponds, marshy areas, burrowed pits and poorly or unregulated irrigation channels are the important contributing factors of the disease transmission.

Maximum prevalence of malaria is found in warm and humid environment and mostly seen in July to November, in India. Optimal temperature and humidity for the development of parasite is 20° to 30°C and about 60 percent humidity. Rainfall provides opportunities for mosquito breeding and may give rise to epidemics. Garden pool, irrigation channels, burrow pits, favors breeding of mosquitoes and man-made malaria results.

Vector of malaria is female anopheles mosquito which is having about 45 species. Among them *Anopheles* culicifacies is common in rural areas and *Anopheles stephensi* is common in urban areas. They have different resting habit, breeding habit, biting time and resistance to insecticides.

Pathology

Malarial parasite enters human host as sporozoites which migrates from the peripheral blood into the liver and reticulo-endothelial tissue within 60 minutes of mosquito bite. In liver, exoerythrocytic multiplication occurs and sporozoites become hepatic schizonts which ruptured to release thousands of merozoites into the blood stream. The number of merozoites produced from a single sporozoite varies considerably with the infecting species. Some hepatic forms of schizonts persist and remain dormant in the hepatocytes and may cause relapse.

Once the parasites enter the RBC they do not reinvade the liver. Merozoites penetrate the RBC and pass through the stages of trophozoite (signet ring and mature form) and schizont. The infected erythrocyte rupture and release morozoites into the circulation which infect fresh RBCs. The cycle is repeated for 48 to 72 hours. In this erythrocytic phase, the infected individual becomes symptomatic with paroxysms of high fever. Fever with paroxysms corresponds to the development of the parasite in the RBCs. The peak of fever coincides with the release of merozoites into the blood stream. When RBCs are ruptured, various substances like hemozoin pigments and parts of unused cytoplasm are released with merozoites, which induce paroxysm and other pathological changes like tissue pigmentation, anemia, fatty degeneration and hyperplasia of reticuloendothelial system.

Clinical Manifestations

The typical paroxysmal attack of malarial fever found in three stages, i.e. cold stage, hot stage and sweating stage followed by an afebrile period.

The onset of *cold stage* is usually found with lassitude, headache, nausea, anorexia, pain in the limbs and chilly sensation followed by rigors within an hour. Then body temperature rises rapidly to 39° to 41°C with severe headache, vomiting, restlessness, weakness and rapid pulse. In early stage the skin feels cold and later it becomes hot. Duration of this stage is 1/4 to one hour. Parasites are usually found in the blood in this stage. Chills and rigors may not be found in infancy and early childhood.

In the *hot stage*, patient feels too much hot and put off clothing. The skin is flashed, hot and dry. Headache becomes intense with full pulse and rapid respiration. Nausea usually diminished with presence of excessive thirst. This stage last for 2 to 6 hours.

In the *sweating stage*, body temperature rapidly reduces to normal with profuse sweating. Skin feels cool and moist. The pulse rate becomes slower. The patient feels relieved and fall asleep. This stage last for 2 to 4 hours.

The febrile paroxysms occur every 3rd or 4th day depending upon the type of parasite involved. The classical 3 stages may not be always found. Diarrhea, vomiting, pain abdomen, convulsions and coma may be found in some children. The relapse of the disease is common and is characterized by enlargement of spleen and secondary anemia. Febrile herpes is common in all malarial patients.

Neonatal malaria is not common in endemic areas due to transplacental passage of maternal antibody (IgG). Congenital malaria may occur due to transmission of malarial parasite from the mother or due to infected blood transfusion or by acquired infection due to mosquito bite.

In endemic areas and in some children the clinical presentations of malaria may be masked or atypical. Clinical features may vary in benign tertian disease caused by *P. vivax* and in malignant tertian disease caused by *P. falciparum*. *P. ovale* and *P. malariae* infection clinically behave just like *P. falciparum*.

Malignant malaria is also known as cerebral malaria and manifested with sudden or gradual onset of irregular fever, delirium, convulsions and unconsciousness with alteration of reflexes. Prognosis of untreated cerebral malaria is fatal. Loss of corneal reflexes and retinal hemorrhage indicate poor prognosis. Falciparum malaria may also be presented with hemolytic jaundice, circulatory failure and shock. The mortality is much greater than in other forms of malaria. Survived children may have complications of major neurological problems.

In some children, severe malaria may be manifested as GI illness with marked vomiting, diarrhea, dehydration, electrolyte imbalance, dark green and brownish stool. The complications of severe malaria include jaundice, severe anemia, pulmonary edema, renal failure due to acute tubular necrosis, hemoglobinuria, shock in black water fever, rupture spleen and chronic malaria.

Diagnosis

History of illness and clinical examination are the most important criteria of diagnosis. Laboratory investigations include—(a) peripheral blood smear examination (thick and thin film) to detect presence of malarial parasite and its type, (b) routine blood examination for Hb% (usually low), WBC count (shows leukopenia), bilirubin and gammoglobin level (both raised) (c) fluorescent antibody technique to detect species specific antibody (IgG) and (d) bone marrow examination.

Management

The specific treatment consists of antimalaria drugs with the recommended drug regimen by national antimalarial program. The drug regimen mentioned specific treatment schedule for high risk areas, low risk areas and for severe and complicated malaria. Chloroquine and primaquine are recommended as presumptive and radical treatment with planned dose per kg of body weight and for specific duration. Severe and complicated cases are to be hospitalized for treatment. Choice of antimalarial drug for these cases is quinine in parenteral route and then in oral route, as early as possible. Injectable form of artemisinin derivatives may be used for severe and complicated malaria only. Chloroquine resistant *P. falciparum* cases are treated with sulfalene/sulfadoxine and pyrimethamine, which should be given cautiously.

Symptomatic management should be done with antipyretics and adequate fluid therapy, orally or with IV fluid. Anticonvulsive drugs and steroids may be needed. Blood transfusion may be required in severe anemia. Other complications should be detect and to be managed accordingly.

Good nursing care should be provided with rest, skin care, tepid sponge, increased fluid intake, balanced diet and hygienic measures. Emotional support and involvement of the parent with necessary instructions are important aspect of care.

Prognosis

Prognosis is generally good with early diagnosis and prompt treatment. With the presence of complications, outcome may vary. Malnutrition and other associated problems may also be found.

Preventive Measures

Preventive measures of malaria include management of malaria cases in the community with early diagnosis. Interruption of malaria transmission with improvement of environmental condition and housing are important measures. Vector control is the primary approach to control malaria especially in endemic area. The important preventive measures are residual spray with DDT (or malathian or fenitrothion or oil), anti larval measures, reduction of mosquito breeding sites, elimination of water collection, good drainage system, individual protection by bed nets, repellents, protective clothing with long sleeve, mosquito coils etc. Chemoprophylaxis is helpful. Malaria vaccines are under development and still in experimental stage. National antimalaria program stressed on different approaches and strategies for malaria control through primary health care.

Lymphatic Filariasis

Lymphatic filariasis is caused by the infection with three closely related nematode worms, i.e. *Wuchereria bancrofti*, *Brugia malayi* and *Brugia timori*. They are transmitted to human by the infective vector mosquito bites.

Lymphatic filariasis is a global problem. It is a major public health problem in India. The problem is increased every year due to gross mismanagement of the environment. The disease is endemic all over India both in urban and rural areas.

Epidemiology

There are at least '8' species of filarial parasites, specific to man. Among them *W. bancrofti, B.malayi* and *B. timori* are responsible for lymphatic filariasis and the others causing nonlymphatic filariasis, usually not found in India.

Man is the definitive host and mosquitos are the intermediate host of the filarial parasite. The adult worms are usually found in the lymphatic system of man. The female worms are about 50 to 100 mm long and males are about 40 mm long. The female worms give birth to microfilariae, about 50,000 per day. The microfilariae (Mf) circulate in peripheral blood via the lymphatics. Adult worms can survive about 15 years and microfilariae can survive for a year or more.

The vector, mosquito picked up the Mf from the infected person during biting and blood feeding. In the vector, the Mf developed into larval stage, i.e. exsheathing, first stage larva, second stage larva and third stage larva. The mosquito cycle is approximately 10 to 14 days with optimum conditions of temperature and humidity. In the human cycle the infective larvae develop into adult male and female worms.

The microfilariae shows a characteristic nocturnal periodicity, i.e. they appear in large number at night and retreat from the blood stream during day time. This is adapted from the nocturnal biting habits of vector mosquitoes.

The source of infection is the person with circulating Mf in the peripheral blood. In late obstructive stage of filarial disease, the Mf are not found in the blood.

Man is a natural host and all ages are susceptible to infection. In endemic areas, filarial infections has been found even in infants aged less than 6 months. The disease is usually associated with urbanization, industrialization, migration of people, illiteracy, poverty and poor sanitation.

The favorable climate influences the mosquito breeding and their longevity. Maximum prevalence observed for culex quinquefasciatus (previously known as culex fatigans) at temperature 22° to 38°C and humidity 70 percent.

Poor drainage system promotes profuse vector breeding in polluted water. Inadequate sewage disposal and lack of town planning also facilitates the breeding of the vector mosquitoes. The common breeding places are soakage pits, poorly maintained drains, septic tanks, open ditches, burrow pits and cesspools.

All three types of filarial infections are transmitted to man by the bites of infective mosquitoes. The vector of Bancroftion filariasis is culex quinquefasciatus and for Brugian filariasis, it is Mansonia mosquitoes (*M. annulifers* and *M. uniformis*). Mansonia mosquitoes breed in presence of aquatic plant such as pistia stratiotes. These mosquitoes cannot breed in the absence of these plant.

Incubation period is 8 to 16 months. This period may be longer in some cases.

Clinical Manifestations

The disease manifestations range from asymptomatic state to acute or chronic obstructive lesions. Only a small portion of infected individual exhibit clinical signs. Two distinct clinical types of manifestations are lymphatic filariasis caused by the parasite in the lymphatic system and occult filariasis caused by an immune hyperresponsiveness of the human host, e.g. tropical pulmonary eosinophilia.

Lymphatic filariasis can be described in four stages: (a) asymptomatic amicrofilaraemia, (b) asymptomatic micro-filaraemia, (c) acute stage of manifestation and (d) stage of chronic obstructive lesions.

Asymptomatic amicrofilaraemia is difficult to diagnosis. Because with the presently available diagnostic facilities, it is not possible to detect whether the individual has detectable infections or free from infections, although has some degree of exposure to infective larvae.

Asymptomatic microfilaraemia stage is an important source of infection in the community. These carriers are usually detected by night blood examination and their blood is positive for Mf.

The acute stage is manifested with filarial fever, delirium, lymphangitis, lymphadenitis, lymphedema of the various parts of the body and epididymoorchitis in male. There is acute inflammation of lymph glands and vessels. This episode can recur frequently, even 10 times a year and subsides spontaneously over 7 to 10 days in each episode.

The chronic stage usually develops 10 to 15 years from the onset of first acute attack. Fibrosis and obstruction of lymph vessels lead to permanent structural damage and manifested as elephantiasis, hydrocele, chyluria and lymphadema. In chronic Bancroftian filariasis, elephantiasis may affect the legs, scrotum, arms, penis, vulva and breasts. The prevalence of chyluria is usually very low. In Brugian filariasis genitalia are rarely involved and other features are same as Bancroftian type.

Not all elephantiasis is caused by lymphatic filarial infections, it may be due to obstructions following tuber-culosis, tumors, surgery or irradiation.

Ocult filariasis developed due to hypersensitivity reaction to filarial antigens and usually manifested as tropical pulmonary eosinophilia with paroxysmal nocturnal cough, dyspnea, fever, wheeze, fatigue and weight loss.

Diagnosis

The diagnosis of filariasis is confirmed by domonstration of microfilaria in the thick blood film collected at night or in body fluids (urine, hydrocele fluid) or in tissue. Adult worm can be identified in the lymph nodes. Monoclonal antibodies have been used to detect and quantify filarial antigents in serum, urine and other body fluids in persons with lymphatic filariasis. Membrane filter concentration (MFC) methods and DEC (Diethylcarbamazine) provocation test can also be done to detect Mf. Chest X-ray helps to diagnose pulmonary eosinophilia.

Management

The specific drug for the treatment of lymphatic filariasis is Diethyl carbamazine (DEC). This drug is effective for both adult worm and microfilariae. The dose is 3 to 6 mg/kg/day for 14 days. Repeated course of treatment may be needed for complete cure. Pulmonary eosinophilia can be treated with DEC, 7 to 10 mg/kg/day for 2 to 3 weeks.

Ivermectin, a macrolide antibiotic, may be effective against Mf. It is given in a single oral dose of 200 to 400 µg/kg. This drugs therapy is associated with high recurrence rates after 6 months of treatment in bancroftian infections.

Symptomatic measures include rest in acute stage, analgesics, antipyretics, antiallergic agents and antibiotics to control secondary bacterial infection and filarial septicemia. Surgery may be needed in filarial abscess and in some case plastic surgery may be required. Elevation of affected part and bandaging with ichthyol—in glycerine are useful to relieve pain and inflammation.

Prognosis

Prognosis of filaria depends upon phase of disease during initiation of treatment, available treatment facilities and presence of complications.

Preventive Measures

Prevention of filariasis can be best done by mosquito control through antilarval measures, environmental management, sewage disposal, use of mosquito nets and increasing community awareness about mosquito control measures.

Mass treatment with DEC in endemic area with annual single dose or use of DEC medicated salt as a special form of mass treatment can be used for filaria control. Common salt medicated with 1 to 4 g of DEC per kg is used. Diagnosis of clinical cases of filaria and appropriate treatment to reduce the morbidity is also an important control measures along with reduction of transmission and interruption of transmission cycle.

Kala-Azar (Visceral Leishmaniasis)

Leishmaniasis are a group of protozoal diseases caused by *Leishmania donovani* transmitted to man by the bite of female phlebotomine sandfly. The most important form found in Indian population is kala-azar or visceral leishmaniasis. It is a chronic infection of the reticulo-endothelial system characterized by irregular fever of long duration, hepatosplenomegaly, malnutrition, anemia and progressive emaciation. It is also termed as black sickness due to characteristic grey pigmentation of skin, seen in some patient.

Other forms of leishmaniasis are cutaneous leishmaniasis (CL), mucocutaneous leishmaniasis (MCL), anthroponotic cutaneous leishmaniasis (ACL), zoonotic cutaneous leishmaniasis (ZCL), post-kala-azar dermal leishmaniasis (PKDL), etc. The majority of the leishmaniasis are zoonotic involving wild or domestic mammals (rodent, canines). Indian kala-azar is considered as nonzoonotic infections.

Leishmaniasis is widely distributed throughout the world and found in endemic form in about 88 countries. Co-infection of visceral leishmaniasis and AIDS is emerging due to spread of AIDS pandemic mainly in Southern Europe.

Indian Kala-azar is found near Ganges and Brahmaputra regions in the forms of both epidemics and endemics. At present maximum number of cases are found in 36 districts of Bihar and 10 districts of West Bengal.

Cutaneous leishmaniasis is distributed in the dry north-western states of India from Amritsar to Kutch.

Both cutaneous and visceral diseases occur in India but Kala-azar is by far the most important leishmaniasis in our country.

Epidemiology

The causative agent of kala-azar is *L. donovani*, a intracellular parasite. There are at least 19 different leishmania parasites which cause human infections. The life cycle of the parasite is completed in two different host, a vertebrate (human) and an insect (sandfly). In human, it occurs in an amastigote form called "Leishmania bodies" (LD) and in insect as flagellated promastigote. The parasite lives in the reticuloendothelial system of human host.

Indian Kala-azar is considered as a nonzoonotic infection with man as a sole reservoir. There is a variety of animal reservoirs, e.g. dogs, jackals, foxes, rodents and other mammals.

Mode of transmission of kala-azar is from person to person by the bite of female phlebotomine sandfly, *P. argentipes*, which is a highly anthropophilic species. Transmission of kala-azar also may occur by blood transfusion or contamination of bite wound or by contact when the insect is crushed during the act of feeding. Cutaneous leishmaniasis is transmitted by *P. papatasi* and *P. sengenti*.

After infective blood feeding the sandfly becomes infective in 6 to 9 days. The incubation period in man is ranging from 10 days to 2 years with an average of 1 to 6 months.

Kala-azar can occur in all age groups including infants. The peak age is 5 to 9 years. Males are affected twice than female.

Movement of the people (migrants, laborers, tourists) from endemic area to nonendemic area can result in spread of infection. Recent resurgence of kala-azar in West Bengal is the extension of epidemics in Bihar (1977), by the movement of infected persons. The disease occurs in poorest people and in those who are working in farming practices, forestry, mining and fishing with risk of bitten by sandflies.

Kala-azar is mostly found in plains and does not occur in high altitudes. It has high prevalence during and after rains. The disease is mainly found in rural areas with favorable environment for breeding of sandfly. Sandfly breeds in the cracks and crevices in the soil and building, tree holes, caves, etc. Transmission occurs by the bite of the vector female sandfly especially at night in overcrowding and illventilated environment.

Clinical Manifestations

Entering in the human host the parasite carried by the blood circulation to distant organ like liver, spleen, bone marrow and causes marked hyperplasia of reticuloendothelial cells which produces clinical features.

The disease is characterized by gradual or insidious onset of intermittent or irregular prolonged low grade fever, which may have double rise in a day. The patient may have headache, vomiting, malaise, and toxic features. Rapid enlargement of spleen in 2 weeks of time is the characteristic feature. Spleen enlarges up to umbilicus or even beyond it. Hepatomegaly occurs slowly. Chronic cases are presented with progressive anemia, loss of weight, pigmentation of the skin of face, hands, feet and abdomen. Falling and brittle hair, malnutrition, jaundice, lymphadenopathy may be associated manifestations. In Infant, the disease is manifested as acute onset with high fever, rigors and vomiting. It is often severe and fatal.

Complications

The common complications of kala-azar are penumonia, dysentry, cancrum oris (gangrenous stomatitis), gingivitis,

severe hemorrhage (epistaxis, gum bleeding), agranulocytosis and malnutrition.

Post-kala-azar dermal leishmaniasis (PKDL) may occur in 5 to 10 percent of cases after 6 months to one year of apparent cure of kala-azar. This condition is characterized by hypopigmented macular patches on the extensor surface of the limbs, sides and back of the trunk and side of face. The patches may be erythematous and nodular lesion. These cases are considered as rich reservoir of infections.

Diagnosis

Clinical features are important clue for diagnosis of kala-azar. The confirmatory tests are blood and bone marrow examination for presence of LD bodies, or demonstration of the parasite LD bodies in the aspirates of the spleen, liver, bone marrow, lymph nodes or the skin (in case of CL).

The aldehyde test of Napire is a simple test widely used in India for the diagnosis of kala-azar. Other laboratory diagnostic tests include Chopra antimony test, complement fixation test, counterimmune electrophoresis, ELISA test, direct fluorescent antibody test, polymerase chain reaction (PCR) test, direct or latex agglutination test etc. Blood examination shows leucopenia, anemia, reversed albumin - globulin ratio, increased ESR and IgG.

Management

The specific management of kala-azar is done with pentavalent antimony compound. Sodium antimony gluconate (SAG) 20 mg/kg IM once daily is given for 30 days (40 days in antimony resistant areas). The common used drugs are urea stibamine or neostibasine. These drugs are preferably given intravenously. A course of 15 or 12 injections are given of the above drugs. Close monitoring of the therapy is very important. The drugs which can be used in resistant to SAG or relapse cases are stibamine, hydroxystibamidine pentamidine, aminosidine amphotericin and interferon gamma.

Supportive management should be provided with good nutritious diet, vitamin and mineral supplementation, good oral hygiene and skin care. Splenectomy may be needed in some cases with poor response to drug therapy.

Prognosis

With adequate treatment 90 percent cases can be cured. Untreated cases may have fatal outcome in 2 years. Some cases are said to have spontaneous cure (about 13–20%). Emergence of drug resistance (both primary and secondary) may be related to delay in diagnosis and inadequate treatment. Relapse and complications are common.

Preventive Measures

Primary prevention of kala-azar can be done by control of source of infection and vector sandfly eradication. Early detection and treatment of all cases should be done intensively. The reservoir of infection (e.g. patients of post kala-azar dermal leishmaniasis) should be treated with repeated course of drug therapy.

Vector control can be done by spraying of residual insecticides in the interiors of houses, windows, doors, crevices in the walls, damp and poorly ventilated places, animal shelters and all places up to a height of 6 feet from the floor level (as the sandfly has short flying range). DDT is the first choice of insecticides and should be sprayed two rounds per year at 1 to 2 g/sq. meter. BHC is the 2nd choice of insecticides.

Sanitarory measures for elimination of breeding places (i.e. cracks of mud or stone walls, rodent burrows, removal of firewood, bricks or rubbish around houses), location of cattle sheds and poultry at a fair distance from human dwellings and improvement of housing and general sanitation are important. Dog and rodent control are also useful to prevent animal reservoir.

Personal protection by avoiding sleeping on floor, using fine-mesh bed nets and insect repellents also very helpful. Health education should be given to provide information about preventive measures. There are no drugs for personal prophylaxis.

Giardiasis

Giardiasis is an intestinal infestation with a protozoal flagellate, i.e. *Giardia lamblia*. It is commonly found in children with malnutrition and immunodeficiency conditions. It is considered as an important cause of morbidity in infancy and childhood and even leading to the fatal outcome, if not treated appropriately.

Pathology

The infection is transmitted by the ingestion of cysts through contaminated water, food or directly from person to person contact. Each cyst liberates four trophozoites and colonize in the duodenum and jejunum. They attach to the brush border of the intestinal epithelial cells and multiply. The powerful sucking disk of the trophozoite causes mechanical irritation and damage to the microvilli of the small intestinal mucosa, resulting in deficiency of disaccharidases in the enterocytes.

Pancreatic damage may occur which can cause extraintestinal steatorrhea, poor tryptic activity and deficiency of enterokinase secretion. Fat malabsorption may occur due to bacterial over growth in the duodenum and upper jejunum and deconjugation of bile salts liberating bile acids.

There is reduction of secretory IgA in duodenal aspirates and depressed 'T' cell functions.

Clinical Manifestations

Most of the infections remain as asymptomatic carrier. In symptomatic children, incubation period is one to two weeks. The clinical features may be found in acute infections as sudden onset of explosive watery foul smelling diarrhea. Other features include abdominal distension, flatulence, epigastric cramps, nausea and poor appetite. There will be no blood or mucus in stools. The illness usually continue for 3 to 4 days and self limiting in normal immunocompetent children.

Subacute onset is presented as recurrent mild to moderate symptoms. There may be constipation in between loose foul smelling stools. Abdominal distension, nausea and flatulence are usually present but abdominal cramps are not present.

Persistent diarrhea may develop in 30 to 50 percent children. Other problems of chronic giardiasis are lactose malabsorption, steatorrhea, failure to thrive, nutritional deficiency conditions and transient ulcerative colitis.

Diagnosis

History of illness, physical examination for presence of clinical features and stool examination help in diagnosis. Stool examination for 3 successive or alternate days specimens show presence of cyst (85% detection rate). Examination of duodenal aspirate (Enterotest) helps to detect *G. lamblia*. Endoscopic brush cytology and intestinal biopsy are useful diagnostic method. Fecal antigen ELISA test help to detect the parasite in stool. Antigiardia antibody titres, especially IgM, elevation indicates acute infection.

Management

The children suffering from giardiasis are usually managed by OPD treatment. The specific treatment includes metronidazole therapy, 15 mg/kg/day in 3 divided doses for 10 days or tinidazole 50 to 75 mg/kg a single dose or 20 mg/kg/day in divided dose for 5 days. Furazolidone 6 to 8 mg/kg/day in 3 divided doses for 7 to 10 days is also effective. Other drugs like mepacrine, secnidazole, albendazole or ornidozole, also can be used for the treatment of this condition.

Symptomatic management of diarrhea and abdominal colic need special attention. Spices, chillies, pulses and milk can aggravate diarrhea and abdominal colic, those items should be avoided in diet. Liberal diet with adequate calories and protein should be provided. Vitamin supplementation especially vitamin 'A' may be helpful. Children with resistant symptomatic giardiasis need repeated courses of an antigiardial agent as such or in different combination.

Preventive Measures

Improving awareness by health education is the most important preventive measures. Instruction should be given about proper disposal of sewage, consumption of safe food and water, improvement of personal and environmental hygiene, avoidance of open field defecation and adequate treatment of infected cases and carriers. Breastfeeding protects the infants and young children from giardiasis.

Intestinal Amebiasis

Amebiasis is a protozoal infection caused by *Entamoeba hystolytica*. It is relatively less common in infancy and childhood. It is commonly found as intestinal infection but may also cause systemic manifestations. The route of entry of the infection is by contaminated food and water or by food handlers, or direct contact with infected stools. Rodents, flies and cockroaches also can transmit the infection by carrying cysts and contaminating food and drink. Asymptomatic hyman cyst carriers are the principal reservoirs of infection. It is found in about 15 percent of Indian population.

Epidemiology

The causative agent of amebiasis is *E. hystolytica*. It exists in two forms—vegetative (trophozoite) and cystic forms. Trophozoites dwell in the colon where they multiply and encyst. The cysts are excreted in stool. The trophozoites are short lived outside the human body. They are not important in the transmission of the disease. The cysts are infective to man and remain viable and infective for several days in stools, water, sewage and soil in the presence of moisture and low temperature. The cysts are not affected by chlorine in the amounts normally used in water purification, but they are killed if dried, heated (55°C) or frozen.

The immediate source of infection is the stool containing cyst. Most infected individuals remain symptom free and are healthy carriers of the parasite. The greatest risk is associated with carriers engaged in the preparation and handling of food. Mode of transmission is feco-oral route and vector borne. Sexual transmission may occur among homosexuals by oral-rectal contact. Incubation period is about 2 to 4 weeks or longer.

Amebiasis is frequently a household infection. When an individual in a family is infected, others in the family may also be affected. It is more closely related to poor sanitation and socioeconomic status. The use of night soil for agricultural purposes favors the spread of the disease. Epidemic waterborne infections may occur, if there is heavy contamination of water supply (sewage seepage). Raw contaminated vegetables especially from fields irrigated with sewage polluted water can readily spread infection. Hand to mouth transmission may occur directly by contaminated hands and finger nails with viable cyst.

Pathology

E. hystolytica enters the human body in trophozoite form which excyst in the small intestines and float in the intestinal contents. They are carried to the large intestine and invade the intestinal mucosa resulting tissue destruction in the form of inflammatory response and ulceration. They mainly settle in the colon due to slow passage of colonic contents.

The infection can reach the liver through the portal circulation and may cause amebic liver abscess, usually found in right lobe of the liver. The liver abscess may be single or multiple with chocolate colored, viscid, usually sterile and nonpathogenic contents. The abscess may regress or rupture or disseminate. The condition can be complicated by transdiaphragmatic rupture of liver abscess which may cause amebic emphyema and pulmonary amebiasis. The infection may cause amebic hepatitis or may spread to lung, brain, genitourinary system or skin. In swimmers, the free living amebae in the water, can cause meningoencephalitis through olfactory neuroendothelium.

Clinical Manifestations

Intestinal amebiasis may remain asymptomatic. Incubation period may vary from 2 weeks to months. Acute amebic infection may be manifested with dysentery, low grade fever, abdominal cramps, tenesmus and stool with mucus and blood. The child may present with intermittent diarrhea without blood and mucus with diffuse tenderness in the cecal or rectosigmoid area. Constipation may be found due to spasm of large intestine.

Complications

Intestinal amebiasis may be complicated with amebic liver abscess, amebic hepatitis, intestinal obstruction, intussusception, performation of the colon, peritonitis, rectal ulcer, rectal fistula, rectal prolapse, chronic colitis and extraintestinal amebiasis including involvement of lungs, brain, spleen and skin. Amebiasis carries substantial morbidity and mortality. It is a potentially lethal disease. Reinfection is very common.

Diagnosis

History of illness and clinical examination help in diagnosis. Laboratory investigations is useful to confirm the diagnosis and plan of management. Examination of fresh specimens of stool for 3 consecutive days sample is performed to detect *E. hystolytica*, cysts or trophozoites in stool sample. Smear from ulcerated area of the rectal mucosa may be examined to detect the infection.

Sigmoidoscopy followed by aspiration of mucosal lesions or biopsy is valuable in symptomatic patients. Examination of aspirate of liver abscess may be performed to confirm the complicated condition. Chest X-ray, liver scan or USG abdomen help to diagnose liver abscess and lung complications. Blood examination shows leukocytosis, anemia and increased alkaline phosphatase in chronic intestinal amebiasis. Serological tests (ELISA, IHA, CIE) can be done to detect extra-intestinal amebiasis.

Management

The most common effective drug used for treatment of amebiasis is the metronidazole. It can be used in both intestinal and systemic amebiasis. Tinidazole is another drug which can also be used for the treatment of amebiasis. These drugs may be given in combination of diloxanide furoate. Metronidazole is given as 20 to 50 mg/kg per day in three divided doses for 10 to 14 days after meal, tinidazole 50 to 60 mg/kg/day in three divided dose for 3 days and diloxanide furoate 20 mg/kg/day in three divided doses for ten days, for intestinal infections. These drugs is effective for elimination of both trophozoites and cyst.

Other drugs recommended for treatment of amebiasis are imidazole, ornidazole, secnidazole and paromomycin.

Treatment of complications should be done accordingly. Liver abscess should be treated as like as intestinal amebiasis and aspiration to be done in case of failure to respond to medical therapy.

Preventive Measures

Prevention of amebiasis can be achieved through prevention of contamination of water, food, vegetables and fruits with human stools.

Safe disposal of human excreta and sanitary practice of washing hands after defecation and before eating are crucial aspects in the prevention of amebiasis. Protection of water supply from fecal contamination is equally important. Practice of water filtration and boiling are more effective than chemical treatment of water against amebiasis.

Food hygiene and protection of foods and drinks from fecal contamination are the important measures. Uncooked vegetables and fruits can be disinfected with aqueous solution of acetic acid (5–10%) or full strength vinegar. Thorough washing of fruits and vegetables with detergents in running water can also remove the amebic cysts. Vegetables, especially those eaten raw, from fields irrigated with sewage polluted water needs special treatment before consumption. Handwashing and short nails are important personal protection for amebiasis. Food handlers are major transmitters of amebiasis, they should be periodically examined, treated and educated in food hygiene practices. Early diagnosis and treatment of infected cases are effective to control the spread of infection. Health education to the general public to create awareness is the most important preventive aspect of the condition.

Cryptosporidiosis

Cryptosporidium, an intestinal protozoa is an important agent of self limiting watery diarrhea in the patient of HIV/AIDS or congenital immunodeficiencies.

The mode of transmission is feco-oral route from person to person or through contaminated water and food. Cryptosporidium resides in the jejunum and may invade the colon and the biliary tract.

The incubation period of the disease is 2 to 7 days. The infection is presented with acute watery diarrhea, vomiting and abdominal cramps, which usually recovers in 10 to 14 days spontaneously. The disease can be complicated with loss of weight, malnutrition, cholecystitis, pancreatitis, papillary stenosis and persistent diarrhea.

Laboratory diagnosis is difficult, stool examination and mucosal biopsy help in identification of oocytes by special acid fast staining method.

No specific treatment is required. Symptomatic management by fluid-electrolyte balance, adequate nutrition and antiemetics are useful. The cause of immunosuppression or immunodeficiency condition should be treated for better prognosis. Hygienic measures to be followed.

Worm Infestations (Helminthiasis) (Fig. 14.1)

Helminthic infestations in children is a major public health problem caused by ineffective disposal of human excreta.

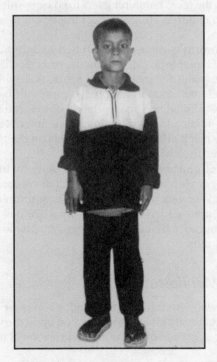

Fig. 14.1: Malnourished child with multiple worm infestations

The common helminths found in adult or sexual forms in the human body are round worms (*Ascaris lumbricoides*), pinworms or thread worms (*Enterobius vermicularis*), hook worms (*Ancylostoma duodenale* and *Necator americanus*) and tapeworms (*Taenia saginata* or *Taenia solum*). Helminthiasis in human in caused by three group of worms, i.e. nematodes (round worms, pinworms, hookworms), cestodes (tapeworms) and trematodes (fishworms or flukes).

Round Worms (Ascariasis)

Ascaris lumbricoides is a nematode, mostly known as round worm. It is most common helminthic infestation. It lives in the lumen of small intestine. The adult female roundworm measures 20 to 40 cm and the male 12 to 30 cm in length. Each female round worm produces 2,40,000 eggs per day. The eggs are excreted in the feces and in the external environment they become infective in favorable conditions. On ingestion of mature egg by the human host (definitive host), it hatches out in the duodenum to release larvae. The larvae penetrates the intestinal wall and are carried to liver then to the lungs through blood stream. In the lungs they break through the alveolar walls and migrate into the bronchioles, then coughed up through the trachea and reswallowed to reach the small intestine, where they become mature into adult worms in 60 to 80 days. The life span of an adult roundworm is between 6 and 12 months and maximum 1.5 to 2 years.

Man is the only reservoir of infection. The infective material is the feces containing fertilized eggs. Infection rates are high in children, they are most important disseminators of infection.

Roundworm is the soil-transmitted helminth. Clay soils are most favorable for development of eggs. Eggs remain viable in the soil for months and years. Soil pollution due to open field defecation is the most important factor. Small children who have no regular habits of defecation, pollute the house floor and surrounding areas. Infective eggs can then easily reach other children who play on the ground and contaminate their hands and food.

Mode of transmission is feco-oral route by ingestion of infective eggs with food or soil or drink or by contaminated hands and fingers. The period of communicability is continued until all fertile female worms are destroyed and stools are negative of round worm eggs. Incubation period is about 2 months.

Clinical Manifestations

The child with roundworm infestations may be asymptomatic. The clinical presentations depend upon the wormload, location or migration of *larvae* and deprivation of nutrients of the host.

The common features are pain abdomen, abdominal distension, nausea, cough, loss of weight, growth failure, anemia, vitamin deficiencies, bruxism and voracious appetite. The associated problems are pica, sleeplessness, irritability, urticaria, fever, eosinophila and diarrhea.

Ascariasis may produce intestinal obstruction (by worm mass) or gangrene or perforation, obstructive jaundice (blockage of ampulla of vater or common bile duct), appendicitis, pancreatitis, ascaris encephalopathy, liver abscess and peritonitis. Protein loss due to ascaris infestations may cause kwashiorkor.

Migration of larvae through the lungs may result in ascaris pneumonia (Loeffler's syndrome). Larvae in the circulation may cause convulsion. Features like retinoblastoma may result from involvement of eye. Hepatosplenomegaly may also develop.

Diagnosis

History of illness and passage of snakelike worm in stool or vomiting is important diagnostic criteria. Clinical examination and stool examination for round worm eggs are useful to confirm the diagnosis.

Management

The commonly used effective anthelmintics are single dose albendazole (15 mg/kg) or mebendazole (100 mg) twice daily for 3 days irrespective of patient's age. Levamisole single dose with 2.5 mg/kg or single dose of pyrantel pamoate 10 mg/kg body weight may also be used.

Piperazin cirtate is ideal drug for eradication of round worm infestation. It is given in a dose of 100 to 150 mg/kg for one or two days at night before sleep in the form of syrup or tablets or granules. The drug paralyses the worms, so the child should pass stools within 12 hours of intake of piperazine.

Preventive Measures

Prevention of round worm infestation can be done by interrupting its transmission. Sanitary disposal of human excreta, reduction of fecal contamination of the soil, provision of safe drinking water, food hygiene, good personal hygiene, improving habits of hand washing before eating and after defecation, avoidance of open field defecation are important means of prevention. Special attention to be taken for foods such as salads and vegetables or raw food items to prevent spread of infestation. Avoidance of pica and playing on contaminated soils and dusts are also effective measures.

Health education to the general public about the use of sanitary latrines, improvement of personal and environmental hygiene and changing of behavioral patterns especially on preventive measures are significant aspect of prevention.

Secondary prevention can be done by effective drug therapy of the human reservoir and mass treatment with periodic dewarming at intervals of 2 to 3 months. Sanitary improvement combined with mass treatment are the best preventive measures of roundworm infestations.

Pinworm or Threadworm (Oxyuriasis)

Infestation with *Enterobius vermicularis* (Oxyuris vermicularis) is commonly known as pinworm or thread worm. It is very common parasitic infestations of infants and young children. The worm does not multiply inside the human body. The gravid female travels to the perianal region at night to lay eggs causing perianal itching. Each egg measures 30 to 60 mcm and matures after 6 hours in a larva, which can survive for about 20 days.

Eggs are carried under fingernails contaminated during perianal scratching or through contaminated clothing, bed linen and dust to infect the human host by autoinfection. Man is only natural host or definitive host of pinworms.

The eggs hatch in the small intestine and migrate to the cecum, where they mature into adult worms. Female worms usually die after laying eggs. Eggs are resistant to disinfectants and remain infective for long time. The development of mature female worm to become capable of laying eggs takes about two months from the ingestion of eggs.

Clinical Manifestations

Majority of children may have no complaints. The infected child may present with vague general symptoms like poor appetite, loss of weight, teeth grinding, abdominal pain, nausea, vomiting and diarrhea.

Pruritus ani is the important feature. It occurs due to crowding of gravid females at the anus which produce intense pruritus. Scratching may cause secondary infection. In female child, vulvovaginitis may be found. The infected child may also present with irritability, restlessness, sleep disturbances, enuresis and masturbation. Rarely the condition may be complicated with appendicitis and salpingitis.

Diagnosis

History of passage of worms and other features are diagnostic. Routine examination of stool usually missed to detect the pinworm eggs, because eggs are generally not passed in the stool. Eggs can be demonstrated by examination of early morning perianal swab, before the child has passed stool. Cellophane-tape or transparent scotch tape technique can be done to detect the eggs. Eggs can be demonstrated in finger nail dirt in about 1/3 of cases.

Management

The specific anthelmintics used for the treatment of pinworm are albendazole, 10 to 14 mg/kg in single dose or mebendazole 100 mg can also be used once only. Other useful drugs are piperazine and pyrvinium. Prognosis is good with the treatment. Reinfection may occur and need repeated courses of treatment for complete eradication of the worms.

All the members of the family should be investigated and preferably treated simultaneously to prevent cross infection and reinfection. Short clean nails and wearing of tight underwear should be promoted. Crotamitone (antipruritic antiseptic) cream should be applied on perianal region to allay irritation and scratching to prevent autoinfection.

Preventive Measures

Simple measures are useful to prevent pinworm infestations. The preventive measures include maintenance of personal hygiene, careful hand washing with soap and water after defecation and before meal, keeping short nails, cleaning nails with soap and old tooth brush, treatment of all infected family members, wearing of tight pants to the children, laundering of infected clothing, etc. Health education about the preventive measures are important aspect of management.

Hook Worms (Ancylostomiasis)

Hookworm is a nematode causing intestinal infestation in human by two species, i.e. *A. duodenale* and *N. americanus*. It is widely prevalent in rural areas and slums. *A. duodenale* is mainly found in north India and *N. americanus* in South India. Another species *A. ceylanicum* has been reported from a village near Kolkata.

Hookworms live in the small intestine mainly in jejunum and remain attached to the intestinal villi. Male worm is 5 to 11 mm long and female worm is 9 to 13 mm long with dorsally curved anterior end or hook. One female *A. duodenale* produces about 30,000 eggs and one female *N. americanus* produces about 9,000 eggs per day.

Eggs are passed in the feces and on warm, moist soil they hatched larva after 1 to 2 days. Newly hatched larva moults twice in the soil and become infective thus able to penetrate skin within 5 to 10 days.

Infection occurs when the larva enters the body through the skin of bare-footed individual. Larvae of *A. duodenale* are also infective by mouth. Entering the human body the larvae migrate via lymphatics and blood stream to the lungs. From the alveolar spaces they travel up the bronchi and trachea, then coughed up and reswallowed to reach small intestines, where they mature and become capable to survive for one to four years.

Human host is the only reservoir and definitive host of the worm. Infective material is the stool of infected individual. Immediate source of infection is the soil, contaminated with infected larvae.

Hookworm is common in agricultural areas. Damp, sandy or friable soil with decaying vegetation is suitable for survival of the larvae. Moisture and rainfall are favorable environmental factors. Direct sunlight can kill the larvae. Soil pollution by open field defecation, using same place for defecation, going barefoot, farming practices using untreated sewage are significant factors causing spread of infection. The social factors like illiteracy, ignorance and low standard of living contribute towards the hookworm infestations.

Mode of transmission of hookworm infective larvae is usually by skin penetration in barefooted individual. The worm may also transmit by oral route with direct ingestion of infective larvae via contaminated fruits and vegetables.

The incubation period for *N. americans* is about 7 weeks and for *A. duodenale*, it varies from 5 weeks to 9 months.

Clinical Manifestations

The clinical features of hookworm depend upon wormload. Adult worms suck blood and cause loss of blood from the left over feeding site. The infected child presents with progressive anemia, loss of appetite, epigastric pain, perverted taste, pica and black colored stools. Diarrhea and constipation may also present. At the site of skin penetration (feet, buttocks) of infective larvae, ground itch may be found as an irritant papulovesicular rash or even as cutaneous larva migrans. Hookworm infection causes chronic blood loss and depletion of body's iron stores leading to iron deficiency anemia.

The infected child may be complicated with malabsorption, malnutrition, growth retardation, gross hypochromic anemia with hypoproteinemia causing edema even anasarca and cardiac failure.

Hookworm may be found in infants and presented as nausea, vomiting, restlessness, diarrhea with blood stool, malena and anemia. Infant can be rarely infected by vertical transmission especially when mother is suffering from hookworm.

Diagnosis is confirmed by examination of stool for hookworm ova and occult blood. Eosinophilia may be found in blood examination.

Management

The specific treatment of hookworm infestation includes albendazole 10 mg/kg single dose or 5 mg/kg daily for 3 days orally. It has 80 to 100 percent effectiveness. Other drugs also can be used for the treatment of hookworm like mebendazole (100 mg twice daily for 3 days) or pyrantel pamoate or Bephenium hydroxynaphthoate (alcopar) or Levimisole.

Correction of anemia should be done with iron therapy and blood transfusion in severe anemic patients. Nutritious diet with iron rich foods and treatment of complications are essential aspects of management. Supportive care with hygienic measures and follow-up should be emphasized.

Preventive Measures

Prevention and control of hookworm infection involves sanitary disposal of feces, periodic case finding and treatment of all infected persons, treatment of anemia and health education. The preventive measures include simple habits of improved personal hygiene, avoiding contact of contaminated soil by using foot wear, use of sanitary latrine for the sanitary disposal of feces to prevent soil pollution, change in farming practices, that is not to use raw feces or untreated sewage as fertilizer and improving use of health facilities for diagnosis and treatment. Community involvement through health education is an important aspect of prevention of hookworm infestations.

Tapeworms (Teniasis)

Tapeworms are cestodes commonly found in children as pork tapeworm (*Taenia solium*) and beef tapeworm (*Taenia saginata*). Other tapeworms are dwarf tapeworms (*Hymenolepis nana*) and zoonotic cestodes (*Echinococcus granulosus* and *Echinococcus multilocularis*). Man gets *T. solium* and *T. saginata* infestations through ingestion of cysticerca in contaminated food and echinococcus through ingestion of eggs. Diphyllobothrium latum infection occurs through ingestion of cyst in fresh water fish.

T. solium infection is endemic in India and in many countries. Human cysticercosis, caused by *T. solium* is a far more important public health problem than human teniasis.

T. saginata occurs almost all over the world where beef is eaten. There is moderate prevalence in India, Southern Asia and other countries.

T. solium and *T. saginata* pass their life cycles in two vertebrate hosts. In man, (definitive host), the adult parasites live in the small intestine. The adult *T. saginata* measures 5 to 12 meters in length and may be up to 24 meters. *T. solium* measures 2 to 6 meters.

The larval stage of *T. saginata* (cysticercus bovis) mainly occurs in intermediate host cattle. The pig is the main host for the larval stage of *T. solium* (cysticercus cellulosae). But man may also be infected. This may result in muscular, ocular and cerebral cysticercosis. The adult stages of these worms may persist for several years in infected humans.

Mode of transmission of tapeworms are: (a) consumption of infective cysticerci in improperly cooked meat of infected pork (pig) or beef, (b) ingestion of unwashed raw vegetables, food and water contaminated with eggs and

(c) reinfection by regurgitation of eggs from the small intestine by retroperistalsis (rare).

The infected child usually passed 1 to 2 cm long segments or proglottides in stool or crawl over perianal area. Tapeworm eggs passed in the stool, that swallowed by beefs or pigs. In the infected pigs/beefs, the larvae penetrate intestinal wall and get encysted in muscle and other tissues, which is consumed by the man who gets infection thereafter. *T. solium* consists of a scolex with sucker and hooks by which they attach to intestinal wall.

In infected human, the eggs disintegrate and the infective stage (larvae) leave the intestine by blood stream via the hepatic portal system and are dispersed throughout the body, where they develop to form cysticerci. In about two months time, the larvae mature into cysticerci. When they develop in the CNS (neurocysticercosis), represent a serious threat to the individual with a variety of pathological changes. The common target organs for cysticerci are brain, muscle and subcutaneous tissue.

Clinical Manifestations

Most of the infected individuals remain asymptomatic. The symptomatic children may present with headache, abdominal pain, abdominal distension, recurrent diarrhea and growth failure inspite of voracious appetite. History of passing proglottides in stool or crawling over the perianal area may be present.

Carriers of this worms have increased risk of developing cysticercosis due to repeated autoinfection. Cysticercosis can be found any where in the body caused by the infection with larvae of *T. solium*. Cysticercosis of the brain are only symptomatic and presented with convulsions or inflammation. Active neurocysticercosis may manifest as intracranial hypertensive syndrome, epilepsy, focal neurological deficit and alteration of level of consciousness. Brain tumor, hydrocephalus, meningitis or psychiatric illness may also develop.

The clinical features related to *T. saginata* infection are similar as *T. solium* with exception of less chance of developing cysticercosis.

Diagnosis

The diagnosis of tapeworm is confirmed by stool examination for eggs or examination of proglottids or motile segments passed in the stools. Neurocysticercosis is diagnosed by CT scan or MRI. CSF examination and blood for ELISA test are supportive to confirm the condition.

Management

Management of both tapeworms can be done with praziquental 10 mg/kg in a single dose. Other drugs which can be used are mepacrine, niclosamide, albendazole or mebendazole. For neurocysticercosis, praziquental (PZQ) 50 mg/kg/day in 3 divided dose for 2 to 3 weeks or albendazole 15 mg/kg/day in three divided doses for 28 days can be administered.

Symptomatic and supportive treatment should be provided depending upon the presence of symptoms and complications. Surgical interventions may be needed in symptom-producing cysticercosis.

Preventive Measures

The preventive measures of tapeworms include treatment of infected persons, meat inspection, consumption of meat with proper cooking, adequate sewage treatment and disposal and creating awareness about preventive aspects by health education. Health education messages should include adequate cooking of meat, thorough washing of raw vegetables and fruits, proper housing and feeding of pigs, prevention of pollution of food, water and soil with human feces and improving hand washing practices.

Hydatid Disease (Echinococcosis)

Human echinococcosis occurs due to infection with larvae of Echinococcus granulosus or *E. multilocularis*. Other species like *E. oligarthus* or *E. vogeli* also can infect human and may cause the disease. Echinococcus species are small tapeworms. Dog is the definitive host and sheep, cattle or goats are intermediate host. Basically the tapeworms have 'dog-sheep' life cycle, with man as an accidental intermediate host. Man does not harbour the adult worms.

The adult worms are found in dogs and other carnivores. The adult tapeworm commonly lives in the small intestine of dogs (definitive host) for 2 to 4 years. The eggs are passed in the stool and contaminate soil, vegetation and drinking water. Sheep, cattle and other host become infected when they ingest contaminated vegetation. Ingested eggs hatch in the intestine and the larvae migrate to various organ of the body in sheep, and develop hydatid cyst. The life cycle is completed when the sheep (cattle) visera containing hydatid cyst are eaten by the dogs. Infected dogs begin to pass eggs about 7 weeks after the infection.

Human infection is acquired usually in childhood through contact with infected dogs. The infection occurs by ingestion of eggs of Echinococcus with food, water, or unwashed vegetables contaminated with feces of infected dogs. Infection can also take place while handling or playing with infected dogs, e.g. hand to mouth transfer of eggs or by inhalation of dust contaminated with infected eggs. The disease is not directly transmissible from person to person.

Eggs are ingested by the man and larvae are hatched in the intestines, penetrate mucosa and are carried to the target organs. The important target organs are liver and lungs where larvae develop into characteristic unilocular or multilocular cyst, known as hydatid cyst. It can also occur in kidney, eyes, bones, spleen, peritoneum and brain. It takes several years to grow the hydatid cyst. It is more common where sheep and cattle are raised.

Clinical Manifestations varies on the site and number of cysts. Large cyst may cause pressure symptoms (e.g. jaundice in liver cyst). Lung cyst may present with chest pain, hemoptysis and respiratory distress.

Diagnosis is established based on the history of residence, close association with dogs and presence of slow-growing cystic tumor. X-ray of the affected part, USG, CT scan, ELISA test and Casoni test help to confirm the diagnosis.

Management is done with albendazole therapy 15 mg/kg/day in 3 divided doses for 14 to 28 days for four courses with 15 days drug free interval in between two courses. Surgical removal of the large solitary cyst may be required after albendazole therapy.

Preventive measures include health education about the avoidance of handling of stray dogs, isolation and treatment of infected dogs and preventing dogs to become infected by eating dead animals and infected viscera at slaughter houses.

Other Helminthic Infestations

- *Trichuris trichiura (whipworm)* transmitted by ingestion of embryonated eggs in contaminated food, drinks and hands or indirectly through flies and other insects.
- *Stronglyoides stercoralis* infects human through skin contact with contaminated soil by infective filariform larvae or by autoinfection.
- *Dracunculus medinensis (guineaworm)* infection is acquired by drinking contaminated water that contains crustaceans.
- *Schistoma mansoni* or *S. hematobium* cause Schistosomiasis or blood fluke (flatworm). This infestation may occur through penetration of intact skin by cercariae. Snails are the main primary intermediate host.
- *Trichinosis* or infection with *Trichinella spiralis* occurs due to ingestion of undercooked meat contaminated with infective larvae.

Respiratory Diseases

15

- Acute Respiratory Infections
- Bronchiectasis
- Emphysema
- Atelectasis
- Pleural Effusion
- Empyema

- Pneumothorax
- Lung Abscess
- Bronchial Asthma
- Drowning and Near-drowning
- Cystic Fibrosis

INTRODUCTION

Respiratory diseases are very often found in children, especially the respiratory infections. It is one of the leading causes of morbidity and mortality in young children. Respiratory problems are responsible for a large proportion of pediatric admissions and outpatient attendance.

The important risk factors associated with respiratory diseases include malnutrition, low birth weight, climatic variations especially in winter and rainy season, overcrowding house, poor ventilation, air pollution, lack of environmental sanitation and poor socioeconomic conditions.

The common clinical features related to respiratory diseases are cough, dyspnea, expectoration, chest indrawing, chest pain, cyanosis and respiratory sounds like wheezing, stridor, grunting and snoring. Apnea, air hunger and flaring of alae nasi may also present. In chronic cases hemoptysis, clubbing and associated cardiac or neurological symptoms may be found.

Special diagnostic procedures in the patients with respiratory diseases can be done to confirm the diagnosis. They include ABG analysis, blood examination (eosinophil, Ig viral antibody, etc), examination of body secretions (sputum, nasal cytology, throat swab, tracheal secretions, bronchial aspiration), radiology (chest X-ray, barium swallow, CT scan) MRI, USG, Skin test (Mantoux test and BCG test for TB, Casoni

test for hydatid cyst, test for allergens), direct laryngoscopy, pulmonary function tests (spirometry), bronchoscopy, thoracentesis, lung biopsy, pilocarpine iontophoresis for sweat chloride in cystic fibrosis, etc.

ACUTE RESPIRATORY INFECTIONS

Acute respiratory infections (ARI) and its complications are most frequent conditions of acute illness in infants and children. In India, ARI is one of the major causes of childhood death. It is also one of the major reasons for which children are brought to the hospitals and health facilities. About 13 percent of inpatient death in pediatric wards is due to ARI. The proportion of death due to ARI in the community is much higher as many children die at home. Most children have 3 to 5 attacks of ARI in each year. Many of these infections run their natural course without specific treatment and without complications.

Definition

Acute respiratory infections is an acute infection of any part of the respiratory tract and related structures including paranasal sinuses, middle ear and pleural cavity. It may cause inflammation of respiratory tract anywhere from nose to alveoli with a wide range of combinations of symptoms and signs. It includes all infections of less than 30 days duration, except the infection of the ear lasting less than 14 days. The incidence of ARI is highest in young children, especially below 5 years of age and decreases with the increasing age.

Classification

I. Depending upon the site of infections of respiratory tract, ARI can be classified as follows:
   a. *Acute upper respiratory infections:* These include common cold, rhinitis, nasopharyngitis, pharyngitis and otitis media.
   b. *Acute lower respiratory infections:* These include epiglottitis, laryngitis, bronchitis, bronchiolitis, penumonias.
II. Depending upon the anatomical involvement of lung the classification include the followings:
   a. *Bronchopneumonia:* Patchy involvement of lungs.
   b. *Lobar pneumonia:* One or more lobes of lung involved.
   c. *Pneumonitis or interstitial pneumonia:* Alveoli or interstitial tissue between them affected.
III. Depending upon the severity of infections, the ARI and pneumonia can be classified as follows (WHO recommendation):
   a. For the children within 2 months to 5 years of age
      • No pneumonia
      • Pneumonia (not severe)
      • Severe pneumonia.
      • Very severe disease.
   b. For the infant less than two months of age
      • No pneumonia
      • Severe pneumonia
      • Very severe disease.

Majority of ARI deaths in children are due to pneumonia. Pneumonia is the infection of the lung parenchymal tissue. There is consolidation of alveoli or infiltration of the interstitial tissue with inflammatory cells. Pneumonia may occur as primary infection or secondary to acute bronchitis or upper respiratory tract infections. The causative organisms of the infections include the followings:
• Bacterial: *Pneumococcus, Staphylococcus, Streptococcus, H. influenzae, Klebsiella, M. tuberculosis, E. coli, H. pertussis.*
• Viral: Influenza, measles, chickenpox, respiratory syncytial virus (RSV).
• Mycoplasma: *Mycoplasma pneumoniae.*
• Fungal: Candidiasis, coccidioidomycosis, histoplasmosis, blastomycosis.
• Protozoal: *Pneumocystis carinii, Toxoplasma gondii, E. hystolytica.*
• Rickettsial: Typhus

• Miscellaneous: Aspiration pneumonia (amniotic fluid in newborn, vomitus, drowning, foreign body), chemical pneumonia (due to kerosene oil poisoning), hypostatic pneumonia, Loeffler pneumonia, etc.

Clinical Manifestations

The clinical features of ARI depend upon age of the children, site and severity of infections, causative organism, general health and associated medical conditions.

Common manifestations of ARI are nasal discharge (watery or mucoid), cough, fever, malaise, anorexia, sore throat, irritability, chest pain, chills, tachycardia, respiratory distress, ear problems, etc.

Upper respiratory infections may present as dry cough with postnasal discharge, purulent nasal discharge and inflammation of tonsils, pharynx and glands.

Acute bronchitis: Usually present with fever, dry cough (worst at night), wheezing and mild constitutional symptoms. Cough becomes productive after 5 days. Some tachypnea is often present. On auscultation bronchi and coarse crepitation are found.

Acute bronchiolitis: It is manifested as severe illness with severe dyspnea and prostration. Cough is either absent or mild. Mild to moderate fever is usually present. It is common in infant and present with marked dyspnea, air hunger, flaring of alae nasi and cyanosis. Chest retraction, wheezing, dehydration and respiratory acidosis are usually found. Crepitation and diminished breath sound are detected on auscultation.

On the basis of WHO recommendation, the features of lower respiratory infections can be grouped as follows:
a. Only cough and cold indicates no pneumonia.
b. Fast breathing, i.e. increased respiratory rate with the presence of cough and cold indicates pneumonia (not severe).

   Fast breathing is diagnosed when the respiratory rate is as below:
   • 40 breaths per minute or more in a child with 1 to 5 years of age.
   • 50 breaths per minute or more in a child with 2 to 12 months of age.
   • 60 breaths per minute or more in a child less than 2 months of age.
c. Chest indrawing with or without fast breathing indicates severe pneumonia.

   Other signs which may present in severe pneumonia include nasal flaring, cyanosis, grunting or wheezing (soft musical noise when child breath out due to swelling and narrowing of small airways of the lungs)
d. Very severe disease is indicated by the presence of danger signs like inability to drink, excessive drowsiness, stridor

in calm child, grunting, wheezing, cyanosis, apnea, fever or hypothermia, abdominal distension, and convulsions.

Diagnostic Measures

Careful examination of clinical features, details history taking and auscultation of chest sound help in diagnosis of ARI and pneumonia. Only in complicated cases, blood for TC, DC, ESR and chest X-ray can be done.

Complications

Complications of ARI include pleural effusion, emphysema, atelectasis, empyema, lung abscess, bronchiectasis, pyopneumothorax and pneumatocele.

Otitis media, chronic sinusitis, pericarditis, congestive cardiac failure, respiratory failure and paralytic ileus may also develop. Metastatic spread may cause meningitis, septic arthritis and osteomyelitis.

Management

Treatment depends upon type of illness, severity of infections and associated complications. The standard treatment for childhood ARI is recommended by National ARI Control Program especially for primary health care setting.

a. The child with 'no pneumonia' can be treated at home with home remedies for symptomatic treatment (fever and cough) and does not require antibiotic therapy.

b. The child with 'pneumonia' can be treated in outpatient department (OPD) with oral antibiotics and other symptomatic treatment like antipyretic and bronchodilator.

c. The child with 'severe pneumonia' should be hospitalized urgently and requires parenteral antibiotics with symptomatic treatment.

d. The child with 'very severe disease' needs immediate hospitalization and to be treated with parenteral antibiotics, oxygen therapy, antipyretics, bronchodilators and other supportive care.

The effective antibiotic therapy is given with cotrimoxazole, penicillin, ampicillin, cloxacillin, gentamicin, amoxicillin, chloramphenicol, erythromycin or cephalosporin (cefotaxime or ceftriaxone). Bronchodilators like deriphyllin or salbutamol may be needed.

Supportive general measures include bedrest, propped up position, warmth, isolation, suctioning to remove secretions from tracheobronchial tree, adequate fluid and dietary intake, humid environment, hygienic measures, clearing of air passage and nose, monitoring of child's condition (vital signs, O_2 saturation, pulse oximetry), postural drainage, chest physiotherapy and treatment of complications.

In complicated cases, surgical interventions may be needed, e.g. aspiration in case of empyema, closed chest drainage in case of pyopneumothorax and ventilatory support in case of respiratory failure.

Prognosis

Prognosis is good in early diagnosis and early initiation of treatment in appropriate time. Staphylococcal pneumonia carries worst prognosis. Complicated cases may have fatal outcome.

Nursing Management

Nursing Assessment

To determine the severity of infection and respiratory problems, initial assessment to be made and thereafter continuous monitoring of the child's condition is essential throughout the course of illness.

Initial history of present complaints and history of illness help to assess the need for priority interventions. Details history of different aspects to be collected when the child's condition becomes stable. Duration of illness, age of the child, previous illness, presence of associated symptoms, and any treatment taken before, are very important along with routine history.

Physical examination to be done including percussion and auscultation to diagnose the extent and severity of infections. Respiratory pattern, associated signs and symptoms, features of complications to be evaluated carefully. Thorough general and systemic examination to be performed.

Nursing Diagnosis

Nursing assessment helps to document nursing diagnosis. It should be recorded clearly, because it is very essential for further nursing management. The common nursing diagnoses for the child with ARI can be:

- Ineffective airway clearance related to inflammation, obstruction or secretions of respiratory tract.
- Ineffective breathing pattern related to inflammatory process.
- Fluid volume deficit related to fever, anorexia and vomiting.
- Fatigue related to increased work of breathing.
- Anxiety related to respiratory distress and hospitalization.
- Parental role conflict related to illness of the child.

Nursing Interventions

In general, nursing interventions for a child with ARI include the followings:

- Provision of bed rest with comfortable position and head up.
- Administration of oxygen therapy and clearing of air passage by removing secretions.
- Maintenance of warm, humid and well-ventilated environment.
- Maintenance of adequate hydration by oral or parenteral fluid and recording of intake and output.
- Provision of adequate nutrition by breastfeeding or dietary intake. Nasogastric tube feeding may be necessary. If the child is having airway obstruction, breast sucking is usually withheld to prevent aspiration and suffocation.
- Practising safe measures for prevention of accidents and other infections.
- Monitoring of child's condition continuously with immediate recording.
- Provision of frequent change of position (2 hourly). Chest physiotherapy and postural drainage may be useful to prevent complications and for early recovery.
- Administration of prescribed medications and recording of treatment given (antibiotic, antipyretic, bronchodilator, etc.)
- Giving tepid sponge to treat fever.
- Maintenance of personal hygiene and elimination.
- Explanation and reassurance to the parent and child about treatment plan and prognosis. Involving parent in child care as possible.
- Arrangement of play materials, in recovery phase for diversion and recreation and to reduce anxiety and tension related to hospitalization.
- Planning for discharge from hospital and home care. Health education to the parent and family members for home care, follow-up and prevention of further attack.

Preventive Measures of Acute Respiratory Infections

Acute respiratory infections (ARI) can be prevented by modification of risk factors related to respiratory infections and other diseases. Family members and parents need to be informed about the followings:

- Good hygienic practices related to personal and environmental hygiene.
- Appropriate handling and disposal of respiratory secretions of the infected individuals.
- Isolation of the infected patients and to take precautions to prevent spread of infections.
- Maintenance of warm, well ventilated environment.
- Avoiding synthetic clothing and exposure of skin.
- Special protection during weather variation to prevent cold.
- Maintenance of nutritional status with exclusive breastfeeding up to 4 to 6 months, weaning from 4 to 6 months and balanced diet thereafter. Adequate hydration to be maintained.
- Immunization to be completed as per schedule.
- Use of home remedies for cough and cold, e.g. tulsi, honey, basak, zinger, hot drinks, etc.
- Regular health check-up for detection of deviation from normal health and growth and development, nutritional status and associated problems.
- Avoiding harmful practices related to child care during illness or in wellness.

Sample Nursing Process of a Child with ARI

Ramu, is a 8 months old infant, admitted in pediatric ward with severe respiratory distress having cough and cold for 5 days.

Nursing assessment includes both subjective and objective data with the information of history of illness from parents and findings of physical examination.

The infant is having fever, inability to suck the breast and no urine for 8 hours. On examination the infant is having temperature 102°F, respiration 70 breaths per minute, heart rate 160 beats per minute, and body weight only 5 kg. There is chest indrawing, wheezing sound on expiration and drowsiness. Parents are very anxious. See page 263 for the sample nursing process on ARI.

BRONCHIECTASIS

Bronchiectasis is a chronic and permanent dilatation of the bronchi and bronchioles. It develops due to complete obstruction by inflammation, infections or inhalation of foreign body. Incomplete obstruction of bronchi may result in obstructive emphysema. Obstruction may develop due to collection of thick mucus in case of chronic bronchitis, bronchial asthma or cystic fibrosis. The infections which can cause bronchiectasis are measles, staphylococcal pneumonia, whooping cough, tuberculosis, sinusitis, etc.

Infections and obstruction lead to damage of the bronchial wall as formation of cavitation and tissue destruction. It causes segmental areas of collapse, which exert negative pressure on the damaged bronchi leading them to dilate. Collapse, emphysema and pneumonia usually accompany bronchiectasis.

The bronchial dilation may be found as cylindrical or fusiform or saccular type. The most common site of dilation is left lower lobe. Right lower lobe may be affected due to foreign body and middle lobe due to tuberculosis. It is usually unilateral. History of bronchial occlusion and inflammation for a prolonged period leads to the development of the condition. When the occlusion is significant, there results collapse distal to and dilation proximal to the site of obstruction. Prolonged suffering, further progression of the

Nursing process of a child with ARI

- Identification data
- History of illness
- Findings of physical examination and laboratory investigations
- Date and time

Assessment	Nursing diagnosis	Planning	Implementation	Evaluation
Database				
• Fast breathing as respiration 70 breaths/min • Chest indrawing • Presence of wheezing	• Ineffective breathing patterns related to inflammatory process	• To improve breathing pattern for adequate ventilation	• Placing the infant in prop-up position with pillow on mother's lap. • No supine position. Removing nasal secretions by suctioning. • Giving oxygen therapy. • Administering medications as prescribed. (antibiotics, antipyretics and bronchodilators) • Monitoring infant's condition and respiratory status. • Arranging ventilatory support, if necessary in respiratory failure.	• Respiratory distress reduced partially. Respiration 60 breaths per minute. • Nasal passage clear. • Chest indrawing till present.
• Fever as body temperature 102°F • No urine passed for 8 hours • Refusal of feeding	• Fluid volume deficit related to fever and poor feeding	• To promote adequate hydration and to maintain fluid electrolyte balance	• Administering IV fluid at prescribed rate with Arolyte-p. • Withholding oral feeds to prevent aspiration. • Allowing clear oral fluid when respiratory status improve. • Managing fever by tepid sponge and syp. Paracetamol. • Recording intake and output.	• Urine passed normally after one hour of IV fluid therapy • Temperature 100°F
• Drowsiness • Weakness • Lethargy	• Fatigue related to increased work of breathing	• To promote adequate rest	• Gentle handling during nursing care and organizing care when the child is awake, not disturbing sleep. • Provision of calm and quite environment. • Encouraging mother to provide warm, comfort and safety.	• The baby is sleeping and responding to stimuli.
• Anxious parents	• Anxiety related to respiratory distress and hospitalization of infant.	• To reduce anxiety of the parents.	• Explaining the treatment plan and procedures according to the level of understanding of the parents. • Observing the infant at regular interval and recording the findings. • Maintaining oxygen therapy, IV infusion and medication as prescribed. • Answering questioning to the parents and encouraging to ask questions. • Involving the parent in care of the infant.	• Mother looks less anxious and asks questions about care of the infant.
• Poor feeding • Body weight of the infant is 5 kg • Weaning not yet started only addition of diluted cow's milk	• Alteration of nutrition, less than body requirements	• To provide adequate nutrition	• Encouraging oral feeding when infant's respiratory distress is reduced. • Instruction for continuation of breastfeeding and adequate weaning foods, e.g. fruit juice, mixed rice and daal mashed potato, mixed khichdi with vegetables, etc. • Maintaining cleanliness and food hygiene.	• Infant takes small amount of expressed breast milk and orange Juice.
• Poor personal hygiene • No immunization	• Knowledge deficit related to care of infant	• To improve knowledge about child care by health teaching.	• Instructing and explaining the mother about hygienic measures, weaning, warmth, immunization, prevention of ARI by home remedies, regular health check-up and medical help whenever necessary.	• Mother maintains cleanliness and listen the instructions carefully and ensure that she will try to follow the advice.

Note: The sample nursing process is not inclusive of all needs of the infant and parents. Additional nursing diagnoses that can be included are as follows:
- Alteration of comfort related to painful procedures.
- Altered growth and development related to illness.
- Fear related to unfamiliar environment of hospital.
- Potential to superadded infection related to low immunity power in respiratory infections and malnutrition.

lesion along with repeated infections ultimately produce classical clinical pictures.

Clinical Manifestations

The onset of the condition is usually insidious with persistent or recurrent cough. There is foul smelling and productive cough with copious mucopurulent sputum having postural relationship. Fever and recurrent attacks of respiratory infections are common. Afterwards the child may present with dyspnea, wheezing, cyanosis, poor, general condition, exhaustion, anorexia, poor weight gain, hemoptysis and clubbing, in advanced stages. On auscultation, localized crepitations and leathery rales may be heard. Trachea and mediastinum are shifted towards the affected site.

Diagnosis

History of illness and physical examination help in clinical suspicion. Chest X-ray shows honeycomb appearance of affected part with increased bronchovascular marking extending towards the base of the lung and mediastinal shift. Bronchoscopy, bronchography and CT scan help to assess the extent of involvement and need for surgery. Bacteriological study with culture and sensitivity of respiratory secretions and sputum help to detect presence of infections or other problems.

Management

Management of bronchiectasis is performed with appropriate systemic antibiotic therapy, especially in acute exacerbation. Clearing of secretions and exudates from airpassage and breathing exercise with postural drainage are essential measures. Improvement of general health and treatment of associated symptoms with bronchodilators, expectorant may be required for some children. Associated medical conditions, e.g. tuberculosis, should be treated with antitubercular therapy. Surgical resection of the affected lobe may be needed, when the condition is not responding with medical treatment for one year.

Bronchiectasis can be prevented by prompt and adequate management of pulmonary infections and immunization against measles and pertussis. Accidental aspiration of foreign body should be prevented and need immediate medical attention when it happens.

Complications

Emphysema, atelectasis, cor pulmonale, brain abscess, amyloidosis are important complications which may develop in bronchiectasis.

Prognosis

Prognosis is usually good with adequate management in early stage. In few cases, the condition may improve significantly and clinically with medical treatment alone, during adolescence.

Nursing Management

Nursing management should emphasize on the following aspects with special attention:

- Assessing respiratory status, signs of complications, general health and ABG analysis.
- Providing rest, comfort and warm comfortable environment.
- Administering oxygen therapy.
- Maintaining airway clearance by removal of secretions.
- Assisting in breathing exercise and postural drainage.
- Allowing increased fluid intake and humid atmosphere.
- Providing frequent mouth care and other hygienic measures.
- Maintaining well-balanced dietary intake with high calorie, high protein diet in small frequent feeding.
- Organizing diagnostic procedures.
- Administering prescribed medications and other therapy.
- Assisting in preoperative and postoperative care whenever needed in surgical interventions.
- Reducing parental anxiety and providing necessary information and health education.

EMPHYSEMA

Emphysema results from distension and rupture of the alveoli due to the loss of elasticity of the lung tissue with resultant air trapping. Emphysema can be classified as follows:

a. *Obstructive emphysema:* It occurs due to partial occlusion of bronchus or a bronchiole in case of atelectasis, bronchial asthma, lung infections, bronchiolitis, miliary tuberculosis, mucoviscidosis, tumors, foreign body aspiration, etc.

b. *Compensatory emphysema:* It occurs when normal lung tissue expands to fill up the areas of collapsed lung segments, e.g. in pneumonia, empyema, atelectasis, pneumothorax, etc.

c. *Congenital lobar emphysema:* It is found in neonates and young children resulting from severe respiratory distress.

d. *Familial emphysema:* It is found especially in female young child as progressive dyspnea, which is inherited as autosomal recessive trait.

Clinical Manifestations

The clinical features of emphysema depend upon the area of lung tissue involved. The common features are progressive dyspnea, tachypnea, cough, wheeze, chest retraction, cyanosis, etc.

Management

Management of the condition depend upon the cause of emphysema. Symptomatic relief is important with oxygen therapy, bronchodilators, mucolytic agents, and antibiotics. Interstitial emphysema can be treated by conservative management. Congenital lobar emphysema should be managed with lobectomy.

Supportive nursing care is essential with need-based nursing interventions. Continuous monitoring of child's condition is required with special emphasis on respiratory functions. The nursing interventions should include routine care with rest, prop-up position, clear airway, increased oral fluid intake, adequate diet, avoidance of bronchial irritants (e.g. smoking), oral hygiene specially after inhalation of medications, chest physiotherapy, breathing coughing exercise, postural drainage, administration of medications with necessary precautions, care during surgery and necessary health teaching to parents.

ATELECTASIS

Atelectasis is the collapse or airless condition of the lung with incomplete expansion. The whole or part of the lung fails to expand. It can be lobar or lobular atelectasis. It is found as congenital or primary atelectasis and acquired or secondary atelectasis.

Congenital atelectasis is common in preterm or LBW baby. There is failure of alveolar expansion due to immaturity of the respiratory muscles or abnormalities of the alveolar ducts or any pulmonary disorders.

Acquired or secondary atelectasis develops from bronchial obstruction due to foreign body, excessive secretions, mucus plugs, tumors, enlargement of heart or lymph nodes. It may be produced by large pleural effusion, pneumothorax, tension cyst, intrathoracic SOL, or after prolonged general anesthesia for thoracic or abdominal surgery. It may occur as postoperative complications due to hypoventilation or in poliomyelitis or postdiphtheric paralysis.

Clinical Manifestations

The clinical features depends upon extent of collapse and seriousness or type of onset. The common manifestations are fever, tachypnea, dyspnea, cyanosis, chest pain, chest retractions and decreased chest wall movement. On examination, mediastinal shift to the affected side, elevation of diaphragm of the affected hemithorax and compensatory emphysema are found. On auscultation, breath sound is diminished or absent over the affected area. Percussion note may impaired.

Diagnosis

History of illness and findings of clinical examination help to assess the condition. Chest X-ray and bronchoscopy help to confirm the diagnosis.

Management

Management of atelectasis includes the treatment of specific cause of the condition. Postural drainage and chest physiotherapy are important measures. Bronchoscopic aspiration can be done in persistent cases.

Special considerations in nursing interventions should include continuous assessment of respiratory functions, pulse oximetry, arterial blood gas (ABG) analysis, incentive spirometry and intermittent positive pressure breathing support, as prescribed. Deep breathing and coughing exercise to be encouraged. Analgesics can be administered to reduce pain. Adequate fluid intake, humidified air and clearing of air passage to be ensured. Explanation, reassurance and necessary health education to be given along with routine nursing care.

Complications

The common complications of atelectasis are bronchietasis, fibrosis and infections.

Prognosis

Atelectasis has good prognosis. Prolonged illness may result due to persistent atelectasis and poor prognosis may found in massive bacterial atelectasis.

PLEURAL EFFUSION

Pleural effusion is the collection of fluid in the thoracic cavity between visceral and parietal pleura. It is less common in children below 5 years. Small effusion rarely produces symptoms or definite physical signs and usually detected by X-ray. Large effusion may cause respiratory distress, chest pain and fever. The fluid that accumulates in the pleural cavity may be transudate, exudate, serous, sanguineous, sterile, purulent or chylous.

Serous pleural effusion is commonly develop due to tuberculosis. Hemothorax may develop as a result of trauma, malignancy or hemorrhagic diseases. Chylothorax usually rare in childhood, may occur due to injury of thoracic duct or filaria. Purulent effusion (empyema) is common in children due to complications of various infections which are not treated appropriately.

Clinical Manifestations

The clinical features of pleural effusion include high fever, cough, chest pain on affected side that worsens on deep breathing and coughing, reflex abdominal pain in case of basal effusion and weight loss. The onset is usually subacute.

On examination, decreased chest movements on affected side, mediastinal shift to the opposite side, fullness of the intercostal space, pleural rub, decreased breath sounds, dull percussion note, decreased vocal resonance are usually found.

Diagnosis

History of illness, findings of physical examination and chest X-ray help to diagnose the condition. X-ray chest shows a uniform opacity with a curved upper border of fluid line which may become horizontal when air is also coexisting. There is definite mediastinal shift to the opposite healthy side. Diagnostic pleural fluid aspiration to assess the nature of fluid by biochemical and cell study with culture and sensitivity confirms the diagnosis. Straw colored fluid with lymphocytic response indicates tuberculosis.

Management

Management of pleural effusion should be done according to the specific cause. Specific chemotherapy along with symptomatic and supportive measures should be provided. Relief of respiratory distress can be done by therapeutic thoracentasis for the removal of collected fluid, especially in case of large pleural effusion. Special care should be taken during thoracentesis.

Complications

Pleural adhesion and pleural thickening may develop as complications, which interfere with re-expansion of diseased lung.

EMPYEMA

Empyema is the collection of thick pus in the pleural cavity. It is also termed as pyothorax. It may develop directly from lungs or from neighboring structure or through blood. It is fairly common in infancy.

The most common organism is the *Staphylococcus*. Other responsible causative organisms are *Pneumococcus*, *Streptococcus*, *H. influenzae*, etc. Empyema may develop following pneumonia, lung abscess, pulmonary tuberculosis, chest injury, suppurative lung disease, septicemia and due to metastatic spread of suppurative foci from distant lesions such as osteomyelitis.

Clinical Manifestations

History of measles or staphylococcal infections anywhere in the body may found in case of empyema. Many children do not have any symptoms of empyema, but they may have growth failure and some nonspecific symptoms like fever and diarrhea. These cases are detected during clinical check-up.

The specific presenting features of empyema include fever, cough, respiratory distress, chest pain, cyanosis and toxemia. In case of prolonged suffering the child may present with loss of weight, clubbing, anemia and other features of malnutrition.

Chest signs are found as diminished movement of the affected side, mediastinal shift to the opposite healthy side, widening and dullness of the intercostal spaces, dull percussion note and diminished air entry.

Diagnosis of the condition is confirmed by chest X-ray and diagnostic pleural aspiration for biochemical and bacteriological examination.

Complications

The complications of empyema are bronchopleural fistulas, pyopneumothorax, lung abscess, purulent pericarditis, osteomyelitis of ribs, septicemia, meningitis, arthritis, etc.

Management

Management of empyema should be done with appropriate antibiotic therapy, intercostal drainage and symptomatic measures.

Antibiotic therapy should be started as early as possible and to be continued for 3 to 4 weeks. Commonly used antibiotics are penicillin, cloxacillin, ampicillin, chloramphenicol or newer antibiotics, e.g. cephalosporins (cefazolin, cephalexin), etc.

Continuous closed intercostal drainage is strongly recommended for the management of empyema rather than the multiple aspirations of the pleural cavity.

Surgical drainage after thoracotomy may be needed to remove the collection, in case of severe respiratory difficulty, or in loculated pus or in the presence of marked mediastinal shift and when there is no improvement of the condition even after 3 to 4 weeks of medical management.

Symptomatic measures include antipyretics, analgesics and nutritional supplementation. Supportive nursing care include bed rest, semi-Fowler's position, oxygen therapy, more intake of fluid, protein-rich diet, breathing exercise, administration of drugs as prescribed, emotional support and health teaching. Special attention to be taken for care of water seal intercostal drainage with aseptic technique, maintenance of patency and necessary precautions regarding dislodging of drainage tube. Continuous monitoring of child's condition and chest drainage, along with recording of necessary information are important nursing responsibilities. Other routine nursing interventions should be provided according to priority need.

Prognosis

Empyema is a serious respiratory disease. With the use of appropriate antibiotic therapy, the prognosis is usually good. Some long-term complications may develop in some children especially in delayed initiation of management.

PNEUMOTHORAX

Pneumothorax is the collection of air or gas in the pleural space. It may develop due to rupture of subpleural or mediastinal nodes through the parietal pleura.

Pneumothorax is usually occur along with fluid (hydropneumothorax), with blood (hemopneumothorax) and purulent materials (pyopneumothorax).

It may occur spontaneously as spontaneous pneumothorax (due to trauma or pathological process) or be introduced deliberately as artificial pneumothorax.

The causes of pneumothorax in neonates are mainly the vigorous resuscitative procedures and staphylococcal infections. In infancy, the common causes are infections (staphylococcal, pertussis) and iatrogenic problems (thoracentesis, tracheostomy). In older children, the common causes of pneumothorax are tuberculosis, empyema, rupture of emphysematous bleb and foreign bodies

Clinical Manifestations

The clinical presentations of the condition are dyspnea, cyanosis, chest pain, mediastinal shift to healthy side, and hyper-resonant percussion note. Flat percussion indicates presence of fluid. Resonance above the level of the fluid with a clear cut level may be obtained in case of hydropyopneumothorax.

Diagnosis of the condition is confirmed by history of illness, thorough clinical examination, chest X-ray and pleural puncture with removal of small amount of air.

Management

Management of pneumothorax should be done promptly after confirmation of diagnosis. Relief of cardiorespiratory embarrassment is very important and should be done with closed chest tube drainage. Management of the underlying cause should be done, after the acute phase is over. Symptomatic and supportive care should be provided for better outcome.

LUNG ABSCESS

Lung abscess is a common complication in the children with bacterial pneumonia, especially due to *Staphylococcus aureus* and *Klebsiella*. It may develop as a single abscess or multiple abscess. Single abscess is usually develop due to pneumonia, tuberculosis or foreign body and occasionally following rupture of amebic liver abscess into the lung or due to superadded infection of hydatid cyst. Multiple abscesses usually may develop due to pneumonia, tuberculosis, cystic fibrosis, fungal infection, leukemias, agammaglobulinemia, etc.

The pathological changes include necrosis, liquefaction and inflammation in the surrounding lung tissue. When an abscess fails to resolve, it may cause pleurisy, pleural effusion or empyema.

Clinical Manifestations

The clinical presentations of lung abscess may be acute or may be detected as chronic abscesses. Acute abscesses usually develop during the course of staphylococcal pneumonia which may resolve spontaneously with appropriate treatment. Chronic abscesses are manifested insidiously with fever, persistent cough, foul smelling sputum, dyspnea, chest pain, pallor, anorexia and lethargy. Patient may have clubbing of fingers, if remains untreated over a prolonged period of time.

The diagnosis of the condition is confirmed by chest X-ray and USG. X-ray chest shows characteristic opacities and the cavities with fluid levels. The characteristic breath sound is also diagnostic.

Management

Management of lung abscess is done with appropriate antibiotic therapy, breathing exercise and postural drainage. Symptomatic management of the problems need specific attention. Surgical resection of affected lobe is done if medical measures fail to resolve the condition. Surgical drainage of the abscess is now obsolete.

BRONCHIAL ASTHMA

The word 'asthma' means struggling for breath. It is chronic inflammatory disorder of the lower airway due to temporary narrowing of the bronchi by bronchospasm, manifested as dyspnea (usually expiratory), wheezing and excessive cough. The peak incidence is found in 5 to 10 years of age. Boys are more sufferer than girls. The condition may be caused by allergy, infection or psychological factors, either alone or in combination. Allergic asthma is the most common in children.

Etiological Factors

Bronchial asthma is multifactorial. There are some excitatory factors and predisposing factors.

Predisposing factors: The important predisposing factors of bronchial asthma are: (a) heredity, with a family history of asthma or some other allergic disorder and (b) labile and over conscientious nature.

Excitatory factors

a. Allergy to certain foreign substances produce allergic or extrinsic asthma.
   i. Inhalation of pollen, wool, feather, animal hair, cotton seeds, smoke, powder and dust (especially house dust with mite, dermatophagoides pteronyssinus)
   ii. Ingestion of foods, like egg, some fish, meat, chocolate, wheat, some vegetables (brinjal), etc. and food additives.
   iii. Drugs, like aspirin or penicillin products.
b. Respiratory infections.
c. Worm infestations.
d. Change in climate.
e. Emotional disturbances due to stress, anxiety, tension, fear and conflict.
f. Excessive fatigue, exhaustion and exercise.

Classification

Bronchial asthma can be classified as allergic or extrinsic asthma and nonallergic or intrinsic asthma. Intrinsic asthma is uncommon in children.

Allergic or extrinsic asthma: It is produced by a hyperimmune (IgE) response to the inhalation of specific allergen (pollen, dust, feather, etc). The children with extrinsic asthma usually have positive skin test to the offending allergen and a positive family history of allergy.

Nonallergic or intrinsic asthma: It is produced in response to unidentified or nonspecific factors (triggers) of the environment. No hyperimmune response is produced. There may be positive family history. These children have irritable and hyper-reactive airway. Inhalation of irritants like cigarette smoke, odor of soap and perfumes, air pollution may induce the episodes of bronchospasm and wheezing. Exercise, drugs, change in temperature, atmospheric pressure, viral respiratory infections, emotional stress and excitement are also significant triggers of asthma.

In most children, the cause of asthma cannot be specifically identified as extrinsic or intrinsic. It can be mixed type.

Pathophysiology

The major pathological changes resulting airway obstruction in bronchial asthma are: (a) inflammation and edema of the mucous membrane, lining the airways, (b) increased secretions and accumulation of thick, tenacious mucus, inflammatory cells and cellular debris, within the bronchi and bronchioles, and (c) spasm of the smooth muscle of the bronchi. These processes interfere with ventilation and produce the clinical features. Several biochemical and mechanical events contribute to bronchial smooth muscle contraction and airway narrowing.

Recent studies show that all asthmatics have a common basic disorder, which may be associated with some type of IgE reaction, but the exact mechanism remains obscure. Inflammation of lower airway is considered to be the basic pathology.

The significant defect appears to be in neuromechanisms, in antigen-antibody reaction and bronchial inflammation for a patient with bronchial asthma.

Neuromechanisms involve stimulation of vagus nerve and beta-adrenergic and parasympathetic receptors by intrinsic triggers leading to bronchoconstriction and hypersecretion of mucus.

Antigen-antibody reaction is stimulated by extrinsic triggers. The antigen combines with IgE causing the mast cell to degranulate and release chemical mediators. These chemical mediators act on bronchial smooth muscle to cause bronchoconstriction, on dilated epithelium to reduce mucociliary clearance, on bronchial glands to cause mucus secretion, on blood vessels to cause vasodilation and increased permeability and on leukocytes to cause a cellular infiltration and inflammation. Late phase reactions include influx of eosinophils, neutrophils, lymphocytes and monocytes.

Bronchial inflammation occurs in initial and late phase reactions caused by antigen-antibody response and noxious environmental stimuli. Inflammation may cause bronchial hyper-reactivity by mast cell activation. Platelet activation factor (PAF) may formed by the inflammatory cells leading to bronchial hyperactivity.

Clinical Manifestations

The acute asthmatic paroxysmal attack is usually begins suddenly at night. The onset may be gradual. The sudden attack occurs usually due to exposure to allergens. An episode of asthma may be preceded by nasal congestion, rhinitis, sneezing, coughing and upper respiratory infections. It may be preceded by 'asthmatic aura' as tightness of chest, restlessness, itching, polyuria and mental excitement.

The typical attack of asthma is characterized by marked dyspnea, bouts of cough and expiratory wheezing. Nasal flaring with subcostal and intercostal retractions are apparent. Restlessness, sweating, exhaustion, tachycardia, cyanosis and pallor are usually present. The child looks anxious and pale and can speak only in difficulty. Abdominal pain and vomiting may found in intense cough. Many chidren get relief of dyspnea following vomiting. The attack may subside after one or two hours.

The child may suffer with the attacks generally for a period of 2 to 7 days. Then there may be symptom free intervals for several months. Short interval between attacks affect the child's general health and emotion. In chronic cases and severe asthma, the chest becomes barrel-shaped with increased anteroposterior diameter.

Status Asthmaticus

It is most intractable form of the asthmatic paroxysms, where wheezing continues for hours to days, in spite of administration of bronchodilators. It is a severe form of asthma in which the airway obstruction is unresponsive to usual drug therapy. It is a medical emergency and should be treated with intensive care.

There is tachypnea, labored respirations with suprasternal retractions and use of accessory muscles of respiration. Diminished breath sounds, distressing cough, decreased ability to speak in phrases or sentences, anxiety, irritability, fatigue, headache, impaired mental functioning, diaphoresis, muscle twitching and somnolence are common presenting features. Tachycardia and elevated blood pressure is found. Heart failure and death from suffocation usually develop. The attacks may suddenly terminate with copious expectoration and may lead to serious complications or death.

Complications

The most common complication of bronchial asthma is emphysema. Other complications include, severe hypoxemia, cardiac arrhythmias, atelectasis, pneumothorax, pneumo-mediastinum, bronchiectasis, cor pulmonale, respiratory failure and congestive cardiac failure. Psychological problems and chronic invalidism may develop. Prolonged use of steroids may complicate the condition. Tuberculosis, growth retardation, poor academic achievement, disturbed family functions, and alteration of parent child relationship are long-term sequelae.

Diagnosis

The condition can be diagnosed clinically with presenting features for prompt initiation of management. History of illness should be taken in details especially for allergy, infections, foreign body aspiration, ascariasis, filariasis, etc. Physical examination to be done thoroughly with auscultation of chest signs. The important findings are marked decrease of air flow and feeble breath sound. The chest is hyper-resonant because of excessive air trapping. The child presents with recurrent attacks of wheezing (i.e. a prolonged whistling sound heard at the mouth during expiration). Presenting cough generally worsen after exercise. Chronic spasmodic cough may suggest occult asthma.

Different investigations are to be done to assess the underlying cause and severity of the condition. These investigations include pulmonary function test, absolute eosinophil counts, chest X-ray and allergy test (skin test and RAST or radioallergosorbent test).

Management

Childhood asthma should be managed therapeutically for the prevention of acute attacks and maximum control of symptoms alongwith maintenance of growth and development. Medications, chest physiotherapy, exercise, counseling, avoidance of allergens and irritants are important aspect of management.

During acute attack, the management is done to control the paroxysm through relief from bronchospasm and inflammation. The commonly used drugs are bronchodilators (beta-2 adrenergic agents, theophylline) and steroids along with additional supportive and symptomatic measures.

During the period in between attacks, attempts should be made to detect the offending allergen, to avoid that and if possible to hyposensitize the patient with allergen, as the interim measures. 'Asthma preventers' (ketolifen, cromoglycate, steroid) may be used in chronic asthma to prevent the acute exacerbation. Since infection is an important excitatory factors, it should be controlled and sites of infection to be detected for complete elimination.

Drug therapy: Drug therapy in bronchial asthma help the child in rest, sleep, normal physical activity including regular school attendance, with minimum side effects and less or no hospitalization. It promotes bronchodilation, reduces inflammation and removes bronchial secretions.

The drugs commonly used for the treatment of bronchial asthma are as follows:

a. Beta-2 adrenergic agonists—Salbutamol, Terbutaline, Formoterol, Salmeterol.
b. Methylxanthines—Theophylline, Aminophylline.
c. Corticosteroids—Beclomethasone, Budesonide Predni-solone, Adrenaline.
d. Disodium cromoglycate.
e. Anticholinergics—Atropine derivative such as Ipratro-pium bromide.
f. Ketotifen.
g. Other drugs—For the management of acute asthma like IV infusion of magnesium sulfate, ketamine, inhalation of helium-oxygen mixture and frusemide are under investigation. In steroid dependent cases of asthma, high dose of IV immunoglobin can be used. In refractory cases, methrotrexate can be given as steroid sparing agents. Leukotriene antagonists also have shown good results for control of mild to moderate acute asthma. Antihistaminics are not usually advised in cases of asthma but potent histamine antagonists selective for H_1 receptors (cetirizine) inhibit early bronchoconstriction. These all drugs can be delivered orally, parenterally or through various inhalation devices.

Additional measures

a. Mild tranquilizers to remove anxiety and emotional stress.
b. Expectorants to remove excessive secretions.
c. Antibiotics to treat infections.

d. Oxygen therapy in severe respiratory distress and cyanosis.
e. IV fluid therapy for maintenance of fluid electrolyte balance and to correct metabolic acidosis.
f. Comfortable prop-up/sitting position to relief respiratory distress.
g. Calm and quiet environment to provide rest and supportive measures with good nursing care.

In Case of Status Asthmaticus

Immediate hospitalization is required considering the condition as medical emergency. Management of such patient should be done with aminophylline or theophylline infusion, IV corticosteroid and beta-adrenergic aerosol therapy with continuous monitoring by pulse oximetry, ABG analysis, etc. The child may need ICU care with ventilatory support.

Interim management in between asthmatic attacks:
a. Identification of offending allergens and to avoid and to hyposensitize the allergens.
b. Treatment of focal infections, e.g. tonsillitis, adenoiditis, nasal polyps, sinusitis, etc.
c. Chest physiotherapy, postural drainage and breathing exercise.
d. Change of environment to avoid environmental allergens and psychological stress.
e. Regular follow-up, thorough medical supervision and continuation of prescribed drugs to prevent acute exacerbation and recurrent attacks.
f. Psychotherapy and counseling of the family and the child at child guidance clinic or by professional person.
g. Parental education about long-term, home-based care, constant supervision, emotional support, continuation of medications, regular follow-up and care at acute attack.

Long-term, home-based care: The objectives of long-term care are to prevent acute episodes of respiratory distress, due to bronchial obstruction and to reduce the number of visit to clinic or hospital. Parental support and health education are important to promote growth and development and well-being of the child with involvement of parents towards self-management plan.

Long-term treatment should be planned according to the severity of chronic asthma. Best inhaler device should be selected among those available. Treatment can be stepped up or down. The need for treatment should be reviewed every 8 to 12 weeks. The control of asthma is assessed on symptom frequency, improvement in activity, growth and development level and school attendance. Health education is vital for effective long-term home-based care. The following instructions to be given:
- Provision of dust free environment.
- Avoidance of the allergic situation which can create allergic reactions, e.g. foods, smoke, perfumes, etc.

- Administration of prescribed medications with exact dose of drugs and necessary precautions.
- Observation of side effects and serious complications for prompt and appropriate action.
- Promotion of breathing and coughing exercises 3 to 4 times/day (blowing bubbles, deep breathing).
- Encouragement of active play like running, jumping, dancing, climbing, etc.
- Maintenance of consistent discipline, love and affection, active and productive life.
- Arrangement of regular health supervision and prevention of acute attacks.

Nursing management: Nursing care of children with asthma involves skilfull assessment and innovative approaches to assist the child toward optimal respiratory functioning, growth and development. During acute phase of illness and in hospitalized care, following interventions are required:
a. *Evaluating respiratory status and patient's general condition*—Frequent assessment of respiratory pattern, cyanosis, breath sounds, vital signs, cerebral functions, etc. The findings to be recorded along with laboratory and other investigations.
b. *Providing emotional support and necessary instructions*—Calm and quiet approach, trusting relationship, explanation, reassurance, play and recreation and parental participations are important aspects.
c. *Positioning*—Comfortable sitting position and supporting with pillow or leaning forward with support may be allowed to relief respiratory distress.
d. *Administering oxygen therapy*—Humidified oxygen should be given with nasal cannula or face mask.
e. *Administering medications*—Drugs can be given orally, parenterally or through inhalation devices. The available inhalation devices are: (i) Metered dose inhaler (MDI), (ii) Spacehaler (space device inhaler). (iii) Dry powder devices (Rotahaler, spinhaler, Turbuhaler) and (iv) Nebulizers. These devices should be used with appropriate technique. Usually instructions are given along with the devices.

For IV medications child's condition must be closely monitored. Syringe pump or infusion pump should be used for continuous IV drug therapy. Recording should be done accurately.
f. *Administering fluid therapy*—During asthmatic attack, child is usually having less fluid intake, abdominal discomfort, vomiting and increased insensible loss due to hyperventilation which leads to fluid and electrolyte imbalance. IV fluid should be given to prevent these problems. Intake and output chart to be maintain strictly.
g. *Maintaining adequate dietary intake*—Clear liquids to be given in small amount frequently. Forced feeding and large amount may lead to abdominal discomfort and vomiting. Potentially allergic foods to be avoided. Irritating spicy and gas forming food items also should be

omitted from the diet. Balanced diet should be planned to provide adequate nutrients for maintenance of health and to promote growth when the acute phase is over.

h. *Providing rest and sleep*—Adequate rest and sleep should be provided to relief from labored respiration. Gentle approach and minimum disturbances during nursing care are important.

i. *Maintenance of hygienic measures*—Routine hygienic care, dust free safe environment, prevention of accidents and promotion of safety measures, aseptic technique, care of bladder and bowel should be ensured.

j. *Supporting parents and family members*—Emotional support, allowing parents to participate in child care, discussion of treatment plan, answering questions and explanation are important supportive measures along with related health education.

Prognosis

Prognosis of bronchial asthma depends upon frequency, severity and duration of attacks. Asthma is not fatal unless severe complications are developed. Occasionally, a child with status asthmaticus may have fatal outcome. Childhood asthma may continue to adult life as long-term chronic illness. Relatively the condition has good prognosis.

Various Inhalation Devices

a. *Metered dose inhaler (MDI):* This aerosol therapy for asthmatic children need good hand to lung co-ordination and understanding of instructions. It is used for children more than 6 years of age. The drugs appropriate for administration by MDI are beta-2 adrenergics (salbutamol, terbutaline), steroids (beclomethasone, budesonide), atropine derivatives and cromoglycate sodium. The dose is administered by taking a puff for 5 to 7 seconds, which can be repeated after a gap of one minute. The action begins within 5 minutes. Side effects of the drugs are minimized.

b. *Space device inhaler (spacehaler):* It can be used for infants and younger children. The capacity of available space inhaler is 150 mL for infants and young children and 750 mL for children aged 4 years or more. The drug is administer through a mouthpiece of the spacer. It has to be attached to the MDI. A facemask can be attached to spacer for the small children. Bronchodilators and steroids can be administered effectively with this devices.

c. *Dry power devices (rotahaler, spinhaler, turbuhaler):* Rotahaler is used for steroids and beta-2 adrenergics. Spinhaler for cromoglycate and turbuhaler for prophylactic steroid therapy. These devices do not need patient's co-operation and may be useful for children below 5 years of age.

d. *Nebulizers:* Nebulization comprises passage of gas at high velocity, leading to formation of particles of a specific size (5 to 25 microns). It is suitable in very sick patients with acute asthma and in very young infants and children who are not in a position to synchronize. It can be used by oxygen instead of air compressor and to deliver the drugs directly to the lungs. Drugs available for nebulization are beta-2 adrenergics, steroids, cromoglycate and atropin derivatives. Nebulization is done for a period of 5 to 10 minutes at a time or as needed. Second nebulization can be done after 2 minutes with a maximum 6 doses. Maintenance dose at 4 to 6 hours interval for 2 to 3 doses is required.

DROWNING AND NEAR-DROWNING

Drowning means submersion in water leading to death within 24 hours. Near-drowning means when the individual manages to survive after successful resuscitation for 24 hours following submersion in water, no matter whether he/she dies or survives later. If the individual dies later, the term near drowning with delayed death is used.

A vast majority of the drownings are accidental. Infants drown when left unattended. Adolescents drown during swimming because they overestimate themselves.

Aspiration, laryngospasm or breath holding are contributing for most of the death. Hypoxemia, metabolic acidosis and transient hypercarbia are major pathological changes occur following drowning. Respiratory obstruction and asphyxia leading to death may occur with or without water being aspirated while the individual is submerged. Dry drowning with no aspiration of fluid occurs only in 10 percent of those who drown. Acute laryngospasm and asphyxia being the cause of death for them. The wet drowning with aspiration of fluid into the lungs occurs in 90 percent of all victims.

Salt water or sea water drowning causes hypertonic water to get into the alveoli leading to shift of fluid from vascular bed into the lungs resulting in hemoconcentration, hypovolemia and pulmonary edema with decrease ventilation.

Fresh water drowning (river, pond, lake) alters the surface tension properties of pulmonary surfactant and leads to unstable alveoli, atelectasis and hypoxemia. There is hemodilution and hypervolemia, as the fluid is drawn into the blood vessels. Pulmonary edema and hyperkalemia may develop due to hemolysis of RBCs as a result of drop in hemoglobin and hematocrit.

Clinical Manifestations

Patients with near-drowning can be grouped into three categories depending upon their severity of illness.

The patients may be conscious and awake, they are grouped as category 'A'. The victims of category 'B' may found with respiratory distress cyanosis, stupor and hypothermia. Category 'C' patients are comatosed with apnea and respiratory failure following the event.

Management

Initial resuscitation should be done with basic life support measures (mouth-to-mouth breathing, closed cardiac massage). Category 'A' and 'B' require supportive care. Category 'C' patients require advanced life support measures. Oxygen therapy, diuretics, sodium bicarbonate and bronchodilators can be administered depending upon the presenting features. Hypothermia should be managed by adequate warming. Other symptomatic and supportive management are useful for better prognosis. There is no value of steroids and prophylactic use of antibiotics. Serious neurological sequelae may occur in some cases of near drowning. Health education about the prevention of drowning or near-drowning is important nursing responsibility.

CYSTIC FIBROSIS

Cystic fibrosis (CF) is a fatal autosomal recessive disease that manifests itself in multiple body system. It affects lungs, pancreas, urogenital system, skeleton and skin. It is a major cause of severe chronic lung disease in children.

The name cystic fibrosis is derived from the characteristic histological changes in the pancreas. It is also known as mucoviscidosis.

This condition leads to chronic obstructive pulmonary disease, frequent lung infections, deficient pancreatic enzymes, osteoporosis and abnormally high electrolyte concentration in sweat.

Clinical Manifestations

In neonates, it may present as meconium ileus. In infancy and early childhood, this condition may present with pulmonary symptoms like cough, nasal obstruction, rhinorrhea, shortness of breath, cyanosis, hemoptysis, wheezing and exercise intolerance. The manifestations are in relation to the congestion and block of the respiratory passages with thick secretions.

These children may suffer with recurrent bronchiolitis, bronchitis, pneumonia, bronchiectasis, nasal polyposis, chronic lung disease and respiratory failure.

This condition may also present with recurrent or chronic diarrhea with steatorrhea, pancreatitis, and pancreatic exocrine deficiency causing intestinal malabsorption of fats, protein and carbohydrate. Other problems such as gallbladder diseases, peptic ulcer, malnutrition, failure to thrive, arthritis, delayed puberty, diabetes, aspermia and azoospermia may also be found in this condition.

Complications

Atelectasis, pneumothorax and corpulmonale are common complications in cystic fibrosis.

Diagnostic Evaluation

History of illness, presence of typical family history, physical examination of the child and Sweat chloride test (>60 mEq/L) are important to diagnose the condition. DNA studies are considered as the important approach to diagnose cystic fibrosis.

Management

Individualized and continued treatment is necessary throughout the life.

Assessment of specific problems and appropriate symptomatic management are helpful to prevent complications and to promote healthy survival of the children.

Continuous emotional support and guidance must be provided to the family and the child.

Respiratory care includes intermittent aerosol therapy, mucolytic agents, bronchodilators, antibiotics, anti-inflammatory agents, mist inhalation and postural drainage.

Management of diarrhea, steatorrhea, malabsorption and other gastrointestinal problems should be performed adequately to prevent further complications.

Nutritional support should be provided with increased caloric intake, supplementation of fat-soluble vitamins and pancreatic enzyme replacement. Frequent feeds, gavage feeding or even gastrostomy feeding is required for the child suffering from CF.

Genetic counseling and gene therapy can be arranged, whenever possible.

Early diagnosis with treatment of complications and other organ dysfunctions are important aspect to promote long term survival of these children.

Nursing Management

Nursing care with rest, reassurance, hygienic care, skin care, more fluid intake and well-balanced high calorie diet with fat soluble vitamins should be provided.

Chest physiotherapy, deep breathing and coughing exercise should be given to help to mobilize secretions along with prescribed medications.

Observations and recording for respiratory signs, weight, nature of stool and abdominal symptoms are significant nursing responsibilities.

Prognosis

Male children survive much longer than females. Anticipated survival for sufferer of this condition is about 30 years.

Diseases of Gastrointestinal System and Liver

16

- Diarrheal Diseases
- Dysentery
- Malabsorption Syndrome
- Ulcerative Colitis
- Hypertropic Pyloric Stenosis
- Esophageal Atresia with Tracheoesophageal Fistula
- Gastroesophageal Reflux Disease
- Intestinal Obstruction
- Acute Abdomen
- Appendicitis
- Hirschsprung's Disease

- Anorectal Malformations
- Umbilical Malformations
- Hernia
- Rectal Prolapse
- Pancreatitis
- Jaundice (Icterus)
- Hepatomegaly
- Extrahepatic Biliary Atresia
- Liver Abscess
- Indian Childhood Cirrhosis

INTRODUCTION

Gastrointestinal problems are very common in childhood. Numbers of medical and surgical problems are found among children. GI disturbances are influenced by problems of liver and pancreas. Digestion, absorption and metabolism are the combined actions of gastrointestinal and hepatopancreative system. Functions of GI systems are also related to combined actions of many functional systems. Disturbances in any one, affects GI system leading to various problems. For example, diarrhea develops due to increased overload of fluid from small intestines into the colon following maldigestion and active secretions. Defect of intestinal mucosal immunity may lead to intestinal infections. Intestinal obstruction follows loss of normal intestinal motility. Problems of digestion and absorption may cause abdominal complaints, failure to thrive and weight loss.

Gastrointestinal problems are manifested commonly with vomiting, diarrhea or constipation, pain abdomen, anorexia, nausea, abdominal distension, etc. Problems of maldigestion

and malabsorption are presented as poor general health and growth retardation. Fluid electrolyte imbalance, circulatory disturbances, renal disorders, GI bleeding, nutritional deficiency diseases may develop in association with GI disorders.

Liver diseases are manifested with common symptoms like jaundice, itching, abdominal pain, dark colored urine, clay-colored stool, abdominal distension and fluid retention. Nonspecific features like nausea, vomiting, malaise and neuropsychiatric symptoms like confusion, alteration of sensorium, sleep disturbances are commonly found. There may be hepatomegaly, endocrinal abnormalities and renal dysfunction in addition with liver disease.

Special diagnostic procedures related to GI diseases include, barium meal, endoscopy, esophagoscopy, mucosal biopsy, pH monitoring, stool examination, enzyme estimation, USG, abdominal X-ray, etc. Investigations for liver diseases include liver function tests, liver biopsy, enzyme analysis, barium swallow, USG, plain X-ray abdomen, CT scan, MRI, radionuclide scanning, cholangiography, ERCP (Endoscopic retrograde cholangio-pancreatography), etc.

DIARRHEAL DISEASES

Diarrheal diseases rank among the top three causes of childhood death in the developing countries. On an average a child suffers from about 12 episodes of diarrhea, 4 such episodes occurring during the very first year of life. Existance of malnutrition makes the child very much vulnerable to diarrheal diseases.

Diarrhea is defined as the passage of loose, liquid or watery stools, more than three times per day. The recent change in consistency and character of stool rather than number of stools is more important. Especially in children one large amount watery motion may constitute diarrhea.

'Acute diarrhea' is an attack of loose motion with sudden onset which usually lasts 3 to 7 days but may last up to 10 to 14 days. It is caused by an infection of the large intestine, but may be associated with infection of gastric mucosa and small intestine. The term 'acute gastroenteritis' (AGE) is most frequently used to describe acute diarrhea.

Chronic diarrhea is termed when the loose motion is occurring for 3 weeks or more. It is usually related to underlying organic diseases with or without malabsorption.

Diarrhea with watery stools and visible blood in the stools is called as dysentery.

Persistent diarrhea refers to the episodes of acute diarrhea that last for 2 weeks or more and may be due to infective origin.

Epidemiology

Diarrhea is a major public health problem in India, among children below the age of 5 years. About one-third of total hospitalized children are due to diarrheal diseases and 17 percent of all deaths in indoor pediatric patients are related to this condition. The morbidity rate in terms of diarrhea episodes per year per child under the age of 5 years is about 1.7. Diarrheal diseases cause a heavy economic burden on health services.

Agent Factors

Diarrhea is mostly infectious. A large numbers of organism are responsible for acute diarrhea. The infectious agents causing diarrhea with enteric infection include the followings:

- *Viruses:* Rotavirus, adenovirus, enterovirus, norwalk group viruses, measles virus, etc.
- *Bacteria: Campylobacter jejuni, E.coli, Shigella, Salmonella, Cholera vibrio, Vibrio parahemolyticus,* etc.
- *Parasites: E. histolytica, G. lamblia, Cryptosporidium, H. nana, malaria,* etc.
- *Fungi: Candida albicans.*

Diarrhea may occur due to spread of infection by parenteral route from other infections like pneumonia, tonsilitis, upper respiratory infections, otitis media, urinary tract infection, etc. Other important causes of diarrhea are related to dietary or nutritional factors, e.g. over feeding, under feeding or malnutrition, food allergy and food poisoning. Some drugs (antibiotics) also can cause diarrhea.

Noninfectious causes of diarrhea are congenital anomalies of GI tract, malabsorption syndrome, inflammatory bowel disease, immunodeficiency conditions, inappropriate use of laxative and purgatives, emotional stress and excitement.

Reservoir of infection: Man is the main reservoir of enteric pathogens, so most transmission originates from human factors. For some enteric pathogens and viral agents animals are important reservoir.

Host factors: The disease is the most common in children especially those between 6 months to 2 years. The incidence is highest during weaning period, i.e. 6 to 11 months of age. It occurs due to combined effects of reduced maternal antibodies, lack of active immunity and introduction of contaminated food or direct spread through child's hands. Diarrhea is more common in artificial feeding, specially with contaminated cow's milk or unhygienic preparation of tin milk. Malnourished children are more prone to diarrhea. Malnutrition leads to infection and infection leads to diarrhea, which is a vicious cycle, as diarrhea is a major contributor of malnutrition. The predisposing factors of diarrhea include prematurity, immunodeficiency conditions, lack of personal hygiene, inadequate food hygiene, incorrect infant feeding practices, illiteracy, poor socioeconomic status, etc.

Environmental factors: Bacterial diarrhea is more frequently occur in summer and rainy season, whereas viral diarrhea (specially rotavirus) found in winter. Diarrheal diseases are commonly seen in unhygienic environment.

Mode of transmission is mainly feco-oral route. It is water-borne, food-borne disease or may transmit via fingers, fomites, flies or dirt.

Types of Diarrhea

Secretory Diarrhea

It is caused by external or internal secretagogue (cholera toxin, lactase deficiency). It has tendency to be watery, voluminous and persistent, even if no oral feeding is allowed. There is decrease absorption and increased secretion.

Osmotic Diarrhea

It is due to ingestion of poorly absorbed solute (alcohol, sorbitol) or maldigestion or a small bowel defect. It tends to be watery and acidic with reducing substances.

Motility Diarrhea

It is associated with increased or delayed motility of the bowel. There is decreased transit time or stasis of bacteria leading to overgrowth.

Pathophysiology

The pathogenic organisms produce diarrhea in the susceptible host with following mechanisms:

a. Adhesion to the intestinal mucosal wall by localized or diffuse adherence, e.g. enteropathogenic *E. coli* infection.
b. Elaboration of exotoxin as in secretory diarrhea, e.g. enterotoxigenic *E. coli*, *Vibrio cholerae* infection.
c. Mucosal invasion as in exudative diarrhea, e.g. entero-invasive *E. coli*, *Shigella*, *Salmonella* infection.

Diarrhea results in dehydration and dyselectrolytemia due to loss of water and electrolytes in loose stools. Diarrheal fluid losses are mainly from extracellular fluid (ECF) compartment, i.e. from blood, interstitial fluid and secretions. Due to loss of sodium in loose motions there is fall in osmolality of ECF which leads to fluid movement from ECF to ICF. This is manifested as loss or impairment of skin elasticity. Depletion of ECF compartment leads to reduction of blood volume which results in peripheral circulatory failure, oliguria, anuria, renal failure and shock.

Loss of potassium in stools results in hypokalemia and presented as abdominal distension hypotonia and ECG changes. Loss of bicarbonate in stools leads to acidemia with acidotic deep and rapid respiration.

Diarrheal loss of nutrients, presence of anorexia and inadequate food intake result in undernutrition and susceptibility to further infections. Impaired intestinal absorption causes loss of macro- and micronutrients, leading to deficiency conditions. There is loss of vitamin 'A' during diarrheal episodes.

Clinical Manifestations

The clinical presentations of diarrheal diseases may vary with severity, specific cause and type of onset.

Dehydration is the important life-threatening feature which is usually associated with diarrhea. It should be assessed accurately for the appropriate management. Assessment of diarrheal dehydration is given in Table 16.1.

Diarrhea stools are usually loose or watery in consistency. It may be greenish or yellowish-green in color with offensive smell. It may contain mucus, pus or blood and may expelled

Table 16.1: Assessment of dehydration

		A	B	C
1.	Ask about			
	• Diarrhea	– Less than 4 liquid stools per day	– 4 to 10 liquid stools per day	– More than 10 liquid stools per day
	• Vomiting	– None or a small amount	– Some	– Very frequent
	• Thirst	– Normal	– Greater than normal	– Unable to drink
	• Urine	– Normal	– A small amount and dark	– No urine for 6 hours
2.	Look at			
	• Condition	– Well, alert	– Restless, irritable or sleepy, unwell	– Lethargic or unconscious, floppy
	• Eyes	– Normal	– Sunken	– Very sunken and dry
	• Tears	– Present	– Absent	– Absent
	• Mouth and tongue	– Moist	– Dry	– Very dry
	• Breathing	– Normal	– Faster than normal	– Very fast and deep
3.	Feel			
	• Skin pinch	– Goes back quickly	– Goes back slowly	– Goes back very slowly
	• Pulse	– Normal	- Faster than normal	- Very fast, weak or cannot feel
4.	Decide degree of dehydration	– The patient has *no signs of dehydration*	– If the patient has two or more signs including at least one sign there is *some dehydration*	– If the patient has two or more signs including at least one sign there is *severe dehydration*

with force, preceded by abdominal pain. Frequency of stools varies from 2 to 20 per day or more.

The child may have low-grade fever, thirst, anorexia with intermittent vomiting and abdominal distention. Behavioral changes like irritability, restlessness, weakness, lethargy, sleepyness, delirium, stupor and flaccidity are usually present. Physical changes like loss of weight, poor skin turgor, dry mucous membranes, dry lips, pallor, sunken eyes, depressed fontanelles are also usually found. The vital signs are changed as low blood pressure, tachycardia, rapid respiration, cold limbs and collapse. There is decreased or absent urinary output. Convulsions and loss of consciousness may also present in some children with diarrheal diseases.

Diagnosis

Physical examination with through history of illness and assessment of degree of dehydration are important diagnostic criterias for prompt initiation of management.

Stool examination can be done for routine and microscopic study and identification of causative organisms. Blood examination can be performed to detect electrolyte imbalance, acid-base disturbances, hematocrit value, TC, DC, ESR, etc. The suspected associated cause should be ruled out for adequate management.

Management

Rehydration Therapy

The management of diarrhea in a vast majority of children is best done with ORS (Oral Rehydration Salts) solution and continued feeding. Replacement of fluids by rehydration therapy is the principal measure. It can be provided by ORT (Oral rehydration therapy) or intravenous fluid therapy. Table 16.2 shows standard formulation of ORS as recommended by WHO and approved by Government of India.

Instruction

- To be diluted in one liter of potable water.
- Mix entire content of the packet in one liter of water
- ORS solution to be used within 24 hours of preparation.

Table 16.2: Ingredients of oral rehydration salts

Component	Content per liter water
• Sodium chloride	3.5 gm
• Potassium chloride	1.5 gm
• Sodium citrate	2.9 gm
• Glucose anhydrous	20.0 gm

Oral rehydration therapy means drinking of solution of clean water, sugar and mineral salts to replace the water and salt lost from the body during diarrhea, especially when accompanied by vomiting, i.e. gastroenteritis. ORT is beneficial in three stages of diarrheal disease, i.e. (a) Prevention of dehydration (b) rehydration of the dehydrated child and (c) maintenance of hydration after severely dehydrated patient has been rehydrated with IV fluid therapy. ORT is provided with ORS solution and home available fluid (HAF), i.e. fruit juices, tender coconut water, dal-soup, sarbat (with sugar, salt and lemon), weak tea, etc.

a. The child with loose motion having *no dehydration* can be treated at home. There are three rules for treating diarrhea at home, which should be explained to the mother. The rules are:
    - Give the child more fluids than usual to prevent dehydration, with HAF and ORS, until the diarrhea stops.
    - Give the child plenty of food to prevent undernutrition. Continue breastfeeding frequently. Offer food at least 6 times a day with cereals, pulses, vegetables, meat or fish, vegetable oil, fresh fruit juices or mashed banana, etc.
    - Take the child to the health worker/health center, if the child does not get better in 3 days or develops any of the followings many watery stools, repeated vomiting, marked thirst, eating or drinking poorly, fever or blood in the stool.

Demonstration of ORS preparation and how to give ORS to the child are very important responsibility of the nurses. ORS packets should be available easily or to be supplied from the health center.

b. When the child is having diarrhea with *some dehydration*, management should be done under supervision of health worker with ORS. The approximate amount of ORS solution to be given in the first 4 hours are as follows:
    - Age less than 4 months or weight less than 5 kg—200 to 400 mL.
    - Age 4 to 11 months or weight 5 to 7.9 kg—400 to 600 mL.
    - Age 12 to 23 months or weight 8 to 10.9 kg—600 to 800 mL.
    - Age 2 to 4 years or weight 11 to 15.9 kg—800 to 1200 mL.
    - Age 5 to 14 years or weight 16 to 29.9 kg—1200 to 2200 mL.
    - Age 15 years or older or weight 30 kg or more to 2200 to 4000 mL.

After 4 hours of rehydration therapy the child should be reassess for degree of dehydration. If there is no signs of dehydration the child should be managed at home with necessary instructions to the mother. If the signs of severe dehydration have appeared the child should be admitted in the hospital for IV fluid therapy. During ORS therapy, if the child is having puffy eyelids, then ORS should be stopped and plain water and breastfeeding to be given.

c. The child with *severe diarrheal dehydration* should be treated quickly. Intravenous fluid to be started immediately with Ringer-lactate solution 100 mL/kg, (or, if not available, normal saline to be used). If the patient can drink, ORS to be given by mouth about 5 mL/kg/hour. Ringer-lactate to be infused at first 30 mL/kg in one hour and then 70 mL/kg in 5 hours for infants. In older children, it should be given first 30 mL/kg in 30 minutes and then 70 mL/kg in 2.5 hours. The patient should be reassess every one to two hours. More rapid I/V fluid to be given if hydration is not improving. When the patient's condition improves, gradually I/V fluid to be stopped, then ORS and Oral feeding to be given according to child's tolerance.

Symptomatic Management

Symptomatic management of vomiting, fever, convulsion and abdominal distension to be done with specific drugs. Supportive nursing care to be provided with routine and need-based care.

Chemotherapy

Routine use of antibiotics is not favored by the experts. Bacterial or protozoal diarrhea can be treated with specific drugs. Ampicillin, nalidoxic acid, norfloxacin, ciprofloxcin, furazolidine, metronidazole can be used.

Dietary Management

Dietary management is a vital aspect of treatment for the children with diarrheal diseases. Diet to be planned to prevent malnutrition and allow normal nutritional requirement. Food items may include energy rich food with rice, potatoes, wheat, pulses, vegetables oil, curd, fish, meat, fruits and vegetables. Foods rich in fats and sugar, high fiber content foods and soft drinks should be avoided. Breastfeeding to be continued during diarrheal episodes even along with ORS. Cereal mixture like rice-milk, dalia- sagu, or khichri can be given to the infants more than 6 months of age. Hygienic measures to be followed during preparation and serving of foods. If the infant is nonbreast-fed, cow's or buffalo's milk should not be diluted with water. Feeding to be given in small quantity frequently, every 2 to 3 hours.

Nursing Management

Nursing management to be done based on nursing assessment. It includes appropriate history of illness, thorough physical examination and assessment of dehydration. Nature and frequency of stools, type of onset, length of illness and associated symptoms to be evaluated to formulate the nursing diagnoses. The important nursing diagnoses are:

- Fluid volume deficit related to diarrhea.
- Risk for cross-infection related to infective loose motions.
- Potential to altered skin integrity related to frequent passage of stools.
- Altered nutritional status, less than body requirement related to malabsorption and poor oral intake.
- Fear and anxiety related to illness and hospital procedures.
- Knowledge deficit related to causes of diarrhea and its prevention.

Nursing Interventions

- Restoring fluid and electrolyte balance by ORS, IV fluid therapy, intake and output recording and checking of vital signs.
- Prevention of spread of infection by good hand washing practices, hygienic disposal of stools, care of diapers, general cleanliness and universal precautions.
- Preventing skin breakdown by frequent change of diaper, keeping the perianal area dry and clean, avoiding scratching and rubbing of irritated skin and use of protective barrier cream.
- Providing adequate nutritional intake by appropriate dietary management.
- Reducing fear and anxiety by explanation, reassurance, answering questions and providing necessary informations.
- Giving health education for prevention of diarrhea, home management of diarrheal diseases, importance of ORS, dietary management, hygienic practices, medical help, etc.

Preventive Measures

The important preventive measures are improvement of food hygiene, personal hygiene and environmental hygiene. These include safe water, adequate sewage disposal, hand washing practices, clean utensil, avoidance of exposures of food to dust and dirt, fly control, washing of fruits and vegetables, etc. Avoidance of bottle feeding is most significant practice needed for prevention of diarrhea. Boiling or filtering to be practiced for safe drinking water.

Prevention of LBW and prematurity, exclusive breast-feeding, appropriate weaning practices, balanced diet, immunization are significant aspects of child care which prevents malnutrition and diarrheal episodes.

Complications

The life-threatening complication of diarrhea is dehydration and its consequences. Other complications are hypovolemic shock, renal failure, paralytic ileus, thromboembolism, CCF, convulsions, overhydration, super-added infection, hypoglycemia, consumptive coagulopathy, toxic megacolon, malnutrition, growth retardation and mental subnormalities.

Prognosis

Prognosis of diarrheal diseases depends upon age, nutritional status, causative factors, severity of illness, presence of complication and initiation of management.

- Mortality is higher in neonates and infants than the older children.
- Malnourished children are having poor prognosis and greater mortality.
- Antibiotic resistant type *E. coli* and *Shigella* cause very severe illness and poor prognosis.
- Presence of severe dehydration, electrolyte imbalance and pneumonia have poor prognosis.
- Early diagnosis with prompt and appropriate management helps in good prognosis.

DYSENTERY

Dysentery is characterized by passage of blood, mucus and pus in loose stools accompanied by fever, crampy abdominal pain and tenesmus (false desire to pass stools). The onset is usually sudden and may associated with toxemia and exhaustion. This condition is different than the passage of blood per anus due to anal or rectal lesions.

Dysentery is one of the major public health problem in India. It is found in two forms, i.e. (a) bacterial or bacillary dysentery and (b) protozoal or amebic dysentery.

Bacillary Dysentery (Shigellosis)

Bacillary dysentery is an acute infection of the large intestine caused by the bacteria of genus *Shigella*. The disease is more common in children below 10 years of age. It is prevalent throughout the world and more endemic in tropical countries among the people living with poor sanitation.

Epidemiology

The causative agent is *Shigella*, a nonmotile, nonflagellate rodshaped organism. It is subdivided into 4 groups— (1) Group-A, *Shigella shiga* or *dysenteriae*, (ii) Group-B, *Shigella flexneri* or *paradysenteriae*, (iii) Group-C, *Shigella boydii* and (iv) Group–D, *Shigella sonei*. There are about 30 serotypes of Group A, B, C and D which are responsible for serious disease.

These organisms affect the children living in the place with poor sanitation. Severity of disease depends upon general health and nutritional status of the child. It is more severe in debilitated child.

The disease is found mainly in late summer. The mode of transmission is feco-oral route which is influenced by poor personal hygiene, lack of environmental hygiene causing breeding of flies, consumption of contaminated water, ice, milk and other foods. The disease spreads through carriers or mild cases specially by food-handlers. Incubation period is 1 to 7 days with an average of 4 days.

Pathology

The organisms enter through contaminated food and water and then invade and penitrate the epithelial cells of the intestine. They multiply in the submucosa and lamina propria. Local inflammation and superficial ulcer develop mainly in the colon which may bleed and produce clinical features.

Clinical Manifestations

The clinical features may present with mild bowel upset to fulminant dysentery with toxemia and dehydration. The onset is acute with fever, abdominal colic, vomiting, tenesmus and diarrhea with blood, mucus and pus. The child may have headache, drowsiness, weakness and prostration. The condition may be complicated with fluid-electrolyte imbalance, shock, coma and convulsions.

The *diagnosis* is confirmed by routine stool examination which shows pus cells and RBCs. Stool culture helps to detect the offending organism. Blood examination reveals marked leukocytosis.

Management

The specific antibiotic therapy to be administered with sensitive drugs, i.e. ampicillin, cotrimoxazole, nalidixic acid, ciprofloxacin, etc. for 5 to 7 days.

The symptomatic management includes IV fluid therapy, antipyretics, antispasmodics and antiemetics. ORS is important for those having no vomiting. Antimortility drugs may decrease frequency of motions but delay excretion of *Shigella* and are best avoided. Blood transfusion may be needed.

Planning of diet for this patient is very important. Buttermilk, rice water, albumin water, apple juice, carrot juice may be allowed in acute stage. Gradually soft food to be given as frequent small amount feeding with boiled rice, eggs, vegetables, etc. The young children should have frequent breastfeeding.

Preventive Measures

Consumption of safe water, maintenance of good personal hygiene and food hygiene along with improvement of environmental sanitation are the essential aspects of preventive measures. Control of carriers and treatment of the infected child should be done promptly. Health education is very important for creating awareness about the preventive measures of dysentery because no vaccine is available till now.

Complications

Various complications may develop in a case of dysentery. They include rectal prolapse, anemia, hypoproteinemia, malnutrition, arthritis, pneumonia, otitis media, vaginitis, hemolytic uremic syndrome, Reiter's syndrome and chronic shigellosis.

Prognosis

Prognosis is usually good in early diagnosis, prompt treatment and absence of complications. Less blood in stools, fewer stools, no fever and normal activity in first two days indicate better response to therapy.

Amebic Dysentery

See Chapter 14 for detail.

MALABSORPTION SYNDROME

Malabsorption syndrome is a group of disorders marked by subnormal absorption of dietary constituents and thus excessive loss of nutrients in the stools, which may be a defect in digestion or a mucosal abnormality or lymphatic obstruction. It is characterized by the association of chronic diarrhea, abdominal distension and FTT.

The clinical features develop due to poor absorption of nutrients in the small intestine particularly absorption of fats. Poor absorption of other nutrients including carbohydrates, minerals and proteins may also occur.

Causes

Malabsorption occurs due to several causes including gall-bladder and pancreatic diseases, lymphatic obstruction, vascular impairment and bowel resection. It is related to mild-to-moderate steatorrhea and may found in PEM, iron deficiency anemia and intestinal parasitosis. Severe steatorrhea is found due to cystic fibrosis, celiac disease and tropical sprue.

Clinical Manifestations

Malabsorption syndrome is presented with chronic diarrhea, abdominal distension and failure to thrive. Other associated features are flatulence, anorexia, fatigue, loss of weight and direct consequence of malabsorption which leads to malnutrition and growth failure. Chronic diarrhea is presented as abnormal stools which continues or recurrently occurs over several months. Stools may be loose and bulky in celiac disease, pasty and yellowish in exocrine pancreatic insufficiency. It may be liquid as water and mistaken for urine in infants with congenital chloride diarrhea or passed with noise and flatus is case of sugar intolerance. Non-specific chronic diarrhea in toddlers is presented as mucus containing, foul smelling stools.

Malabsorption and chronic diarrhea is manifested in three major categories, i.e. impaired digestion, intestinal malabsorption and carbohydrate malabsorption.

Impaired Digestion

Impaired digestion due to exocrine pancreatic insufficiency also results in chronic diarrhea and malabsorption. It also occurs due to cystic fibrosis, lipase deficiency, bile-duct atresia and Crohn's disease. It is manifested as frequent loose pasty, greasy stools with undigested fat and offensive cheesy smell. Massive steatorrhea occurs most frequently in exocrine pancreatic insufficiency.

Intestinal Malabsorption

Intestinal malabsorption can be presented with chronic diarrhea as loose or liquid stools, often with an acidic smell. These patients have steatorrhea abnormal D-xylose test and abnormal intestinal histology. This condition is usually associated with celiac disease, food protein sensitivity (cow's milk, wheat, etc.), giardiasis, immunodeficiency, tropical enteropathy, malnutrition and bacterial overgrowth.

Carbohydrate Malabsorption

Carbohydrate malabsorption may be presented as chronic diarrhea due to fermentation. It occurs due to congenital deficiency of mucosal enzymes for digesting mono- or disaccharides. It is presented with liquid acidic loose stools which is usually passed with flatus. Volume of stools is variable.

Investigations

History of illness and characteristic stool are suggestive of diagnosis. General health and appearance are important clue. The diagnosis is confirmed by repeated routine stool examination, fecal fat studies, D-xylose test, intestinal biopsy, and specific testes like sweat chloride test for cystic fibrosis, exocrine pancreatic function test in steatorrhea, serology for celiac disease, breath analysis for carbohydrate malabsorption and lactose tolerance test, etc. Radiology like barium meal study help to detect structural problems. Serum IgA, antigliadin antibodies represent reliable screening test for celiac disease.

Management

Management depends upon underlying cause and promotion of adequate nutrition intake considering the specific defect. Symptomatic control of diarrhea is desirable.

In celiac disease, a strict gluten free diet is the cornerstone of management. Rice and maize are nontoxic and act as wheat substitutes.

In cystic fibrosis, the diet is introduced gradually with simple nutrients which are tolerated. Diet should be planned with food items rich in protein and sugar. Vegetable fats rich in polyunsaturated fatty acid are preferred to the animal fats. Pancreatic supplements, antacids, sodium bicarbonate and antihistamine are essential. Suitable antibiotics, additional salt during summer months and prostaglandin analogue are used. Breathing exercises with chest physiotherapy are encouraged to prevent pulmonary complications. Gene therapy is now available for cystic fibrosis.

Treatment of carbohydrate malabsorption consists of excluding glucose and galactose from diet. A period of intravenous nutrition is usually indicated in serious cases.

Nursing Management

Nursing management should be planned according to findings of nursing assessment. The important assessment includes daily intake and output, daily weight, vital signs, serum electrolytes and GI functions as frequency and characteristics of stools with other related clinical features. Nursing interventions should emphasis on:

- Improvement of nutritional status by appropriate diet planning and supplementation of deficient nutrients or substituting them.
- Restoration of fluid and electrolyte balance by oral and parenteral therapy.
- Continuous monitoring and recording of patient's condition.
- Relief of pain by medications, Fowler's position and comfort. Analgesics, antiflatulents and antidiarrheal agents are administered as prescribed.
- Maintenance of skin integrity specially of perianal area (drying, application of ointment locally).
- Health education to the parent about general cleanliness, nutrition, hydration, danger signs, home care and follow-up for necessary medical help.
- Relief of fear and anxiety about long-term illness and hospitalization by appropriate explanation, reassurance and necessary support.

ULCERATIVE COLITIS

Ulcerative colitis is a chronic inflammatory bowel disease (IBD) with overwhelming gastrointestinal presentations and some systemic manifestations. Other IBDs are Crohn's disease or regional ileitis and intermediate colitis.

Ulcerative colitis is a chronic diffuse nonspecific inflammation of the colonic mucosa. It is manifested as recurrent bloody diarrhea and begins in childhood and adolescence. It may also involve rectal mucosa. The exact cause is not known. The disease may occur due to immunological abnormalities in genetically vulnerable children. Psychosomatic factors seems to play an important role in the clinical course of the disease.

Clinical Manifestations

The onset of the disease may be insidious or acute with high fever, prostration and fulminant bloody diarrhea with copious mucus. Other manifestations are fecal urgency and frequency, tenesmus, abdominal cramps, anorexia and weight loss. Abdominal tenderness and distention may present. Extra intestinal features (less common in children) include arthritis, erythema nodosum, pyoderma, iritis, hepatitis, hemolytic anemia, etc.

The disease may be complicated with peritonitis, intestinal perforation, megacolon, anal fistula and colo-rectal cancer (due to pseudo polyp). The child may found with FTT, nutritional deficiencies and growth retardation. The disease is characterized by recurrent exacerbations and asymptomatic during remissions over months to years.

Diagnosis

The diagnosis of the disease is confirmed by details history of illness, clinical examination, stool examination, barium enema, proctoscopy, sigmoidoscopy or colonscopic examination with mucosal biopsy.

Management

Management of ulcerative colitis is done with steroid therapy as anti-inflammatory drugs, sulfasalazine and immuno-suppressive drugs like 6 - MP, azathioprine, cyclosporine, with steroid sparing effects. Blood transfusion and tranquilizers may be needed for some children.

Nutritional support is very important in treatment of children with the disease. High calorie low-residue diet with liberal amount of fluids, vitamins and minerals supplementation is required.

Supportive care include skin care (especially perianal area), psychotherapy, weight recording, regular follow-up with necessary health education.

Surgical management may be needed, if the condition is not responding to medical management and in complications like perforation, and colonic cancer.

HYPERTROPIC PYLORIC STENOSIS

Hypertropic pyloric stenosis is one of the common surgical problems in infancy. It may be familial and usually found in first born male child.

Hypertropic pyloric stenosis is a marked and progressive overgrowth or enlargement of circular muscle fibers of pylorus causing partial or total obstruction of the stomach outlet due to narrowing of the lumen (Fig. 16.1).

Etiology

The exact cause of hypertropic pyloric stenosis is not yet fully understood. Previously it was thought to be a congenital problem. But it is now known that the condition is not a congenital problem but an acquired condition.

The etiological factors are considered as maternal stress in last trimester, elevated prostaglandin level, deficiency of nitric acid and immature pyloric ganglion cells with abnormal muscle innervation. The local enteric innervation is involved and primarily argyrophilic nitrergic neurons are affected.

Pathology

The circular musculature of the pylorus is thickened and increased in size as the shape and size of 'Olive'. The pyloric muscles become elongated and enlarged causing narrowing of the lumen. Stomach becomes dilated. Gastric emptying become delayed.

Clinical Manifestations

Clinical onset of the condition usually found in 3 to 12 weeks of age. Initially occasional regurgitation may be found. Gradually vomiting increases in frequency and intensity. The

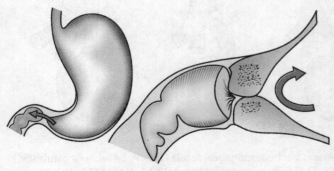

Fig.16.1: Hypertropic pyloric stenosis

characteristic projectile nonbilious vomiting occurs forcefully within 30 minutes of feeding. Vomitus contains milk and gastric juices but it may be blood stained and coffee ground in color.

The child presents with other classical features like constant hunger, irritability, failure to thrive with loss of weight, constipation, decreased quantity of stools and urine output. The child is usually lethargic with shallow respiration. Starvation diarrhea as greenish stools, jaundice and gastric hemorrhage occasionally may be present. Dehydration due to lack of fluid intake is a common feature.

The important clinical findings include epigastric fullness with visible peristalsis in the upper abdomen from left to right and a palpable olive shaped firm mass (2–3 cm) in epigastrium or right hypochondrium.

Complications

The common complications are fluid and electrolyte imbalance (especially alkalosis and dehydration), hematemesis, jaundice and tetany.

Diagnosis

History of illness and clinical examination is diagnostic. Plain X-ray abdomen, barium meal X-ray, USG, help to confirm the diagnosis. Blood examination for Hb%, serum electrolyte and urine examination may be done before surgery.

Management

There is no medical management of the condition. Surgical management is the choice. *Ramstedt's pyloromyotomy* is done at the age of 4 to 5 weeks after the initial conservative management of dehydration and dyselectolytemia. In case of pylorospasm, gastric lavage with normal saline, atropine methyl nitrate and metoclopramide may be used.

Nursing Management

Preoperative nursing management should emphasis on maintenance of fluid and electrolyte balance along with nutritional intake by breastfeeding, if not contraindicated. Relief of parental anxiety and routine preoperative care are important. Nasogastric aspiration may be needed to reduce vomiting. During feeding, baby should be placed in upright position on slightly right side. Small frequent feeding to be given. Gentle handling of the baby is essential. Measures to be taken for prevention of hospital acquired infection. Continuous monitoring of infants condition is very important. Recording of vital signs, hydration status, body weight, vomiting, stool, urine and signs of complications should be done frequently. Parental involvement in baby care to be promoted, especially for hygienic care.

Postoperative nursing management should be done with basic postanesthetic care and routine care of an operated patent. Special attention to be provided on oral feeding, usually after 8 to 12 hours of surgery, small frequent feeds with expressed breast milk to be started in a stepwise manner. Initially feeding can be started with 1 or 2 teaspoon of clear solution (5% glucose) given every 2 hours for about 8 hours, after the child comes out of anesthesia, provided the baby does not start vomiting. After feeding baby should be placed with elevating the head for 45 to 60 minutes and on the right side of the baby.

Routine postoperative care to be provided with warmth, feeding, wound care, medications, hygienic care, emotional support to parents and health education with discharge advice for continuation of care at home and for follow-up. Baby is usually discharged on 3rd or 4th postoperative day. Prognosis is good, if operated timely before complications start. Postoperative complications may develop as infections, fluid-electrolyte imbalance, persistent obstruction and duodenal perforation.

ESOPHAGEAL ATRESIA WITH TRACHEOESOPHAGEAL FISTULA

Esophageal atresia (EA) is failure of the esophagus to form a continuous passage from the pharynx to the stomach during embryonic development. It is usually asociated with tracheoesophageal fistula (TEF). TEF is an abnormal connection between trachea and esophagus. These disorders are commonly found among premature or LBW infants and mothers having polyhydramnios. Congenital heart diseases or other GI anomalies may present along with these conditions.

Etiology

The exact cause of these anomalies is not known in most cases. Some factors influencing the incidence of the problems are heritable genetic factor, teratogenic stimuli and intra-uterine environment.

These anomalies may develop due to aberration or deviations of the septum between the espohagus and trachea or altered growth of septum between them. TEF results due to failure of growth along the septum and EA develops due to deficient growth of the dorsal wall. The failure of proper separation of the embryonic channel into the esophagus and trachea occurs during 4th and 5th weeks of gestational life.

Pathophysiology

The baby with TEF and EA is unable to swallow effectively which results in accumulation of saliva or feeds in upper esophageal pouch and aspiration in respiratory passage. Gastric secretions may regurgitate through distal fistula. Abdominal distention occurs due to air entering the lower esophagus through the fistula and passing into the stomach during crying. Respiratory distress may develop due to gastric distention and elevation of diaphragm.

Classification

EA with TEF can be classified as follows (Figs 16.2A to E):

a. Type-I: EA without fistula (8%). It is second most common type. There is no connection of esophagus to trachea. The upper (proximal) segment and lower (distal) segment of esophagus are blind.

b. Type-II: EA with TEF (upper). It is rare and found in less than 1 percent of all cases. Upper segment of esophagus open into trachea by a fistula. The distal or lower segment is blind.

c. Type-III: EA with TEF (lower) (80-90%). It is the most common type. In this condition, proximal or upper segment of the esophagus has blind end. The distal lower segment of esophagus connects into trachea by a fistula.

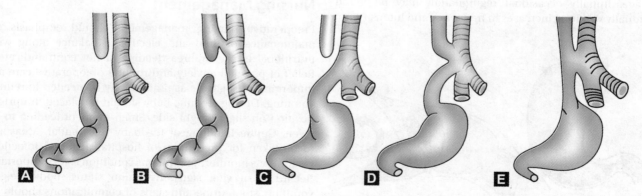

Figs16.2A to E: Five most common types of esophageal atresia (EA) and tracheoesophageal fistula (TEF): A. EA without fistula (8%); B. TEF (upper) with EA (1%); C. TEF (lower) with EA (80–90%); D. TEF both upper and lower (1%); E. H type TEF (4%)

d. Type-IV: EA with TEF both upper and lower segment. It is also rare (less than 1%). There is EA with fistula between both proximal and distal ends of trachea and esophagus.

e. Type-V: H-type TEF. It is found in about 4 percent of all cases and not usually diagnosed at birth. Both proximal/ upper and distal/lower segments of esophagus open into trachea by a fistula. No EA present.

Clinical Manifestations

The clinical features appear soon after birth. The baby presents with excessive salivation, (blowing bubbles), constant drooling, large amount of secretions form nose, coughing, gagging, choking and cyanosis. Intermittent unexplained cyanosis occurs due to laryngospasm caused by aspiration of accumulated saliva in blind pouch.

On the very first feed, after first or second swallow, the infant coughs, chokes or fluid returns out through nose and mouth. The infant struggles for breath and cyanosis occurs. Only abdominal distension and poor feeding may found in some infants.

Diagnosis

Clinical presentations arouse a strong suspicion. Simple technique can be done to diagnose the condition with plain catheter. Inability to pass catheter through nose or mouth into the stomach indicates blind pouch or atresia. Precautions to be taken to prevent coiling of catheter.

Antenatal diagnosis of the condition can be done by USG. Postnatal diagnostic procedures include USG, plain X-ray abdomen, chest X-ray or passing of radiopaque catheter through esophagus and confirming the anomalies by X-ray. Bronchoscopy also help to confirm the diagnosis. ECG and Echocardiogram can be done to detect associated cardiac anomalies.

Management

Immediate Management

Immediately after diagnosis, the infant should be managed with propped up position (30° angle) to prevent reflux of gastric secretion, and nothing per mouth, airway clearance O_2 therapy, IV fluid therapy, nasogastric tube aspiration nasogastric tube to be kept *in situ* and suctioning to be done frequently to prevent aspiration. The blind pouch to be washed with normal saline to prevent blocking of tube with thick mucus.

Gastrostomy is done to decompress the stomach and to prevent aspiration and afterwards to feed the infant.

Supportive care should include maintenance of nutritional requirements and warmth, prevention of infections, antibiotic therapy, respiratory support, detection and treatment of complications, continuous monitoring of patients condition, chest physiotherapy and postural drainage.

Surgical Management

The surgical correction of defect is done by end to end anastomosis with excision of the fistula by right posterolateral thoracotomy followed by intercostal chest drainage. This is done when the infant has more than 2 kg body weight and no pneumonia present and the baby is clinically stable.

Surgical correction can be done in stages with division of fistula. Gastrostomy is performed in initial stage followed by esophageal anastomosis or colonic transplant after one year. This staging is done in small premature or very sick neonates or with other associated congenital anomalies.

Other surgical interventions include cervical esophago-stomy, esophago-coloplasty and esophago-gastroplasty.

Nursing Management

Nursing assessment is very important to detect the condition immediate after birth or at first feed. Risk factors to be excluded by details history of the condition. Clinical features and problems to be assessed promptly for life-saving measures.

The important nursing diagnoses include the followings:

Preoperative
- Risk for aspiration related to esophageal abnormality.
- Risk for fluid volume deficit related to inadequate oral intake.
- Parental anxiety related to congenital anomalies of the neonate.

Postoperative
- Ineffective airway clearance related to surgical inter-ventions.
- Altered nutrition, less than body requirements related to inadequate oral intake.
- Pain related to surgical interventions.
- Risk for infections related to hospital procedures.
- Risk for injury related to complex surgery.
- Impaired tissue integrity related to postoperative drainage.
- Risk for altered parenting related to prolonged illness.
- Knowledge deficit related to home based long-term care.

Nursing Intervention

Nursing interventions are performed based on nursing diagnoses.

Preoperative interventions should emphasis on:

- Preventing aspirations by positioning, suctioning and nothing per month, thus reducing chance of respiratory infections.
- Preventing dehydration by IV fluid, intake and output recording, monitoring of vital signs and child's general health.
- Preventing infections by infection-control measures.
- Reducing parental anxiety by emotional support.

Postoperative interventions should emphasis on:

- Maintaining clear airway.
- Providing adequate feeding by IV fluid and/or gastro-stomy feeding.
- Reducing pain by analgesics and comfort measures.
- Maintaining chest tube drainage with necessary precautions.
- Preventing infections by general cleanliness, hygienic measures and administering antibiotics.
- Monitoring child's condition and detecting problems for early interventions.
- Stimulating parent-child bondage by parental partici-pation in care of the infant.
- Improving knowledge by necessary health education, encouraging questions and explaining the answers.

GASTROESOPHAGEAL REFLUX DISEASE

Gastroesophageal reflux (GER) is malfunction of the distal end of the esophagus resulting spontaneous effortless return of stomach contents into the esophagus.

It may be physiologic, below the age of one year, due to inadequate development of lower esophageal pressure regulation. After the age of one year, the GER can be considered as pathological and usually associated with inappropriate transient relaxation of lower esophageal sphincter. It may occur along with swallowing and pharyngeal contractions.

The cause of GER is mostly undetermined. The causes can be delayed neuromuscular development, physiological immaturity, cerebral defects, increased abdominal pressure and obesity. The associated conditions which can cause GER are supine position, coughing and wheezing in case of cystic fibrosis, bronchopulmonary dysplasia, asthma, indwelling orogastric or nasogastric tube, medications like theophyllin and mechanical ventilations.

Clinical Manifestations

The clinical features of GER vary in infants and older children.

In infants, the features are unexplained vomiting immediate after feeding, regurgitation, rumination, refusal to eat and features of dehydration. The infants also presents with irritability, excessive crying, sleep disturbances, arching and stiffening. Respiratory symptoms like cough, wheeze, stridor and pneumonia may found. Loss of weight or failure to gain weight is usual feature.

In older children features are noncardiac chest discom-fort, upper abdominal discomfort, chronic cough, stridor, nocturnal asthma, dysphagia, anemia, hemetemesis or melena.

Diagnosis

History of feeding behavior, presenting signs and symptoms are essential for diagnosis.

Barium swallow, esophageal pH monitoring, technetium scintigraphy, esophageal manometry, endoscopy and eso-phageal histology are useful diagnostic evaluation procedure to confirm the disease.

Management

Management to be planned to alleviate and relieve the symptoms and prevent complications. Medical and surgical management may be required.

Medical Management

1. *Positioning:* It helps to reduce the amount of reflux.
   a. Infants younger than 6 months should be placed on right lateral position during sleep, head of the crib should be raised at least 6 inches. The infant may also be held upright.
   b. Older children should be placed in head raised to 30° to 45° angle position. Avoid recumbent position after meal for at least 3 hours. Upright of semi-upright position during awaking is helpful.
2. *Feeding:* Special precautions to be taken during feeding of infants and older children.
   a. Infants to be given thickened feed in small amount frequently followed by appropriate positioning, to prevent the reflux.
   b. Older children should be allowed nothing per month 2 hours before bed time. Low fat diet, spicy and acidic foods (onion, citrus products, apple juice, tomato), esophageal irritants (chocolate, peppermint, passive smoke) and carbonated beverages should be avoided. Avoidance of obesity, tight or constricting clothing and NSAIDs at bedtime are also important measures. Chewing gum can be allowed to stimulate parotid secretions which increases esophageal clearance.
3. *Medications:* Antacids H_2-receptor antagonists (cimetidine), prokinetic drugs (metoclopramide) and proton pump inhibitors (omeprazole) can be given alone or in combination.

Surgical Management

If medical management fails even after 3 to 6 months course or in case of intractable respiratory disease, surgery is indicated.

Fundoplication (Nissen's operation) is most popular method. A gastric wrap procedure is done. Wrapping of the fundus around the lower esophageal sphincter (a 360° wrap) completely prevent reflux episodes.

Antroplasty or pyloroplasty may also be performed in some cases. Gastrostomy may be needed for feeding purposes or temporarily to decompress the stomach.

Nursing Management

Special nursing interventions to be performed as follows:
a. Preventing aspiration by positioning and appropriate feeding technique.
b. Maintaining fluid and electrolyte balance by IV fluid therapy, (whenever needed), intake and output recording and estimation of electrolyte level.
c. Providing adequate nutritional intake.
d. Continuous monitoring of vital signs, assessment of features of complications and necessary investigations.
e. Reducing fear of eating and modifying feeding schedule.
f. Providing preoperative and postoperative care as for abdominal surgery of children.
g. Providing emotional support.
h. Giving health education regarding, positioning, feeding, home-based care and follow-up.

Complications

The complications related to GER are associated with frequent and sustained reflux of acid gastric content. The possible complications are aspiration pneumonia, chronic esophagitis, failure to thrive, anemia, asthma, sudden infant death syndrome (SIDS), esophageal stricture and hiatal hernia.

INTESTINAL OBSTRUCTION

Intestinal obstruction is an interruption in the normal flow of intestinal contents through the intestine. The obstruction may occur in small or large intestine. It may be complete or partial obstruction and may be due to mechanical or paralytic cause. It may be found as congenital anomalies or as acquired conditions.

Causes of Intestinal Obstruction

Congenital Intestinal Obstruction

It is found as following conditions:

Intestinal atresia: Atresia of the intestine most commonly found in the duodenum. Other sites of obstruction are ileum, jejunum and colon. It can be found at multiple sites and may be complete or incomplete.

Malrotation of gut: It is incomplete rotation of the gut during intrauterine life (12th week), so that cecum comes to lie below pylorus, root of mesentery becomes very narrow, ascending and transverse colon become mobile and vulnerable to twisting in a clockwise direction. The rotation abnormalities are of two kinds: (a) Ladd's bands from the cecum pass to the posterior abdominal walls compressing the second part of duodenum and (b) the unfixed mesentery allow the small bowel to twist around it.

Meconium plug syndrome: Obstruction of lower colon by a thick plug of meconium, found in neonates.

Meconium ileus: It occurs due to inspissated putty like meconium plugging the lumen of the terminal ileum and cause obstruction. It occurs in lack of pancreatic enzymes and mucoviscidosis (cystic fibrosis).

Annular pancreas: The head of the pancreas compress the second part of the duodenum giving rise to an extrinsic form of obstruction.

Mickel's diverticulum: It is an occasional sacculation or appendage of the ileum, derived from an unobliterated yolk stalk. Diverticulum is circumscribed pouch or sac occurring normally or created by herniation of the lining mucus membrane through a tear in the muscular coat. Mickel's diverticulum is the most common remnant of the vitello-intestinal duct and situated in the anterior mesenteric border of the ileum anywhere from 10 cm to 1.2 m from the ileocecal junction. It may remain asymptomatic and may becomes symptomatic before 2 years of age. It can be complicated with bleeding, intestinal obstruction, inflammation as dirverticulitis and umbilical fistula.

Hirschsprung's disease or congenital megacolon. (see later on page no. 289).

Acquired Intestinal Obstruction

The important causes of acquired intestinal obstruction are:
1. *Intussusception:* It is telescoping of intestinal wall into itself. It is found as invagination or slipping of one part of intestine into another part just below it. In children, the most common site is ileocecal region (Fig. 16.3.)
2. Volvulus or twisted loop of intestine commonly occurs in sigmoid colon (Fig. 16.4.)
3. Tumor or hematoma as intrinsic or extrinsic to intestine.
4. Hernia and strangulation.
5. Stricture or stenosis of the intestine.
6. Inflammatory diseases—Ulcerative colitis, Crohn's disease, appendicitis.

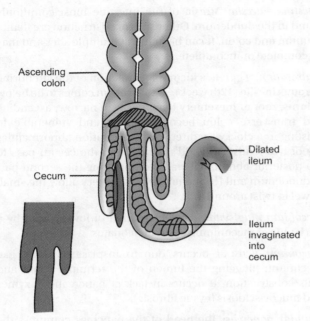

Fig.16.3: Intussusception

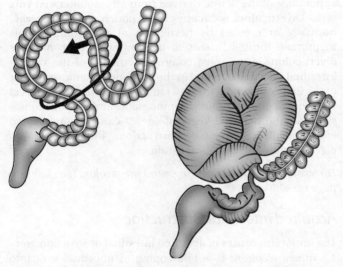

Fig.16.4: Volvulus of sigmoid colon (the counter clockwise twist)

7. Foreign body (e.g. coin) or fecal impaction or polyp.
8. Worm mass (commonly round worms) and amebiasis.
9. Paralytic ileus due to toxic or traumatic disturbances of autonomic nervous system leading to ineffective peristalsis by reduced motor activity.

Pathology

Obstruction leads to accumulation of gases and secretions above the blockage causing increase in intraluminal pressure. Venous pressure of the affected area increases leading to circulatory stasis and edema. Bowel necrosis and gangrene may develop due to tissue anoxia and compression of the arterial supply. Peritonitis develops due to passage of bacteria and toxins across the intestinal membrane.

Clinical Manifestations

The child with intestinal obstruction usually presents with abdominal colic (cramps), abdominal distension, bilious vomiting, absence of flatus and no passage of stool. Fever, drowsiness, dehydration and toxicity are also found in these children. There is increased bowel sound, which may reduce gradually. Minimal diffuse tenderness of abdomen may also present. The child may manifest with shock and respiratory distress.

There may be rectal passage of bloody mucus (red-currant jelly stool), sausage-shaped lump palpable in upper abdomen (in early stage) and cervix-like mass and blood in rectal examination. These features are diagnostic of intussusception.

Diagnosis

History of illness and physical examination help in clinical diagnosis. The diagnosis is confirmed by X-ray abdomen and chest, barium enema, proctoscopy, sigmoidoscopy or USG. Blood examination shows reduction of sodium, potassium and chloride level, elevated WBC count (in case of necrosis, strangulation and peritonitis) and elevated serum amylase level.

Management

Initial Management

Initial management is done with IV fluid therapy to correct fluid and electrolyte imbalance, and nasogastric suctioning to decompress the bowel. Analgesics and sedatives are administer to reduce pain and to provide comfort. Antibiotics to be given to treat and prevent infection. Causes and complications to be detected early and necessary management is planned to treat them promptly.

Surgical Management

Surgical management is done to relieve the obstruction. Laparotomy followed by specific surgery to be done.

a. Resection of bowel is done, for obstructing lesions or strangulated bowel, alongwith end-to-end anastomosis.
b. In malrotation of gut, cutting of Ladd's band and lengthening of the roots of the mesentry is done.
c. Enterotomy is performed for removal of foreign bodies in the intestine.
d. Closed bowel procedures may be done to reduce volvulus and intussusception or incarcerated hernia. Conservative hydrostatic reduction is performed in case of intussusception. Hypertonic enema is given to relieve the obstruction due to round worms mass.

Nursing Management

Nursing assessment to be done to detect the nature and location of pain, presence or absence of abdominal distension, flatus, vomiting, stools, obstipation, bowel sound, etc. General condition of the child should be assessed thoroughly especially vital signs, intake, output and level of consciousness. The following *nursing diagnoses* require special attention.

- Pain related to intestinal obstruction and abdominal distension.
- Risk for fluid and electrolyte imbalance related to vomiting, poor intake of fluid and diarrhea.
- Ineffective breathing related to abdominal distension.
- Potential to shock related to toxicity.
- Fear and anxiety related to severity of illness.
- Ineffective coping related to life-threatening symptoms.
- Knowledge deficit related to long-term care.

Nursing interventions should emphasize on the following aspects:

a. Providing rest and comfort.
b. Relieving pain by analgesics.
c. Maintaining fluid and electrolyte balance by IV fluid therapy and recording of intake and output.
d. Providing adequate respiration by relieving abdominal distension through nasogastric tube aspiration.
e. Reducing fear and anxiety by explanation reassurance and answering questions.
f. Maintaining normal bowel elimination.
g. Providing basic preoperative and postoperative care and administering prescribed medications.
h. Promoting effective coping with hospitalized care.
i. Giving informations and instructions for home-based long-term care.

ACUTE ABDOMEN

Acute abdomen is a common problem found in children due to various reasons. It requires immediate diagnosis and prompt management. Delay in initiation of management leads to serious complications.

Acute abdomen is an abnormal condition in which there is sudden and abrupt onset of severe abdominal pain lasting for 3 to 4 hours or more. It is also known as surgical abdomen.

Common Causes of Acute Abdomen

Related to Gastrointestinal System

i. Obstructive lesions—Intussusception, strangulated hernia, roundworm mass, bands, tumors, volvulus.
ii. Inflammatory lesions—Acute enteritis, acute appendicitis, nonspecific enterocolitis.

Related to Hepatobiliary System

i. Obstructive lesions— Gall stone, choledochal cyst.
ii. Inflammatory lesions—Acute hepatitis, acute acalculous cholecystitis.

Related to Urinary System

i. Obstructive lesions—Hydronephrosis, renal calculi.
ii. Inflammatory lesions—Acute pyelonephritis, acute cystourethritis.

Related to Pancreas

Acute pancreatitis, pseudopancreatic cyst.

Related to Reproductive System

Torsion of the testis in male, pelvic inflammatory disease (PID) in female.

Abdominal Pain with Uncertain Mechanism

Diabetes mellitus, mesenteric adenitis, measles in prodormal and eruptive stage, acute rheumatic fever at onset of disease.

Extra-abdominal Causes

Acute lower lobe pneumonia, pleurodynia (paroxysmal pain in the intercostal muscle), osteomyelitis of the spine, herpes-zoster infection, inflammation of muscle, tendons and joints adjacent to the abdomen.

Diagnosis

Details history of illness with presenting features are diagnostic of the condition. The history should include type and site of abdominal pain, presence of abdominal distension, types of vomiting (bilious or nonbilious), alteration of bowel habit, presence of jaundice, etc. Other details history related to past illness and present complaints are also important for the diagnostic evaluation.

Thorough physical examination to be done to assess the presence of dehydration, jaundice, tenderness and rigidity of abdomen, abdominal distension, exaggerated or absent bowel sound, absence or presence of liver dullness, etc. Rectal examination to be performed to identify problems of the area. Body weight and vital signs also to be checked.

Special investigations like X-ray abdomen, chest X-ray, USG and laboratory studies of blood, urine and stool to be done to diagnose the exact cause.

Management

1. Initial conservative management to be done with resuscitation of the child from shock and metabolic acidosis (if present). Intravenous fluid therapy, nasogastric tube aspiration, analgesics, antibiotics and other symptomatic treatment to be provided. Continuous monitoring of vital signs and abdominal signs along with other complicating features are needed.
2. Surgical interventions or medical management to be done according to the specific cause of acute abdomen. Supportive nursing care to be provided according to specific problem. Preoperative and postoperative management to be done according to nature of surgery.

APPENDICITIS

Appendicitis is the inflammation of the vermiform appendix caused by the obstruction of the intestinal lumen. It may occur due to fecalith, infection, stricture, foreign body or tumor. It is common surgical emergency in childhood and usually found in age group of 5 to 15 years.

Pathophysiology

Obstruction of the intestinal lumen results in edema, infection and ischemia. Collection of secretion inside the lumen leads to distension and pressure on the intramural blood vessels. Inflammation leads to ulceration and gangrene. Necrosis and perforation usually occur due to intraluminal tension. Ruptured appendix followed by peritonitis may develop following inflammatory changes:

Clinical Manifestations

Initially the child presents with classical triad symptoms of periumbilical pain followed by vomiting and fever. The pain usually starts in epigastrium and colicky in nature.

Later, within 2 to 12 hours pain shifts and localizes at right lower quadrant or McBurney's point in right iliac fossa and increases in intensity.

There may be some variations of site of pain depending upon the position of the appendix. In retrocecal appendix, pain may radiate to the right flank which may be mistaken as ureteric colic. In pelvic appendix, pain may radiate to lower abdomen. In appendicular perforation, pain becomes generalized. In peritonitis, the pain usually present over whole of the lower abdomen.

Other presenting features are anorexia, nausea and constipation. Diarrhea may occur occasionally. Rebound tenderness and involuntary guarding with generalized abdominal rigidity are found during abdominal examination. Positive Psoas sign and Rovsing's sign are suggestive of appendicitis.

Complications

The appendicitis can be complicated with ruptured appendix, intestinal perforation, paralytic ileus, peritonitis, pelvic abscess and subphrenic abscess.

Diagnosis

The diagnosis of acute appendicitis is done on the basis of detailed history and thorough clinical examination. Other investigative methods are useful in case of any doubt.
- Urine examination to be done to exclude urinary problems.
- Blood examination shows moderate leukocytosis.
- Abdominal X-ray helps to identify the presence of fecalith or perforation or intestinal obstruction.
- USG abdomen helps in the diagnosis of ruptured appendix or abscess formation.

Management

The treatment of acute appendicitis is mainly appendectomy and necessary symptomatic and supportive management. There is no role of conservative management, as the chance of perforation and peritonitis are very high in children.

Appendicular mass should be treated with IV antibiotics, fluid therapy and analgesics. Interval appendectomy is done if the mass undergoes resolution. Otherwise immediate exploration is indicated when fever and appendicular mass persist with increased abdominal pain.

Nursing interventions should emphasize on the basic preoperative and postoperative care including special attention on pain management and prevention of infections. Parents should be involved in care of the child. Emotional support to the child and parents is important in relation to surgery. Instructions and necessary informations should be given regarding continuation of care after discharge with special attention of operative area and follow-up.

HIRSCHSPRUNG'S DISEASE

Hirschsprung's disease is also called as congenital aganglionic megacolon. It occurs due to congenital absence of the parasympathetic ganglionic nerve cells, both in muscle layer or submucosal layer of distal colon and rectum, which result in extreme dilatation of the colon. It involves varying length and even the whole of the colon. Most commonly affect part is the rectosigmoid colon (Fig. 16.5).

The disease occurs due to unknown etiology and may be found as familial illness with genetic predisposition. It is commonly found in male child and about one in 5,000 births.

Pathophysiology

The disease develops due to an arrest in embryonic development affecting the migration of parasympathetic nerves in the intestine occurring before the 12th week of gestation.

The intrinsic ganglionic cells are absent in muscle layer (Aurbach's plexus) and in the submucosal layer (Meisner's plexus) of the intestine. These result in lack of coordination of the peristalsis causing functional obstruction with dilatation and hypertrophy of the proximal normal ganglionic colon.

Rectosigmoid colon is the most commonly affected and known as short segment disease. The long segment disease is less common which extend to the upper descending colon and possibly the transverse colon.

No peristalsis occurs in the affected part and it becomes spastic, contracted and narrowed. So no fecal material passes through it, thus leading to accumulation of fecal material above the affected portion. The colon, proximal to

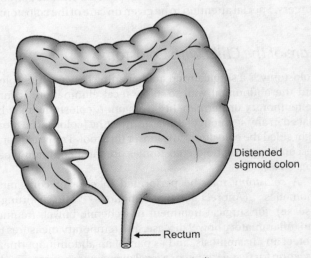

Fig.16.5: Hirschsprung's disease

Distended sigmoid colon

Rectum

the narrow affected part, is dilated and filled up with fecal material and gases. There is hypertropy of the muscular coat. Ulceration of mucosal layer may develop especially in neonates. Evacuation of fecal material and gases is prevented due to failure of internal rectal sphincter to relax, resulting abdominal distention and constipation.

Clinical Manifestations

Clinical presentations of Hirschsprung's disease depend upon the degree of involved part. The features vary in neonates and older children.

In neonates, the symptoms appear at birth of within 7 days. The baby usually presents with delayed passage of meconium. There may be no passage of meconium in the first 2 days of life with bile stained or fecal vomiting, abdominal distension and constipation. Sometimes, overflow type of diarrhea and dehydration may found in these children. The neonate may present with features of intestinal obstruction or failure to thrive.

In older children, the symptoms are not prominent at birth. The short segment disease is more common. The presenting features are history of obstipation (intractable constipation) at birth, progressive abdominal distension and visible peristaltic activity. Other features are anorexia, abdominal discomfort, irritability and constipation unresponsive to conventional remedies. The child usually present with absence of will to defecate and fecal soiling. There may be diarrhea alternating with constipation and presenting as ribbon-like, fluid-like or pellet stools.

The child may be complicated with gross malnutrition, anemia and failure to thrive. Many children present with mild constipation and related symptoms.

Diagnosis

History of illness and physical examination are very important clue in diagnosis of the conditon. Rectal examination is supportive to exclude aganglionic part which reveals a tight anal sphincter and empty rectum followed by an explosive gush of stool and flatus.

Plain X-ray abdomen helps to reveal severe gaseous distention of the bowel with multiple fluid levels and absence of air in the rectum. Ingestion of radioopaque markers measure intestinal transit time.

Barium enema shows a transition zone between the proximal dilated normal innervated colon and the distal narrow aganglionic colonic area.

Anorectal manometry reveals absence of relaxation reflex of internal sphincter in response to transient rectal distension.

Biopsy of rectal or colonic tissue demonstrates absent or reduced number of ganglionic nerve cells. It is definitive diagnostic measure for the disease.

Management

Definitive management is performed by surgical interventions for removal of the aganglionic, nonfunctioning and dilated segment of the colon, followed by end-to-end anastomosis to improve the functioning of internal rectal sphincter and to establish continuity between rectum and the proximal segment.

Initially, after confirmation of the diagnosis, a colostomy or ileostomy is performed in the normal ganglionic part to decompress the intestine, to divert the fecal materials and to provide rest to normal colon.

The *reconstructive surgery* is done by the following three techniques:
1. Swenson's operation or abdominoperineal pull through.
2. Duhamel's operation or retrorectal transanal pull through.
3. Soave's operation or endorectal pull through.

The optimal age for these operation is 6 to 8 months after temporary colostomy or 12 to 15 months of age or untill the child's weight is 7 to 9 kg.

In the older children, where the symptoms are not severe, management should be done by repeated enemas with isotonic saline, stool softeners and low residue diet.

In case of enterocolitis and extremely ill child, initial management should be done to resuscitate the child with the following measures:

(a) IV fluid therapy (b) nasogastric tube aspiration (c) antibiotic therapy (d) colonic irrigation with saline solution and (e) surgical decompression by colostomy followed by definitive surgery.

Complications

The serious complication of the condition is enterocolitis. It is due to proliferation of bacteria in the colonic lumen which presents with severe toxemia. There is abdominal distension, profuse watery diarrhea mixed with blood, vomiting, lethergy, fever and shock. Treatment of this conditon should be done aggressively, otherwise mortality is very high.

Other complications of the disease include bowel perforation, intestinal obstruction, hydroureter or hydronephrosis, failure to thrive and multiple nutritional deficiencies. Water intoxication may occur, if tap water enema is given to the patient.

Postoperative complications may develop as enterocolitis (within 2 years of surgery), leaking of anastomosis, colostomy related problems, pelvic abscess, temporary constipation, intestinal obstruction (due to adhesions, volvulus or intussusception), infections, hemorrhage and shock.

Nursing Management

Nursing management should be planned based on details nursing assessment and nursing diagnosis. Nursing assessment should include details history related to illness, bowel habit, feeding habit and related clinical problems. Neonatal assessment is an important step to diagnose this condition especially regarding passage of meconium, presence of constipation, characteristics of stools, enema or suppositories needed or not, presence of abdominal distention, etc. In older children, failure to thrive, malnutrition along with constipation are important features which help to formulate nursing diagnosis for planning care.

Nursing Diagnoses

The important nursing diagnoses before surgery are:
- Constipation due to aganglionic colonic segment.
- Altered nutrition, less than body requirement due to poor intake of food.
- Ineffective breathing and discomfort related to abdominal distention.
- Pain related to intestinal obstruction.
- Dehydration related to diarrhea and vomiting.
- Shock related to complication like enterocolitis.
- Fear and anxiety related to life-threatening and chronic illness.
- Knowledge deficit related to health maintenance in long-term illness.

The important nursing diagnoses after surgery are:
- Risk of complications related to postoperative period.
- Risk of infections of surgical wound.
- Discomfort related to postoperative abdominal distension.
- Ineffective family coping related to care of the child with colostomy.

Nursing interventions should be performed based on the above nursing diagnosis like other patients with abdominal surgery. Special attention to be given on care of the colostomy.

Care of the Child with Colostomy

Colostomy is a surgically created opening between the colon and the abdominal wall to allow fecal elimination. It may be temporary or permanent diversion. A colostomy may be placed in any segment of the large intestine (colon). The more right sided the colostomy, the looser the stool. Transverse and descending or sigmoid colostomies are most common types (Fig. 16.6.).

A *colostomy* may be performed in case of congenital anomalies (Anorectal malformations, Hirschsprung's disease), for surgical treatment of ischemic bowel, trauma, and inflammatory bowel disease, as a temporary measures to protect an anastomosis, and as part of an abdominoperineal resection for rectal cancer or a fecal diversion for unresectable cancer.

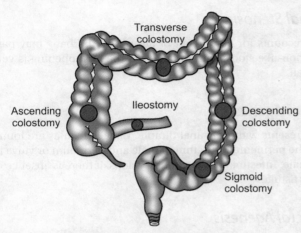

Fig.16.6: Placement of fecal ostomies

An *ileostomy* is usually formed at the terminal ileum of the small bowel and is placed usually in the right lower quadrant of the abdomen. Stools from an ileostomy drains average 4 to 5 times per day and harmful to skin. It is usually required as temporary or permanent measure in ulcerative colitis, Crohn's disease, congenital defect and trauma.

The word 'ostomy' is often used interchangeably with the word 'stoma', i.e. part of the intestine that brought above the abdominal wall. It becomes the outlet for discharge of intestinal contents. It is normally pink-red moist, bleeds slightly when rubbed, no feeling to touch, stool functions involuntary and postoperative swelling gradually decreases over several months. Stoma can be classified as end-stoma, double - barrel stoma and loop stoma.

Standard of Care Guidelines

1. Prepare the parents and child (if possible) preoperatively by explanation about the colostomy, stoma characteristics and ostomy management with a pouching system.
2. Determine the site of colostomy before operation by the specialist ostomy nurse.
3. Prepare the child as for general abdominal surgery.
4. Support the family and the patient with psychological considerations of ostomy surgery.
5. Monitor the stoma color and amount of stoma discharge postoperatively at every shift. Record and report any abnormalities.
6. Assess hydration status and prevent dehydration.
7. Change the pouching system over the ostomy to avoid leakage and protect the peristomal skin. Pouching system should be properly fitted over the stoma.
8. Assess the peristomal skin during change of pouching sustem for skin breakdown, allergy, infections, etc. and all findings to be recorded.

9. Teach the parents or caregiver about routine pouch emptying (when it is 1/4 to 1/3 full), cleansing skin and stoma and change of pouching system. Care of the reusable bag, prevention and treatment of skin excoriation around the stoma are of primary concern. Demonstrate these techniques to the parents.
10. Instruct the parent about the control of gas and odor of colostomy. Care during bathing and travel with attention to clothing should be informed.
11. Inform the parents about increased fluid intake, diet, possible complications, necessary medical help, follow-up, good hygiene, safety measures and promotion of normal growth and development of the child.
12. Prepare and explain about the next definitive surgical procedures or colostomy closure as indicated. Encourage to verbalize feelings. Explain that colostomy irrigation is not a part of management in small children. It should be done only in preparation for diagnostic tests or surgery and occasionally for the treatment of constipation.
13. Refer the child to ostomy support group or ostomy association, if available.

ANORECTAL MALFORMATIONS

Anorectal malformations (ARMs) are developmental deformities of the lower end of the alimentary tract, i.e. the anorectal canal. Some of the deformities are very minor, others are profound and affect the adjacent genitourinary and skeletal structures. The term imperforate anus is used to describe all congenital abnormalities of the anorectal canal or in location of the anus within the perineum.

The exact cause of these malformations is not known. It occurs due to arrest in embryonic development of the anus, lower rectum and urogenital tract at the 8th week of embryonic life.

Approximately 40 percent of neonates with ARMs have associated congenital anomalies like Down's syndrome, congenital heart disease, undescended testes, renal abnormalities, esophageal atresia and neural tube defect.

Classification of ARMs

A. Classification of ARMs can be done into three groups in the infants without a normal anus.
   1. **With a visible abnormal opening of the bowel:**
      a. Anal stenosis
      b. Anoperineal fistula.
      c. Anovestibular fistula in female.
   2. **With an invisible but manifested opening of the bowel:**
      a. Rectovaginal fistula in female.
      b. Rectourethral fistula in male.
      c. Rectovesicular fistula.

3. **No manifested opening of the bowel:**
   a. Persistent anal membrane.
   b. Rectal atresia.
B. Anorectal malformations can be classified into two groups on the basis of levator ani muscle, which is the main muscle of fecal control—
   1. *Supralevator or high anorectal malformations:* When rectum terminates above the levator ani muscle, which is found as rectal atresia, rectoprostatic fistula and rectovaginal fistula. About 30 percent of children with high ARMs or associated genito-urinary fistula achieve bowel continence.
   2. *Translevator or low anorectal malformations:* When rectum terminates below the levator ani muscle, e.g. in anocutaneous fistula and anovestibular fistula. About 90 percent of children with low ARMs achieve bowel continence.

Clinical Manifestations

Anorectal malformations are usually diagnosed immediately after birth by the person conducting the delivery or within hours by the caregivers.

The important presenting features are abnormally formed or no anal opening and absence of meconium or presence of fistula with passage of stool through the fistula. In female baby the fistula may present between rectum and vagina or perineum. In male baby the fistula is commonly found between rectum and urinary tract or perineum. Presence of meconium in urine may be found in some children. Progressive abdominal distension and vomiting may present. Rectal tube cannot be inserted into the rectum during examination.

The specific features for specific anomalies (Figs 16.7A to D) are as follows:

Imperforate Anal Membrane

Infant fails to pass meconium. Greenish bulging membrane is seen on examination. Bowel and sphincter return to normal after excision.

Anal Stenosis

It accounts for 10 percent of all ARMs. The baby may pass ribbon-like stools with difficulty as the anal opening is very small.

Anal Agenesis

It presents with only anal dimple. Usually fistulas are found to the perineum or urethra in male and perineum or vulva in female. Intestinal obstruction develops, if there is absence of any fistula.

Rectal Agenesis

This condition accounts for 75 percent of all ARMs. It presents with fistula. In male baby, fistula may communicate with posterior urethra and in female with upper vagina. Associated major congenital malformations are common.

Rectoperineal Fistula

It is found as small orifice in the perineum, usually anterior to the center of the external sphincter. In male baby it is found close to the scrotum and in female the vulva.

Rectovaginal Fistula

It presents with a communication between rectum and vagina and stool passed through the vagina.

Diagnosis

Physical examination of the neonates is the most important diagnostic measure of ARMs. USG helps to locate the rectal pouch. X-ray with inverted infant (upside down position), i.e. invertogram or Wangensteen-Rice X-ray is useful to locate rectal pouch which can be performed only after the infant is 24 hours of age. Urinary fistula can be diagnosed by urine examination for presence of meconium and epithelial debris.

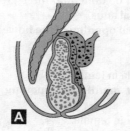 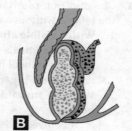 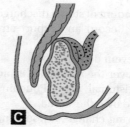 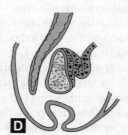

Figs 16.7A to D: Anorectal malformations. A. Anal stenosis; B. Imperforate anal membrane; C. Anal agenesis; D. Rectal agenesis

Micturating cystourethrogram (MCU) can be done to detect urinary abnormalities.

Management

The reconstructive surgery is done to correct or repair the congenital malformations. It depends upon the type of anomalies and sex of the infant.

In case of low ARMs, rectal cutback anoplasty or Y-V plasty is done for male infants and dilatation of fistula with definitive repair or perineal anoplasty is performed for female infants.

In case of high ARMs, initial colostomy is done in the neonatal period followed by definitive reconstructive surgery as posterior sagittal anorectoplasty (PSARP) at the age of 10 to 12 months or when the infant is having 7 to 9 kg body weight. Colostomy closure is done after 10 to 12 weeks of successful definitive surgery.

Nursing Management

Basic preoperative and postoperative care should be provided as for abdominal surgery. Special interventions in preoperative period should include maintenance of warmth, fluid and electrolyte balance and general stability of the infant. Measurement of abdominal girth is important before surgery. Special care to be provided for colostomy.

In postoperative period, prevention of skin breakdown around colostomy wound and prevention of infections are important measures. Maintenance of fluid and electrolyte balance and routine postoperative care to be provided after colostomy and definitive surgery. Emotional support for family coping and demonstration of colostomy care are essential aspects of nursing management. Health education to be given about continuation of care at home, diet modification, prevention of fecal impaction, bowel habit training and need for medical help.

Complications

The common complications of ARMs are urinary tract infection, intestinal obstruction, fecal impaction, colostomy related problems, recurrence of fistula, anal stenosis and postoperative complications.

Prognosis

Prognosis of ARMs depends upon type of anomalies, presence of associated malformations, operative skill, presence of neuromuscular fecal control and general health of the infant. Most children lead normal live and become normal adults. It some children fecal control may be achieved untill the age of 10 years. Toilet training is possible after definitive surgery.

UMBILICAL MALFORMATIONS

Several anomalies are found at the umbilicus. These can be grouped into the followings:
A. Abnormalities related to vitello-intestinal duct.
B. Umbilical hernia.
C. Examphalos and gastroschisis.

Abnormalities Related to Vitellointestinal Duct

1. *Patent Vitellointestinal Duct (PVID):* It is found as fecal discharge at umbilicus, especially when the communicating tract is wide. There may be just serous and mucoid discharge or it may be infected in case of narrow communicating tract. PVID may present as cyst or polyp. Vitellointestinal fistula may be found as umbilical discharging sinus due to persistence of the entire vitello-intestinal duct. Recurrent attacks of omphalitis indicate presence of fistula or sinus.

   These conditions can be managed by laparotomy followed by excision of whole tract of PVID.
2. *Patent urachus:* It may remain asymptomatic or may present with watery discharge at umbilicus with urine smell. It may be associated with lower urinary tract obstruction especially in posterior urethra. In some cases, the opening of urachus at umbilicus is closed and may form bladder diverticulum or urachal cyst. The diagnosis of the condition is confirmed by USG, CT scan or MCU. Surgical interventions is required to manage the condition.
3. *Umbilical granuloma:* It presents as a pink-red mass in umbilicus at the 2nd or 3rd week of life, when the umbilical cord falls off. It occurs in case of chronically infected umbilicus. There is usually serosanguinous or blood stained discharge from raw tissue in umbilicus.
   This condition can be managed with chemicals like silver nitrate or copper sulfate applications. It may required excision and electric cautery.
4. *Umbilical polyp or adenoma:* It is a true mucosal remnant of vitellointestinal or omphalo-mesentric duct. It is usually asymptomatic but may connect with a cyst or sinus, or band to the small intestine. There may be serous or hemorrhagic discharge. Management is done with surgical excision and repair of base of umbilicus.

Umbilical Hernia

Umbilical hernia is the protrusion of intestine or omentum through the fascial defect in the umbilicus due to imperfect closure or weakness of the umbilical ring. It is one of the common problems in infants and seen in one among 6 to 8 infants.

Normally, by the 10th week of gestational life, midgut returns to the abdominal cavity and abdominal wall begins to close. Each lateral body wall folds medially and closes at the center. The central region of closure is the umbilicus.

The defect is more common in low birth weight babies and in congenital anomalies like trisomy 13 to 18 and Hurler syndrome. The defect may be 1 to 5 cm in diameter. It may be associated with diastasis recti (divertication of abdominal recti muscles).

Spontaneous closure of umbilical hernia is very common and occurs in almost 90 to 95 percent of cases by the age of 3 to 5 years. Surgical correction is indicated, if the defect persists beyond 3 to 5 years and further increases in size or gets strangulated. In recurrent attacks of incarceration, even if the fascial defect is less than 1 cm or if the defect becomes larger than 2 cm, then surgical intervention is required.

Conservative management has no role in the treatment of umbilical hernia-like strapping by adhesive or placement of coins over the protrusion. These measures may cause skin ulceration or perforation. In some infants, hernia becomes more tense during crying and when the child stops crying, the hernia is reduced easily. Parents need explanation and support in these cases.

Paraumbilical hernia may occur when herniation of peritoneal contents found either above or below the umbilical cicatrix. It does not close spontaneously and must be surgically repaired.

Exomphalos (Omphalocele)

Exomphalos is the herniation of the abdominal organ through a wide open umbilicus. The herniated contents are covered with shiny avascular sac which is externally formed by amnion and internally by yolk sac with Wharton's jelly in between. The opening is present in the umbilical cord. The contents of the sac are mostly liver and varying amount of intestine. Exomphalos should be differentiated from umbilical hernia which is covered by skin. Larger defects are termed as exomphalos.

This condition is usually associated with other anomalies in about 50 percent of cases. The most common associated anomalies are trisomy 13, 18 or 21 and Beckwith - Weideman syndrome (omphalocele, macroglossia, macrosomia and microcephaly). Cardiac, genitourinary and skeletal anomalies are frequently found along with this anomaly. Intestinal anomalies like malrotation of gut, Mickel's diverticulum and intestinal atresia may also present is association with this condition.

Complications

Omphalocele may be complicated with rupture of sac, evisceration of bowel loops, infections, sepsis, hypothermia and hypovolemia (due to evaporative water loss)

Management

The definitive management of the defect is done by surgical repair of the abdominal wall and reposition of the herniated contents into the peritoneal cavity. Surgery can be done in stages depending upon the size of the defect.

Preoperative management should include nasogastric tube aspiration to prevent intestinal distention and covering of sac and its contents by sterile plastic sheet directly to prevent evaporative loss of fluid. Wet saline sponges should not be used to cover the sac. Supportive measures should include IV infusion, warmth, breast feeding, oxygen therapy and mechanical ventilation, if required. Basic preoperative and postoperative care to be provided along with routine nursing care same as abdominal surgery. Prognosis depends upon severity of associated anomalies.

Gastroschisis

Gastroschisis is characterized by herniation of the abdominal viscera through a defect in the abdominal wall to the right of the umbilical cord and through the rectus muscle. A tear occurs at the base of umbilical cord. Umbilicus may remain well formed without any opening. Unlike in exomphalos, there is no membrane covering the exposed bowel and no gastroschisis sac. Usually the small intestine or part of colon eviscerates. The abdominal cavity is underdeveloped, as most of the viscera have remained outside. Liver, spleen or stomach also may eviscerates.

Surgical intervention is done to reposit the abdominal viscera either by creating skin flaps or making an artificial silo followed by closure of abdominal wall. The exposed bowel is loosely covered with saline soaked pads and the abdomen is wrapped in a plastic drape in preoperative period. Supportive measures should include prevention of infection, maintenance of warmth, ventilatory support, maintenance of fluid and electrolyte balance and provision of total parenteral nutrition along with routine care.

HERNIA

Hernia is the protrusion or projection of an organ or a part of an organ through the abnormal opening in the wall of the cavity that normally contains it. Hernia of abdominal organs are more common.

Causes

Hernia develops due to various causes. It may be congenital or acquired. Hernia may result due to—(a) failure of certain normal opening to close during development, (b) weakness due to debilitating illness and injury, (c) prolonged distention due to tumors or obesity and (d) increased intra-abdominal pressure due to straining and coughing.

Common Hernias in Children

Inguinal Hernia

It is a common problem in infants and children requiring surgical repair. It is frequently found in male and preterm infants. Right sided inguinal hernia is more common (60%) than left sided (30%) and bilateral (10%) type. It has familial tendency and results from persistence of the patency of processus vaginalis accompanying the spermatic cord. An intermittent swelling in the inguinal or inguinoscrotal area appears particularly on crying or straining. It can be indirect or direct inguinal hernia.

Indirect inguinal hernia occurs due to weakness of the abdominal wall. The hernial sac protrudes through internal inguinal ring into the inguinal canal and often descend into the scrotum. Herniotomy should be done to manage the problem and to prevent obstruction and strangulation.

Direct inguinal hernia develops when the hernial sac protrudes through abdominal wall in the region of Hesselbach's triangle, a region bounded by the rectus abdominis muscle, inguinal ligament and inferior epigastric vessels. It is rare in children (1% or less). Repair of the posterior wall of the inguinal canal is required to managed this problem. Repair is a difficult procedure.

Female children may also have inguinal hernia. The canal of Nuck undergoes the same obliteration as the processus vaginalis in boys. Girls have a 20 percent incidence of sliding hernias containing ovary and fallopian tube. These should be promptly repaired because there is a risk of ovarian torsion in the inguinal canal. If a female child has bilateral inguinal hernia, sex chromatin and/or chromosomal analysis should be done to rule out testicular feminization syndrome.

Congenital Diaphragmatic Hernia (CDH)

It is herniation of abdominal contents into the thoracic cavity due to developmental defect in the diaphragm. The herniation occurs usually through the posterolateral foramen of Bochdalek on left side (80%). It is more common is females. This condition results in severe respiratory distress and should be considered as dire emergency. Most of the cases are symptomatic at birth. The infant presents with profound respiratory distress within first hour of life with scaphoid abdomen. Auscultation of peristaltic sounds inspite of breath sound on the affected side helps to confirm the diagnosis. Heart sounds are displaced with mediastinal shift.

Few cases (5–25%) may become symptomatic beyond neonatal period and usually present with recurrent chest infections. It may be associated with pulmonary hypoplasia, esophageal atresia, omphalocele, malrotation of gut, cardiovascular lesions, etc.

The diagnosis of CDH is confirmed by chest X-ray which shows intestinal loops in the chest cavity. Blood gas analysis helps to assess the presence or extent of hypoxia and acidosis. Antenatal diagnosis is possible by USG. The condition is suggested by the presence of polyhydramnios.

Immediate management after diagnosis is significant aspect to save the life. Initial management should be done with endotracheal intubation and intermittent positive pressure ventilation with adequate oxygenation. Mask ventilation to be avoided because it will distend the stomach and cause more respiratory distress. Maintenance of warmth, nasogastric tube aspiration to decompress stomach, IV fluid therapy, mechanical ventilation correction of acidosis, and continuous monitoring of child's condition with ABG analysis are important supportive measures.

Surgery is done for reduction of herniated content into the abdominal cavity and repair of diaphragmatic defect. Timing of operative intervention should be decided depending upon the clinical condition of the particular infant. Specialized care for thoracic surgery should be provided to the infant with ventilatory support.

Hiatal Hernia

Hiatal hernia or partial thoracic stomach is the herniation of cardiac end of the stomach through the esophageal hiatus of the diaphragm. The infant is presented with regurgitation or vomiting (may be blood stained), dehydration and aspiration pneumonia. Failure to thrive and anemia are usually found.

Diagnosis is confirmed by barium-meal study. Surgical repair is indicated in persistent vomiting, esophagitis, hematemesis, melena, frequent aspiration and impending stricture. Conservative measures may be useful with propped-up position, thickened feed and antacids. The surgery of choice for hiatal hernia is the Nissen type of fundoplication.

Epigastric Hernia

It is protrusion of intestine through an opening in the midline in the linea alba above the umbilicus. It requires surgical correction.

Femoral Hernia

It is herniation of intestine through the femoral ring. It is a rare condition and found in female child between 5 and 10 years of age. The hernia is usually small irreducible as most of the swelling is composed of a fibrofatty tissue. It should be differentiated from inguinal hernia. The diagnosis is made on the situation of the swelling below the inguinal ligament and lateral to the pubic tubercle. Operation should be done as early as possible.

RECTAL PROLAPSE

Rectal prolapse is the abnormal descent of the mucous membrane of the rectum through the anus. It is common between 3 and 5 years of age.

The precipitating factors are increased intra-abdominal pressure due to constipation, bloody diarrhea, frequent passage of stools, rectal ulcer, prolonged squatting, severe malnutrition and loss of ischiorectal fat. The support structures, i.e. sphincters and muscles are weakened leading to rectal prolapse.

There is usually blood stained stools. Prolapse can be partial or complete. It may be associated with spinabifida, exstrophy of bladder or may be found after anoplasty in ARMs.

Management should be done with reduction of prolapsed part and correction of precipitating factors. Prevention of constipation, correction of malnutrition and management of worm infestations are important measures. Perineum strengthening exercises and dietary modification are essential. In severe cases strapping of the buttocks is done after reduction of the prolapse. Surgical intervention (Rectopexy) may be needed in intractable cases to repair the sphincter. Thiersch's operation and Ripstein procedure are done whenever indicated. Sclerosing injection (5% phenol in glycerine) can be injected into submucosa of the rectum.

PANCREATITIS

Inflammation of the pancreas is a unique condition in which the pancreatic proenzymes are activated by enzymes found in certain bacteria and leukocytes leading to autodigestion of the pancreatic tissue. It occurs more often in adolescent boys. It can be found as single or recurrent episodes and acute or chronic problem.

Causes

There are variety of factors which can cause pancreatitis. The important causative factors are:

a. Blunt injury of abdomen which influences the inflammatory changes.
b. Infections like mumps, hepatitis, rubella, coxsackie virus infections and Reye's syndrome can lead to inflammation of the pancreas.
c. Biliary abnormalities or disorders, like gallstone, choledochal cyst and anomalous insertion of the common bile duct are sometimes responsible for recurrent pancreatitis.
   - Other causes include metabolic disorders (hypercalcemia, hyperlipidemia), SLE, periarteritis nodosa, drug reactions (especially valproic acid, prednisolone, thiazides, etc.)

- In some cases no specific cause is found, which can be due to hereditary or idiopathic.

Clinical Manifestations

The clinical presentations of pancreatitis include very severe abdominal pain accompanied by prostration, fever, nausea, vomiting and discomfort. It is uncommon cause of abdominal pain but may be very serious. Pain may be in the epigastric region or below and may radiate to the back. The abdomen feels full and tender. Bluish discoloration around the umbilicus may found due to hemorrhage. Shock may complicate the condition due to loss of blood. Pancreatic pseudocyst may form and present as an abdominal mass.

Diagnosis

Elevated levels of amylase in serum or urine are diagnostic. If serum amylase is not elevated, then amylase-creatinine ratio is calculated and if found to be more than 5, it is suggestive of pancreatitis. There may be hemoconcentration. leukocytosis, hypocalcemia, coagulopathy and eleveted levels in liver function tests. Blood glucose level is elevated and glycosuria is revealed. Plain X-ray abdomen may show calcification. Ultrasonography and CT scan are helpful for diagnose the condition and related pathology.

Management

Problem of the management is mainly supportive and symptomatic. It should include complete bed rest, nothing per mouth, IV fluid therapy, nasogastric aspiration, oxygen therapy, analgesics, antibiotics, antacids and treatment of complications (metabolic acidosis, shock). Good nursing care is very important measure for better prognosis. Surgical intervention may required especially in case of pseudocyst, pancreatic necrosis, gallstone, etc.

Complications

Pancreatitis may be complicated with pulmonary infiltrates, pleural effusion, hemorrhage with hypovolemic shock, acute renal failure, pancreatic ascites, abscess, or pseudocyst, multiple organ dysfunction syndrome, biliary tract obstruction and pancreatic fistula.

JAUNDICE (ICTERUS)

Jaundice is an important and common symptom of liver disease. It is a clinical term used for the yellowish discoloration of the mucous membrane and skin due to increased blood bilirubin level. The clinical features of jaundice usually vary according to various age group. Many newborn manifests jaundice when serum bilirubin levels are high, i.e. 4 to 5 mg/dL. In older children jaundice is usually found when bilirubin level reaches above 2 mg%.

Pathophysiology

The elevation of bilirubin may occur due to the following conditions:

1. Excessive hemolysis leads to hemolytic or prehepatic jaundice.
2. Damage of liver parenchyma resulting disturbances of bilirubin metabolism and bilirubin excretion. The disturbances occur in transferring of bile pigment after conjugation into the bile capillary or by obstruction of bile pigment in the liver (intrahepatic cholestasis) or from being excreted through the bile duct due to cholangitis. These leads to hepatocellular jaundice which is the most common type found in clinical areas.
3. Interference with the excretion of bile due to obstruction in the bile ducts, e.g. congenital obliteration of bile ducts.

Common Causes of Jaundice in Children

1. Physiological jaundice in neonates.
2. Hepatitis.
3. Hemolytic jaundice—ABO and Rh incompatibility, mismatched blood transfusion, septicemia, thalassemia.
4. Obstructive jaundice—Extrahepatic biliary atresia, cholelithiasis, cholecystitis.
5. Cirrhosis of liver.
6. Portal hypertension.

Investigations

Details history of illness and physical examination help to detect the cause. Laboratory investigations to exclude the exact cause of jaundice include estimation of direct and indirect bilirubin, hemoglobin percentage, blood grouping and typing, reticulocyte count, Coombs' test, examination of peripheral blood smear, stool examination, liver function tests and other specific test for suggestive etiology. Hepatic imaging, endoscopic retrograde cholangio pancreatography (ERCP), Radionuclide scanning, MRI, etc. also help to diagnose the exact cause.

Management

Management of a child with jaundice primarily directed towards the etiology. Special supportive nursing care is very important and includes rest, skin care, dietary restriction of fat, spices and fried food, intake of more carbohydrate,

maintenance of hygienic measures, care of bladder and bowel, prevention of injury and bleeding, emotional support and health education.

HEPATOMEGALY

Hepatomegaly, the enlargement of liver is found alone or with splenomegaly as the manifestation of some systemic disease. It is a clinical sign, not a disease. Just palpable liver does not necessarily signify hepatomegaly. Any enlargement of the liver more than 3 cm below the costal margin with sharp lower edge and some degree of firmness should be considered as abnormal.

Causes of Hepatomegaly

Liver may be enlarged due to some pathological causes like inflammation, fatty infiltration, kupffer's cell hyperplasia, hepatic congestion, cellular infiltration in malignancies and storage of metabolites. Hepatomegaly may found in some apparent conditions or due to some actual pathology.

Apparent Hepatomegaly

The apparent (but not true) hepatomegaly is found in following conditions:

a. Relaxation of abdominal musculature in severe PEM, rickets, amyotonia congenita, etc.
b. Increased intrathoracic pressure in emphysema, pneumothorax, pleural effusion, empyema, subphrenic abscess, etc.
c. Thoracic deformity.
d. Abnormalities in position of liver, i.e. hepatoptosis or generalized visceroptosis.

Actual Hepatomegaly

The actual hepatomegaly is found in the following conditions:

a. *Infections* like infective hepatitis, serum hepatitis, malaria, kala-azar, amebiasis, amebic hepatitis, infectious mononucleosis, typhoid fever, bacterial septicemia, tuberculosis, syphilis, toxoplasmosis, ascariasis, hydatid disease, liver abscess, etc.
b. *Hemolytic anemias:* Thalassemia major, sickle cell anemia.
c. *Fatty infiltration:* PEM (mainly in kwashiorkor), severe infections, diarrhea, diabetes mellitus, hypervitaminosis, corticosteroid therapy, tetracycline toxicity, cystic fibrosis.
d. *Cirrhosis:* Indian childhood cirrhosis of liver, veno-occlusive disease of liver, neonatal hepatitis, biliary atresia, galactosemia, Wilson's disease, cystic fibrosis.
e. *Hepatic congestion:* CCF, pericardial diseases, Budd-Chiari syndrome.

f. *Myelo proliferative diseases:* Leukemia, myelofibrosis.
g. *Neoplasms:* Hepatomas, lymphomas, Hodgkin's disease, neuroblastoma.
h. *Metabolic/storage diseases:* Glycogen storage disorders, amyloidosis, Wilson's disease, lipidoses, mucopolysaccharidoses.
i. *Miscellaneous:* Sarcoidosis, hemangiomas, congenital cyst.

The common causes of hepatomegaly in the newborn are heart failure, hemolytic diseases, biliary atresia, neonatal hepatitis, congenital syphilis, galactosemia.

In infant and older childen the common causes are hepatitis, Indian childhood cirrhosis (ICC), tuberculosis, PEM, amebiasis, hepatomas, leukemias and hypervitaminosis 'A'.

Investigations

Details history of illnes and thorough clinical examination is useful to identify the cause. Laboratory investigations, like liver function test, blood examination and specific test for suspected cause are helpful to diagnose the cause. Ultrasonography, X-ray abdomen are essential investigative procedures.

Associated clinical manifestations which aid in diagnosis of hepatomegaly are:
- PEM—Fatty infiltration of liver.
- Jaundice—Chronic liver disease.
- Engorged neck veins and raised jugular venous pressure—Constrictive pericaritis.
- Skin rash—Histiocytosis.
- Microcephaly or hydrocephalus—Intrauterine infections like toxoplasmosis, cytomegalic inclusion disease.
- Cataract and mental retardation—galactosemia.
- Kayser–Fleischer ring over the cornea—Wilson's disease.
- Enlargement of spleen—Infections (like malaria, kala-azar, tuberculosis, toxoplasmosis) and cellular infiltrations (leukemia, lymphoma, thalassemia).

EXTRAHEPATIC BILIARY ATRESIA (EHBA)

Biliary atresia is obliteration or hypoplasia of one or more components of the bile ducts due to arrested development in fetal life resulting in persistent jaundice, liver damage, ranging from biliary stasis to biliary cirrhosis and progressive portal hypertension with splenomegaly.

Usually there is absence or atresia of the extrahepatic ducts and the common bile duct. In some instances, there is also absence of intrahepatic ducts. Gallbladder may be absence or distended with bile if the obstruction is distal.

The *cause* of biliary atresia may be due to developmental aberration of bile duct system in early period of gestation or may be related to autoimmune reaction, or intrauterine viral infection or ischemia. It may occur following neonatal hepatitis:

Clinical manifestations are mainly persistent progressive obstructive jaundice with pale putty like clay colored stools due to absence of bile pigment in the stools. Jaundice is usually not present at birth but appear within 2 to 3 weeks of life. The skin color deepens and becomes bronze olive green. Urine becomes dark in color due to heavily excretion of bile pigments. The liver is enlarged and due to biliary obstruction. Cirrhosis and portal hypertension may develop. Spleen also becomes enlarged. In advanced cases, hepatic failure, bleeding disorders, esophageal varices, generalized cachexia due to nutritional failure are found.

The diagnosis is confirmed by operative cholangiogram (before 8 weeks of age), USG, scanning and liver biopsy. Delay in corrective surgery beyond 3 months of age complicates the problem and liver biopsy at that time may show intracellular and intracanalicular cholestasis, inflammatory cell infiltration, interstitial fibrosis, degeneration and proliferation of ducts and even giant cell formation.

At present *four anatomic types of EHBA* are recognized.
- Type – I: Atresia of common bile duct.
- Type – II: Atresia of common hepatic duct.
- Type – III: Atresia of porta hepatis.
- Type – IV: No patent bile ducts at porta hepatis.

Management of EHBA is done by surgical exploration and correction of the defect, within one or two months of age. Symptomatic treatment with vitamin 'K', vitamin 'D', antihistaminics, antibiotics, diuretics may be needed in inoperable cases.

Kasai hepatic portoenterostomy is performed as surgical interventions in selected cases for extrahepatic biliary atresia.

In intrahepatic biliary atresia, cholysteramine may be useful to reduce bilirubin level and itching.

Prognosis is poor in untreated and inoperable cases. Average period of survival being 1.5 to 2 years. Survival period is longer in intrahepatic type rather than extrahepatic type. With early surgery, 40 to 50 percent long-term survival is reported in case of EHBA.

LIVER ABSCESS

Liver abscess may found as single or multiple abscess and may be amebic or pyogenic or due to echinococcal cyst. Fungal infection also may cause liver abscess in immunocompromised subjects.

Amebic Liver Abscess

Amebic liver abscess is due to *E. histolytica* and commonly found in adults but may also be found in children though infrequent. The *clinical features* include irregular fever, chills, painful tender swelling over the right hypochondrium or the epigastrium. History of dysentery may or may not be present. Jaundice may present in some cases. Laboratory investigation shows polymorphonuclear leukocytosis. Chest X-ray usually shows elevation of right hemidiaphragm. USG and CT scan are useful to confirm the diagnosis.

Management is done with antiamebic drugs—metronidazole 20 to 50 mg/kg/day for 7 days in combination with chloroquine. Needle aspiration of the abscess (in case of large abscess) or open surgical drainage may be done.

Pyogenic Liver Abscess

Pyogenic liver abscess is usually due to infections like *Staphylococcus, Streptococcus, E. coli, Pseudomonas*, etc. It may be found as solitary abscess or multiple abscesses. The predisposing factors include immunocompromised conditions (ALL, chronic granulomatous disease, steriod therapy, measles), malnutrition, typhoid fever, skin infections, trauma, aplastic anemia and ventriculoperitoneal shunt. In neonates, it may occur in umbilical vessel catheterization, prematurity, supportive umbilical thrombophlebitis, peritoneal abscess, skin infection, septicemia and surgery for necrotizing enterocolitis.

Clinical features of pyogenic liver abscess include spiky fever, chills, rigors, anorexia, nausea, vomiting, abdominal distention, abdominal pain in right upper quadrant, lassitude and tenderness over hepatic area. Diagnosis is confirmed by USG, CT scan, or radionuclide scans and culture-sensitivity of aspirated fluid for the abscess.

Management of liver abscess include appropriate chemotherapy, percutaneous needle aspiration and open surgical drainage. Supportive and symptomatic management are important. Following prompt diagnosis and appropriate management pyogenic abscess resolves in over 6 weeks.

The pyogenic liver abscess may be complicated with pleuropulmonary involvement, peritonitis, subphrenic abscess, abscess-duodenum fistula, pericardiac effusion and Budd-Chiari syndrome.

INDIAN CHILDHOOD CIRRHOSIS

Indian childhood cirrhosis (ICC) is a disease peculiar to the Indian infants and children, usually occurs between 6 months and 4 years of age. It may also found in Indian subcontinent and West Indies.

It is a progressive disease with abdominal distension, marked irritability, unexplained irregular low-grade fever, hepatosplenomegaly with hepatic failure, ascites and jaundice.

Epidemiology

The disease is prevalent all over India in some particular communities. Male children are 4 times more sufferer than female. The first born child is at greater risk. Large number of cases belongs to the low middle class family of rural areas with vegetarian food habits. There is familial predisposition of the disease. At present, there is remarkable decline in the incidence of ICC, which appears to be related to declining practice of use of copper or brass utensils for boiling milk.

Etiology

The following factors are considered for etiopathogenesis of ICC:

a. Hepatotoxic agents: Hepatotoxic harmful agents like guttis or *Aspergillus flavus* that grow on ground nuts, maize and rice may cause ICC though the cause and effect relationship is not fully understood. Use of copper utensils for boiling milk or cooking food and early weaning with milk supplement before the age of 3 months may have some influence for occurrence of ICC.

b. Metabolic defects: These may cause ICC specially disturbed lactose, zinc, copper and magnesium metabolism.

c. *Immunological disturbances:* These are found in high-levels of circulating immune complexes which can cause immune mediated injury of the liver.

d. *Genetic factors:* Familial occurrence of ICC points the possibility of underlying genetic factor along with environmental factors.

e. *Nutritional factors:* Previously it was believed that malnutrition was an important cause of cirrhosis. At present, it does not seem to play a clear role in its pathogenesis.

f. *Viral infections:* ICC has been thought to be a consequence of neonatal hepatitis or infective hepatitis. Though there is some objections of this hypothesis.

No single factors seems to be the cause of ICC. Multiple factors are responsible for occurrence of the disease. The role of nutrition and viral infection is considered as remote.

Pathology

There is variation of size of the liver and color which ranges from gray to frank green, due to the disease process. The basic pathologic change is the diffuse liver damage by way of degeneration going on to necrosis and replacement fibrosis. The capsule shows patchy thickening and the surface is finely nodular. The microscopic study shows marked hepatocyte damage as degenerative changes in the cytoplasm. Kupffer's cells show mild degree of proliferation. Gross pericellular fibrosis in the hepatic lobules are found. Intracellular hyaline called as Mallory's hyaline are seen. There is gross excess of copper and copper associated protein (orcein).

Clinical Manifestations

The onset of the disease can be insidious or acute. There are three arbitrary stage in insidious onset which tend to merge each other.

The children with ICC may present with irritability, disturbed appetite, abdominal distension, chalky and pasty stools with constipation or diarrhea and mild fever. Progressive growth failure usually present in spite of adequate diet. Within few months to a years, there is hepatomegaly, jaundice and features of portal hypertension including splenomegaly, ascites, hematemesis, anemia, prominent superficial abdominal veins and thrombocytopenia. There may be high incidence of intravascular hemolysis. In the terminal stage, the child becomes apathetic, emaciated with deep jaundice. Liver is usually gross enlarged with protuberant abdomen. The child generally have hepatic failure and intercurrent infections which may be fatal. Duration of illness may be 6 months to 3 years.

Acute onset ICC may present with sudden appearance of jaundice, fever, clay colored stools and hepatomegaly. Hepatic coma may develop rapidly leading to fatal outcome of the disease. Some children may become symptomatic for variable period and again reappearance of features may found which behave like ICC of insidious onset.

Diagnosis

The important diagnostic approaches are liver biopsy (may not be feasible if prothrombin time is prolonged). Cupriuresis test may be performed by oral administration of D-penicillamine, using urinary copper/creatinine ratio as the index parameter, sensitivity and specificity with positive and negative values are obtained.

Management

Few cases of ICC improve spontaneously and survive without specific treatment.

D-penicillamine therapy is used as copper-chelating agent from the liver, which impoves the survivals. Immunomodulating agents like levamisole, corticosteroids, gammaglobulins may also be used. Symptomatic treatment should be done especially for infections and vitamins and minerals deficiency.

Supportive care should be provided as rest, diet with good quality proteins, IV glucose drip, oxygen therapy, antibiotics therapy (neomycin) and good nursing care. Hepatic coma or precoma should be detected early for prompt management.

Nursing interventions should provide special attention on improving nutritional status, promoting of activity tolerance, protecting skin integrity, preventing injury and bleeding, and expert care for unconscious patients, if needed.

Exchange transfusion may be effective to remove circulating toxins. In case of portal hypertension causing hematemesis, *Sengstaken tube* may be of help to control esophageal bleeding. Portocaval anastomosis may be done to relieve the portal hypertension and complications of hypersplenism.

Preventive management should be emphasized with continuing breastfeeding up to six months and avoiding boiling of milk in copper or copper alloy pots. Increasing public awareness about the preventive measures is important regarding lowering of copper intake through copper-rich food, water and utensils.

Prognosis

Despite the best of efforts, ICC invariably had a fatal outcome in the past. Recently, survival of some cases are reported.

Heart Diseases in Children

17

- Fetal Circulation
- Congenital Heart Disease
- Congestive Cardiac Failure
- Acute Rheumatic Fever

- Rheumatic Heart Disease
- Infective Endocarditis
- Cardiomyopathy in Children

INTRODUCTION

The most common heart diseases in children are congenital heart disease and rheumatic fever with its consequences. Congestive cardiac failure is a common pediatric emergency, with its different etiology than that of adults. Other heart diseases which may found in infants and children are cardiomyopathy, myocarditis, paroxysmal atrial tachycardia, sick sinus syndrome, Takayasu arteritis (pulseless disease), pericardial diseases and hypertension.

Common clinical features of cardiac diseases include chest pain, tachycardia, bradycardia, dyspnea, cyanosis, palpitation, sweating during feeding, fatigue, squatting position, orthopnea, feeding difficulty, clubbing, edema, chest deformity, engorgement of neck veins, hepatomegaly, etc. History of illness, clinical examination, cardiac examination and auscultation are very important aspect of diagnostic evaluation before the planning of investigations.

The investigations to detect the cardiac problems and to confirm the diagnosis include X-ray studies, ECG, echocardiography, MRI, radionuclide angiography, cardiac catheterization, ABG analysis, complete hemogram, urinalysis, etc.

FETAL CIRCULATION

Knowledge about fetal circulation is absolutely necessary for proper understanding of congenital heart diseases. The fetal heart assumes its four-chambered shape by the end of six weeks of fetal life. Growth of fetal heart occurs with increasing age of the fetus. But there are four different anatomical structures present in fetal circulation which differentiate it from the neonatal circulation in extra uterine life. These structures are ductus venosus, foramen ovale, ductus arteriosus, and umbilical (hypogastric) arteries. Other characteristic differences of fetal circulation include the followings:

- Placenta is the site of gaseous exchange and excretion of fetal waste and provides a low resistance circuit.
- Intracardiac and extracardiac shunts are presents in fetal circulation.
- Lungs take oxygen from blood rather than supplying it. Very small amount of blood flows to the lungs from the right ventricular output. Lungs secrete a fluid into the respiratory passage, thus right ventricle has to pump blood against higher resistance than left ventricle.
- Liver receives the highest percentage of oxygen and nutrients from maternal circulation.

Fetus receives oxygenated blood (80% oxygen saturation) from the placenta by umbilical vein, which enters the fetus at the umbilicus. The umbilical vein carries the blood to the liver and given off branches to the left lobe to supply the oxygenated blood and receives the deoxygenated blood from the portal vein. Most of the umbilical venous blood by-passes the liver through the ductus venosus and enters in the inferior vena cava, then to the right atrium of the heart. Inferior vena cava also contains the deoxygenated blood from lower extremities and the structures below the diaphragm. So there is mixing of blood and reduction is oxygen saturation.

From the right atrium (70% oxygen saturation), one-third of the inferior vena caval return enters the left atrium through the foramen ovale and rest two-thirds mixes with venous return from superior vena cava and flows to the right ventricle.

In the left atrium, there is mixing of blood received from right atrium with the small amount of venous blood returning from the lungs through the pulmonary veins. From left atrium, blood flows to the left ventricles which is then pumped in the ascending aorta and arch of the aorta to supply heart, head, neck and upper extremities.

The right ventricular blood is pumped into the pulmonary trunk and a small amount of the blood enters the pulmonary circulation. The major portion of the blood from the right ventricle via the pulmonary trunk, bypasses the non-functioning lungs through the ductus arteriosus into the descending aorta and mixed with the small amount of blood from aortic arch which then supply to the lower extremities and other structures below the diaphragm.

The deoxygenated blood leaves the fetus by the two umbilical arteries, branches of internal iliac arteries, to reach the placenta for oxygenation and recirculation.

Figures 17.1A and B, shows the diagrammatic representation of fetal circulation with four sites of shunts.

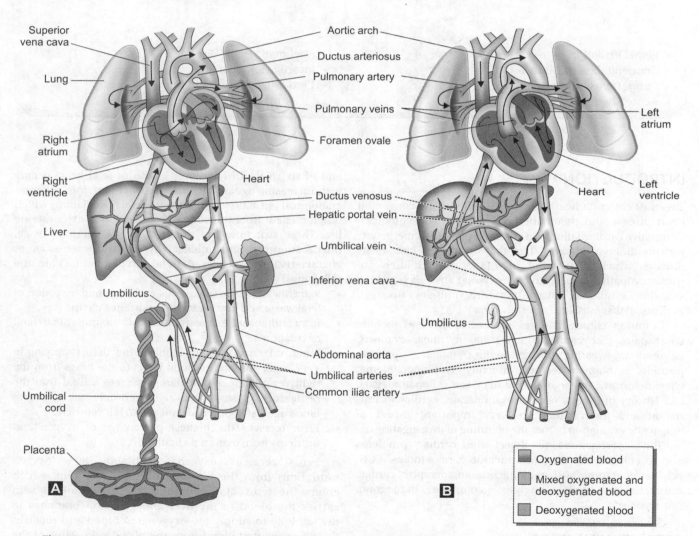

Figs 17.1A and B: (A) Fetal circulation before birth; (B) Changes to the fetal circulation at birth *(For color version, see Plate 6)* *(Source: Ross and Wilson. Anatomy and physiology by Churchill Livingstone: Elsevier)*

Changes of Fetal Circulation at Birth

There are profound changes occur in the fetal circulation soon after birth due to cessation of placental blood flow and initiation of respiration. The major changes are as follows:

- *Closure of the umbilical arteries:* It occurs due to clamping and cutting of the umbilical cord. The functional closure is almost immediate and actual obliteration takes about 2 to 3 months. The distal parts form the lateral umbilical ligament and proximal part remains open as vesicle arteries.
- *Closure of umbilical vein:* It occurs a little later than arteries, allowing few extra volume of blood (80-100 mL) to be received by the fetus from the placenta. The umbilical vein form the ligamentum teres, after complete obliteration.
- The ductus venosus collapses and becomes ligamentum venosum afterwards. The blood flows through the ductus venosus disappears by the 7th day of neonatal life.
- Foramen ovale closes due to increased pressure in the left atrium and decreased pressure of right atrium. It happens due to expansion of lungs with enhancement of pulmonary blood flow and loss of placental circulation. Anatomical closure of foramen ovale occurs over a period of months to years when septum primum and septum secundum become firmly adherent.
- The functional closure of ductus arteriosus may occur soon after birth with the initiation of respiration and satisfactory pulmonary circulation. Expansion of lungs leads to increased left heart pressure and lowering the pulmonary vascular resistance which leads to fall in a pulmonary arterial pressure. So there is reversed flow of blood through the ductus arteriosus from aorta to pulmonary artery. Increased oxygen saturation of blood results in constriction of musculature of the ductus which is enhanced by the action of prostaglandins and leads to closure of ductus arteriosus. The structural obliteration of the ductus arteriosus takes places about 1 to 3 months.

Within one to two hours following birth, the cardiac output is estimated to be about 500 mL per minute and the heart rate varies from 120 to140 per minute.

CONGENITAL HEART DISEASE

Congenital heart disease (CHD) is the structural malformations of the heart or great vessels, present at birth. It is the most common congenital malformations. The exact number of prevalence is not known.

Etiology

The exact cause of CHD is unknown in about 90 percent of cases. Heredity and consanguineous marriage are important etiological factors. Genetic disorders and chromosomal aberrations (Trisomy-21, Turner's syndrome) are also known to predispose congenital heart disease. Other associated factors responsible for CHD include fetal and maternal teratogenic infections (rubella), teratogenic drug (thalidomide) intake, alcohol intake by the mother and irradiation in first trimester of pregnancy, maternal IDDM, high altitude, fetal hypoxia, birth asphyxia, etc.

Classification

Congenital heart disease (CHD) can be grouped into three categories:

1. *Acyanotic CHD:* There is increased pulmonary blood flow due to left to right shunt. It includes:
   - Ventricular septal defect (VSD)
   - Atrial septal defect (ASD)
   - Patent ductus arteriosus (PDA)
   - Atrioventricular canal (AVC)
2. *Cyanotic CHD:* There is diminished pulmonary blood flow due to right to left shunt. It includes:
   - Tetralogy of Fallot (TOF)
   - Tricuspid atresia (TA)
   - Transposition of great arteries (TGA)
   - Truncus arteriosus.
   - Hypoplastic left heart syndrome.
   - Total anomalous pulmonary venous return.
   - Eisenmenger syndrome or complex.
3. *Obstructive lesions*
   - Coarctation of aorta.
   - Aortic value stenosis.
   - Pulmonary valve stenosis.
   - Congenital mitral stenosis.

The most common congenital heart diseases are discussed below.

Ventricular Septal Defect (Fig. 17.2)

A ventricular septal defect (VSD) is an abnormal opening in the septum between right and left ventricles. It is the most common acyanotic congenital heart disease with left to right shunt. It is found approximately 25 percent of all CHD. The size of defect can be small or large. Large VSDs can be restrictive or nonrestrictive type. Number of defects can be single or multiple. VSD can be found as perimembranous or muscular.

Pathophysiology: There is flow of oxygenated blood from high pressure left ventricle to low pressure right ventricle through the VSD. Increased right ventricular and pulmonary arterial pressure leads to pulmonary over circulation. Increased venous return to the left heart results in left heart dilation. Long standing pulmonary overcirculation causes change in pulmonary arterial bed resulting increased pulmonary vascular resistance, which can reverse the shunt from right to

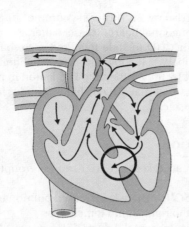

Fig. 17.2: Ventricular septal defect

left. This complicated condition is known as Eisenmenger's complex. The child with this condition presents with cyanosis and surgical correction of VSDs is not possible in this stage.

In case of a restrictive VSD (under 0.5 cm²) higher pressure in the LV is able to cause only a limited left to right shunt. In case of nonrestrictive VSD (large, usually over 1 cm²), magnitude of the shunt from left to right is, therefore, limited at birth due to higher pulmonary vascular resistance. In next few weeks, with the reduction in resistance, the shunt magnitude increases. VSD becomes symptomatic when the shunt magnitude becomes quite large.

Clinical manifestations: Small VSDs are asymptomatic. In large defects, symptoms develops within one to 2 months of age. The manifestations are recurrent chest infections, feeding difficulties, tachypnea, exertional dyspnea, pale, delicate looking, tachycardia, excessive sweating associated with feeding, poor weight gain, failure to thrive, hepatomegaly, biventricular hypertrophy and CCF.

The characteristic loud pansystolic murmur heard maximal down the left sternal border, usually accompanied by the thrill. The functional diastolic murmur may present.

Diagnostic evaluation: History of illness, physical examination and auscultation of harsh systolic murmur and pulmonary second sound (p_2) are important for diagnosis of the condition. Chest X-ray shows enlargement of the heart and increased pulmonary vascular marking. ECG reveals biventricular hypertrophy. Two-dimensional echocardiogram with Doppler study and color flow mapping are performed to identify the size, number, site of defect and associated problems.

Management: In small VSD, usually no medical management is required. Surgical repair may be indicated in some cases. Prevention of complications is very essential measures. Spontaneous closure of VSD occurs in 30 to 50 percent cases with small defects.

In large VSD, initial management of associated problems like CCF and endocarditis, should be done with appropriate treatment. Early surgical repair is planned after management of complications.

Surgery is done as one-stage or two-stage operation. One-stage operation with patch closure of VSD by open-heart method can be performed. Two-stage approach is done with first stage, to band the pulmonary artery to restrict pulmonary blood flow by closed-heart method. Second stage operation is done to patch close the VSD and remove the PA band. Surgery is contraindicated in shunt reversal.

Long-term prognosis after corrective surgery is excellent. Expert nursing management is important during surgical interventions and in complications. Long-term follow-up and monitoring of ventricular functions are important measures to promote excellent prognosis.

Complications: The common complications of VSD are CCF, recurrent respiratory tract infections, infective endocarditis, Eisenmenger's syndrome, pulmonary stenosis, pulmonary hypertension and failure to thrive. Postoperative complications after thoracic surgery may be life-threatening for the child.

Atrial Septal Defect (Fig. 17.3)

Atrial septal defect (ASD) is an abnormal opening between right and left atria resulting left to right shunting of blood. It accounts for 9 percent of all CHDs.

Types: There are three types of ASDs:
1. *Ostium secundum ASD:* It is the most common type of ASDs. An abnormal opening in the middle of the atrial septum presents due to abnormal development of the septum secundum.

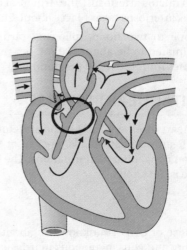

Fig. 17.3: Atrial septal defect

2. *Ostium primum ASD:* It presents as an abnormal opeing at the bottom of the atrial septum due to improper development of the septum primum. There may be increased association with cleft mitral valve and atrioventricular defects.
3. *Sinus venosus ASD*: It is an abnormal opening at the top of the atrial septum. There may be increased association with partial anomalous pulmonary venous connection.

Pathophysiology: There is flow of oxygenated blood from higher pressure left atrium to lower pressure right atrium across the ASD resulting volume overload to right ventricles and right ventricular dilation. Thus increased blood flow to lungs leads to elevated pulmonary artery pressure.

Clinical manifestations: Ostium secundum and sinus venosus ASDs are usually asymptomatic. The manifestations due to ostium primum ASD depend upon the associated defects.

The child may have recurrent chest infections, dyspnea on exertion, easy fatigability, bulging of the chest, poor weight gain, cardiac enlargement and CCF.

Diagnostic evaluation: Auscultation of heart sound is important diagnostic approach. In ostium secundum ASD, soft systolic flow murmur heard best at the left upper sternal border. It is preceded by a loud first sound and may be radiated to the apex and back. Pulmonary second sound p_2 is widely split and fixed. In ostium primum ASD, systolic murmur heard best at the lower left sternal border because of mitral regurgitation.

Chest X-ray shows right atrial and ventricular dilation and increased pulmonary marking. ECG demonstrates right ventricular hypertrophy and right axis deviation. Two-dimensional echocardiogram with doppler study and color flow mapping and cardiac catheterization are useful approach for detection of problems and associated complications.

Management: Surgical closure of the defect is planned in early childhood to prevent further complications. CCF and arrhythmias should be managed medically. Antibiotic prophylaxis is necessary during dental procedures, if needed.

Repair of the defect is done by suture closure or pericardial patch repair by open heart surgery. Result of surgical interventions are gratifying. Supportive nursing care is very important.

Complications: The complications of ASD may include infective endocarditis, pulmonary arterial hypertension, CCF, growth retardation and postoperative complications after surgical repair.

Patent Ductus Arteriosus (Fig. 17.4)

It is the persistent vascular connection between the pulmonary artery and the aorta. Functionally, the closure of ductus arteriosus (which is normally present in fetal life) occurs soon after birth. When ductus arteriosus remains patent and open

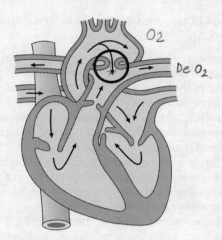

Fig. 17.4: Patent ductus arteriosus

after birth, the blood flows in the ductus from the aorta to the pulmonary artery due to higher pressure in the aorta.

Patent ductus arteriosus (PDA) is common in preterm infants who weigh less than 1.5 kg. It is the more common type in female baby and occurs approximately 11 percent of all CHDs.

Pathophysiology: In PDA, there is left to right shunt as blood flows from aorta (higher pressure) to pulmonary artery (lower pressure) leading to pulmonary overload. Thus oxygenated blood of systemic circulation flows back to pulmonary circulation resulting in increased vascular pressure in the pulmonary tree and volume load on left heart. In severe degree PDA, pulmonary vascular disease and pulmonary hypertension may occur.

Clinical manifestations: The clinical presentations of PDA depend upon the size of ductus and its patency. Small and moderate size PDA are usually asymptomatic. Symptomatic cases manifested with tachypnea, bounding pulse and Corrigan pulsation in the neck. Dyspnea and frequent respiratory infections usually found. There is increased systolic pressure and low diastolic pressure with wide pulse-pressure. Precordial pain, hoarseness of voice, feeding difficulties, slow weight gain or growth failure and CCF are common features of a child with PDA.

Diagnostic evaluation: History of illness and physical examination help in diagnostic evaluation. Auscultation of heart sound reveals continuous murmur (machinery murmur) heard at second left intercostal space or below the left clavicle or lower down, i.e. at left sternal border. There may be paradoxical splitting of P_2.

Chest X-ray shows cardiomegaly and increased pulmonary vascular marking. Two-dimensional echocardiogram with Doppler study and color flow mapping and cardiac catheterization can also be done to detect the extent of problems. ECG reveals left arterial dilation and left ventricular hypertrophy.

Management

- *Medical management:* In symptomatic patient with PDA, Indomethacin, 0.1 to 0.25 mg/kg/dose/I/V—over 30 minutes very slowly is administered, every 12 to 24 hours for 3 doses, for pharmacological closure of ductus arteriosus. Antiprostaglandin agents, aspirin, ibuprofen and mefanamic acid can also be used.

  Supportive care is provided with rest, adequate intake of calorie for weight gain and promotion of normal growth and development with routine care. Emotional support to the parents are essential.

  Conservative management of CCF and other associated complications should be done with appropriate treatment.

- *Surgical management:* Transection or ligation of patent ductus arteriosus via a lateral thoracotomy, a closed heart intervention is performed. It is done preferably between 3 and 10 years of age in asymptomatic patients and in symptomatic patients, it should be done irrespective of age and in the presence of pulmonary hypertension. The result of surgery is excellent. Preoperative and postoperative care for thoracic surgery to be provided with all precautions.

Complications: A child with PDA can have complications like CCF, infective endocarditis, pulmonary hypertension and pulmonary vascular occlusive disease. Rarely, calcification of ductus, thromboembolism, rheumatic heart disease and Eisenmenger syndrome may develop.

Tetralogy of Fallot (Fig. 17.5)

Tetralogy of Fallot (TOF) is the most common cyanotic congenital heart disease. It accounts for 6 to 10 percent of all CHDs. This condition is characterized by the combinations of four defects: (1) pulmonary stenosis, (2) ventricular septal defect, (3) overriding or dextroposition of the aorta, and (4) right ventricular hypertrophy.

Pathophysiology: Due to structural defects, there is right to left heart shunt causing cyanosis. The most vital abnormalities are pulmonary stenosis and VSD (generally perimembranous variety). Obstruction of blood flow from the right ventricle due to pulmonary valve stenosis results in shunting of deoxygenated blood through the VSD into the left ventricle, then to the aorta causes cyanosis. Degree of cyanosis depends upon the degree of right ventricular outflow tract obstruction and the size of the VSD. Outflow obstruction can also occur due to infundibular hypertrophy and supravalvular stenosis. Right ventricular hypertrophy develops due to the obstruction. Finally the condition is complicated by persistent arterial unsaturation, poor pulmonary vascularity, polycythemia to compensate cyanosis and increased blood viscosity resulting thrombophlebitis and formation of emboli. Minimum right to left shunt in small obstruction causes mild form of TOF and termed as pink or acyanotic tetralogy of Fallot.

Clinical manifestations: Clinical features of TOF depend upon size of VSD and degree of right ventricular outflow obstruction. Blue baby or cyanosis of lips and nailbeds with dyspnea is found initially with crying and exertion in neonates especially when the ductus arteriosus begins to close.

As the infant grows, other presenting features are observed, i.e. hypoxic-anoxic or blue (hypercyanotic) spells, which occur due to cerebral anoxia. The spell consists of irritability, dyspnea, cyanosis, flacidity with or without unconsciousness. The spell is also termed as Tet-spell, and found in the morning soon after awakening, during or after feeding and painful procedures. The child feels comfortable in squatting posture or in lying down position. Slow weight gain and mental slowness are found. By the age of two years, the child usually develops clubbing. CCF is unusual in infants and children suffering from TOF.

Diagnostic evaluation: Details history of illness and thorough clinical examination are important diagnostic approach. Auscultation of soft or harsh systolic ejection murmur heard best at the upper left sternal border in third space. P_2 is usually single.

Chest X-ray shows poorly vascularized lung fields, a small boot-shaped heart (due to RVH) and concavity of the pulmonary artery segment. There may be right aortic arch.

ECG shows right axis deviation and RVH. Two-dimensional echocardiogram and cardiac catheterization help to detect structural abnormalities, degree of obstruction and coronary artery pattern.

Management

- *Medical management:* The child with TOF should be managed for cyanosis, hypoxic spells and other associated complications. Oxygen therapy, correction of

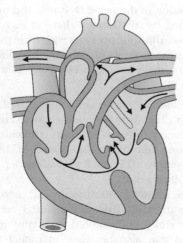

Fig. 17.5: Tetralogy of Fallot

dehydration, anemia, antibiotic therapy, supportive nursing care and continuous monitoring of child's condition are very important measures.

Hypoxic spells should be managed by placing the baby in knee-chest position, sedatives, oral propranolol therapy, IV fluid, treatment of acidosis, oxygen therapy and administration of IV vasopressors (phenylephrine, methoxamine). Oxygen therapy during the spells has limited value. Planning for surgical correction of defects should be done as soon as the child starts having spells. Parents should be taught about the immediate care at home during the spells and necessary medical help.

Neonates with severe TOF, may be benefited from prostaglandin E$_1$ (IV) which causes dilatation of the ductus and allows adequate pulmonary blood flow. It should be administered immediately on diagnosis of cyanotic CHD.

- *Surgical management:* Surgical interventions can be planned as palliative surgery or definitive correction in one stage repair. One stage repair may be contraindicated in abnormal coronary artery distribution, multiple VSDs, hypoplastic branch of pulmonary arteries and small infant with less than 2.5 kg body weight.

Palliative surgery is performed by different techniques as Modified Blalock-Taussig (BT) shunt, Potts operation or Waterson's operation.

Definitive correction is performed by direct vision open heart surgery for patch closure of VSD and relief of right ventricular obstruction. Total correction carries a mortality of 15 percent. Long-term follow-up of the survived cases is very essential to monitor child's condition and early detection of complications.

Survived child may show complete disappearance of cyanosis, clubbing and improvement in growth and development. Specialized nursing care is essential for these children before and after surgery.

Complications: Hypoxic spells, Tet spell, polycythemia and CCF (rare) may develop in children with TOF. Postoperative complications include sudden death due to cardiac arrhythmias, exercise disability, complete heart block and operative complications.

Transposition of Great Arteries (Fig. 17.6)

Transposition of great arteries (TGA) occurs when the pulmonary artery originates from the left ventricle and the aorta originates from the right ventricle. It is an embryologic defect caused by a straight division of the bulbar trunk without normal spiralling. It accounts 5 to 10 percent of all CHDs. It occurs predominantly in males. Incidence is significantly high in the history of diabetes in grandparents and the babies having large birth weight.

It is the most important cause of cyanosis at birth and responsible for most of the mortality from cyanotic CHD in the first year of life. It may be associated with other defects

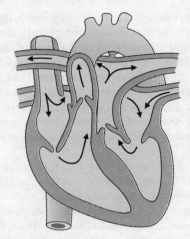

Fig. 17.6: Transposition of great arteries

like VSD, ASD, PDA, pulmonary stenosis and coarctation of aorta.

In TGA, there are two independent circuits of circulation, life can only be maintained postnatally, if some communication between systemic and pulmonary circulation exists. Such communication is provided with VSD, ASD, PDA or collateral circulation resulting mixing of oxygenated and deoxygenated blood and causing cyanosis.

Clinical manifestations: The neonate with TGA is presented with severe cyanosis, appearing soon after birth. Afterwards, dyspnea, metabolic acidosis, severe hypoxia and CCF are found. The condition may complicated with multiorgan ischemia, cardiomegaly and growth failure. Clubbing may develop in few months.

Diagnosis is confirmed by auscultation of heart sound, radiology, ECG, cardiac catheterization and angiocardiography.

Management: Medical management of the condition is done with IV prostaglandin E$_1$, (PGE$_1$), digoxin, diuretics and iron therapy. Severe hypoxia can be treated with balloon atrial septostomy. Supportive nursing care is important.

Surgical management is planned depending upon the associated defects. Arterial switch operation, Restelli's operation, Beffe's operation are the different methods, can be performed to offer best results.

Tricuspid Atresia

Tricuspid atresia (TA) is the congenital absence of tricuspid valve resulting no communication between the right atrium and the right ventricle. So the total systemic venous return enters the left heart by means of foramen ovale or an ASD, resulting cyanosis.

This condition is characterized by small right ventricle, large left ventricle and diminished pulmonary circulation. Blood from right atrium flows to left atrium and mixes with oxygenated blood which is returning from lungs. Left ventricle receives the mixed blood and pumped into the systemic circulation. Lungs may receive the blood from three routes, i.e. VSD, PDA, and bronchial vessels. The size of VSD and the presence and severity of pulmonary stenosis determine the degree of cyanosis with which most subjects present in early months.

About 30 percent cases of tricuspid atresia may have associated TGA. Pulmonary blood flow in these cases is usually increased and may cause early CCF.

In 90 percent cases of tricuspid atresia, pulmonary blood flow is decreased and presented as early onset cyanosis. The diagnosis is confirmed by chest X-ray, ECG, echocardiogram and cardiac catheterization.

Medical management of tricuspid atresia is done with PGE_1 infusion (IV), intubation and ventilatory support (if needed) with other supportive and symptomatic care.

Surgical management is planned depending upon the level of pulmonary blood flow. Blalock Taussig (BT) shunt and pulmonary artery banding is performed in neonates. Bi-directionl Glenn shunt is done for the infants and modified Fontan operation is preferred at the age of 2 to 5 years. Postoperative complications may include pleural effusion, vena caval syndrome, thromboembolism, supraventricular arrhythmias and left ventricular dysfunction.

Intensive care is required for promoting survival of the children in preoperative and postoperative period. Parents need support and involvement in planning and providing the necessary interventions to the child.

Aortic Stenosis

Congenital aortic valve stenosis (AoS) is an obstructive cardiac lesion, constitutes about 8 percent of all CHDs. It may be valvular, subvalvular and supravalvular.

Valvular stenosis accounts for 75 percent of the cases of aortic stenosis. It results from either an unicuspid or a bicuspid aortic valve. The bicuspid aortic valve results in significant obstruction when the valves become thicker and relatively immobile with fused commissures that does not open completely. Aortic stenosis may occur due to hypoplastic aortic valve annulus.

Subvalvular stenosis is found as three types, i.e. discrete membranous, fibromuscular and idiopathic hypertropic.

Aortic valve stenosis is the most common form of left ventricular outflow tract obstruction. It is a progressive lesion and occurs more often in boys. Additional left heart obstruction may be found, i.e. coarctation of aorta and mitral valve stenosis.

Clinical manifestations: Most patients with aortic stenosis have no manifestations except easy fatigability, exercise intolerance, dizziness and syncope. Symptomatic neonates present with severe CCF, tachypnea, faint peripheral pulse, poor perfusion, poor capillary refill, cold skin, poor feeding and metabolic acidosis. In older children, manifestations are chest pain on exertion, decreased exercise tolerance, dyspnea, pulmonary edema, shortness of breath, fatigue, dizziness, light headedness, palpitations, arrhythmias, syncope and sudden death. The condition may be complicated with bacterial endocarditis and left heart failure.

Diagnosis is confirmed by X-ray chest, ECG, ecocardiography, serial catheterization and cineangiography.

Management: Management of aortic stenosis in neonates is done with PGE_1 infusion, ventilatory support (if needed) with intubation, aortic balloon valvuloplasty by cardiac catheterization and surgical procedure as valvotomy. The older children is managed by close monitoring of child's condition by regular follow-up and restriction of intense exercise and anerobic exercise like competitive sports, athletics, strenuous exercises and weightlifting. Surgical interventions in older children are done as aortic balloon valvoplasty, valvotomy and aortic valve replacement. Postsurgery follow-up is very important to prevent complications, especially in valve replacement. Intensive care to be provided during surgery and thereafter. Parents need details informations about long term care.

Postoperative complications include aortic regurgitation and failure of replaced valve to work indefinitely. The result of surgery in discrete membranous subvalvular aortic stenosis are better than valvular type.

Coarctation of Aorta (Fig. 17.7)

Coarctation of aorta (CoA) is a distinct narrowing or a long segment hypoplasia of the aortic arch, usually distal to the subclavian artery. The narrow aortic lumen may exist as

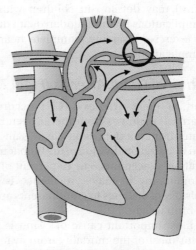

Fig. 17.7: Coarctation of aorta

preductal or postductal obstruction depending upon the position of the obstruction in relation to the ductus arteriosus. The lesion produces an obstruction to the blood flow through the aorta causing increased pressure and workload of the left ventricle. The constriction is found in the shape of a sharp indentation involving the anterior, lateral and a posterior wall of the aorta. The aorta immediately distal to the coarctation is often dilated. Collateral vessels grow and bypass the coarctation to perfuse the lower body parts.

The condition is more commonly found in male and may accompany with other defects like VSD, PDA, tubular hypoplasia of the aortic isthmus and bicuspid aortic valve. It is a common association in Turner syndrome.

Clinical manifestations: The clinical features of CoA depend upon type of the defect and usually become evident after the closure of PDA. In the neonates, the presenting features are severe CCF, poor perfusion, tachypnea, acidosis and absent femoral pulses. In older children, it may be asymptomatic with normal growth and development. But overgrowth of upper limbs and hypertension in the upper extremities with absent of weak femoral pulse may be suggestive of the defect.

Other manifestations include fatigue, cramps, intermittent claudication, headache, weakness and exertional dyspnea. The condition may be complicated with hypertension, CCF, cerebral hemorrhage, encephalopathy and bacterial endocarditis.

Diagnosis of the condition can be confirmed by chest X-ray, barium swallow, ECG, M-mode ecocardiography, cardiac catheterization and angiocardiography. 'Barium swallow demonstrated 'E' sign. The first arch of the 'E' is due to dilatation of aorta before the coarctation, the second is due to poststenotic dilatation and middle due to the coarctation itself.

Management: Medical management of the condition is done with PGE_1 infusion, antibiotics and prevention and treatment of complications. Surgical intervention is planned in 3 to 5 years of age after management of systemic hypertension and other associated complications. Corrective surgery is performed as resection of constricted area and end-to-end anastomosis. Subclavian flap repair and Dacron patch repair can be preferred. Chances of development of recoarctation in later life are considerably reduced. Survival of the child depends upon the presence of complications and long-term care provided to the children.

If CCF develops in neonatal period or early in infancy, death is a rule, unless vigorous treatment is offered. If no CCF occurs, the child may do well without surgery throughout the childhood and adolescence.

Nursing Management of the Children with Congenital Heart Diseases

Nursing management aims at early diagnosis and management of the problems with prevention of complications and genetic counseling.

Nursing Assessment

Detail history of present complaints, history of illness, birth history, family history and development history are specially significant.

Anthropometric measurements help to assess the severity of problems and associated growth failure. Measurement of weight, length/height, head, chest and arm circumference are essential aspects of assessment to be done and recorded.

Assessment of vital signs, oxygen saturation, skin color (pink, cyanotic, mottled), mucous membrane (dry or cyanotic), peripheral pulse (rate, symmetry, quality), edema, capillary refill, cold to touch, clubbing, chest wall deformity, level of activity and consciousness, respiratory pattern, heart sound, feeding behavior, intake and output, sleep pattern, etc. are all important to plan and implement nursing care. Laboratory findings and other investigation reports to be reviewed to identify the problems.

Nursing Diagnoses

The important nursing diagnosis in care of the children with CHDs are as follows:
- Impaired gas exchange related to disturbed pulmonary blood flow.
- Decreased cardiac output related to reduced myocardial functions.
- Activity intolerance related to hypoxia.
- Altered nutrition, less than body requirements related to excessive energy demands required by increased cardiac workload.
- Risk for infections related to chronic illness.
- Fear and anxiety related to life-threatening illness.
- Knowledge deficit related to long-term problems and prevetion of complications.

Nursing Interventions (Based on above Nursing Diagnoses)

- Relieving respiratory distress by semi-up right position, clearing oral and nasal secretions, oxygen therapy, administering prescribed medications, (diuretic, bronchodilators) and prevention of aspiration with continuous monitoring of respiratory pattern. (ABG analysis, respiratory status).

- Improving cardiac output by uninterrupted rest, minimum exercise (as play and other activities of daily living), maintaining normal body temperature and comfortable environment, administering medications (digoxin, anti-hypertensive) and monitoring child's condition (vital signs, heart sound).
- Improving oxygenation and activity tolerance by conti-nuous monitoring by pulse oximetry, oxygen therapy (by face mask or nasal cannula) and emotional support with physical rest.
- *Providing adequate nutrition:* The child should be provided with small frequent feeding. Oral feeding should be limited to 15 to 20 minutes. Nasogastric tube feeding may be needed to provide extra calories, when oral feeding is not possible. The older children may required high calorie diet according to likes and dislikes. Feeding intolerance should be observed. Daily weight recording and maintenance of intake and output chart are compulsory. Adequate fluid intake should be allowed unless contraindicated.
- Preventing infections by avoiding exposure to infections and infected person, good handwashing practices, maintaining general cleanliness and hygienic measures, completion of immunization schedule, early detection and treatment of upper respiratory infections and GI infections.
- Reducing fear and anxiety by explanation, reassurance and answering questions of the child, parents and family members. Informing about available facilities and support services.
- Teaching about health maintenance and follow-up according to the level of understanding and child's problem are important. Instructing about adequate diet, rest, immunization, prevention and control of infections, regular medical and dental check-up. Teaching the parent and family members about signs and symptoms of complications and emergency care especially in hypoxic spells, dehydration, pulmonary edema, CCF, cardiac arrest, etc. Encouraging the parents to treat the child as in normal manner by avoiding overprotection, overindulgence and rejection. Promoting growth and development and avoiding projection of fear, anxiety and stress. Information to be given regarding available medical facilities, community health nursing services and social support for rehabilitation.

CONGESTIVE CARDIAC FAILURE

Congestive cardiac failure (CCF) is a common pediatric emergency. It is also termed as congestive heart failure (CHF). It indicates inadequate cardiac output.

Congestive cardiac failure can be defined as "inability of the heart to maintain an output at rest or during stress, necessary for the metabolic needs of the body (systolic failure) and inability to receive blood into the ventricular cavities at low pressure during diastole (diastolic failure)". It is a syndrome due to various anatomical or pathological causes. Systolic failure is much more common clinical problem.

Etiology

Congestive cardiac failure may result due to congenital heart disease and also due to acquired heart diseases like acute rheumatic fever, rheumatic heart disease, myocarditis, hypertension, cardiomyopathy and paroxysmal supra-ventricular tachycardia. Noncardiovascular diseases, like chronic pulmonary disease, respiratory infections, anemia, nephrotic syndrome, iatrogenic fluid over load, also may cause CCF.

Pathophysiology

Decreased cardiac output leads to inadequate supply of oxygen and nutrition to the tissue. To meet the metabolic demands of the body the heart rate increases to enhance cardiac output which results to increase stroke volume (cardiac output = heart rate × stroke volume). The systemic vascular resistance increases to maintain blood pressure. Reduced blood flow to the kidneys decreases glomerular filtration rate and tubular reabsorption increases, causing sodium and water retention leading to edema and diminished urine output. Thus cardiac output decreases further. Increased venous pressure due to poor contraction of failing heart results in venous congestion and edema. Pulmonary system becomes congested. In chronic long-term illness, myocardial failure, myocardial hypertrophy and chamber dilation lead to progressive heart failure.

Clinical Manifestations

The clinical features of CCF are related to impaired myocardial functions, pulmonary congestion and systemic venous congestion.

Impaired myocardial function is presented as tachycardia, poor peripheral perfusion with weak peripheral pulses and cool extremities, pallor, easy fatigability, excessive perspiration, restlessness and exercise or activity intolerance.

Pulmonary congestion is manifested as tachypnea, cyanosis, chest retractions, nasal flaring, grunting, non-productive persistent cough and pulmonary edema with dyspnea at rest (orthopnea) or on exertion.

Systemic venous congestion is presented as hepatomegaly, peripheral edema, scrotal and orbital edema, oliguria, water weight gain, neck vein distension, abdominal discomfort, anorexia and feeding difficulties.

Diagnostic Evaluation

Details history of illness and physical examination including palpation of weak peripheral pulses with cold extremities, poor capillary refill, palpable liver are useful for diagnosis. Auscultation of heart reveals gallop rhythm, systolic flow murmur and tachycardia. Auscultation of lungs reveals crackling and wheezing sound. Chest X-ray shows cardiac enlargement and pulmonary congestion.

Management

Management of CCF is aimed at correction of inadequate cardiac output. This can be achieved by reducing cardiac work, augmenting myocardial contractility, improving cardiac performance by reducing heart size and correcting the cause of heart failure.

Management of the child with CCF to be done with bedrest in propped up position (45°) and restricting activities. Oxygen therapy is important to improve tissue oxygenation.

Sedative should be administered to manage restlessness and to reduce anxiety. Digitalis is the most important drug for the management of CCF. It should be administered with calculated dose in stat and maintenance purpose. Diuretics (frusemide) is given orally or parenterally (0.5–1.5 mg/kg). Potassium–sparing mild diuretics (amiloride, spironolactone) is also used in a dose of 1 to 4 mg/kg/day. Potassium supplement to be given during digitalis therapy, Iron supplement may be needed for correction of anemia. Antibiotic should be given to treat co-existing infection. Vasodilator and ACE inhibitors can be given to reduce cardiac work.

Diet should be planned with low salt for sodium restriction and to be given in small amount frequently. It may be difficult to maintain to low-salt diet in infants. Correction of anemia may be done by improving iron containing food intake whenever needed.

Supportive nursing care should emphasize on skin care and other hygienic measures, prevention of infections and fluid-electrolyte imbalance, diet, administration of medications with necessary precautions, continuous monitoring of child's condition, maintenance of intake-output and other records.

Emotional support and health teaching with necessary instructions should include dietary and activity restrictions, features of complications, drug intake, prevention of complications, daily hygienic care, and measures for prevention of infections and injury of edematous skin, need for emergency medical help and regular follow-up.

Correction of underlying cause of CCF should be seriously considered. Surgically manageable cases should be identified early and appropriate referral is needed for adequate management. Refractory CCF cases should be re-evaluated for appropriate treatment. Ultrafiltration or dialysis may required in renal shutdown. Cardiac transplantation with or without mechanical support may prove life saving in some cases.

Prognosis

Prognosis in case of CCF depends upon the cause and available treatment facilities. Early diagnosis and initiation of treatment promote better prognosis. The child with associated complications like metabolic acidosis, lower respiratory infections and arrhythmia, may cause poor prognosis. Long-term suffering may lead to failure to thrive and growth retardation.

ACUTE RHEUMATIC FEVER

Acute rheumatic fever (ARF) is an acute autoimmune collagen disease occurs as a hypersensitivity reaction to group-A beta hemolytic streptococcal infection. It is characterized by inflammatory lesions of connective tissue and endothelial tissue. It affects heart, joint, blood vessels and other connective tissue. It is the most important acquired heart disease in children and commonly found in 4 to 15 years of age with incidence rate 5.0/1000 approximately.

The predisposing factors of ARF are genetic predisposition, temperate climate, winter season, unhygienic living conditions, overcrowding in the family, poor dietary intake and increasing immunological response.

The etiology of rheumatic fever is not clear, but there is strong association with beta hemolytic streptococcal sore throat.

Pathophysiology

The exact etiopathogenesis of ARF is not well understood. Preceding streptococcal infection may not always clinically manifest. It is considered as a sort of hypersensitivity reaction. There is an antigen-antibody reaction usually following streptococcal sore throat. Antistreptococcal antibody titer elevated in majority of the patients, although the streptococci have never been isolated from rheumatic lesions in joints, heart or in the blood-stream.

The autoantibodies attack the myocardium, pericardium and cardiac valves. Aschoff's bodies (fibrin deposits) develop on the valves, especially on the mitral valve and leading to permanent valve dysfunction. Severe myocarditis may result dilation of the heart and heart failure.

The antibodies may react with striated muscle, vascular smooth muscle and nervous tissue resulting joint inflammation, involuntary movements as chorea and lesions in blood vessels and other connective tissues.

Clinical Manifestations

The clinical features of acute rheumatic fever can be grouped as major, minor and essential manifestations or criteria, as described in modified Jones criteria (Revised) for diagnosis of rheumatic fever.

Major Manifestations or Criteria

Carditis: It is an early manifestations of rheumatic fever as pancarditis, i.e. pericarditis, myocarditis and endocarditis. It is evidenced as presence of significant murmur, ECG changes, cardiac enlargement, friction rub, pericardial effusion and features of heart failure.

Polyarthritis: It is usually flitting or migratory type of joint inflammation with pain, decreased active movements, warm, tenderness, redness and swelling. Two or more joints are affected. Commonly knees, ankles and elbows are involved, but sometimes smaller joints may also be affected.

Chorea: It is purposeless involuntary, rapid movements, usually associated with muscle weakness, incoordination, involuntary facial grimace, speech disturbance, awkward gait and emotional disturbances.

Subcutaneous nodules: It is found as firm painless nodule over the extensor surface of certain joints, (elbows, knees and wrists), occiput and vertebral column.

Erythema marginatum: It is pink macular nonitching rash, found mainly over trunk, sometimes on the extremities but never on face. It is transient and brought out only by heat and migrates from place-to-place.

Minor Manifestations or Criteria

- *Fever:* Increase in body temperature is common findings. It rarely goes above 39.5°C.
- *Arthralgia:* Pain in the joints occurs in about 90 percent of cases. It presents along with arthritis.
- Previous attack of rheumatic fever or rheumatic heart disease. This is applicable for a second attack of rheumatic fever.
- ECG changes with prolonged P-R interval is considered as minor criterion. It is not diagnostic of carditis.
- Elevated ESR or presence of C-reactive protein may be considered as minor criteria.

Essential Criteria

- Elevated antistreptolysin-O (ASO) titer indicates previous streptococcal infection (normal 200 IU/mL).
- Positive throat swab culture may show streptococcal infection (sore throat, scarlet fever, etc.)

Other Manifestations

Other features which may found in case of ARF include precordial pain, abdominal pain, headache, easy fatigability, general weakness, tachycardia, malaise, sweating, vomiting, skin rash, erythema nodosum, epistaxis, anemia, pleuritis, weight loss, etc.

Diagnostic Evaluation

- The presence of two major or one major and two minor criteria plus evidence of a preceding streptococcal infection is essential for labeling a case as rheumatic fever.
- Doppler echocardiography is considered as an important diagnostic approach.
- Artificial subcutaneous nodule test.
- Endomyocardial biopsy showing Aschoff's nodules or histiocytes confirms the diagnosis. It is not quite useful as a routine diagnostic procedure.
- Chest X-ray shows cardiomegaly and heart failure.
- Electrocardiography.
- Blood test for ESR, ASO-titer, WBC counts (leukocytes).

Management

- Bedrest is important in the management of children with rheumatic fever. It is needed for at least 6 to 8 weeks till the rheumatic activity is disappeared.
- Nutritious diet to be provided with sufficient amount of protein, vitamins and micronutrients. Salt restriction is not necessary unless CCF is present. Avoid rich spicy food.
- Antibiotic therapy, penicillin is administered after skin test to eradicate streptococcal infection. Initially, procaine penicillin 4 lacks units deep IM, twice a day is given for 10 to 14 days. Then the long-acting benzathine penicillin 1.2 mega units every 21 days or 0.6 mega unit every 15 days to be given. Oral penicillin 4 lakhs units (250 mg), every 4 to 6 hours for 10 to 14 days can be also given. Erythromycin can be used in penicillin sensitive patients.
- Aspirin is administered as suppressive therapy to control pain and inflammation of joints. The dose of aspirin is 90 to 120 mg/kg/day in 4 divided doses. It may be needed for 12 weeks. The dose can be modified for the individual patients. Aspirin should not be given in empty stomach. Antacid to be given just prior to or with the aspirin.
- Steroid (prednisolone) therapy is given as suppressive therapy along with aspirin. The initial dose is 40 to 60 mg/day or 2 mg/kg/day in 4 divided doses, for 7 to 10 days. Then the dose is reduced to 1 mg/kg/day. It should be tapered off gradually over 12 weeks period and used for patients having carditis with or without CCF.
- Management of chorea can be done with diazepam or phenobarbitone.
- Treatment of complications, if present, especially for CCF should be done. Symptomatic care to be provided accordingly.

- Good nursing care with emotional support to the child and parents is as important as the medication.

Nursing Management

Nursing assessment is vital for the care of the child with rheumatic fever. It should include special attention to vital signs, cardiac monitoring (ECG, heart sound), pain assessment and other associated problems.

Important nursing diagnoses are (a) decreased cardiac output related to carditis (b) pain related to polyarthritis (c) risk of injury related to involuntary movements in chorea, (d) anxiety related to disease process, (e) knowledge deficit related to long-term treatment and prognosis of the acquired heart disease.

Nursing Interventions

Nursing interventions should emphasize on the followings along with routine care:

Improving cardiac output by:
- Providing rest as long as rheumatic activity and heart failure persist. In milder cases light indoor activity is allowed.
- Organizing nursing care with uninterrupted rest and modifying activities.
- Maintaining normal body temperature by managing fever.
- Providing bland diet with adequate nutrition and fluid intake with salt restriction in case of CCF.
- Administering medication as prescribed with necessary precautions.
- Monitoring cardiac functions, intake-output and features of improvement or deterioration.

Relieving pain by:
- Administering anti-inflammatory analgesics as prescribed and assessing features of aspirin toxicity.
- Providing comfortable position and support to the inflamed joints.
- Arranging diversional activities and play materials according to age and choice of the child.

Protecting the child from injury by:
- Removing hard and sharp objects from the child's reach.
- Assisting the child in feeding, ambulation and other fine motor activities and channelization of the stress.
- Administration of drugs to control the chorea.
- Explaining about self-limiting course of the condition and importance about physical and mental rest.

Health teaching for maintenance of health and prevention of complications:
- Explaining the duration of treatment, its importance and compliance, activity restriction, follow-up, continuation

of school performance and improvement of living standard.
- Instructing about preventive measures.

Prevention of Rheumatic Fever

- Primary prevention can be achieved by educating the people to avoid streptococcal sore throat and elimination of predisposing factors of the disease. Treatment of streptococcal pharyngitis with penicillin or other medications can be useful measure to prevent primary attack of rheumatic fever.
- Secondary prevention of the disease can be done by early detection, adequate treatment and prevention of recurrences of rheumatic fever. Long acting penicillin therapy should be continued every 15 days or 21 days for at least 5 years from the last attack of rheumatic fever or up to 18th birth day, whichever comes earlier. Parents should be made aware about the continuation of treatment, medical help and follow-up.

Complications

Chronic rheumatic heart disease is the most common complications with involvement of mitral valve as mitral incompetence or mitral stenosis. Aortic involvement may be observed as aortic incompetence.

Heart failure, infective endocarditis, pericardial effusion and permanent cardiac damage are also common complications of rheumatic fever.

Prognosis

Prognosis of rheumatic fever depends upon the age, presence of heart lesions, stage of detection of the disease, available treatment facilities and number of previous attacks. Prognosis is worst in patients with carditis in early childhood.

RHEUMATIC HEART DISEASE

Rheumatic fever may have complications as valvular involvement resulting the diseases of mitral, aortic and tricuspid valves. The common rheumatic heart disease includes mitral regurgitation and mitral stenosis. Aortic valve and tricuspid valvular disease include mainly aortic and tricuspid regurgitation.

Mitral Regurgitation or Incompetence

Mitral regurgitation is the backflow of blood from the left ventricle into the left atrium resulting from imperfect closure of the mitral valve. It is the most common complication of acute or recurrent rheumatic carditis.

There is left ventricular dilation and hypertrophy along with shortening and thickening of the chorda tendinae. Back pressure into the pulmonary system results in right ventricular hypertrophy and CCF. Left atrial enlargement with atrial arrhythmias, pulmonary edema and pulmonary hypertension may develop in long-term illness with this condition.

The patients may present with easy fatigability, exertional dyspnea due to reduced cardiac output and palpitation due to atrial arrhythmias. Increased pulse rate, wide pulse pressure, downward and outward shifting of apex beat are important features.

The most important auscultatory finding is a moderately low blowing pansystolic murmur at the apex. It may be transmitted to the left axilla, to back and upwards. A systolic thrill is usually felt at the mitral area. Echocardiography (ECG) and chest X-ray are important diagnostic measures.

Medical management is done for controlling of CCF, penicillin prophylaxis against future recurrence of rheumatic fever and prevention against infective endocarditis.

Surgical management of mitral regurgitation includes mitral valve repair or replacement of it by prosthetic valve. Surgery is indicated in more than 55 percent cases with refractory CCF, pulmonary hypertension and progressive cardiomegaly. Surgical repair is the choice in pediatric patients, and done in sophisticated cardiothoracic centers with specialized care facilities.

Mitral Stenosis

Mitral stenosis is the narrowing of the mitral orifice obstructing free flow of blood from the left atrium to the left ventricle. Mitral opening gets tight due to progressive sclerosis of the base of the mitral ring. It develops relatively late in children with rheumatic carditis. It is less common than mitral regurgitation and commonly found in male children.

In moderate to severe cases, there is left atrial dilation and hypertrophy which results in back pressure in pulmonary system leading to right ventricular hypertrophy and CCF.

The child with mitral stenosis presents with dyspnea on exertion or even at rest or as paroxysmal nocturnal dyspnea and palpitation, Tiredness, cough, hemoptysis and peripheral cyanosis may present. Pulmonary edema, atrial fibrillation and atypical angina may also develop but in less frequency. Infective endocarditis may occur. On examination, distended neck veins, weak peripheral pulses, palpable RV impulse and prominent precordium are found.

Diagnosis is confirmed by important auscultatory findings, ECG, ecocardiography and chest X-ray.

Medical management of a patient with mitral stenosis is done with rest, digitalis, diuretics, activity restriction, salt restriction in diet, penicillin prophylaxis for recurrence of rheumatic fever and prevention of infective endocarditis.

Surgical management is performed as closed mitral valvotomy (mitral commissurotomy), if the heart failure does not respond to medical management. Surgery is done in absence of carditis. Severely damaged valve can be replaced by prosthesis. Mitral valve replacement needs lifelong anticoagulant therapy. Balloon mitral valvoplasty is another surgical technique can be done for mitral stenosis.

Postoperative complications include restenosis, CCF, bleeding disorders and arterial embolization.

Aortic Regurgitation or Incompetence

Aortic regurgitation is the backflow of blood into the left ventricle due to an incompetent aortic valve. It is less frequent than mitral regurgitation. It occurs due to sclerosis of aortic valve resulting shortening, distortion and retraction of the cusps leading to inadequate closure. Left ventricular hypertrophy, pulmonary edema and CCF developed as consequence of the condition.

In chronic and severe cases, the clinical presentations include palpitations, exercise intolerance, exertional dyspnea, even paroxysmal nocturnal dyspnea and anginal pain. Characteristic rapid water-hammer pulse, bounding corrigan pulsation of corotid arteries, wide pulse pressure, early diastolic murmur and cardiac enlargement are important features present in case of aortic regurgitation. Chest X-ray, ECG and clinical examination along with history of illness help in diagnosis.

Medical management of aortic regurgitation is done with diuretics, digoxin, salt restriction in diet and vasodilators like ACE inhibitors and antiarrhythmic agents.

Surgical management is done in the form of aortic valvotomy or aortic valve replacement by prosthetic valve and homograft. Valve replacement should be planned before the child develops CCF.

Tricuspid Regurgitation

Tricuspid regurgitation is the backflow of blood from the right ventricle into the right atrium. It is found in about 20 to 50 percent cases of rheumatic heart disease. There are no specific symptoms of this condition. It is a common accompaniment of mitral stenosis and mitral incompetence.

Physical signs related to tricuspid regurgitation include prominent "V" waves in jugular veins in neck, systolic pulsations of liver and a pansystolic murmur in lower left sternal border. On examination signs of mitral stenosis and pulmonary hypertension are usually found. ECG and echocardiography help to diagnose the condition.

Management is done with decongestive therapy (digitalis, diuretics) and treatment of associated problems. Surgery is done with various procedures. Mitral valve replacement is required when the tricuspid regurgitation is associated with mitral incompetence. Balloon mitral valvoplasty can be done when the condition is associated with mitral stenosis. Tricuspid annuloplasty or repair may also be performed.

INFECTIVE ENDOCARDITIS

Infective endocarditis is the inflammation of the endocardium, the inner lining of the heart. It occurs due to bacterial and fungal infection and as serious complication of congenital heart disease and rheumatic (valvular) heart disease.

Infective endocarditis should be considered as medical emergency, since it can damage valves, myocardium and other vital organs like brain and kidneys.

The most common infecting organism is *Streptococcus viridans*. Other causative agents are *Staphylococcus aureus*, *E. coli, Pseudomonas aeruginosa* and some other gram-negative bacilli. Pathogenesis depends upon virulence of the infective organism. Involvement of cardiovascular system and presence of an immunological reaction to infection are responsible to produce clinical features.

Infections usually occur over the endocardium of the valves or in the mural endocardium as well as endothelium of the blood vessels. Bacteria are deposited on the endocardium and are covered by fibrin and platelets forming vegetations on the surface of the endocardium or in the endocardium itself. Most commonly, there is involvement of the heart valves or inner lining of the cardiac chambers.

Bacteremia may occur from the infections like furuncles, otitis media, septicemia, valve replacement, cardiac or urinary catheterization, dental extractions and osteomyelitis. Drug addicts (especially parenteral route users) are prone to endocarditis.

Clinical Manifestations

The onset of infective endocarditis may be acute or subacute. The infected child presents with low-grade fever, chills, rigor, night sweating, general weakness, malaise, anorexia and weight loss. Joint pain and diffuse myalgia may present. Initially features of cardiovascular involvement may be absent. Appearance of features of heart failure, abnormal heart sound and splinter hemorrhages (under nails and conjunctiva) are found. Clubbing, petechiae, anemia and splenomegaly are usually present. Osier nodes (tender erythematous nodules over the pulp of finger tips) may be seen in some patients. Hematuria, GI bleeding, CNS embolism indicate cardiovascular involvement. Janeway lesion as nontender erythematous patches over palms and soles also may found in some cases.

In acute form of the disease, manifestations appear early and progress rapidly with features of mitral and aortic regurgitation.

Complications

Infective endocarditis can be complicated with valvular damage or perforation and rupture of chordae tendinae, vasculitis, glomerulonephritis, renal insufficiency, CCF, systemic embolism, pulmonary embolism, mycotic embolism, ruptured valsalva sinus, brain abscess, splenic or mesenteric abscess, osteomyelitis, acquired VSD, obstructive valve disease due to large vegetations and heart block.

Diagnostic Evaluation

- History of unexplained fever for 7 to 10 days in a known case of heart disease and clinical features of the condition are important diagnostic measures.
- Diagnosis is confirmed by positive blood culture.
- Echocardiography helps to localize the vegetations in advanced cases.
- ECG and immunological investigations are also useful to diagnose the condition in advanced cases.
- Blood examination shows elevated WBC count and ESR, with reduced Hb% and platelet count.
- Urine examination shows microscopic hematuria in most of the cases.
- Radionuclide tests found to be useful in the identification of endocarditis.

Management

Management of infective endocarditis should be started as early as possible using heavy dose of antimicrobial agents for a long period to treat current episodes and to prevent relapse of the condition.

Appropriate antibiotic therapy to be administered for 4 to 6 weeks. Selection of antibiotics should be done on the basis of culture and sensitivity report. The commonly used antibiotics are penicillin in massive dose, gentamicin, streptomycin, cefezolin, ampicillin, coxacillin, amikacin, vancomycin, etc. Antifungal agents like amphotericin-B, 5-fluorocytosine to be used in fungal endocarditis.

Symptomatic and supportive nursing care are important towards better prognosis. Patient should be nursed with bedrest in calm, quiet environment in high Fowler's or orthopneic position. Assisting in activities of daily living, and use of commode to reduce cardiac workload need special attention. Monitoring of vital signs, cardiovascular status, renal function, signs of embolic phenomenon, drug toxicity, etc should be done frequently. Administration of medication with necessary precautions and arrangement of laboratory investigations are important aspect of management. Emotional support with necessary instructions and health teaching are important nursing responsibilities. Ambulation and permitted activity with necessary restrictions should be explained. Features of relapse, need for follow-up, importance of continuation of treatment and possible complications with prognosis should be informed. Parents and children should be encouraged to express their feeling and necessary support. Prevention of the condition should be discussed.

Prevention

Prevention of endocarditis can be promoted in the susceptible children with the following measures:

- Appropriate oral and dental hygiene with improvement of general cleanliness.
- Aseptic precautions for any invasive procedures and surgical interventions (especially cardiac surgery and cardiac catheterization)
- Vigorous and prompt treatment of any local infections in patients with known valvular or congenital heart disease.
- Antibiotic prophylaxis for susceptible patients before and after surgical procedures including tooth extraction and other dental procedures, or surgery of respiratory, genitourinary and gastrointestinal systems.

Prognosis

Infective endocarditis is a life-threatening disease with mortality rate about 20 to 25 percent and high morbidity. Complications are found in 50 to 60 percent of the cases.

CARDIOMYOPATHY IN CHILDREN

Definition

Cardiomyopathy is the abnormalities of the myocardium in which there is impairment of the contractility of cardiac muscles. It includes any disease that affects the heart muscle resulting diminished cardiac performance.

The child with cardiomyopathy may present with asymptomatic condition. Common symptoms are shortness of breath, chest pain, orthopnea and other symptoms of CHF. Patients may have ventricular arrhythmias, palpitation, syncope or sudden death.

Etiological Factors

The possible etiological factors are familial or genetic cause, infections, deficiency states (selenium), metabolic abnormalities and collagen vascular diseases.

In children most of the cases of cardiomyopathy are considered as primary or idiopathic, in which the causes are unknown and the cardiac dysfunction is not associated with systemic disease. They may be due to abnormalities of the cell function of the cardiac myocyte.

Some known causes of secondary cardiomyopathy are drug toxicity (antineoplastic), hemochromatosis (excessive iron store), Duchenne muscular dystrophy, Kawasaki disease, collagen disease and thyroid dysfunction.

Types of Cardiomyopathy

Dilated Cardiomyopathy

It is most common type found in children and also known as idiopathic dilated cardiomyopathy (IDC). This condition is characterized by ventricular dilation with greatly decreased contractility and weakness of the heart muscle. Cause of this disease is mainly uncertain or may be due to familial inheritance or due to viral infection and toxic exposure.

Idiopathic dilated cardiomyopathy is manifested with CHF, tachycardia, dyspnea, hepatosplenomegaly, poor growth, fatigue and dysrhythmia. Chest radiography, echocardiography, cardiac catheterization with endomyocardial biopsy are usually helpful to diagnose the condition, to identify the cause and to manage appropriately.

Hypertrophic Cardiomyopathy

It is characterized by an increase in heart muscle mass without an increase in cavity size usually in left ventricle. There is excessive and disorganized growth of myofibrils and impaired filling of heart with reduction in the size of ventricular cavity.

Half of these patients have familial inheritance. Infant of diabetic mother may have this condition, which may resolve with time.

Clinical features usually present in school-aged children or in adolescents. Common symptoms are anginal chest pain, dysrhythmias, syncope and sudden death. The child may present with CHF in infancy with poor prognosis. Diagnosis is confirmed by chest X-ray and ECG. Echocardiography is most helpful to identify septal hypertrophy and an increase in LV wall thickness with small LV cavity.

Restrictive or Constrictive Cardiomyopathy

It is rare condition in children. This condition is caused by endocardial and myocardial disease or both due to lack of flexibility of ventricular walls. It may found in case of hemochromatosis and amyloidosis. Thrombus formation and embolic events are common. Elevation of pulmonary vascular resistance may occur. The child usually present with CHF.

Congestive Cardiomyopathy

It is mainly found in myocardial disease associated with enlargement of left ventricle of the heart and CHF.

Secondary Cardiomyopathy

This condition is usually associated with well-defined systemic disease, like inflammation, toxic chemicals, metabolic abnormalities and inherited muscle disorders.

Therapeutic Management

- Treatment should be done according to the specific cause.
- Aim of treatment is management of CHF and dysrhythmias.
- Digoxin, diuretics and aggressive use of afterload reduction agents have been found to be helpful for dilated cardiomyopathy.
- Beta-blockers or calcium channel blockers have been used for hypertrophic cardiomyopathy.
- Careful monitoring and treatment of dysrhythmias are essential.

- Anticoagulants may be given to reduce the risk of thromboembolic events.
- IV inotropic support with dobutamine for several days has been successfully used for worst heart failure and signs of poor perfusion.
- For severely ill patient mechanical ventilation, oxygen therapy, IV afterload reduction agents (nitroprusside) are useful.
- Heart transplantation may be indicated in patients who have worsening symptoms, especially in IDC, despite medical therapy.
- General supportive therapy should include rest, weight control, avoidance of strenuous physical exercise, salt-restricted diet, vasodilators, ACE inhibitors, etc.
- Problem oriented nursing management is important for better prognosis of the condition.

Childhood Blood Dyscrasias

18

- Anemia
- Iron Deficiency Anemia
- Megaloblastic Anemia
- Hereditary Spherocytosis (Congenital Hemolytic Anemia, Familial Acholuric Jaundice)
- Sickle Cell Anemia
- Aplastic Anemia
- Thalassemia (Cooley's Anemia, Mediterranean Anemia)
- Hemophilia
- Leukemia
- Bleeding Disorders/Purpura
- Disseminated Intravascular Coagulation
- Immunodeficiency

INTRODUCTION

Blood formation begins in the 4th week of gestation. During the first 6 months of fetal life, liver produces majority of the blood cells and at term bone marrow carried on this function. During period of growth, all the bone marrows produce blood cells, but afterwards, hemopoiesis is limited to the epiphysis (i.e. the end of long bone), vertebra and certain flat bones. In childhood, during extra demand many organs (other than liver and spleen), lymph nodes and other reticuloendothelial tissues of the body produce additional blood cells (extramedullary hemopoiesis).

Blood is composed of RBCs, WBCs, platelets and plasma. RBC has hemoglobin, the oxygen carrying pigment. Hemoglobin is made up of iron pigment (heme) and protein (globin). The globin molecule is made up of two pair of polypeptide chains, each chain having a heme group. The hemoglobin of a normal adult is HbA and is composed of two alpha and two beta chains. Fetal hemoglobin is HbF and represented as $alpha_2$ and $Gamma_2$.

White blood cells (WBCs) are concerned with invading antigen and production and transportation of antibody. Platelets take part in the formation of thrombus and arrest bleeding. Normal hematological levels varies with age and sex. Levels below the lower limit need investigation for detection of underlying cause.

Diagnostic Procedures

These are related to blood disorders should include the followings:

a. Blood examination for complete blood count, hematocrit values, PCV, MCV, MCHC, MCH, TLC, DLC, ESR, cell morphology (reticulocytes, anisocytes, poikilocytes, microcytes), hemoglobin percentage, etc.
b. Bone marrow cytology.
c. Blood enzyme analysis.
d. Serum level of iron, ferritin, transferrin, lead, bilirubin, clotting factors, antibody titer, immunoglobin, etc.
e. Osmotic fragility test.
f. Hemoglobin electrophoresis.
g. Radiological investigations.
h. DNA analysis

Common blood diseases among children include different types of anemias, coagulation disorders, hemorrhagic diseases and leukemia.

ANEMIA

Anemia is the most common blood disorder in infant and children, especially of poor socioeconomic group. Anemia is defined as the reduction in the number and quality of circulating red blood cells when the hemoglobin content is below the normal level for particular age, resulting in decreased oxygen carrying capacity.

World Health Organization (WHO) proposed the cut-off points of Hb level for different age groups for the diagnosis of anemia.

a. Children 6 months to 6 years—11 g/dL
b. Children 6 years to 14 years—12 g/dL
c. Above 14 years—Male—13 g/dL
   —Female—12 g/dL

At all ages the normal mean corpuscular hemoglobin concentration (MCHC) should be 34. Values of MCHC below 34 indicate hypochromic RBC, which usually found in iron deficiency anemia.

According to the statistical report 2005 to 2006, anemia status by Hb level among Indian children age aged 6 to 59 months is found as below:

- Mild anemia (10.0–10.9 g/dL)—26.3 percent
- Moderate anemia (7.0–9.9 g/dL)—40.2 percent
- Severe anemia (less than 7 g/dL)—2.9 percent

Any anemia (Hb level less than 11 g/dL) is found in 69.5 percent children.

WHO Grading of Anemia

- Hb level between 10 g/dL and cut off point—Mild anemia for age.
- Hb level between 7 g/dL to 10 g/dL—Moderate anemia.
- Hb level below 7 g/dL—Severe anemia.

Clinical Grading of Anemia

According to clinical observations, the grading of anemia is done as follows:

- Pallor observed in conjunctiva and mucous membrane only—Mild anemia.
- Pallor observed in skin—Moderate anemia.
- Pallor observed in palmar creases along with skin and mucous membrane—Severe anemia.

Causes of Anemia

Red blood cells (RBCs) and hemoglobin are normally formed and destroyed at the same rate. But when formation of RBC and hemoglobin is decreased and their destruction is increased then anemia develops. The oxygen carrying capacity and CO_2 removing capacity are decreased. There are various causes of anemia but in some cases causes can be idiopathic.

Causes of anemia can be described as follows:

a. *Impaired of RBC production:* Impaired of RBC production due to deficiency of hemopoietic factors in nutritional deficiency (nutritional anemia)

The most common nutritional anemia is iron deficiency anemia. Other nutritional deficiency conditions causing anemia are folic acid deficiency, vitamin B_{12} deficiency, vitamin B_6 deficiency and vitamin C deficiency.

b. Increased destruction of RBCs (hemolytic anemia)
  1. Hemolysis due to intrinsic factors
     i. Abnormal hemoglobin synthesis—thalassemia, sickle cell disease.
     ii. Enzymatic defect—Glucose-6-phosphate—dehydrogenase deficiency.
     iii. Abnormalities in RBC membrane or structural defects of RBC—Hereditary spherocytosis.
  2. Hemolysis due to extrinsic factors
     i. Infections—malaria, kala-azar.
     ii. Antibody reaction—Rh or ABO isoimmunization, autoimmune hemolytic anemia, lupus.
     iii. Drugs—Primaquine, phenacetin, phenytoin.
     iv. Poisoning—Lead.
     v. Burns
     vi. Splenomegaly.
c. Increased blood loss (hemorrhagic anemia)
  1. Acute—Trauma, epistaxis, bleeding diathesis (leukemia, purpura, hemophilia), hemorrhagic disease of newborn and scurvy.
  2. Chronic—Hookworms, bleeding piles, chronic dysentery, esophageal varices.
d. Decreased RBC production (bone marrow depression)
  1. Primary—Hypoplasia or aplasia, Fanconi anemia.
  2. Secondary—Irradiation, infections, chronic illness like nephritis, leukemia and other neoplastic diseases, tuberculosis, liver disease, hypothyroidism and drug therapy (chloramphenicol, sulfas)

Classification of Anemia

Anemia can be classified according to the RBC morphology into three groups.

1. Microcytic hypochromic anemia—It occurs in iron deficiency anemia and ineffective RBC production (thalassemia, lead poisoning).
2. Normocytic normochromic anemia—It is found in impaired cell production and hemolysis.
3. Macrocytic anemia—It develops due to:
  a. Megaloblastic erythropoiesis—in nutritional deficiency (Vitamin B_{12} Folates, protein), drug toxicity (methotrexate, phenytoin) and malabsorption.
  b. Nonmegaloblastic erythropoiesis—in chronic hemolytic anemia, liver disease, hypothyroidism.

Clinical Manifestations

The early symptoms of anemia are fatique, listlessness and anorexia. Late symptoms may include pallor (skin, nail bed, mucous membrane), weakness, vertigo, headache, malaise and drowsiness. Other features are sore tongue, gastro-intestinal problems, tachypnea, shortness of breath on exertion, tachycardia, palpitations, etc. Jaundice, petechiae and ecchymosis may present in some cases. Hepatomegaly may be associated feature in hemoglobinopathies and liver disorders. Enlarged lymph gland may be found in leukemia, infections, malignancy and myeloproliferative disorders.

Complications

Complications of anemia usually found as circulatory collapse and shock, CCF, cardiac enlargement, systemic or local infections, growth retardation, mental retardation or sluggishness with decreased attention span and intelligence, delayed puberty, etc.

Management

Medical management of anemia depends upon the specific cause of the condition.

Anemia due to excessive blood loss should be treated accordingly. Acute blood loss needs immediate control of bleeding and to restore blood volume by IV infusion, blood transfusion along with treatment of shock and the cause of bleeding. Chronic blood loss usually produces iron deficiency anemia. The exact cause should be detected and treatment should be planned according to the specific cause.

Anemia due to excessive blood cell destruction requires the identification and treatment of specific hemolytic disorder.

Anemia due to decreased blood cell formation is mainly due to deficiency states and bone marrow disorders. Specific deficiency of iron, folic acid, vitamin B_{12}, etc should be detected and treatment to be done with replacement therapy of specific nutrients. In case of bone marrow depressions, the specific cause (like drugs, toxins) to be identified and treatment to be performed by removal of offending agents.

Nursing Management

Nursing assessment is the corner stone of nursing inter-ventions. It is done by obtaining details history to detect poten-tial causes of the condition. History of present complaints, past illness, chronic diseases, presence of infections, worm infestations, exposure to medications, poisons, dietary habits, behavioral problems like pica and history of familial diseases are important aspects of assessment.

Physical examination to be done to exclude the presence of clinical features like pallor of skin and mucous membrane with other signs and symptoms related to anemia. Assessment of anthropometric data (height, weight, MUAC, skin fold thickness, head and chest circumference), vital signs and

review of laboratory investigations are important to identify the problems and to implement the care.

Sample nursing process for a child with anemia is given on page No. 321.

Raja, a four years village boy, admitted in pediatric ward with fever, edema, cough and loss of appetite. On examination there is pallor, sore in the mouth, weakness, fatigue, tachypnea and tachycardia. The child is having features of malnutrition, 8 kg body weight, Hb% 6 g/dL. History reveals open field defecation, poor dietary intake and repeated respiratory infection.

IRON DEFICIENCY ANEMIA

The most frequent cause of anemia in children is iron deficiency. It causes microcytic hypochromic anemia. The factors resposible for this condition are, inadequate iron storage during intrauterine period, prematurity, twin baby, maternal anemia and inadequate iron intake in diet due to prolonged breastfeeding or feeding with cow's milk, delayed weaning, ignorance about child care, poverty, etc. The disease conditions which can result iron deficiency anemia (IDA) include diarrheal diseases, infections, malabsorption syndrome, hookworm infestations and chronic illnesses.

Preschool age and adolescence are more prone to IDA, due to discrepancy between the demand and supply of iron for rapid somatic growth. Iron requirement is affected during growth period by expansion of blood volume, by the need for increased Hb formation to maintain normal concentration and by the demand of iron for muscular development.

Clinical Manifestations

The child with iron deficiency anemia presents with pallor, irritability, fatigue, tiredness, listless, weakness, anorexia and failure to thrive. There is usually vomiting, diarrhea and respiratory infections for which the child brought to hospital.

On examination, excessive pallor of the skin, conjunctiva and mucous membrane is found. Nails become thin, brittle and flat. The child may have pica and atrophy of tongue papillae. Older children may present with koilonychia. In severe anemia, spleen may enlarge. Cardiac enlargement with soft systolic (Hemic) murmur may be detected. The child may be manifested by unhappiness, lack of co-operation and short attention span with poor school performance.

Complications

The important complications of IDA are CCF, recurrent infections, malabsorption syndrome, growth retardation and mental subnormality.

Nursing process for a child with anemia

	Date and time
• Identification data	
• History of illness in details	
• Findings of physical examination and laboratory investigations	

Assessment day-1	Nursing diagnosis	Planning	Implementation	Evaluation day-2
• Fatigue • Weakness • Hb%—6 g/dL • Tachycardia • Tachypnea • Loss of appetite	• Fatigue related to decreased oxygen supply to the tissues	• To minimize fatigue and to relief respiratory problem	1. Observing the child for vital signs and other related features. 2. Positioning the child in upright posture. 3. Providing need based care and assisting in activities of daily living. 4. Promoting rest and sleep. 5. Allowing foods containing more calories and iron.	• Increase in activity level especially related to self-care.
• Pallor • Edema in lower limbs • Body weight—8 kg • Sore in the mouth • Hookworm ova in stool examination	• Altered nutrition less than body requirements related to inadequate dietary intake and chronic blood loss.	• To provide adequate nutritional intake	1. Providing diet rich in protein and iron according to food preference and availability. 2. Giving small amount frequent feed. 3. Encouraging the child for positive attempt to take food. 4. Administering anthelmintics drugs as prescribed. 5. Giving iron-supplementation in between meals with fruit juices. 6. Informing about side-effects of iron therapy.	• Improved food intake. No side-effects of iron therapy observed.
• Fever • Temperature—101° F • Pulse—140 b/m • Respiration 50 b/m • Cough	• Risk for infection related to general weakness	• To prevent and to treat infections	1. Promoting hygienic measures and general cleanliness. 2. Avoiding exposure to cold and infection. 3. Maintaining aseptic technique and handwashing practices during care. 4. Recording of TPR at 4 hours interval. 5. Arranging the diagnostic tests. 6. Administering prescribed medications (antipyretics, antibiotics)	• No fever • Respiration 40 b/m • Pulse 120 b/m
• Child is crying and irritable • Mother is apprehensive	• Anxiety related to painful diagnostic procedure and fear of hospitalization	• To reduce anxiety and to remove fear	1. Explaining the procedure according to child's level of understanding. 2. Allowing the child to handle hospital equipment used in procedures (torniquets, syringe, empty vials). 3. Allowing mother to remain with the child during procedures. 4. Involving the mother during care of the child. 5. Encouraging parents to ask questions and clarifying doubts.	• The child and mother are co-operative during procedure.
• Body weight 8 kg • Height 90 cm • MUAC 13 cm • Head circumference 50 cm • Chest circumference 48 cm	• Altered growth and development related to decreased energy level and poor general condition	• To promote growth and development of the child and to treat malnutrition	1. Ensuring adequate dietary intake and nutritional rehabilitation 2. Instructing the mother to continue care at home and regular weight check-up. 3. Explaining about importance of improved dietary intake especially low-cost food items, food value, iron and protein containing foods, etc. 4. Encouraging play and other recreational activities.	• Dietary intake increased • Mother is concerned about care of the child and accept the instructions.
• Illiterate mother of poor family	• Knowledge deficit related to child care	• To improve knowledge by health teaching	1. Explaining about importance of food hygiene, general cleanliness, wearing of shoe, use of latrine, prevention of infections and worm infestations. 2. Informing about the signs of deterioration or any complications and available medical help and follow-up. 3. Discussing about support facilities available in the community to improve family income.	• The mother listen the information carefully and ensure to follow at home.

Diagnostic Evaluation

1. Blood examination reveals the followings:
   - Peripheral blood smear shows—microcytic hypochromic RBCs with anisocytosis (abnormal size) and poikilocytosis (abnormal shaped).
   - Reticulocytes count may be normal or reduced.
   - Hb % is usually low. RBC count is reduced.
   - PCV, MCH, MCHC and MCV values are low.
   - WBC and platelets counts are usually normal. Leukocytosis may be found in presence of infections.
   - Serum iron level is low and iron binding capacity is high.
   - Serum ferritin level is decreased.
   - Free erythrocyte protoporphyrin level is increased.
2. Bone marrow study may show absence of hemosiderin or reduced iron granules in sideroblasts.
3. Specific investigations to be done to detect any underlying disease condition for IDA. Dietary history and history of illness along with clinical examination are very useful diagnostic criteria.

Management

Management of IDA consists of detection and treatment of underlying cause:

- Improvement of dietary intake, specially iron and protein containing food should be emphasized.
- Chronic blood loss (rectal polyp, chronic dysentery, ulcerative colitis) should be diagnosed and treated adequately.
- Iron therapy can be administered in oral route, intramuscularly, or IV route as single total dose infusion (TDI), depending upon the child's condition.

   Oral iron therapy is given with elemental iron dose 3 to 6 mg/kg/day in divided doses in between meals. The duration of treatment may vary from 3 to 6 months. Side-effects should be observed and necessary modification may be done as needed. Parenteral iron therapy is indicated in oral intolerance, defective absorption and poor compliance.

- Blood transfusion is indicated only in severe cases of anemia, where Hb% need to be increased quickly.
- Deworming to be done and other symptomatic and supportive care to be provided as required.
- Increasing awareness about prevention of IDA is essential measure that need to be promoted by health education.

Prevention

- Adequate antenatal care for prevention of maternal anemia and iron-folic acid supplementation to all antenatal mother.
- Prevention of preterm delivery or low-birth weight, and control of infections in prenatal, natal and neonatal period.
- Introduction of semi-solid and solid foods from 4 to 6 months of age as complementary feeding.
- Universal immunization to all children to prevent chronic illness.
- Iron-folic acid supplementation to the children and adolescent girls.
- Adequate treatment of parasitic infestations, chronic illnesses and IDA
- Improvement of living condition by avoidance of open-air defecation, practicing environmental sanitation, hygienic measures, wearing of shoes, balanced diet and preventive measures of nutritional deficiencies.

Nursing Management
(*See* Nursing Management of Anemia)

Nursing management of a child with IDA should include rest, diet containing iron and protein rich food, administration of iron therapy (with precautions) and other medications, arranging blood transfusion whenever needed, providing emotional support, monitoring child's conditions (vital signs, elimination, dietary intake, signs of complications, etc.), maintaining hygienic care and giving health education for continuation of care at home, follow-up and prevention of anemia.

MEGALOBLASTIC ANEMIA

The common causes of megaloblastic anemia are deficiency of folic acid and vitamin B_{12} or both. Lack of secretion of intrinsic factor in the stomach and vitamin 'C' deficiency are also responsible for development megaloblastic anemia) Folic acid and vitamin B_{12} act as coenzymes in the synthesis of nuclear protein and essential for erthropoiesis. The megaloblastic anemia is characterized by presence of oval macrocytes and hypersegmented polymorphs in the peripheral blood smear and megaloblasts in the bone marrow.

Folic acid deficiency: It is almost always found along with vitamin 'C' deficiency and/or iron deficiency. It is usually caused by dietary deficiency of the nutrient, use of goat milk for infant feeding, malabsorption syndrome, prematurity, diarrheal diseases and in association with hemolytic anemia and drug therapy with anticonvulsant and antifolic acid agent. Laboratory investigations are diagnostic for the condition.

Vitamin B_{12} deficiency: It may develop due to dietary inadequacy, lack of intrinsic factor in the stomach, inhibition of B_{12} and intrinsic factor complex, malabsorption and infants of B_{12} deficient mothers. The vitamin B_{12} and intrinsic factor complex is necessary for vitamin B_{12} absorption. The deficiency of this complex results in *juvenile pernicious anemia*. The clinical features of the condition include anemia and neurological involvement as ataxia, parasthesia of hands and feet, loss of vibration sensation, absent tendon reflexes, etc. Bone marrow study and serum vitamin B_{12} level estimation help in diagnosis.

Management of megaloblastic anemia is done with administration of deficient folic acid and/or vitamin B_{12} in oral or parenteral route. Vitamin 'C' also need to be administered. Associated causative factors to be managed accordingly. Dietary improvement is very essential.

HEREDITARY SPHEROCYTOSIS (CONGENITAL HEMOLYTIC ANEMIA, FAMILIAL ACHOLURIC JAUNDICE)

It is an inherited chronic hemolytic disease with autosomal dominant inheritance. The basic defect is the deficiency of spectrin and ankyrin, red cell stromal proteins which maintain stability of the erythrocyte membrane shape.) Deficiency occurs due to reduced synthesis of the proteins which makes the RBCs spherical, biconvex and voluminous. These spherical cells are sequestrated within the spleen leading to destruction of the cells.

The condition is manifested as hemolytic anemia, with reticulocytosis, spherocytosis, hyperbilirubinemia and splenomegaly.

The diagnosis of the condition is confirmed by the peripheral blood smear examination to demonstrate microspherocytosis with increased MCHC and osmotic fragility. The only effective treatment is splenectomy, and should be delayed up to 6 years of age. If the surgery is done prior to that age, postsplenectomy septicemia may be fatal. Symptomatic management before the surgical interventions can be done with exchange blood transfusion and folic acid supplementation.

SICKLE CELL ANEMIA

Sickle cell anemia is an autosomal recessive disorder in which an abnormal hemoglobin (Hbs) causes chronic hemolytic anemia, with a variety of severe clinical consequences. This Hbs forms crescent shaped crystals under low-oxygen tension and produces sickle-shaped RBCs) These RBCs tend to impact in the capillaries and cause hemolysis with local anoxemia. Anoxia leads to further sickling. Blockage of the capillaries causes infarction in various tissues and organs (spleen, liver, heart, lungs, brain, bones, GIT, urinary tract and muscles).

The sudden and severe hemolysis in sickle-cell anemia is termed as hemolytic crisis. The sudden onset of symptoms leads to vascular occlusion causing vaso-occlusive crisis.

The clinical features of sickle cell anemia are progressive anemia, mild jaundice, fever, headache (which may shrink later due to repeated thrombosis). Other features include growth retardation, superadded bacterial infections, enlarged heart, and nonhealing ulcer. Sickle cell anemia may be complicated with multisystem disease and may cause death due to organ failure.

Diagnosis is confirmed by the presence of sickle-shaped red cells in peripheral blood smear. Hemoglobin S is detected by electrophoresis. Antenatal diagnosis is possible by chorionic villi sampling. Genetic counseling is needed after prenatal diagnosis.

Management of the condition is done by blood transfusion, parenteral fluid therapy, treatment of infections, analgesics, correction of acidosis and other symptomatic and supportive care. Folic acid and other vitamin supplementation are given. Newer treatment modalities include red cell Hbs concentration reducing agent, membrane active agent and bone marrow transplantation.

APLASTIC ANEMIA

Aplastic anemia is caused by bone marrow depression and involved all the blood elements resulting pancytopenia (insufficient numbers of RBCs, WBCs and platelets) Hemopoietic failure is mediated by activated cytotoxic T cells in blood and marrow. Involvement of only RBCs is termed as hypoplastic anemia. Involvement of granulocytes is known as agranulocytosis and of platelets as thrombocytopenia.

Aplastic anemia can be congenital as Fanconi anemia, Diamond-Blackfan syndrome, Dyskeratosis congenita and TAR syndrome.

Acquired aplastic anemia may occur due to viral infections (HIV, HB, EBV) or bacterial or parasitic infections. It may develop due to infiltration of malignant cells as in leukemia, or due to exposure to radiation, chemicals (DDT) and drugs (chloramphenicol, antimetabolites).

Hypoplasia of the bone marrow may occur due to defect in stem cells or as a result of immune mediated injury by cytotoxic cells.

Clinical features of this condition may be found as progressive and persistent anemia, weakness, easy fatigability, petechiae and ecchymosis. The child may have mucosal bleeding, hematuria, or GI bleeding. Recurrent infections are common due to leukopenia and neutropenia. Intracranial bleeding may occur and presented as headache, irritability, excessive drowsiness, convulsions and unconsciousness. The diagnosis is confirmed by blood examination and bone marrow study.

Management of the condition includes mainly supportive care, bone marrow transplantation and immunotherapy. Treatment of infections and bleeding are important. Blood transfusion and steroid therapy to be given. Children with mild to moderate aplastic anemia can be treated with androgens for 3 to 5 months or more.

THALASSEMIA (COOLEY'S ANEMIA, MEDITERRANEAN ANEMIA)

Thalassemia is a group of hereditary hemolytic anemia characterized by reduction in the synthesis of hemoglobin. It produces hypochromic microcytic anemia due to defective hemoglobinization of RBCs, hemolysis and ineffective erythropoiesis. Thalassemia can be considered as hemolytic and hypoproliferative anemia related to abnormal hemoglobin.

The word 'thalassemia' is derived from the Greek words 'Thalassa' means the great sea. The disease was first described by Cooley in 1925. It was first noticed in patients originating from the littoral countries of the Mediterranean sea. At present the disease has been found in several countries all over the world. The prevalence of the disease in India is high among Gujaraties, Sindhis and Punjabis. There are millions of people as carriers of thalassemia gene and every year thousands of thalassemic children are born in our country (Fig. 18.1).

Pathogenesis

The basic defect is the hereditary inability to synthesis globin polypeptide chain (alpha or beta) which results in ineffective erythropoiesis and hemolysis due to immature, thin RBCs with short life span.

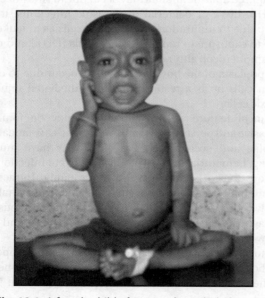

Fig. 18.1: A female child of 11 months with thalassemia

Alpha chain synthesis is reduced due to gene deletion which reduces the level of all three normal hemoglobin A, A_2 and F and causing alpha-thalassemia. Beta-thalassemia is usually caused by point mutations rather than large deletions. Delta-beta thalassemia is due to suppression of both beta and delta chain synthesis with moderate anemia and high HbF. Features of thalassemia usually develop after 6 months of age, when the hemoglobin synthesis switches from hemoglobin F to hemoglobin 'A'. Beta thalassemia is the most common than other types.

Classification

Depending upon the severity of the disease thalassemia can be divided into three groups. Severity of thalassemia depends upon (a) type of mutation affecting beta chain synthesis (b) presence of alpha-chain mutation, (c) effect of gamma-chain synthesis and (d) association of other hemoglobinopathies. The classification of thalassemia are as follows:

Thalassemia Major

It is a severe form of the illness and associated with homozygous state. In this condition, thalassemic genes (beta) are inherited from both parents and synthesis of beta chain is markedly reduced. Erythropoiesis becomes ineffective leading to hemolysis and anemia. Anemia stimulates production of erythropoietin resulting more ineffective erythropoiesis. Expansion of medullary cavity of different bones occur. Extramedullary hemopoiesis leads to hepatosplenomegaly. Iron released from breakdown of RBCs and transfused blood cells, cannot be utilized for hemoglobin synthesis which results in hemosiderosis, i.e. deposition of iron in various organs like liver, spleen, heart, etc. leading to their malfunctions and failure.

Thalassemia Intermedia

It is a state of chronic hemolytic anemia caused by deficient alpha or beta chain synthesis. It is also a homozygous form. The clinical manifestations of this condition are mainly intercurrent illness with exaggeration of anemia and persistent jaundice. These patients may have chronic liver dysfunction, osteoporosis, mild hepatomegaly and chronic anemia.

Thalassemia Minor

It is a mild form of the illness produced by heterozygosity of either alpha or beta chain. It may be completely asymptomatic or may have very mild anemia, mild jaundice and abdominal pain. This condition is usually diagnosed during the family study of a child having thalassemia major. The prognosis of this condition is excellent.

Thalassemia may be found as thalassemia trait which is a asymptomatic form. Thalassemia may also found as alpha thalassemia, hemoglobin-H disease which is presented with hypochromia, microcytosis, red cell fragmentation and fast migrating hemoglobin in electrophoresis.

Clinical Manifestations of Thalassemia Major

Thalassemia major usually manifested at the age of 3 months with progressive pallor, jaundice, hepatosplenomegaly, recurrent respiratory infections, enlargement of lymph nodes and growth failure.

In severe cases facial appearance becomes mongoloid and characterized by bossing of the skull, prominent frontal and parietal eminences with flat vault and straight forehead. Maxilla becomes prominent with exposure of malformed teeth. Bridge of the nose becomes depressed with puffy eyes. Anorexia, poor feeding and abdominal distension may present. Irregular fever may occur due to intercurrent infections, and increased metabolic activity.

Increased pigmentation of the skin found as bronze discoloration due to high level of melanin and hemosiderin. Hypogonadism, poor nutritional status with reduced activity level are common findings. Marked growth retardation is observed. Skeletal changes are marked and pathological fracture may occur due to osteoporosis.

Complications

Thalassemia major can be complicated with CCF, hepatic failure, aplastic crisis, intercurrent infections, gallstone, growth retardation, delayed puberty, hemosiderosis and hemochromatosis. Transfusion related infections (HIV, HB, HC), complications related to iron-chelation therapy, endocrinopathies (diabetes mellitus, hypothyroidism, hypogonadism), skeletal complications and multiorgan dysfunctions (MOD) also may found.

Diagnostic Evaluation

1. Blood examination shows the followings:
   - Hemoglobin percentage—reduced usually 2 to 6 g/dL.
   - RBC count reduced, 2 to 3 million/cmm.
   - Fetal hemoglobin level (HbF) increased.
   - Hematocrit values are reduced, MCV, MCH, MCHC values are low.
   - Reticulocyte count increased or may be low.
   - RBCs in peripheral smear shows—hypochromia, anisocytosis, poikilocytosis, microcytosis, nucleated RBCs and target cells.
   - WBC count may be reduced or sometimes increased.
   - Platelet count is usually normal or increased.

   - Serum bilirubin level is moderately elevated.
   - Serum iron level is high.
2. Bone marrow study shows hypercellular and erythroid hyperplasia.
3. Osmotic fragility test shows decreased fragility.
4. Radiological findings show skeletal changes including thinning of the cortex, widening of the medulla and coarsening of trabeculations due to bone marrow hyperplasia in the long bones, metacarpals and metatarsals. Skull bones show "hair-on-end" appearance due to vertical trabeculae or striations from widening of the diploic space and atrophy of the outer surface of the skull.

Management

Repeated Blood Transfusion

It is given at regular interval to maintain the hemoglobin level at least 10 to 11 g/dL. Interval and amount of blood transfusion depends upon the level of hemoglobin of the child. Usually 10 to 15 mL/kg every 2 to 3 weeks washed packed RBCs are transfused. Special precautions to be taken during transfusion to prevent complications. Transfusion related infections can be prevented by specific protection with immunizing agents. Neocyte transfusion with new RBCs having longer life span can also be given, though it is not being used at present.

Iron Chelation Therapy

Iron chelating agent desferrioxamine (Desferal) is recommended to prevent complications of repeated blood transfusions, i.e. hemosiderosis and hemochromatosis. It is given as continuous subcutaneous infusion in the dose of 25 to 50 mg/kg/day over a period of 8 hours to 12 hours. Special microinfusion pump is used. Usually this therapy is given at night and 5 to 6 nights per week. It is given after 10 to 15th transfusion. Serum ferritin level is maintained between 1000 to 2000 ng/mL. Vitamin 'C' 100 mg/day is given concurrently to enhance the iron excretion. Overdose of this iron-chelating agent may result in growth retardation, visual problems and hearing toxicity. The iron-chelation therapy is very costly.

Intravenous desferrioxamine therapy is indicated in patients with poor compliance and large iron-induced cardiac disease. It is far more expensive than SC therapy.

Oral iron-chelating agent, deferiprone (DFP) is now available with less toxicity. The dose is 75 to 100 mg/kg/day in 2 to 3 divided dose. The common side-effects are joint pain, nausea, vomiting, pain abdomen, etc.

Splenectomy

Splenectomy is indicated when the child need very frequent blood transfusion and develop hypersplenism or big spleen causing discomfort.

Folic Acid Supplementations

Folic acid supplementations are recommended whereas iron therapy and dietary iron should be avoided to prevent more iron deposition.

Supportive Management

Supportive management is important to manage associated problems and to treat complications (like CCF, hepatic failure). Vaccination with hepatitis 'B' to be given to prevent transfusion related infection along with other routine immunization. Emotional support is very essential to the parents and child. Basic supportive nursing care are very important to prevent various complications.

Bone Marrow Transplantation

Bone marrow transplantation is an effective treatment modality with potential of curing thalassemia. Defective stem cells are replaced by normal stem cells. It is extremely expensive and possible in only very selective cases.

New Approaches

New approaches in the management of thalassemia are gene therapy and gene manipulation. In gene therapy, insertion of normal gene is done in the stem cells to correct underlying defect. It is done in two approaches, i.e. somatic and transgenic. In gene manipulation, excess of alpha chains is decreased by increasing the gamma chains.

Nursing Management

Nursing assessment should be done based on subjective and objective data to formulate the nursing diagnoses for the particular child and to implement the nursing interventions.

The important nursing diagnoses for a thalassemic child are as follows:

- Altered tissue perfusion related to abnormal hemoglobin.
- Risk of infection related to anemia.
- Activity intolerance related to anemia, CCF, etc.
- Chronic pain related to skeletal changes.
- Body image disturbances related the bony changes and facial deformities.
- Ineffective family coping related to poor prognosis.
- Knowledge deficit related to child care in long-term chronic illness with hemolytic anemia.

Nursing Interventions

Nursing interventions should emphasized on the following aspects:

- Assessment of child condition to prevent complications that can be done as hospital based or community based (at home).
- Preparation for repeated hospitalization for treatment of the disease and its complications.
- Arrangement of necessary diagnostic measures.
- Administration of blood transfusion and iron chelating agent with appropriate precautions for specific therapy.
- Provision of supportive care with rest, comfort, nutritious diet with restriction of iron containing food. Vitamin supplementation, immunization, hygienic care and other symptomatic care.
- Prevention of infection by aseptic techniques and promotion of general cleanliness.
- Preoperative and postoperative care during splenectomy with necessary health education after the surgery.
- Information regarding treatment plan, prognosis and complications to be given to parent and family members with appropriate explanation.
- Emotional support to the parents and family for effective coping about the stress of the illness.
- Teaching the parent about importance of follow-up, blood transfusion, investigations, signs of complications, dietary restriction, activity modification, recreation, diversion and available treatment facilities.
- Referral and necessary guidance for available support services and community facilities.

Preventive Measures

Antenatal screening in the first trimester of pregnancy by amniocentesis or chorionic villous sampling or fetoscopy help to detect thalassemia in fetal life. Genetic counseling in that respect is very important preventive measure which guide the parent to decide whether to continue pregnancy with thalassemic fetus or to terminate pregnancy (by MTP) of affected fetus.

Carriers can be detected by simple blood examination or by identification of thalassemia gene. Creation of awareness among public regarding detection of thalassemia gene before marriage and marital counseling are also very important preventive aspect.

Prognosis

Prognosis of thalassemia major is poor. Severe anemia and early onset of manifestations have poorer prognosis. Presence of complications also results in poor outcome.

Patients with thalassemia intermedia may continue their life up to 5 to 6 decade. Thalassemia minor may lead near normal life.

HEMOPHILIA

(Hemophilia is an inherited bleeding disorder due to deficiency of plasma coagulation factors) It is primarily found in males but transmitted by female carriers. Hereditary hemophilia may account about 80 percent of cases as sex-linked recessive trait where abnormal gene carried on the X-chromosome. Affected males may pass the gene to female offspring making them carrier. Female baby may be affected rarely only when a female carrier bears the child with a male hemophiliac partner.

Table 18.1 shows probability of transmission of hemophilia in children.

About 20 percent of cases may account as acquired hemophilia due to spontaneous mutation where family history of the illness may not always present for the disease.

Classification

Hemophilia is classified into three groups based on the deficient factors of coagulation.

A. Hemophilia-A (classical hemophilia)—It occurs due to deficiency of plasma factor VIII, the antihemophilic factor (AHF). It accounts for 80 to 85 percent of all hemophilics.

B. Hemophilia-B (Christmas disease)—It results from deficiency of plasma factor IX, the plasma thromboplastin component (PTC). It accounts for about 15 to 20 percent of cases.

C. Hemophilia-C—It results from deficiency of factor XI, plasma thromboplastin antecedent (PTA). It accounts for few cases only.

Hemophilia-'A' can be classified based upon the factor—VIII level in plasma. They are as follows:

a. *Severe hemophilia-A*—In this condition, the factor level is found less than 1 percent of normal value. Patients have tendency of spontaneous bleeding and severe bleeding.

b. *Moderate hemophilia-A*—Factor level remains between 1 to 5 percent of normal. Patients have no spontaneous bleeding and may not have severe bleeding until any trauma occurs.

c. *Mild hemophilia-A*—Factor level is in between 6 to 30 percent of normal. Patients usually lead normal lives and bleeding only occurs in severe injury and surgical interventions.

Pathophysiology

Hemophilia is concerned with absence or decrease of deficient functions of blood coagulation factors leading to excessive, prolonged or delayed bleeding. The basic defect is in the intrinsic phase of the coagulation process. The blood clotting factors are essential for the formation of prothrombin activators which converts the prothrombin to thrombin. The rate of thrombin formation is almost directly proportional to the amount of prothrombin activator available. The rate of clotting process is proportional to the amount of formed thrombin. Clinical manifestations depend upon plasma level of the involved deficient coagulation factors.

Clinical Manifestations

Patient with mild and moderate hemophilia are usually asymptomatic. They may have bleeding after any injury or surgery.

In severe hemophilia excessive bleeding may occur in neonates from umbilical cord. But usually the condition is diagnosed when the child becomes active. The history of illness includes prolonged bleeding after circumcision or tooth extraction or any injury. The child may present with easy bruising, spontaneous soft tissue hematomas, prolonged bleeding from lacerations in the nasal mucosa or oral cavity. Spontaneous bleeding may also be observed.

The important cause of hospitalization is hemorrhages into the joints (hemarthrosis) especially in elbows, knees or ankles. The condition may present along with pain, swelling and limitations of movement (fixed joint) of the involved joint. The child may have spontaneous hematuria, GI bleeding, intracranial hemorrhage or bleeding from any site of the body. But petechiae do not occur in hemophilia.

Diagnostic Evaluation

1. Blood examination shows the following findings:
   • Prolonged clotting time and partial thromboplastin time.

Table 18.1: Probability of transmission of hemophilia in children

Mother's genotype	Father's genotype	Female child			Male child	
		Normal	Carrier	Hemophiliac	Normal	Hemophiliac
• Carrier	• Normal	50%	50%	0	50%	50%
• Noncarrier	• Hemophiliac	0	100%	0	100%	0
• Carrier	• Hemophiliac	0	50%	50%	50%	50%

- Reduced prothrombin consumption.
- Increased thromboplastin level.
- Bleeding time and prothrombin time are normal.
- Assay of specific clotting factors indicates deficient level.

2. X-ray if the affected joints help to detect the severity and complications of hemarthrosis.
3. Gene analysis for antenatal diagnosis of hemophilia.
4. Detection of carrier of hemophilia and DNA studies.

Management

Prompt and appropriate management to be provided by early diagnosis to prevent long-term complications. The specific management include the followings:

1. Replacement of missing coagulation factors is the important aspect of management
   - Factor VIII made from cryoprecipitate or factor VIII concentrate is transfused in hemophilia A.
   - Factor IX made from fresh frozen plasma is administered for hemophilia 'B'.
   - Fresh frozen plasma is given to supply factor XI.
2. Mild to moderate factor VIII deficient hemophiliacs may respond to desmopressin which causes release of factor VIII from the endothelial stores.
3. Fresh whole blood transfusion can be given if the commercially prepared coagulation factors are not readily available.
4. Antifibrinolytics such as aminocaproic acid and tranexamic acid are given for mucosal bleeding to prevent clot breakdown by salivary proteins and to promote hemostasis.
5. Supportive management in case of hemarthrosis should include rest, immobilization of joint, application of local cold (ice bag) and pressure bandage with local application of thrombin powder or foam. Pain can be relieved by analgesic like paracetamol or NSAIDs. Aspirin, indomethacin, and betazolidone are not used as they inhibit platelets function and promote bleeding. Steroid can be used in cases of hemarthrosis.

   Ambulation and exercise can be allowed after the acute phase is over. Later, local heat and physiotherapy should be given to prevent ankylosis of the joint.
6. Home treatment with factor VIII infusion is now becoming popular. Parent and child need to be specially trained for home treatment.
7. Synovectomy can be recommended to remove damage synovium in chronically involved joints.
8. Orthotics can be used to prevent injury to affected joint and help to resolve hemorrhages.
9. Gene therapy is now under research.
10. Prophylactic measures to be taken to prevent complications. Parent teaching is important regarding prevention of injury, avoidance of intramuscular injection, immunization against hepatitis 'B', blood safety measures to prevent transfusion-related-infections (HIV, hepatitis-B and C) and avoidance of drugs like aspirin. Precautions should be taken before any surgical procedures. Prophylactic factor-VIII therapy can be given to prevent morbidity of hemophiliacs.
11. Genetic counseling and antenatal diagnosis should be arranged especially with positive family history of hemophilia.

Nursing Management

Nursing assessment should include details history of illness with family history and history of prolonged bleeding after any injury or surgery. Thorough physical examination to be done to assess the nursing diagnosis and to plan nursing interventions.

A. Important nursing diagnoses include:
   - Risk for volume deficit related to hemorrhage.
   - Pain related to bleeding joints.
   - Potential for bleeding related to deficiency of clotting factors.
   - Impaired physical mobility related to hemarthrosis.
   - Ineffective family coping related to life-threatening illness.

B. Nursing interventions:
1. Assessing the child at frequent interval and recording of findings related to the disease.
2. Preventing hypovolemia by control of bleeding with the following measures:
   - Applying pressure and cold on the area for 10 to 15 minutes even after injection and venipuncture.
   - Placing absorbable gelatin foam or fibrin foam on wound and applying fibrinolytic agent for oral bleeding.
   - Avoiding suturing and cauterization during surgery.
   - Immobilizing and elevating the affected part.
   - Providing rest, comfort and quiet environment.
   - Monitoring vital signs and signs of shock.
3. Administering drugs as prescribed with necessary precautions. Missing factors or blood should be given slowly to minimize transfusion reaction (2–3 mL/min). Packet should be checked for negative test of hepatitis 'B' HIV, etc.
4. Preserving joint mobility by treating hemarthrosis with prescribed drugs, immobilization in a slight flexion position, applying cold and following other instructions of supportive care. Affected joint can be treated with plaster cast if necessary. Preventing weight bearing on the affected joint.
5. Providing protection against injury and bleeding.
6. Teaching the parent and family members about home care, safety measures, regular follow-up, continuation

of school education, avoidance of sports injury and overweight; need for hospitalization, complications, etc.

7. Providing emotional support to cope with the problem and involving parents in routine care of the child.

Complications

Hemophilia may cause numbers of complications. They include:

1. Airway obstruction caused by bleeding into the neck and pharynx.
2. Intracranial bleeding leading to neurological impairment.
3. Intestinal obstruction due to GI bleeding.
4. Compartment syndrome due to compression of nerves by bleeding into deep tissues.
5. Degenerative joint disease, osteoporosis and muscle atrophy due to repeated hemorrhage.
6. Chronic hepatitis and cirrhosis due to contaminated cryoprecipitate.
7. HIV/AIDS due to transfusion related infections.
8. Physical, psychological and social handicaps.

Prognosis

Prognosis of hemophilia patients may vary. Death may occur due to serious hemorrhage and obstructions due to bleeding. Life-span may be uncertain for many hemophiliacs as a result of complications of hemorrhage and blood borne infections. Cripple patients may need rehabilitative services. A normal life span may be possible as a result of advances of management schedule.

LEUKEMIA

Leukemia is the most common type of childhood malignancy characterized by persistent and uncontrolled production of immature and abnormal white blood cells. It is a disease of abnormal proliferation and maturation of bone marrow which interferes with the production of normal RBCs, WBCs and platelets.

About 95 to 98 percent of childhood leukemias are acute type. Mostly the cases are acute lymphocytic leukemia (70–75%) and other variety is acute nonlymphocytic leukemia (about 20%). Chronic myelocytic leukemia and other varieties account for about 4 percent of all cases. Chronic lymphocytic leukemia is very rare in children.

Etiology

The exact cause of leukemia is not clearly understood. The following factors may responsible for the condition.

• Genetic factor is considered as responsible for leukemia. Genetic diseases like Down's syndrome, Fanconi's anemia, Bloom syndrome may predispose the disease.

• Environmental factors contribute in etiopathogenesis of leukemia which include exposure to ionizing radiation, viral infections like Human T-cell lymphoma leukemia virus (HTLV) and Epstein-Barr virus.

Classification

A. Acute lymphocytic leukemia (ALL)
   • Null-cell variety—Having no cellular surface markers and 80 percent belongs to this type.
   • T cell variety—High risk type.
   • B cell variety—High risk type.
B. Acute nonlymphocytic leukemia (ANLL).
C. Chronic lymphocytic leukemia (CLL)—rare in children.
D. Chronic myelocytic leukemia (CML).
   a. Adult type.
   b. Juvenile type (congenital leukemia).

Acute Lymphocytic Leukemia (Fig. 18.2)

Acute lymphocytic leukemia (ALL) is a primary disorder of the bone marrow in which the normal bone marrow elements are replaced by immature or undifferentiated blast cells. It is characterized by anemia, thrombocytopenia and neutropenia specially granulocytopenia.

The incidence of ALL is about 1 in 2,000 live birth. Peak age of onset is 3 to 7 years. The male children are more affected than females. The ALL can be classified on the basis of cell morphology as three subtypes, i.e. L_1, L_2, L_3 (according to French-American-British classification).

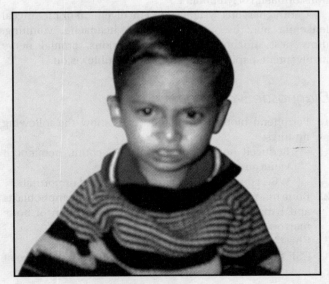

Fig. 18.2: A male child of 3 years with acute lymphocytic leukemia

Pathophysiology

Acute lymphocytic leukemia occurs from growth of abnormal nongranular fragile leukocytes in the blood forming tissues, particularly in the bone marrow, spleen and lymph nodes. Normal bone marrow elements are replaced by the leukemic cells. Formation of RBCs and platelets are decreased causing anemia, prolonged and unusual bleeding, tendency to bruise and petechiae. Normal WBCs are significantly decreased causing susceptibility to infections. Infiltration of leukemic cells into lymph nodes, spleen and liver results in enlargement of lymph glands and hepatosplenomegaly. Expansion and hyperplasia of bone marrow and infiltration of leukemic cells into bone causes joint and bone pain. Nutritional deprivation and generalized weakness occur due to immense metabolic needs of the proliferating leukemic cells.

Clinical Manifestations

Clinical presentations of leukemia depend upon types of leukemic cells. The onset is usually acute or insidious. The ALL is a great imitator with vague and varied signs and symptoms, resembling almost any disease.

The initial manifestations are fever anorexia, malaise, weakness, petechiae, purpura, ecchymosis and bleeding. The child may present with progressive pallor, decreased activity level, weight loss and muscle wasting. The child may complain abdominal pain, bone pain, joint pain and sternal tenderness. Hepatosplenomegaly, hematemesis, melena, hematuria, oral infections are common associated features. Excessive bleeding from nose prick or minor injury or minor operation like tooth extraction may be the first alarming features. Rarely lymphadenopathy may found in T-cell ALL or leukemic transformation of lymphoma.

Central nervous system (CNS) involvement or meningeal leukemia may be manifested with headache, vomiting, drowsiness, unconsciousness, convulsions, cranial nerve involvement, papilledema, blurred or double vision.

Diagnostic Evaluation

1. Peripheral blood examination may show the following findings:
   - Reduced hemoglobin level, RBC count, hematocrit value and platelet count.
   - WBC count may be decreased, elevated or normal.
2. Bone marrow study shows large numbers of lymphoblasts and lymphocytes with hypercellular condition of bone marrow.
3. Chest X-ray helps to diagnose mediastinal mass.
4. CSF study determines CNS involvement with presence of leukemic cells.

Management

The effective treatment is now available for ALL. Specific management of ALL includes chemotherapy, radiation therapy and bone marrow transplantation. Supportive and symptomatic management to be provided to prevent complications like infections, bleeding, anemia, pain, etc. Expert nursing management is important aspect to promote well-being.

Chemotherapy

It is given initially as remission induction then as maintenance therapy and late intensification therapy. The aims of chemotherapy are to eradicate malignant cells and to restore normal bone marrow functions.

a. *Remission induction chemotherapy*—It is administered for 4 to 6 weeks with vincristine, prednisolone, asparginase and adriamycin. These drugs give 95 to 98 percent remission with recommended dose by intensive systemic chemotherapy. This treatment can be carried out for two additional weeks, if normal bone marrow is not achieved. No response at 8 weeks indicates poor prognosis.

b. *Maintenance therapy or systemic continuation*—It is given for 2.5 to 3 years with 6MP (Mercaptopurine) and MTX (Methotrexate) as per recommended dose.

c. *Late intensification or reinforcement therapy*—It is provided with vincristine and prednisolone every 4 weeks.

d. *CNS prophylaxis*—In case of CNS involvement triple therapy is administered in intrathecal route as antileukemic drugs do not penetrate into the CSF. Methotrexate, hydrocortisone and cystosine arabinoside are administered once a week during induction and then every 8 weeks for 2 years. Cranial irradiation can be given in combination with the above drugs.

Complications

A child with ALL can be complicated with infections (lungs, GI tract, skin), bleeding, arrhythmias and heart block. There may be CNS, skeletal and testicular involvement. Urate nephropathy may develop. Complications related to chemotherapy, irradiation therapy and bone marrow transplantation are commonly found.

Prognosis

Initial remission expected to achieve in at least 95 percent children with ALL having specialized treatment. Overall cure rate is 65 to 75 percent. Prognosis becomes poorer with each relapse. Children who are below 12 months of age or older than 9 years carry poor prognosis. Higher initial WBC

count has worse prognosis. The factors contributing to poorer prognosis in Indian children are:
- Poor treatment compliance due to economical problems.
- High incidence of superadded infections.
- Lack of appropriate supportive care.
- Poor tolerance of chemotherapeutic regimen due to associated malnutrition.
- High component of T-cell leukemia and cytogenetic abnormalities.

Acute Nonlymphocytic Leukemia

Acute nonlymphocytic leukemia (ANLL) is responsible for about 20 percent of childhood leukemia. They can be classified as follows:
- M1—Acute myelocytic (no maturation) leukemia.
- M2—Myelocytic (some maturation) leukemia.
- M3—Promyelocytic leukemia.
- M4—Myelomonocytic leukemia.
- M5—Acute monocytic leukemia.
- M6—Erythroblastic leukemia.
- M7—Megakaryocytic leukemia.

Clinical Manifestations of ANLL

Acute nonlymphocytic leukemia can be manifested with anemia, leukopenia and thrombocytopenia. The child presents with progressive pallor, fever, active bleeding, bone pain, GI tract disturbances and gingival swelling due to infiltration of leukemic cells. Some patients may have recurrent infections, hepatosplenomegaly and marked lymphadenopathy. Joint pain and CNS involvement may be found in some children. Orbital swelling producing proptosis may be found in some cases. Diagnosis is confirmed by blood examination and bone marrow study.

Management

Acute nonlymphocytic leukemia is managed with chemotherapy using cystosine-arabinoside continuous IV infusion for 7 days and IV Daunorubicin for 3 days. Over 70 percent of the cases show remission with these drugs. Maintenance therapy is given with rotating combinations of several drugs for up to 2 years. Intrathecal CNS prophylaxis may be indicated in case of CNS involvement. Heparin therapy may be needed is case of DIC and any fatal hemorrhage in M-3 type of ANLL. Supportive treatment with blood, platelet transfusion and intravenous antibiotic therapy may be required. Cranial irradiation and bone marrow transplantation may also be indicated in some cases.

Poor prognosis observed when WBC count is more than 100,000/cmm and extramedullary manifestations are evident. About 30 to 40 percent patients may be cured. Recently with more intensified treatment, prolonged disease free survival has been obtained.

Chronic Myelocytic Leukemia

Chronic myelocytic leukemia (CML) is characterized by increased numbers of myeloid cells in all stages of maturation both in the blood and bone marrow.

Chronic myelocytic leukermia is quite rare in children accounting for 2 to 3 percent of all leukemia. It presents in children as adult and juvenile type. Adult type is most commonly found.

The onset of the disease in insidious with malaise, weakness and progressive massive enlargement of spleen and liver which may reach into the pelvis. Most cases are found in about 10 to 12 years of age. Other presenting features are arthritis, priapism, retinopathy, skin infiltration and unexplained fever.

Blood examination shows anemia, thrombocytosis and excess leukocytic count with remarkable eosinophilia and basophilia. Presence of philadelphia chromosome is very important diagnostic finding. Bone marrow study help to confirm the diagnosis and shows hyperplasia.

Juvenile type CML occurs in children below 2 years of age. It presents with eczema, lymphadenopathy, recurrent bacterial infections and hepatosplenomegaly. WBC count is usually less than 100,000/cmm. Thrombocytopenia is frequently present. Bone marrow study shows monoblastic cells. Philadelphia chromosome is negative. Treatment is done same as ANLL. Response to chemotherapy is discouraging. Bone marrow transplantation gives good result.

Management of adult type CML is done with hydroxyurea or busulfan to keep the WBC count below 100,000/cmm. Splenic radiation, interferon and bone marrow transplantation are also indicated for treatment of CML. Prognosis of CML is very poor. No cure has been reported.

Nursing Management of a Child with Leukemia

Nursing assessment should be done on the basis of subjective and objective data. The important nursing diagnoses are:
a. Anxiety of the parent related to diagnosis of malignant disease.
b. Risk for infections and bleeding related to abnormal bone marrow functions.
c. Pain related to infiltration of leukemic cells.
d. Activity intolerance related to fatigue resulting from disease process.
e. Alternation of body temperature, more than normal due to infections.
f. Altered nutrition, less than body requirement related to anorexia, nausea and gingival ulcers.

g. Alternation of body image related to alopecia, as side effect of chemotherapy.

h. Fear of the child related to various diagnostic and treatment procedures.

i. Knowledge deficit of the parent related to continuation of long-term care.

Nursing Interventions

a. Providing emotional support to the parent to reduce parental anxiety. Encouraging the parents to express their feeling and answering their questions honestly. Necessary informations and instructions to be given to the parents and family members to avail support services, community resources and religious help to adjust with the stress situation.

b. Preventing infections and hemorrhage. The following measures to be followed:
   • Maintaining aseptic technique, hygienic measures, general cleanliness, good handwashing practices, restriction of visitors and taking precautions during any invasive procedures.
   • Administering antibiotics, as prescribed. Oral and IV route to be used. Intramuscular injection should be best avoided.
   • Precautions to be taken during blood transfusion.
   • Avoiding injury. Soft toothbrush can be used for dental care. Soft jelly to be applied for dry lips. Non-irritating mouth wash to be used, no alcohol or H_2O_2 to be used. Breaking of skin and mucous membrane to be avoided.
   • Monitoring vital signs, urinary output, hydration level, signs of infections, bleeding or any other complications.

c. Relieving pain by rest, comfort, minimizing exertion, promoting relaxation and diversion and administering prescribed analgesics.

d. Assisting in activity of daily living (ADL), promoting hygienic care and minimizing disturbance during nursing interventions by gentle approach.

e. Maintaining normal body temperature by tepid sponge in high fever, airy environment, adequate fluid intake, avoiding overclothing and hot environment, administering antipyretics and other prescribed drugs. Recording vital signs 4 hourly. Avoiding use of rectal thermometer.

f. Promoting adequate nutritional intake with high nutritious diet with small frequent feed. Avoiding high salty food, when steroids are given. Antiemetics to be given to prevent vomiting. Diet should be attractive and tasty to promote intake of more amount.

g. Explaining about the change of body image, especially in case of alopecia due to chemotherapy. Ensuring about future change and contacting with people having new hair following alopecia.

h. Reducing fear of the children by allowing parent with them during procedures, improving IPR and allowing play materials.

i. Teaching the parents about health maintenance regarding regular blood testing, chemotherapy or other mode of management, possible complications and their warning signs, necessary medical help and follow-up.

BLEEDING DISORDERS/PURPURA

Bleeding disorder may be congenital or acquired and may be caused by dysfunction in any phase of hemostasis. Hemostasis involves local reactions of blood vessels, multiple activities of the platelets, interaction of coagulation factors, inhibitors and fibrinolytic proteins circulating in the blood. It maintains the dynamic equilibrium between fluidity and coagulation of blood, thus preventing excessive bleeding or thrombosis spontaneously or after a minor trauma.

Common bleeding disorders are thrombocytopenia, immune thrombocytopenic purpura (ITP), disseminated intravascular coagulation (DIC), and von Willebrand disease. Increased bleeding tendency may be found due to purpura or plasma coagulation factor deficiency.

Purpura is characterized by spontaneous bleeding into the skin or mucous membrane due to prolonged bleeding time as manifested with petechiae, a small pinpoint hemorrhage or ecchymosis and large superficial hemorrhages or hematoma. Purpura may be associated with quantitative and qualitative deficiency of platelets or due to impaired vascular integrity. Purpura can be classified as:

a. Thrombocytopenic purpura—When platelet count is decreased.

b. Nonthrombocytopenic purpura—When there is defect in blood vessels or in platelet functions.

Thrombocytopenia

It is a condition due to decreased number of platelets. It is the most common cause of primary hemostatic defect with overt bleeding disorder.

Causes

1. Decreased platelet production—It is found in leukemia, aplastic anemia, myelofibrosis, myelosuppressive therapy and radiation therapy. It may be associated with hereditary disorders like Fanconi's anemia.

2. Increased platelet destruction—It occurs due to infection, adverse drug effects, ITP and DIC.

3. Abnormality or sequestration in spleen.

4. Platelet dilution in RBC transfusion and after hemorrhage.

Clinical Manifestations

Patients with thrombocytopenia may have no symptoms. But when platelet count is less than 50,000/mm³, then petechiae occurs spontaneously with ecchymosis at the site of minor trauma. Bleeding may occurs from mucosa of the nose, GI tract, genitourinary tract, respiratory system and within CNS. Menorrhagia is common in adolescent girls. Excessive bleeding may occur after minor surgery, tooth extraction, etc. Severe blood loss and bleeding into the vital organs are life-threatening conditions.

Diagnostic Evaluation

Diagnosis is confirmed by blood examination. The findings show prolonged bleeding time, prothrombin time and partial thromboplastin time. Platelet count, hemoglobin level and hematocrit values are decreased.

Management

- Initial management is done with platelet transfusion or blood transfusion in severe bleeding.
- Life-threatening bleeding should be managed immediately with specialized approach to control bleeding and to prevent its consequences.
- Identification of the exact cause and specific management to be planned.
- Steroid therapy or IV immunoglobins may be beneficial for some cases.

Nursing management
- Assessment of the patients condition by details history, physical examination, arranging diagnostic tests and reviewing the findings.
- Minimizing bleeding by special precautions during care. Avoiding hard toothbrush, IM injections, use of tourniquets, trauma, nosepricking and rectal procedures.
- Preventing constipation by dietary modifications.
- Restricting activity and exercise to prevent accidental injury.
- Taking precautions during blood or blood product transfusion to prevent anaphylaxis, volume overload and infections.
- Monitoring child's vital signs, intake-output, stool for occult blood, menstrual bleeding flow, etc.
- Instructing the parents and child for avoidance of nose-blowing, nose pricking, use of aspirin and NSAIDs, trauma, etc.
- Teaching about home-based care specially during bleeding, need for medical help and follow-up at regular interval.

Immune Thrombocytopenic Purpura

Immune thrombocytopenic purpura (ITP) was previously known as "idiopathic thrombocytopenic purpura", now it is termed as "immune (autoimmune) thrombocytopenic purpura". It is also known as purpura hemorrhagica and characterized by spontaneous hemorrhages in the skin and mucous membrane. It is one of the most common bleeding disorder resulting from immune destruction of platelets by antiplatelet antibodies.

Definite cause of ITP is not clearly understood, but it seems to be due to autoimmune reactions. History or viral infections may be noticed in some cases. Antiplatelet antibodies (autoantibodies) of both IgG and IgM are directed against the platelet membrane antigen (autoantigen). Thrombocytopenia results from increased destruction of the antibody coated platelets by the reticuloendothelial system in the spleen. The clinical features are developed due to thrombocytopenia, reduced platelet survival, presence of platelet antibodies, and increase number of megakaryocytes in the bone marrow.

Classification of ITP

A. *Acute ITP*—It is more common in childhood, usually following viral infections. There is sudden onset of symptoms associated with thrombocytopenia. Prognosis is good with 80 to 90 percent recovery after 1 to 2 months of suffering. Relapse may occur with infections.
B. *Chronic ITP*—It is less common in children. The onset of symptoms is insidious. No history of viral infection usually detected. Thrombocytopenia is not severe and average course of illness is 6 months. Children with ITP have only 10 to 20 percent chance of natural remission. It may be associated with SLE, thyroid diseases and rheumatoid disease.

Clinical Manifestations

The usual age of onset of the illness is 3 to 8 years. Acute ITP is equally found in boys and girls. Chronic ITP is more common in girls.

The clinical features of ITP include easy bruising following minor trauma, petechiae and bleeding. Petechiae may be found all over the body. Ecchymosis is seen over the anterior surface of lower limbs and over bony prominence. In one-third of cases, bleeding is observed from mucosal surface such as nose and gums. CNS hemorrhage may occur in initial phase of illness. Anemia is proportionate with amount of bleeding. Spleen may be just palpable in one-fourth of the cases.

Severe manifestations may be found as hematuria, GI bleeding, severe nose bleed, menorrhagia, intracranial hemorrhages, etc. Life-threatening complications may arise due to severe bleeding.

Diagnostic Evaluation

- A careful history regarding previous infections, drug therapy, X-ray exposure, use of sprays, exposure to toxins or insecticides should be obtained.
- Thorough clinical examination to be done to exclude the features.
- Tourniquet test or Hess test shows positive findings.
- Blood examination shows reduced platelet count (less than 20,000/cmm in acute ITP and 30,000 to 70,000/cmm in chronic ITP). Lymphocytosis and eosinophilia may present. BT, CT and clot retraction time show abnormal variations. Complete hemogram shows abnormal cells and low hemoglobin percentage.
- Bone marrow study reveals increased number of mega-karyocytes which ruled out the possibility of leukemia and aplastic anemia.
- Platelet antibody assay helps to confirm the diagnosis.

Management

- Supportive management to be provided with blood and platelet transfusion to prevent and treat bleeding episodes.
- Corticosteroid therapy in high dose is given to inhibit platelet antibody production, interaction between platelet and antibodies, prolong platelet survival and improve vascular stability. Usual dose 1 to 2 mg/kg/day of prednisolone for 2 to 3 weeks followed by tapering doses over next 1 to 2 weeks.
- Intravenous immunoglobulin (IV-IgG) is administered with 2 g/kg of total dose to protect platelets antibody.
- Anti-Rh therapy can be used effectively to control the acute bleeding episodes or to increase platelet count before surgery.
- Splenectomy is indicated for the patients not responding to steroids and IV-IgG therapy. About 10 to 15 percent cases of ITP require splenectomy.
- The refractory cases of ITP can be treated with immuno-suppressive drugs like vincristine, azathioprine, cyclophosphamide, etc. Newer treatment modalities like interferon, plasmapheresis have been found effective for these cases.

Prognosis

Recovery is noticed in 85 to 95 percent cases within 6 months. Remaining 10 to 15 percent cases become chronic. In the latter, the cure rate may be 75 percent following splenectomy.

Nonthrombocytopenic Purpura

The Henoch-Schönlein syndrome is the most common non-thrombocytopenic purpura. It is an allergic, anaphylactoid and aseptic vasculitis, with involvement of joints (Schönlein purpura) and/or abdominal viscera (Henoch purpura). It is far less frequent then ITP and found in children between 3 to 12 years of age.

The clinical presentations are found as petechiae, rash, arthritis, signs of acute abdomen, GI bleeding and nephritis with acute renal failure.

Abnormal platelet function is diagnosed by reduced clot retraction or failure of thromboplastin generation. Platelet count is normal. Throat swab culture may show Strep. hemolyticus. ASO titer may be raised.

The disease is self-limiting within 4 to 6 weeks. Corticosteroid therapy is effective alongwith bedrest, adequate nutrition and symptomatic treatment. Complications need early detection and prompt management to prevent fatal outcome. Prognosis may be fatal in renal failure, cerebral or gastrointestinal hemorrhage.

DISSEMINATED INTRAVASCULAR COAGULATION

Disseminated intravascular coagulation (DIC) or consumptive coagulopathy is an acquired thrombotic and hemorrhagic syndrome with abnormal activation of clotting process and acceleration of fibrinolysis. It results in wide spread clotting in small vessels with consumption of clotting factors and platelets. These lead to intravascular fibrin deposition and microvascular occlusion along with bleeding from multiple sites, thrombosis, tissue ischemia, necrosis and hemolytic anemia.

Causes

Several pathological conditions like hypoxia, acidosis, tissue necrosis, endothelial damage and shock can cause DIC. Newborn babies are more vulnerable to DIC due to asphyxia, hypothermia and shock.

A large number of disease conditions may be accompanied by DIC. They include infections, septicemia, leukemia, cyanotic congenital heart disease, thalassemia major, sickle cell anemia, giant hemangioma, SLE, anaphylactic purpura and acute hepatic failure. Major surgery, crush injury, head injury, multiple fracture, burns, snake bite or insect bite and incompatible blood transfusion also may result in this condition.

Clinical Manifestations

Disseminated intravascular coagulation is manifested by generalized bleeding diathesis. Bleeding may start with needle prick or venepucture or surgical incision. It may present as purpura, ecchymosis, petechiae, easy bruising, gum bleeding, epistaxis, subconjunctival hemorrhage, coffee colored vomiting and abdominal pain. Intracranial hemorrhage, acute respiratory distress and peripheral cyanosis may be found. Thromboembolic condition may lead to hematuria, oliguria and acute renal failure. Purpura fulminans may occur due to wide spread thrombotic microvascular occlusion of dermal vessels resulting well-demarcated large patches of ecchymoses with skin infarction. Profound anemia develops due to rapid hemolysis.

In case of chronic DIC, the features are intermittent skin or mucosal bleeds over weeks or months, thrombophlebitis at unusual sites and deep venous thromboembolism.

Diagnostic Evaluation

History of illness and clinical features help to diagnosis the condition for initiation of prompt management of life-threatening bleeding episodes. Laboratory investigations show low platelet count, diminished fibrinogen level, low level of antithrombin-III, heparin cofactor-II, increased level of fibrin split products, presence of RBC fragmentation with schizocytes and reduced prothrombin time (PT) and partial thromboplastin time (PTT).

Management

Identification and treatment of underlying cause is the important aspect of management. Initially treatment of aggravating factors like acidosis, electrolyte disturbances, hypoxia, shock, etc. should be managed promptly. Medications should be given in IV route. Packed cell blood transfusion to be administered to correct anemia. Hydrocortisone and vitamin 'K' will be effective for treatment of purpura.

Fresh frozen plasma or platelet or cryoprecipitate, even fresh blood transfusion are useful as replacement therapy. Platelet count and fibrinogen level should be monitored frequently to maintain safe normal value.

Heparin therapy may be given by continuous infusion when replacement therapy is ineffective in controlling bleeding. Exchange blood transfusion can be helpful for removal of circulating toxin, fibrin split products, activated procoagulants and for supplying replacement factors.

Supportive nursing care should include continuous monitoring of signs of vascular occlusions and patient's general condition, maintenance of IV fluid, oxygen therapy, precautions to prevent injury and bleeding, administration of prescribed medications, avoiding vasoconstriction and dislodging clot, bedrest, change of position, range of motion exercises and maintenance of warmth. Pressure to be applied for 20 minutes at the site of bleeding and topical hemostatic agents to be used to minimize bleeding. Features of internal bleeding to be assessed for prompt management.

Complications

Complications of DIC include pulmonary embolism, acute renal failure, cerebral hemorrage (most common causes of death) and infarction in cerebrum, myocardium and spleen. Hemolytic anemia, GI ulcerations, tissue necrosis and gangrene may also develop.

Prognosis

Mortality rate is high in acute DIC, i.e. about 50 to 85 percent. Highest mortality is found in neonates. Prolonged prothrombin time (more than 1.5 times) and activated partial thromboplastin time indicate poor prognosis.

IMMUNODEFICIENCY

Immunodeficiency is a state of deficient immune response due to impairment of body defence mechanism. It is decreased ability to respond to antigenic stimuli by appropriate cellular immunity reaction.

Types

Immunodeficiency states can be primary or secondary. In primary type, there is no obvious systemic disease for its occurrence, whereas in secondary type, the cause is clearly identified outside the lymphoid system. Secondary (80%) type is more common than primary type (20%).

Primary Immunodeficiency

It is an abnormalities in the development and maturation of immune system resulting in increased susceptibility to infections. It can be classified as follows:

1. Humoral or B-cell defects, e.g. hypogammaglobulinemia.
2. Cellular of T-cell defects, e.g. congenital thymic hypoplasia.
3. Combined B cell and T cell defects, e.g. Wiskott-Aldrich syndrome.
4. Neutrophil defects, e.g. chronic granulomatous disease, congenital splenic defects.
5. Complement defects, e.g. hereditary angioneurotic edema.

Primary immunodeficiency may be suspected in (a) history of recurrent lower respiratory infections, recurrent or persistent diarrhea and failure to thrive (b) recurrent skin infections and fungal infections, (c) severe infections with nonpathogenic organism or opportunistic infections (d) in unexplained leukopenia or lymphopenia and (e) history of death of sibling in early infancy.

Secondary Immunodeficiency

It is an abnormalities outside the lymphoid system. It is usually associated with some aspect of the primary disease which directly affects the immune system. Majority of immunodeficiency states are secondary to other defects.

The important causes of secondary immunodeficiency are viral infections (HIV, measles), severe malnutrition, nephrotic syndrome, severe and chronic systemic infections and drug effects (glucocorticoid, cyclophosphamide, etc). It can be classified as follows:

a. Humoral or B cell defects, e.g. loss of immunological material in case of nephrotic syndrome and protein lossing enteropathy and in infections like malaria, EB virus infections, etc.
b. Cellular or T cell defects, e.g. in nutritional deficiency (PEM, deficiency of iron, zinc, biotin, vitamin 'B' or folate), viral infections, renal failure, chronic granulomatous disease (TB, leprosy).
c. Combined 'B' cell and T cell defects, e.g. bone marrow aplasia, severe/fulminant infections, irradiation, immunosuppressive therapy, etc.
d. Neutrophil defects, e.g. SLE, myeloid leukemia, malnutrition, Down's syndrome, Hodgkin's lymphoma, rheumatoid arthritis, etc.
e. Complement defects, e.g. chronic membranoproliferative nephritis, chronic cirrhosis, severe burns, nephrotic syndrome, lepromatous leprosy, thalassemia, etc.

Common Clinical Presentations of Immunodeficiency States

a. Recurrent infections—Respiratory infections, otitis media, bacterial meningitis, septicemia, *Pneumocystis carinii* pneumonia, etc.
b. Gastrointestinal disturbances—Unexplained diarrhea, malabsorption, recurrent giardiasis, oral thrush, oral apthous ulcer.
c. Recurrent eczema, skin infections, pyoderma.
d. Failure to thrive with unexplained cause.
e. Unusual vaccination reactions following BCG injection.

f. Autoimmune disorders, e.g. rheumatoid arthritis.
g. Malignant diseases, e.g. leukemia.
h. Nutritional deficiency disorders, e.g. PEM, IDA.
i. Parathyroid disorders, e.g. hypocalcemic tetany.
j. Ataxia telangiectasia.
k. Hereditary angioneurotic edema.

Diagnostic Evaluation

Immunodeficiency may be suspected in history of rececurrent infections, multisystem involvement, tonsillectomy, human gamma-globulin therapy and presence of clinical presentations related to the condition. Family history of consanguinity and death due to severe infections to be investigated. Physical examination may show various features, like pyoderma, eczema, fungal infection, stomatitis, perianal excoriation, pallor, etc.

Investigations to be done for the followings:

- Total blood count (TLC, DLC) and WBC morphology.
- X-ray chest.
- HIV testing.
- T cell and B cell rosetting.
- Serum electrophoresis for plasma proteins.
- Serum immunoglobulins estimation.
- Enzyme assay.
- Complement component assays.
- Specific tests like T cell subsets (CD_4, CD_8), Ig subclass, delayed hypersensitivity skin test, hemagglutinin titer, etc.

Management

Management of immunodeficiency states depends upon specific cause of the condition. Special attention for the most common cause, i.e. protein-energy malnutrition, should be considered as vital importance especially in children.

Specific management includes plasma infusion, intravenous immunoglobin therapy, interferon, gamma therapy, antiviral agents,bone marrow transplantation, etc. Symptomatic and supportive treatment are necessary for prolongation of life and prevention of complications.

Genetic counseling is important because majority of primary immunodeficiency conditions are hereditary. Long-term illness with uncertain prognosis may found in some children.

Disorders of Kidney and Urinary Tract

19

- Congenital Abnormalities of the Kidney and Urinary Tract
- Wilms' Tumor (Nephroblastoma)
- Nursing Management of the Child with Urologic Surgery
- Acute Glomerulonephritis

- Chronic Glomerulonephritis
- Urinary Tract Infections
- Nephrotic Syndrome
- Acute Renal Failure
- Chronic Renal Failure
- Care of the Child who Undergoes Dialysis

INTRODUCTION

Disorders of kidney and urinary tract are commonly seen in pediatric units as medical and surgical problems. Congenital malformations, neoplasms, infections, inflammations and progressive impairment of renal functions are common conditions found in children. The important clinical features are abnormal micturition, hematuria, oliguria, dysuria, ureteric colic, enuresis, polyuria and polydipsia. Other features are edema, proteinuria, anemia, hypertension, growth failure, abdominal mass, etc.

Diagnostic evaluation for these problems should include details history of illness, clinical examination, urine examination, blood tests to assess renal functions (creatinine, urea), serum albumin, cholesterol, antistreptolysin O (ASO) titer, glomerular filtration rate (GFR), urinary concentration test and imaging of urinary tract by plain X-ray, intravenous pyelogram (IVP), micturating cystourethrogram (MCU), ultrasonography, radionuclide imaging and renal biopsy, etc.

CONGENITAL ABNORMALITIES OF THE KIDNEY AND URINARY TRACT

Congenital malformations of the kidneys and urinary tract are commonly found in the pediatric surgery units. These problems usually required surgical correction. Some of them are producing no clinical symptoms, but approximately about 25 percent cases of chronic renal failure are due to congenital anomalies. These problems may be associated with other congenital anomalies like trisomy-21, neural tube defects and structural abnormalities of lower limbs.

Congenital anomalies of urinary tract are found in about 8 to 10 percent of children. Common anomalies are mentioned below.

- *Kidney and ureter:* Renal agenesis, renal hypoplasia, horse-shoe kidney, polycystic renal disease, ectopic kidney, duplication of renal pelvis and ureter, congenital renal neoplasm (nephroblastomatosis), hydronephrosis, pelvi-ureteric obstruction, hydroureter or megaureter, ureterocele, ectopic ureteral insertion, etc.
- *Bladder and urethra:* Ectopia vesicae, patent urachus, bladder neck obstruction, posterior urethral valves, neurogenic bladder, hypospadias, epispadias, phimosis, urethral stenosis, meatal stenosis, etc.

Renal Agenesis

Renal agenesis is the absence of kidney due to failure of ureteric bud formation or mesenchymal blastema differentiation of final mesenchymal condensation. It may be unilateral or bilateral and associated with various congenital anomalies. Bilateral renal agenesis with associated malformations is known as Potter's syndrome.

Renal Hypoplasia and Dysplasia

Renal hypoplasia occurs due to reduction of renal mass affecting the nephron. It may be unilateral or bilateral. It is sometimes difficult to differentiate from renal dysplasia which is characterized by disorganization of renal parenchyma with immature nephron and ductal elements resulting in a large or small kidney. Renal hypoplasia may be simple, segmental or oligomeganephric type. Renal dysplasia may be multicystic and sometimes hypoplastic or aplastic. It can be segmental or total and may be associated with urinary tract obstruction.

Horse-shoe Kidney

Horse-shoe kidney develops when lower poles of the kidneys are fused in the midline due to fusion of ureteric buds during fetal development. These kidneys are more vulnerable to develop Wilm's tumor than in general. The child presents with midline firm mass with associated pyuria, albuminuria and vomiting. Diagnosis is confirmed by IVP which shows a single mass with malposition of pelvis and a bridge of tissue. Surgery is indicated when uncontrolled urinary infections result in pyelonephritis.

Polycystic Kidneys

Polycystic kidney is one of the commonest congenital anomalies as inherited autosomal disease. It is a complex syndrome resulting from progressive dilatation of specific portion of the nephron which may arise during development and after completion of development of the nephron due to an adverse hereditary metabolic environment.

There is two distinct type of polycystic kidney, i.e. infantile type (autosomal recessive inheritance) and adult type (autosomal dominant inheritance).

Infantile type presents with palpable bilateral nodular cystic masses with hypertension and progressive renal failure. There may be associated anomalies of liver, lungs, central nervous system (CNS) and chorionic villus sampling (CVS).

Adult type presents with anemia, polyuria, osteodystrophy, hypertension and bilateral palpable nodular renal masses with irregular distribution. This type may not present even before 40 years of age.

Diagnosis of the disease is confirmed by IVP and renal angiography. Management is purely symptomatic. Prognosis is worst in early onset.

Obstructive Lesions of the Urinary Tract

Obstructive uropathy is mainly caused by congenital abnormalities like pelvi-ureteric junction obstruction and posterior urethral valves which may lead to irreversible renal damage. Other congenital causes of obstructive lesions are duplex renal system, neuromuscular bladder dysfunction, meatal stenosis, phimosis, etc. Acquired conditions like renal calculi, trauma, tumor, tuberculosis also may produce the obstruction.

Pelvi-ureteric Junction Stenosis

Pelvi-ureteric junction (PUJ) obstruction is commonly found as unilateral or bilateral stenosis of PUJ causing hydronephrosis. It can be associated with ectopic and horse-shoe kidney. PUJ stenosis may present as a flank mass without any symptoms or with urinary tract infection (UTI) and upper abdominal pain. The diagnosis is confirmed by ultrasound sonography (USG), IVP or renal scan and renal function test. Surgery is indicated for removal of obstruction and to prevent complications.

Hydronephrosis

Hydronephrosis is the dilatation of renal pelvis which may be found as unilateral or bilateral. It may be due to obstruction of urine flow in the distal urinary tract or reflux of urine up the ipsilateral ureter or due to bladder neck obstruction or urethral obstruction. This condition is more common in males than females and more frequently found in left sided kidney.

The patient with hydronephrosis may present with urinary infections or with large abdominal mass. Other features are abdominal pain, failure to thrive, anemia, hypertension, hematuria and renal failure. Diagnosis is confirmed by USG, IVP, MCU, diuretic isotope renography, etc. Management is done by surgical removal of obstruction or pyeloplasty. Percutaneous nephrostomy or nephrectomy may be indicated in complicated cases.

Posterior Urethral Valve

Posterior urethral valves (PUV) almost invariably occur in the male child and most frequent cause of distal urinary tract obstruction. The child present with dribbling of urine, abnormal urine stream, palpable bladder, recurrent urinary tract infections (UTIs), vomiting and failure to thrive. In severe and prolonged obstruction, renal dysplasia and anuria may develop.

Diagnosis of this condition is confirmed by MCU, USG and endoscopy. The valves are found usually at the point of junction of posterior urethra with anterior urethra. There is dilated posterior urethra and enlargement of bladder with vesicoureteric reflux (VUR).

Initially *management* is done with urinary catheterization following aseptic precautions. Definitive management is performed by transurethral destruction of the valvular leaflet by balloon catheter or endoscopic fulguration of the valves, as early as possible after confirmation of diagnosis. Other operative interventions may be indicated in some cases as temporary urinary diversion by cutaneous vesicostomy or bilateral ureterostomies or pyelostomy. Presence of associated complications should be detected and appropriate management to be arranged.

Meatal Stenosis

Meatal stenosis may occur as congenital abnormality. It may be found due to meatal ulcer and scaring, following infection or circumcision and improper hygiene. It can cause lower urinary tract obstruction. Meatal dilatation or meatoplasty may be needed to relieve the obstruction.

Exstrophy of Bladder (*Ectopia vesicae*)

Exstrophy of bladder is a congenital malformation in which the lower portion of the abdominal wall and the anterior wall of the bladder are missing, so that the bladder is everted through the opening and may found on the lower abdomen just above the symphasis pubis, with continuous passage of urine to the outside. It is also termed as 'ectopia vesicae', i.e. malposition or displacement of urinary bladder from its normal position in the pelvis. Exstrophy of bladder usually associated with numbers of congenital anomalies, related to urogenital tract, musculoskeletal system and sometimes of GI system. Male children are more commonly affected.

Clinical Manifestations

This condition is diagnosed on inspection at birth. The child is manifested with constant urinary dribbling through the defect, skin excoriation, infection and ulceration of the bladder mucosa. The child may have ambiguous genitalia and waddling unsteady gait. The condition may be complicated with UTI and growth failure. Cystoscopic examination, X-ray, USG, IVP and urodynamic testing can be done to detect the extent of anomaly and other associated problems.

Management

Exstrophy of bladder can be managed by surgical closure of the bladder within 48 hours. Urinary diversion may be needed in some cases before reconstructive surgery. Complete correction of the malformation can be done in stages by reconstruction of the defect. Orthopedic surgery may be needed in some cases with associated musculoskeletal problems. These interventions should be done by school age.

Supportive nursing care is important before and after reconstructive surgery to prevent complications.

In preoperative period, special attention should be given for protection of bladder area from infections and trauma. These can be obtained by avoiding irritating clothing and linen over the exposed bladder, positioning the infant on back or side, humidifying the exposed bladder by covering

with wet gauze, maintaining aseptic precautions and general hygienic measures along with other routine care. Preparation of parents and child for planned reconstructive surgery is important aspect of nursing care.

Postoperative care should include close monitoring of child's condition, vital signs, features of infections, intake-output, etc. Special attention should be given for care of urinary catheter, its position, drainage and aseptic precautions. The catheter may be placed urethral and/or ureteral. Instruction to be given to parents about necessary precautions for prevention of infection, dislodgement or leakage. Routine postoperative care should be provided to promote early recovery. Necessary information and demonstration to be given to the parents regarding home-based care, follow-up and next probable data of operative interventions, if needed. Teaching about signs of complications and their prevention are important.

Epispadias

Epispadias is the congenital abnormal urethral opening on the dorsal aspect of the penis. Urethra is displaced dorsally due to abnormal development of the infraumbilical wall and upper wall of the urethra. It is usually associated with exstrophy of bladder and ambiguous genitalia. Rarely it may found in female infants.

Classification

Epispadias in male child can be classified as:
- Anterior epispadias with normal continence.
  - Glandular
  - Balanitic or penile.
- Posterior epispadias—associated with incomplete bladder neck and incontinence of urine
  - Penopubic
  - Subsymphyseal

The male infants with epispadias are having short and broad penis with dorsal curvature.

In females, a cleft extends along the roof or entire urethra, involving the bladder neck. Urethra is short and patulous.

Female epispadias can be classified as:
- Bifid clitoris with no incontinence of urine.
- Subsymphyseal with incontinence of urine.

In both male and female, pubic bones are usually found separated, along with epispadias. There is low incidence of associated anomalies. The condition is usually diagnosed at birth. IVP and MCU are performed to detect abnormalities of upper urinary tract, vesicoureteric reflux (VUR) and bladder capacity.

Management

Management of epispadias is done by the surgical correction usually in three stages. First stage operation is done in about

1.5 to 2 years of age for penile lengthening, elongation of urethral strip and chordee correction. Second stage operation is done at least 6 months after first stage for urethral reconstruction. Third stage operation is done about 3 to 4 years of age for bladder neck reconstruction and correction of VUR. Cystoplasty can be done to enhance the bladder capacity after 2 to 3 years of 3rd stage operation.

Supportive nursing care should emphasize on prevention of infections, emotional support for long-term management schedule and routine preoperative and postoperative management. Health maintenance and promotion of growth and development should be emphasized by balanced diet, immunization, hygienic measures and parental guidance.

Hypospadias

Hypospadias is the congenital abnormal urethral opening on the ventral aspect (under surface) of the penis. It is one of the commonest malformations of male children. Undescended testes or inguinal hernia or upper urinary tract anomalies may be associated with hypospadias. It may found in females as urethral opening in the vagina with dribbling of urine.

Classification

Hypospadias can be classified depending upon the site of the urethral meatus.
- *Anterior hypospadias (65–70%):* It may be found as glandular or coronal or on distal penile shaft.
- *Middle (10–15%) penile shaft hypospadias.*
- *Posterior hypospadias (20%):* It may be found on proximal penile shaft or as penoscrotal, scrotal or perineal type.

Problems Related to Hypospadias

A child with hypospadias may have following problems:
- Presence of painful downward curvature of the penis during erection as chordee.
- Due to chordee, there is deflected stream of urine and the child wets his thigh during urination.
- Inability to void urine while standing, in case of penoscrotal, scrotal and perineal hypospadias. It also may found with the penis in the normal elevated position.
- If appropriate management is not done or left untreated, the condition, in later life, interferes during sexual intercourse with difficulty in penetration due to the presence of chordee. Severe forms of hypospadias interferes with reproductive ability as the sperms are deposited outside the vagina due to proximal situation of meatus.
- There can be meatal stenosis, fistula, urethral stricture or stenosis or diverticulum.

Management

Management of hypospadias is done by surgical reconstruction to obtain straight penis at erection, to form urethral tube and urethral meatus at the tip of glans penis.

Meatotomy is done at any age after birth. Chordee correction and advancement of prepuce can be done at the age of 2 to 3 years. Urethroplasty is done 3 to 4 months after chordee correction. The surgical repair should be completed before admission to the school. Operation can be performed as multistage or single stage repair.

Phimosis and Paraphimosis

Phimosis refers to the narrow opening of the prepuce that prevents it being drawn back over the glans penis. The inability to retract the prepuce after the age of 3 years, should be considered as true phimosis. Forcible retraction of the prepuce should be avoided as it may tear and can cause scarring and persistent phimosis.

Phimosis can be congenital or may be acquired due to inflammation of glans or prepuce. Phimosis can predispose UTI. Children with phimosis and recurrent UTI should be evaluated for obstruction of urinary tract or vesicoureteric reflux (VUR).

Circumcision, i.e. excision of the foreskin of the glans penis, is the choice of operative intervention done to treat phimosis. Other measure is the use of betamethasone cream to the narrowed preputial skin for two times daily for 4 weeks. This treatment usually becomes successful as the foreskin becomes soft, elastic and can be retracted gently and gradually.

Paraphimosis

Paraphimosis may develop in phimotic child which also need for surgical management by circumcision or reduction with application of lubricant under deep sedation. Paraphimosis is the retraction of a phimotic foreskin, behind coronal sulcus. It cannot be reduced spontaneously. It results in edematous swelling due to venous stasis causing severe pain. It needs urgent interventions.

Postoperative care after circumcision should include control of bleeding from operated site and prevention of infections. This operation is done as day-care surgery and does not require hospitalization. Parents should be explained about the home-based care and features of complications.

WILMS' TUMOR (NEPHROBLASTOMA)

Max Wilms, German surgeon described this most common renal tumor of childhood. It is associated with chromosomal deletions, especially from chromosomes 11 and 16.

Wilms' tumor is a rapidly developing highly malignant embryonal tumor usually diagnosed within 3 years of age. It is generally unilateral and can be familial in some cases. It may be associated with other congenital anomalies, like hemihypertrophy of the vertebrae, genitourinary anomalies, aniridia, ambiguous genitalia, etc.

This tumor develops within the kidney parenchyma, distorting it and invading the surrounding tissues. The tumor tends to grow in a concentric fashion invading the adjacent renal parenchyma. Characteristically a well developed capsule is present. Hemorrhage, necrosis and calcification may occur rarely. Metastatic spread occurs by lymphatics to the renal hilar, periaortic and pericaval lymph nodes. Distant blood borne metastasis occurs most frequently in the lungs, bone and liver.

Clinical Manifestations

Majority of the affected children present with an asymptomatic abdominal mass, detected during routine examination or by the mother during daily bath or undressing the child. Increasing abdominal girth is important finding. Microscopic hematuria, pain abdomen, fever, pallor, hypertension and superficial venous engorgement may present. Gross hematuria indicates advanced Stage III or Stage IV tumor. On examination large, smooth, fixed, firmed, nontender palpable mass detected in the flank.

Clinical Staging of Wilms' Tumor

This staging helps to determine prognosis and survival of the patients.

- *Stage I:* Tumor limited to kidney and can be fully excised. Renal capsule is intact. Tumor not ruptured and no residual tumor after excision.
- *Stage II:* Tumor extend beyond kidney but can be completely excised. There is regional extension of the tumor by penetration through renal capsule. Vessels outside kidney are either infiltrated or contain tumor thrombus. No residual tumor is apparent beyond the margins of resection.
- *Stage III:* Residual nonhematogenous extension of the tumor confined to the abdomen following surgery. Involvement of hilar, periaortic or other lymph nodes may present. The tumor cannot be completely resectable because of local infiltration into the vital structure.
- *Stage IV:* Hematogenous metastasis to distant organs, i.e. lungs, liver, brain, etc.
- *Stage V:* Bilateral renal involvement which occurs in 5 to 8 percent of the cases.

Diagnostic Evaluation

Clinical suspicion to be supported by history of illness and physical examination. The diagnosis can be confirmed by X-ray abdomen and chest, IVP, USG, CT Scan, MRI, renal function test and urine analysis. Liver function test, bone marrow study and other diagnostic measures help to detect the metastatic spread.

Management

Management of Wilm's tumor depends upon histological findings, clinical staging and metastasis.

Stage I and II Wilm's tumors with favorable histology are usually managed with nephrectomy and chemotherapy for 18 weeks. Stage III, IV and V tumors are treated with nephrectomy, abdominal radiotherapy and chemotherapy for 24 weeks. Preoperative radiotherapy and chemotherapy are indicated in massive tumors. Chemotherapy is usually administered with vincristine, dactinomycin, actinomycin, adriamycin, doxorubicin and cyclophosphamide. Radiotherapy is not given in children below one year of age.

Nursing management should include special care during nephrectomy, radiotherapy and chemotherapy. Reducing anxiety of the parents, by explanation, involvement in child care and teaching long-term home-based care are important nursing interventions to help the family to cope with the situation.

Prognosis

Prognosis of Wilm's tumor depends upon clinical staging, age of the child, size of the mass and histological findings. The disease free survival rates are in Stage I—95 percent, Stage II and III—85 percent, Stage IV—70 to 80 percent and with unfavorable histology 25 to 50 percent. Recurrence of tumor carries bad prognosis.

NURSING MANAGEMENT OF THE CHILD WITH UROLOGIC SURGERY

Basic preoperative and postoperative care to be provided with special attention for the followings:

- Promoting understanding of the parents about the planned surgical interventions by explanation according to level of understanding.
- Preparing for necessary diagnostic procedures.
- Involving the parents in child care.
- Promoting normal urinary functions by monitoring intake and output, care of urinary catheter and drainage tube, (if present), encouraging adequate fluid intake and hygienic measures and observing signs of urinary infections.
- Preventing infections by aseptic precautions, hand washing practices, taking care of wound, administering prescribed antibiotics and other medications, IV fluid therapy, monitoring features of infections and vital signs, etc.
- Providing comfort by rest, sleep, comfortable positioning of operated side with support, administering analgesics,

antspasmodics and organizing diversions and recreations by play and toys.

- Providing adequate nutrition to promote healing and prevent infections along with adequate fluid to promote urinary functions.
- Teaching the parents about related care, prevention of infections and complications, importance of fluid intake, diet, follow-up, available support services and facilities.

ACUTE GLOMERULONEPHRITIS

Acute glomerulonephritis (AGN) is an immune-mediated inflammatory disease of the capillary loops in the renal glomeruli. The antigen—antibody complex deposition within the glomeruli results in glomerular injury which is manifested as hematuria, oliguria, edema and hypertension. Onset of the disease process is relatively abrupt and commonly seen in preschool or in early school age group of male children.

Etiology

There is initial infection of upper respiratory tract (throat) or skin, usually one to 3 weeks before the onset of symptoms. The most frequent causative microorganism is nephrotigenic strains of group-A, beta *Streptococcus hemolyticus* (type-12). Acute post-streptococcal glomerulonephritis (APSGN) is the most common.

Pathophysiology

Streptococcal infection produces an antigen antibody complex which trapped in the glomerular loops and causes inflammatory reaction due to activation of complement. There is proliferation and swelling of the endothelial cells. The changes in the glomerular capillaries diminish the amount of the glomerular filtrate and allow the passage of blood cells and protein into the filtrate. Sodium and water are retained. The damage of glomerular basement membrane may lead to progressive renal failure.

Clinical Manifestations

The clinical presentations may be found in the mild or severe form with rapid onset of symptoms. History of sore throat or pyoderma or scabies or impetigo usually presents in most of the patients.

The child may present with decreased urine output with presence of blood or brown color urine. Edema is manifested as periorbital puffiness, found in the morning. Some patients may have pedal edema and generalized edema. Rapid weight gain usually found due to presence of massive edema. The child may have fever, headache, nausea, vomiting, anorexia, abdominal pain and malaise. Hypertension may present in more than 50 percent cases with sudden onset and may appear during 4 to 5 days of illness.

Clinical features of AGN may present in two phases. Phase-I, with edema and oliguria which persists for 5 to 10 days. In Phase-II, edema reduces and urinary output increases.

Complications

Acute glomerulonephritis can be complicated with congestive cardiac failure (CCF), acute renal failure, hypertensive encephalopathy, persistent hypertension, anemia, growth failure and chronic glomerulonephritis.

Diagnostic Evaluation

History of illness and physical examination help in clinical diagnosis. The confirmation of diagnosis is done by the followings:

Urine Examination

It shows increased specific gravity, smoky dirty brown color urine with reduced total amount in 24 hours. Mild to moderate or severe albuminuria is detected. Microscopic examination reveals presence of red cells, WBCs, pus cells, epithelial cells and granular cast.

Blood Examination

Blood examination demonstrates increased level of urea, creatinine, erythrocyte sedimentation rate (ESR), ASO titer and anti-DNAase 'B'. There is decreased level of Hb%, serum complement and albumin in blood. Hyponatremia and hyperkalemia may occur in persistent oliguria.

Throat Swab Culture

Throat swab culture may show presence of beta-hemolyticus *Streptococcus* in some children.

Chest X-ray

It may show pulmonary congestion.

Management

AGN with impaired renal function as severe oliguria and azotemia needs hospitalization for special attention. Mild oliguric patients with normal blood pressure can be managed at home with OPD-based treatment.

The *management* of AGN should include the followings:

- Bedrest for few weeks to be provided, till urine is free from RBC.
- Diet should be arranged with restriction of protein, salt and fluid intake, till oliguria and increased blood urea level persist. Carbohydrate containing food to be allowed freely. Overhydration and sodium retention may increase blood pressure and lead to left ventricular failure. Fluid intake should be allowed in a

calculated amount (i.e., total amount of previous day urine output in 24 hours plus insensible losses to be allowed to drink on that day). Daily weight recording is important to assess the increase and decrease of edema.

- Administration of antibiotics (preferably penicillin) is needed for 7 to 10 days to treat pharyngitis or pyoderma (if present). Other symptomatic management includes antihypertensive drugs (nifedipine, atenolol) to control blood pressure and its consequences. Sedative-tranquilizer (diazepam) may be needed in case of hypertension, convulsions and encephalopathy. Diuretics is not usually indicated except in association with pulmonary edema and left ventricular failure.
- Dialysis may be needed in renal failure and severe electrolyte imbalance.
- Management of complications like CCF, hypertensive encephalapathy, etc. should be done promptly to prevent life threatening outcome. Dopamine infusion, steroid therapy and respiratory support may be required for some patients.

Nursing Management

Nursing Assessment

Nursing assessment should include special attention for history of sore throat or skin infection along with other history of illness. Physical assessment should be done with emphasize on blood pressure and daily body weight recording, calculation of fluid intake and urine output, assessment of edema, skin conditions and urine testing along with other investigations.

Nursing Diagnoses

Important nursing diagnoses in case of AGN include the followings:
- Impaired urinary elimination related to glomerular dysfunction.
- Fluid volume excess related to altered renal function.
- Activity intolerance related to edema.
- Altered skin integrity related to edema.
- Altered nutrition, less than body requirement, related to albuminuria and GI disturbances.
- Fear and anxiety related to disease processes.
- Knowledge deficit regarding care of the child with renal disease and continuation of care at home.

Nursing Interventions

- Monitoring urinary pattern by maintaining intake-output and testing urine at regular interval.

- Reducing excess fluid volume by restriction of salt and fluid intake. Recording daily weight to assess the level of fluid retention. Every day there should be approximate loss of 0.5 percent body weight. Gain in weight indicates increased edema and fluid retention. Diuretics to be given as prescribed. Antihypertensive drugs to be administered after checking of blood pressure.
- Administering antibiotics other drugs, as prescribed.
- Promoting rest, sleep and comfortable position with gentle approach during nursing procedures. Allowing self care activities when acute stage is over and as per capability of the child.
- Providing skin care with special attention to the edematous part. Preventing drying, scratching and injury. Maintaining cleanliness and general hygienic measures.
- Promoting intake of nutritious diet by allowing carbohydrate foods with restriction of protein and salt in oliguric phase. Normal protein intake to be allowed when urine output become normal. Arranging small frequent easily digestable diet considering child's likes and dislikes. Spicy food to be avoided.
- Providing play material for diversion and recreation especially when acute stage is over. Allowing mother to involve in child care.
- Providing emotional support to parents and family members.
- Teaching the parents about continuation of care and follow-up.

CHRONIC GLOMERULONEPHRITIS

Chronic glomerulonephritis is an advanced, irreversible impairment of renal function with or without symptoms. It may develop as a primary glomerular disease or may occur in SLE, drug induced nephropathies and polyarteritis nodosa.

Pathological changes are found as diffuse thickening of glomerular basement membrane or focal segmental glomerulosclerosis with variable deposition of immunoglobin, complement and fibrin. Glomerular filtration rate is reduced. Mesangial proliferation may occur. In late stages, most glomeruli become sclerosed with tubular, interstitial and vascular changes.

Clinical Manifestations

The condition may remain asymptomatic and may be diagnosed during routine urine examination. The symptomatic patients present with edema, severe hypertension, hematuria, nocturia and persistent anemia. Bone pain, bony deformities and failure to thrive are usually present.

Diagnosis is confirmed by urine and blood examination. Urine analysis shows presence of protein, RBC and cast.

Blood examination shows increased urea and creatinine. USG is helpful to diagnose the condition.

Management

Management of chronic glomerulonephritis can be done with steroid and other immunosuppressive drugs as there is no specific treatment for the condition. Antihypertensive drugs and antibiotics are useful as symptomatic measures. The condition may be complicated with chronic renal failure that should be treated accordingly. Symptomatic and supportive care promote the prognosis.

URINARY TRACT INFECTIONS

Urinary tract infections (UTI) is the presence of infective agents (usually bacteria) that exists anywhere between the renal cortex and the urethral meatus. It is sometimes difficult to determine the exact location of the infections. It may cause irreversible renal damage, especially in association with urinary tract anomalies and vesicoureteric reflux (VUR).

The most common causative organism is *E. coli*. Other organisms are Streptococcus, Staphylococcus, Pseudomonas, etc. The commonest route of entry is the ascending infections from the urethra or may be hematogenous spread. This infection is more common is girls.

The contributing causes of UTI are urinary stasis, congenital anomalies or obstruction of urinary tract (PUJ, bladder-neck obstruction, PUV), VUR, poor perineal hygiene, short female urethra, urinary catheterization, or instrumentation, local inflammation, chronic constipation or infection anywhere in the body.

Pathophysiology

Most commonly UTI are found in lower urinary tract. It may occur as cystitis or pyelonephritis. Inflammation results in urinary retention and stasis. Backflow of urine (reflux) into the kidney may occur though ureter. Inflamed part become edematous, thickened and fibrosed. Ureter and renal pelvis may be dilated. If left untreated, kidney may become small and tissue may be destroyed resulting disturbances of renal functions.

Clinical Manifestations

The onset of symptoms may be abrupt or gradual, even the condition may have no symptoms. The patient usually have moderate to high fever with chills, rigors, convulsions, anorexia, malaise, irritability and vomiting. Urinary symptoms may be found as frequency and urgency, dysuria, dribbling and bed wetting. Urine may be foul-smelling. The child may complain abdominal or flank or suprapubic pain. It may present as acute abdomen. Neonates with UTI may have lethargy, diarrhea, jaundice, poor weight gain and features of sepsis.

Diagnosis

The diagnosis of UTI is confirmed by urine culture and urine analysis (routine and microscopic) by clean catch or sterile urine specimen. Associated congenital anomalies or obstructive uropathies should be detected by USG, MCU, IVP, renal scan etc. Blood examination shows increased total leukocyte count (TLC) and ESR with decreased Hb%.

Management

Management of UTI is mainly done with antibiotic therapy. Specific symptomatic and supportive treatment are essential. Associated congenital anomalies should be detected early for prompt management.

The antibiotic therapy is given with combination of ampicillin and gentamicin or amikacin for 7 to 10 days. Other antibiotics also can be used, i.e. ceftriaxone, cefotaxime, etc.

Supportive measures include management of fever by rest, tepid sponge and/or antipyretics, with large amount of fluid intake. Improvement of personal hygiene (perineal hygiene) is important preventive measure. Frequent emptying of bladder should be encouraged to prevent stasis of urine. Repeat urine culture to be done to discontinue the treatment. The UTI may be complicated with recurrent infections, renal damage and severe VUR.

NEPHROTIC SYNDROME

Nephrotic syndrome is one of the common cause of hospitalization among children. Incidence of the condition is 2 to 7 per 1000 children. It is more common in male child. Mean age of occurrence is 2 to 5 years.

Nephrotic syndrome is a symptom complex manifested by massive edema, hypoalbuminemia, marked albuminuria and hyper-lipidemia (hypercholesterolemia). It can be classified as congenital, idiopathic or primary and secondary types.

Types

Congenital Nephrotic Syndrome

It is rare but a serious and fatal problem usually associated with other congenital anomalies of kidney. It is inherited as autosomal recessive disease. Severe renal insufficiency and urinary infections along with this condition result is poor prognosis.

Primary or Idiopathic Nephrotic Syndrome

It is the most common type (about 90%) and regarded as autoimmune phenomenon, as it responds to immunosuppressive therapy. The subgroups of this type are: (a) minimal change nephrotic syndrome (85%), (b) mesangial proliferative nephrotic syndrome (5%) and (c) focal sclerosis nephrotic syndrome (10%).

Secondary Nephrotic Syndrome

It occurs in children about 10 percent of all cases. This condition may occur due to some form of chronic gomerulonephritis, or due to diabetes mellitus, systemic lupus erythematosus (SLE), malaria, malignant hypertension, hepatitis 'B', infective endocarditis, HIV/AIDS, drug toxicity, lymphomas, syphilis, etc.

Pathophysiology

The pathological changes in nephrotic syndrome may be due to loss of charge selectivity and thickening of the foot plate of the glomerular basement membrane. These result in increased glomerular permeability, which permits the negatively charged protein, mainly albumin to pass through the capillary walls into the urine. Excess loss of albumin results in decrease in serum albumin (hypoalbuminemia). Heavy proteinuria more than 1 g/m² body surface area per day leads to serum albumin level below 2.5 g/dL. As a result of hypoalbuminemia, there is reduction in plasma oncotic pressure. Thus fluid flows from the capillaries into the interstitial spaces and produced edema.

The shift of fluid from the plasma to the interstitial spaces reduces the intravascular fluid volume resulting hypovolemia, which stimulates the renin angiotension axis and volume receptors to secrete aldosterone and antidiuretic hormone. These lead to increased reabsorption of sodium and water in distal tubules resulting edema.

Loss of protein and immunoglobins predisposes infections in the child. Diminished oncotic pressure leads to increased hepatic lipoprotein synthesis, which results in hyperlipidemia. LDL (Low-density lipoprotein) and cholesterol level increased initially, then very low density lipoprotein (VLDL) and triglyceride are also elevated.

Clinical Manifestations

The onset of the disease is usually gradual or it may be acute. The child may present with periorbital puffiness. Edema may be minimal or massive. Profound weight gain within a short period of days or week is found. Dependent edema develops in the ankle, feet, genitalia (scrotum) and hands. The edematous part is soft and pits easily on pressure. Striae may appear on the skin due to overstreching by edema. Fluid accumulates in the body space, resulting ascites, pleural effusion with

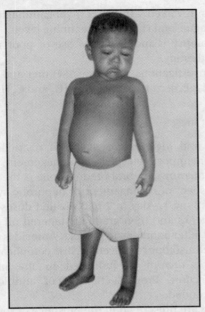

Fig. 19.1: A child with nephrotic syndrome (body weight 15 kg, age 3 years)

respiratory distress and generalized edema (anasarca) (Fig. 19.1). Urine output is reduced in the edematous phase. Urine becomes concentrated with frothy appearance.

GI disturbances usually found as vomiting, loss of appetite and diarrhea. Other features include fatigue, lethargy, pallor and irritability. Hypertension, hematuria, hepatomegaly and wasting of muscle may found in some cases.

Complications

A child with nephrotic syndrome may be complicated with ascitis, pleural effusion, generalized edema, coagulation disorders, thrombosis, recurrent infections of different systems and renal failure. Other complications are growth retardation, calcium and vitamin 'D' deficiency, protein-energy malnutrition and relapse of nephrotic syndrome.

Diagnostic Evaluation

History of illness and physical examination to exclude clinical features help to diagnose the condition clinically. Laboratory investigations to confirm the diagnosis may include the followings:

- Urine examination shows gross proteinuria (2 to 20 g/day), presence of cast, slight hematuria and increased specific gravity.
- Blood examination demonstrates reduced total protein, albumin less than 2.5 g/dL and cholesterol more than 200 mg/dL. Lipoproteins and BUN (Blood Urea-Nitrogen) are increased. Serum albumin and globulin

ratio is reversed. There is hypogammaglobulinemia, hypomagnesemia and low-creatinine level.

- Renal biopsy is indicated in case of poor response to steroid therapy.
- Other investigations show low ASO titer and IgM, raised IgG and IgE, serum complement (C_3 and C_4) is normal.

Management

- *Bedrest* and *high-protein diet* with restriction of fluid intake are important aspects of management.
- *Steroid therapy* with oral prednisolone is the most significant aspect of management of nephrotic syndrome. It is given 2 mg/kg/day in 2 to 3 divided doses for at least 4 to 6 weeks and then gradually tapered off or abruptly stopped, after another 4 to 6 weeks. Antacid is given along with prednisolone to prevent gastric complications.
- *Antibiotic therapy* is indicated in the presence of any infection. Prophylactic use of antibiotic is not recommended.
- *Diuretics* are prescribed in the presence of severe edema and massive ascites. Frusemide 1 to 3 mg/kg/day in 2 divided doses alone or with spironolactone 2 to 3 mg/kg/day in 2 divided doses is given. Rapid fluid loss should not be attempted in 8 to 12 hours. Potassium supplementation to be given along with diuretics.
- *Albumin infusion* (1 g/kg/day) may be given in case of massive edema and ascites. It helps to shift the fluid from interstitial space into the vascular system. Diuretic therapy is given in combination of albumin infusion. Plasma or blood transfusion may be given is some cases to treat hypoalbuminemia.
- *Immunosuppressive drugs* (Levamisole, methotrexate, cyclophosphamide, cyclosporine, chlorambucil) may be administered along with prednisolone in case of frequent (4 or more per year) relapses and in steroid dependent cases.
- *Renal transplantation* is indicated in end stage renal failure due to steroid resistant glomerulosclerosis (focal and segmental).
- Nursing management (see the nursing process on next page).

Prognosis

In early diagnosis and appropriate treatment with steroid therapy and supportive care, about 80 percent children with nephrotic syndrome, recover. About 10 to 15 percent children become complicated with chronic renal failure, and only 2 to 4 percent of cases may have fatal outcome due to infections and coagulation disorders.

Sample nursing process of a child with nephrotic syndrome is given on Page 347.

Ramu, a 4 years old boy, admitted in pediatric medical unit with edema all over the body, less urine output, loss of appetite and lethargy (*see* page no. 347 for details).

ACUTE RENAL FAILURE

Acute renal failure (ARF) is a severe deterioration of renal function, manifested as sudden reduction of urine excretion (less than 1 mL/kg/hr) as oliguria or anuria leading to fluid and electrolyte imbalance and accumulation of metabolic nitrogenous wastes and other biochemical products. It is a life threatening situation.

Etiology

The causes of acute renal failure can be divided into three groups, prerenal, intrarenal and postrenal causes.

Prerenal Causes

These conditions are related to the problems occur in blood supply to the kidney either due to systemic hypovolemia or due to renal hypoperfusion. The important causes are hypovolemia due to diarrheal dehydration, shock, burns, diabetic acidosis, trauma hemorrhage, etc. and CCF.

Intrarenal Causes

These intrinsic renal conditions are related to problems within the kidneys and their functions, causing reduction of GFR, renal ischemia and tubular damage. The important causes are glomerulonephritis, hemolytic uremic syndrome (HUS), renal vein thrombosis, acute tubular necrosis, (due to fluid loss, hemorrhage, shock, nephrotoxic drugs and toxins), DIC, sepsis, interstitial nephritis (due to infections, drugs), etc.

Postrenal Causes

These conditions are related to the problems of the ureter or lower urinary system causing obstruction of urine flow due to obstructive uropathies. The causes include renal calculus, PUV, bladder-neck obstruction, congenital lesion or pus collection in urinary tract or following drug therapy (sulfonamide).

Phases of Acute Renal Failure

Four phases of acute renal failure (ARF) are identified in children depending upon the course of illness.

Initiating Phase

This phase lasts from hours to days with features of renal function impairment.

Nursing process of a child with nephrotic syndrome

• Identification data— • History of illness in details— • Findings of physical examination and investigations—				• Date and Time

Assessment day-1	Nursing diagnosis	Planning	Implementation	Evaluation day-2
• Edema around eyes, feet and genitalia. • Urine output in 24 hours —200 mL. • Body weight 17 kg . • Fluid intake 250 mL in 24 hours	• Fluid volume excess related to fluid accumulation in tissue	• To reduce excess amount of fluid accumulated in tissues	• Providing rest, comfortable position and frequent change of position. • Allowing diet with low salt and high protein (egg, fish, pulse). • Administering prescribed medications- (prednisolone, lasix) orally. • Offering potassium containing food— (orange juice, banana). • Restricting fluid intake. • Maintaining intake-output and body weight chart. • Explaining and reassuring about the treatment plan and involving mother in child care with necessary instruction. • Urine testing for albumin.	• Edema reduced slightly. • Body weight 18 kg. • Urine output 400 mL in 24 hours. • Fluid intake 600 mL in 24 hours.
• Edematous skin • Protein loss in urine (+ +)	• Risk for infection	• To protect the child from infection	• Examining the child for any signs of infections and recording TPR. • Monitoring blood count (TLC, DLC) • Providing skin care, keeping the skin dry and applying body powder for soothing. • Keeping the nails short. • Maintaining general cleanliness and hygienic measures. • Preventing any injury of edematous skin. • Avoiding the contact of two edematous skin (thigh) surface to prevent friction. • Avoiding invasive procedure as possible. • Teaching the mother about skin care and signs of infections and involving the mother during care of the child.	• No signs of infection. • No skin break down. • Hygiene maintained. • TPR Normal.
• Loss of appetite • Proteinuria • Lethargy	• Altered nutrition less than body requirement.	• To improve nutritional status	• Providing small frequent feeding with protein and carbohydrate, considering dietary restriction and child's likes and dislikes. • Providing nutritional supplementation as needed. • Encouraging child to take food.	• Dietary intake increased.
• Anxiety of the parents • Fear of the child	• Altered family process	• To provide emotional support	• Allowing parental involvement in child care. • Allowing play and self-care as tolerated by the child. • Encouraging interaction with other child having chronic illness. • Answering the questions asked by the parents and allowing to express frustration.	• Parents and child express their concern about the illness.
• Inability to take care of the child by the parents.	• Knowledge deficit.	• To improve knowledge about child care by health teaching.	• Discussing about the care after discharge from hospital, regarding rest, diet, hygiene, continuation of medication, need for medical help and follow-up. • Teaching about features of infections, signs of relapse and precautions to prevent complications.	• Mother listen the information and ensure to follow them.

Oliguric Phase

This phase lasts from 5 to 15 days but can be prolonged for weeks. It is shorter in infants and children (3–5 days) and longer in older children (10–14 days). More than 3 weeks duration of oliguric phase indicates irreversible renal damage. It depends upon severity and duration of initial stage causing acute vaso-spastic nephropathy.

Diuretic Phase

This phase lasts for few days and highly variable with mild to severe clinical features.

Recovery Phase

This phase marks the final resumption of normal urine osmolarity, constituents and biochemical alterations in the blood.

Pathophysiology

The cause of renal failure may be different but the end result is renal hypoperfusion and renal outflow obstruction which leads to impairment of renal functions and renal failure.

There is marked reduction of glomerular filtration rate and renal blood flow due to renal vasoconstriction resulting sodium and fluid retention which leads to edema.

Hypertension may develop due to renin-angiotension mechanism caused by arteriolar constriction, increased circulatory overload and sodium retention.

Metabolic acidosis may develop as a result of failure of excretion of hydrogen ions due to reduced functions of nephron and hypercatabolic states, which lead to increased production of acids.

Hyperkalemia may develop due to disturbed sodium and potassium exchange in the distal tubules and increased extracellular potassium level resulting from damage tissue cells, RBCs and hypercatabolic states.

Clinical Manifestations

Clinical presentations of ARF depend upon the underlying cause and duration of the problem. The child may present with severe oliguria or anuria. In some cases, urine output may not be reduced. The child may look remarkably well or extremely sick. This features of underlying cause are usually prominent. Other signs and symptoms include nausea, vomiting, lethergy, dehydration, acidotic breathing, alteration of level of consciousness, irregularities in cardiac rate and rhythm and edema.

Diagnostic Evaluation

The following investigations may help to confirm the diagnosis along with history of illness and clinical findings:

- Blood examination shows raised serum creatinine level as important criteria for diagnosis. Blood urea, electrolytes, pH, bicarbonate and complete blood count are also useful.
- Urine examination reveals proteinuria, hematuria and presence of casts.
- Ultrasonography helps to detect the structural abnormalities, calculi, etc.
- IVP can be done to detect acute tubular necrosis.
- Radionuclide studies can be done to evaluate GFR and renal blood flow distribution.
- Specific investigations to be performed to determine the suspected underlying cause and complications related to ARF.

Management

Management of ARF should be planned on the basis of underlying cause. Correction of dehydration, treatment of shock and hyperkalemia are the immediate concern.

Fluid and electrolyte balance to be maintained promptly. Fluid requirement to be calculated on the basis of previous day urine output in 24 hours and insensible losses (approximately 300 mL/m^2) with other losses (vomiting, loose motion, etc.). Excessive fluid intake is risky. Fluid can be given orally or parenterally depending upon the condition of the patient. 5 percent dextrose is given and no potassium is usually administered or very little can be given depending upon the blood K$^+$ level.

Diet should be planned with low sodium, low potassium, low phosphate and moderate protein (0.6 to 1 g/kg). The recommended calorie requirement is 50 to 60 cal/kg. Liberal amount of carbohydrates and fats can be given along with vitamin and mineral supplementation.

Use of diuretics like mannitol and furosemide is recommended by some authority. Steroids can also be used. In case of presence of complications like anemia, hypertension and CCF, these should be adequately controlled and managed.

Continuous monitoring of patient's condition and identification of complications are important. Complications like fluid-electrolyte imbalance, hyperkalemia, metabolic acidosis, hyponatremia, convulsions, etc. should be detected early for prompt management to prevent fatal outcome.

Dialysis (peritoneal or hemodialysis) is indicated in life threatening complications and should be arranged in following conditions:

- Persistent hyperkalemia, serum potassium level more than 7 mEq/L.

- Congestive cardiac failure.
- Pulmonary edema.
- Severe acidosis, pH less than 7.2, TCO_2 less less 10 to 12 mEq/L.
- Neurological problems due to uremia and hyponatremia.
- Hyperphosphatemia.

Supportive care during dialysis and pre- or postdialysis period are very important. The patient with ARF should be managed by intensive care approach with specialized nursing interventions.

Nursing Management

Nursing Assessment

Assessment should include details history of illness, recent and past illness or injury, and drug therapy or allergy or exposure to toxic substances. Thorough physical examination should be done especially hydration status, cardio-respiratory monitoring, daily weight recording and strict monitoring of intake and output. Necessary laboratory investigations to be arranged to assess the underlying problems.

Nursing Diagnoses

The important nursing diagnoses are:
- Risk of fluid electrolyte imbalance related to impaired renal functions.
- Risk for infection related to alteration of host defense.
- Activity intolerance related to acute illness.
- Altered thought process related to CNS problem.
- Altered nutrition less than body requirement related to GI disturbances.
- Fear and anxiety related to life threatening illness.
- Knowledge deficit related to management of acute renal failure and its consequences.

Nursing Interventions

- Maintaining fluid and electrolyte balance with prescribed IV infusion and maintaining intake and output chart. Monitoring serum electrolytes and features of heart failure.
- Administering prescribed medications with necessary precautions.
- Providing diet with high carbohydrate food, low potassium and low sodium in frequent small amount feeding.
- Providing rest, comfort, change of position, skin care, care of urine drainage (condom drainage may be given) and other hygienic care.
- Preventing infections by aseptic precautions, avoiding urinary catheterization and teaching the parents about infection control measures. Prophylactic antibiotics are

not recommended. Presence of infection to be detected early by continuous monitoring and should be treated accordingly.
- Preventing injury during convulsions and assessing neurological status.
- Providing care for dialysis (see page 347).
- Providing emotional support to the parents, child and family members.
- Teaching about care of the child after discharge at home especially about diet, prevention of infection and follow-up.

Prognosis

Mortality rate of ARF is about 20 to 40 percent which is influenced by the cause and duration of renal failure with severity of pathological changes. Poor prognosis is related to associated sepsis, HUS (hemolytic uremic syndrome), prolonged anemia, cardiac failure, hepatic failure and respiratory failure with delayed initiation of treatment.

CHRONIC RENAL FAILURE

Chronic renal failure (CRF) is a permanent irreversible destruction of nephron leading to severe deterioration of renal function, finally resulting to end stage renal disease (ESRD).

Etiology

The common causes of chronic renal failure below 5 years of age is the congenital renal anomalies and urinary tract malformations. The most common causes in 5 to 15 years age group include glomerular diseases, hereditary renal disorders and renal vascular diseases.

The important causes of CRF can be listed as follows:
- *Glomerular diseases:* Glomerulonephritis, SLE, HUS, familial nephropathy, Henoch-Schonlein purpura, amyloidosis.
- *Congenital anomalies:* Bilateral renal hypoplasia or dysplasia, polycystic kidney.
- *Obstructive uropathy:* PUJ, renal stones, PUV.
- *Miscellaneous:* Bilateral Wilm's tumor, renal vein thrombosis, renal cortical necrosis, renal tuberculosis, reflux nephropathy.

Pathophysiology

Reduction in the renal functions leads to metabolic, endocrinal and hematological disturbances including disturbances of internal homeostatic equilibrium.

Damage of nephron results in hypertrophy and hyperplasia of remaining nephron leading to reduced functions of nephrons to excrete effectively thus resulting azotemia and clinical uremia.

Impaired renal function leads to hyperphosphatemia resulting disturbance of calcium absorption (hypocalcemia) due to inability to vitamin 'D' synthesis. These disturbances produce renal ricket and renal osteodystrophy.

Anemia develops due to disturbance of erythropoietin synthesis. Mild hemolysis and GI bleed also contribute to produce anemia. Excretion of nitrogenous wastes through sweat causes pruritus. Fluid overload leads to edema and hypertension.

Severity of CRF is indicated by GFR. The lower the GFR, the greater the loss of renal function. End-stage renal disease may develop by decline of renal function to an extent that life cannot be continued without dialysis or renal transplantation.

Clinical Manifestations

The clinical features of CRF are variable and not found in chronological sequence. The child may present with initial polyuria, or frequent passage of urine, later oliguria, or anuria develop. Other clinical presentation include increased thirst, decreased appetite, weakness, low energy level, bone pain or joint pain, dryness and itching of skin. The child may have progressive anemia, hypertension and growth retardation.

In late stage, the child manifested with acidotic breathing, hiccough, nausea, vomiting, diarrhea, peripheral neuropathy and convulsions. Purpura, cardiomyopathy, pericarditis and super-added infections may found. The patient may present with unconsciousness or complications like CCF, pulmonary edema, hypernatremia, hyperkalemia and intercurrent infections.

Complications

The complications of CRF include azotemia, metabolic acidosis, electrolyte imbalance, CCF, hypertension, severe anemia, growth retardation and delayed or absent sexual maturation.

Diagnostic Evaluation

The exact cause of CRF to be detected by detail history of illness, clinical examination and laboratory or radiological investigations.

- Blood examination shows decreased level of hematocrit, Hb%. Na^+, Ca^{++}, HCO_3^- and increased level of 'K^+' and phosphorus.
- Renal function test shows gradual increase of BUN, uric acid and creatinine values.
- Urinalysis shows variation in specific gravity increased creatinine level in urine and change in total amount of urine output.
- X-ray chest, hands, knees, pelvis, spine, etc. help to detect bony involvement.
- ECG, IVP, MCU, radionuclide imaging help to detect the extent of complications.

Management

At the initial stage, the management of CRF is planned to retard the progression of the disease by rest, diet, supportive care and symptomatic relief. Later, the treatment of complications, dialysis and renal transplantation to be provided as per need.

Diet should be planned with special attention on maintenance of calorie as per normal requirements. Diet should contain high polyunsaturated fat and complex carbohydrates. Protein intake should be adequate (0.8-1 g/kg/day) with fooditems of high biologic value (egg, milk, meat, fish).

Sodium intake needs to be allowed depending upon the level of impairment of sodium reabsorption, presence of edema, hypertension and azotemia. Potassium balance to be maintained by avoiding potassium containing food. Dairy milk containing high phosphate need to be avoided but calcium supplementation is required. Vitamin B_1, B_2, folic acid, B_6 and B_{12} supplementation to be given. Water restriction is usually not essential except in ESRD and fluid overload.

Correction of acidosis to be done with sodium-bi-carbonate. Hypertension to be managed with antihypertensive drugs. Infection should be managed with least toxic antibiotics. Antihistaminics is given to relief from pruritus.

Correction of anemia can be done with iron-folic acid supplementation, blood transfusion or by human erythropoietin or synthetic erythropoietin. Renal osteodystrophy is managed with low phosphate in diet, antacid therapy (calcium carbonate) and vitamin 'D' supplementation. Correction of calcium and phosphorus imbalance is essential. Growth hormone may be needed to correct growth retardation.

Dialysis (peritoneal or hemodialysis) and renal transplantation are indicated in ESRD.

Nursing Management

Chronic renal failure leads to multi system physiologic crisis. Thorough assessment of all systems are essential to detect the problems and for planning of care. All the nursing diagnoses may be applicable during nursing interventions. Special care to be provided in relation to renal transplant, and dialysis. Routine care should emphasize on maintenance of fluid-electrolyte balance, skin integrity, nutritious diet, ensuring safety from infections and injury, assisting to cope with long-term illness and teaching for continuation of care.

CARE OF THE CHILD WHO UNDERGOES DIALYSIS

Dialysis is the diffusion of solute molecules through a semipermeable membrane, passing from higher concentration to that of lower concentration.

The *purpose of dialysis* is to remove endogenous and exogenous toxins and to maintain fluid-electrolyte and acid-base balance till the renal function recovers. It is a substitute for some excretory functions of kidneys but does not replace the endocrine and metabolic functions.

The *indications of dialysis* in renal failure are as follows:
- Uremic symptoms with neurologic abnormalities
- Persistent hyperkalemia, above 6.5 mEq/L
- Blood urea level more than 150 mg/dL
- Severe acidosis, pH less than 7.2, TCO_2 less than 10 to 12 mEq/L
- Hyperphosphatemia
- Pulmonary edema and CCF.

Methods of Dialysis

- Peritoneal dialysis—It can be done as:
  - Intermittent peritoneal dialysis, or
  - Continuous ambulatory peritoneal dialysis or
  - Continuous cycling peritoneal dialysis.
- Hemodialysis.
- Continuous renal replacement therapy with special procedures like:
  - Continuous arteriovenous hemofiltration.
  - Continuous venovenous hemodialysis.
  - Continuous arteriovenous ultrafiltration.
  - Slow continuous ultrafiltration.

Both hemodialysis and peritoneal dialysis are effective in the management of renal failure. Peritoneal dialysis does not require vascular access and sophisticated equipment. It is easy to perform this procedure.

The following principles should be followed by the nurses during dialysis of pediatric patients.

- *Peritoneal dialysis:* The volume of dialysate should be 30 to 50 mL/kg body weight or 1000 to 1200 mL/m^2. The child should be able to co-operate during the procedure and to perform self-care.
- Hemodialysis
  - Vascular access should be done on suitable peripheral blood vessels depending upon the patient's size.
  - Blood pressure cuff and tourniquets should not be applied to the limb with fistula.
  - Subcutaneous or intramuscular injections should be avoided because the child is receiving anticoagulant therapy, (heparin).
  - Extracorporeal blood volume should be as small as possible. It should not exceed 8 to 10 percent of the child's total blood volume.
  - Efficiency or adequacy of the dialyzer should be noted and blood pump speed to be adjusted accordingly.
  - External catheter should be secured to prevent trauma.
  - Special care for the child during dialysis should be provided by specially trained personnel who is very familiar with the protocol of dialysis and the equipment and machinery being used.

Nursing Interventions

- Preparing the child for the dialysis by explanation and encouraging to express feeling. Allowing to talk to other child who have under gone dialysis.
- Explanation and reassurance to the parents and family members to relief their anxiety so that they can provide support to the child.
- Obtaining informed consent for the procedure.
- Ensuring that all blood examination reports are available with the child before dialysis.
- Protecting the child from infections by strict aseptic technique, hygienic measures, adequate diet with vitamin supplementation, care of wound (if present) and immunization (hepatitis B).
- Maintaining appropriate fluid and nutritional intake by small frequent feeding in regular diet. Fluid and sodium restriction may be needed to prevent fluid overload especially in presence of oliguria and hypertension. Protein should not be restricted as it is important to maintain normal growth and development.
- Assisting during dialysis and following specialized procedures and instructions. Keeping the unit ready for the procedure and preparing the child on the day of dialysis according to the specific protocol.
- Maintaining careful record of temperature, pulse, respiration, blood pressure, intake and output and laboratory investigation reports. Recording body weight before and after each dialysis and continuous monitoring of general condition of the child. All these records are valuable to assess the effectiveness of the therapy and to detect complications.
- Symptomatic and supportive nursing measures before and after dialysis to be provided along with promotion of self-care.
- Teaching the parents and family members regarding dialysis schedule, dietary restriction, medications, prevention of infections, possible complications, available support services, emergency measures, regular follow-up and home-based continued care.

Complications Related to Hemodialysis

- *Complications of vascular access:* Infections, central venous thrombosis or stricture, ischemia of the hand, aneurysm or pseudoaneurysm
- Arteriosclerotic cardiovascular disease, coronary heart disease, CHF, stroke, hypertension
- Disturbances in lipid metabolism
- Intercurrent infections
- Anemia
- Gastric ulcer
- Psychological problems like depression, regression.

Burns and Skin Diseases

20

- Burns in Children
- Common Skin Diseases in Children
- Scabies
  - Superficial Fungal Infections
  - Candidiasis
- Dermatophytosis
- Superficial Bacterial Infections
- Psoriasis
- Acne
- Atopic Dermatitis

INTRODUCTION

Skin diseases are common in children and about 30 percent of pediatric out patient department (OPD) attendance is accounted by these conditions. Skin disorders are associated manifestations of many systemic and hereditary diseases. Detailed history and careful examination help to diagnose the conditions and associated problems.

Primary skin lesions are termed as macules, papules, nodules, vesicles, pustules, wheals, patches, bullae, plaques, etc. The secondary skin lesions include scales, crusts, ulcers, erosions, fissures, atrophy and lichenification.

The most common problem involving skin and its appendages is the burn injury, which need emergency and specialized care.

A vast majority of skin problems can be grouped as follows:
- Infective
  - *Bacterial infection or pyoderma:* Impetigo, folliculitis, cellulitis, furunculosis, erysipelas.
  - *Fungal:* Candidiasis, dermatophytosis.
  - *Parasitic:* Scabies, pediculosis.
  - *Viral:* Warts, molluscum contagiosum.
- *Allergic skin condition:* Atopic dermatitis, urticaria, skin rash.
- *Pigmentary:* Albinism, vitiligo
- *Vascular lesions:*
  - Hemangioma

  i. Port-wine stain or mark (nevus flammeus)
  ii. Capillary hemangioma (strawberry mark)
  iii. Cavernous hemangioma.
  - Telangiectatic angioma (spider nevus).
- *Inherited disorders:* Ichthyosis, psoriasis.
- *Miscellaneous disorder:* Napkin dermatitis, (Intertrigo), miliaria (prickly heat), seborrhea, acne, erythema nodosum, pemphigus, erythema multiforme, etc.

BURNS IN CHILDREN

Burns are common and serious childhood injury causing prolonged effect on growing child with various complications and fatal prognosis. The exact data about the incidence of burn injury is not available. Children are at higher risk of burn injury than adults. Approximately one fourth of burns cases are below 10 years of age, and about 65 percent of burnt children are below 5 years of age. Over 80 percent of burn accidents occur in the child's own home. Scalds from hot liquids constitute maximum numbers and others are due to flame burns, electrical or chemical burns.

The incidence of burns increased during Diwali, festivals and in winter seasons. The children of high-risk for burns include single parent, unsupervised, neglected and less protected child especially of poor socioeconomic group.

Burns are the tissue injury caused by the contact with heat, flame, chemicals, electricity and radiation. The effects of burn injury are not limited to the burnt area, but can cause serious systemic effects depending upon the extent and depth of burns. In children burns are described as—serious with the following conditions:

- Second degree burns with 10 percent or more body surface area injured.
- Burns of face, hands, feet, perineum and joints.
- Burns with presence of other injuries.
- Burns due to electrical energy.

Scalds are important burn injury caused by hot liquids (liquid hot food, hot water, tea, coffee, milk) or steam. It is common in children below 3 years of age.

Electric burns are common in toddlers and adolescents when playing with electrical outlet, extension cord, touching high tension wires, etc.

Open flame burns are common during playing with lighter or at kitchen near stove or over of gasline. It may happen from open fire in winter season or from fireworks during festivals or Diwali. Inhalation burns may occur from fireworks (not from smoke).

Chemical burns is also common in children. Out of curiosity they handle household cleansing chemicals, acids, etc. and get injured.

Pathophysiology

Burn injury involved length, breadth and depth of the affected areas. Length and breadth of the burnt area described as body surface area burnt. Involvement of depth influence the ability to regenerate during recovery period. Burns may injured epidermis or dermis and both. Extent of injury depends upon site and nutritional status of the child, so that same amount of heat energy may have different damaging effects. There are massive changes in postburn period, so severity of burns depends upon extent and depth of injury.

Burns result in serious circulatory changes. There is loss of fluid and fluid shift from intravascular to extravascular compartment due to increased capillary permeability. It leads to hypovolemic shock due to fall in cardiac output. Swelling and edema of burnt area occur due to this changes. Local and systemic inflammatory mediators also contribute to develop severe edema. Ischemia and necrosis occur due to vasoconstriction.

In extensive burns, cardiac output falls within 30 minutes of injury. With appropriate fluid therapy, it returns to normal level within 36 hours. Excessive cardiac strain may develop due to fluid mobilization, progressive anemia, inadequate nutrition and electrolyte imbalance.

Heat energy destroys the cellular elements of blood. Some red blood cells (RBCs) are destroyed immediately and some are permanently affected by the heat. These lead to hemolysis which causes immediate or late anemia. The damage of RBCs are noticed as hemoglobinuria. Higher the depth of burns, more the cellular damage occur.

Burn injury leads to initial rise in white blood cells (WBCs) but leukotaxis and phagocytosis are impaired. Plasma proteins and immunoglobins are reduced resulting increased vulnerability to infections. Breaking of skin barrier, compromised immunocompetence and poor nutritional status influenced more prone to various infections. There is fall in platelet count with abnormal platelet function and fall in fibrinogen level leading to coagulation problems.

Hypovolemia and reduced cardiac output result in decreased renal blood flow and reduced glomerular filtration rate leading to tubular necrosis and renal failure. Hemoglobinuria also may contribute to renal shut down.

Extensive burn injury may cause fatal respiratory complications due to damage of respiratory mucosa by heat or due to severe hypoxia. Damage of mucosa leads to pulmonary congestion, hypostatic pneumonia and respiratory infections.

There are serious metabolic changes due to burn injury. Evaporative fluid loss from burnt body surface can be 6 to 8 liters per day leading to hypermetabolic state. In moderate to severe burns there is negative nitrogen balance and loss of protein. Tissue catabolism is enhanced by release of alpha adrenergic agents, cortisol and catecholamines. Renin angiotension, adrenocorticotropic hormone (ACTH), cortisol, free fatty acid and triglycerides levels are elevated, whereas cholesterol and phospholipids levels are decreased.

As a result of sympathetic nervous system response to trauma, there is decrease peristalsis, which may cause paralytic ileus. Ischemia of gastric mucosa may result duodenal and gastric ulcers, manifested by occult bleeding or life-threatening hemorrhage.

Following burn injury several major immunoglobulins, complement and serum albumin are decreased with depressed cellular immunity. Hypoxia, acidosis and thrombosis of vessels in the wound area impair host resistance to pathogenic bacteria. These immunological disturbances make the patient more susceptible to various infections and wound sepsis.

Classification of Burns in Children

According to Depth of Burn Injury

Superficial Burns (partial thickness burns)
- *Superficial partial thickness burns:* Burn injury involves epidermis and superficial layers of dermis, i.e. up to papillary dermis. The wound usually heals in less than two weeks period of burns.
- *Superficial deep dermal burns:* Burn injury involves beyond papillary dermis and takes more than two week's time for healing.

Full thickness burns: Burn injury involves all layer of skin and sometimes underlying tissues are also destroyed. The wound does not heal normally and needs skin grafting.

According to Extent of Burn Injury

First degree burns: Superficial burns manifested as pink to red discolored area with slight edema. Pain may present up to 48 hours and relieved by cooling. Within 5 days epidermis peels off, pink skin may persist for a week, no scar develops. Healing takes place spontaneously within 10 to 15 days, if not infected.

Second degree burns:

- Superficial second degree burns are presented as pink or red discoloration of the area with blister formation, weeping and edema. Superficial skin layers are destroyed. Wound becomes moist and painful and takes several weeks to heal. Scaring may develop.
- Second degree deep dermal burns are manifested as mottled white and red area become pale on pressure. The area may or may not be sensitive to touch but sensitive to cold air. Hair does not pull out easily. Wound takes several weeks to heal and scar may develop.

Third degree burns: It includes destruction of epithelial cells even fat, muscles and bone. Reddened areas do not blanch with pressure. It is not painful, inelastic and discoloration may vary from waxy white to brown. Eschar develops as leathery devitalized tissue, which must be removed. Granulation tissue develops and grafting is required if the burnt area is larger than 3 to 5 cm. Grafting is done after wound debridement.

First degree and second degree burns are included in partial thickness burns. The third degree burns is considered as full thickness burns.

According to Severity of Burn Injury

Severity of burn injury depends upon total area injured, depth of injury, location of injury, age, general health of the child presence of additional injury or chronic diseases and level of consciousness.

- Minor burns: 10 percent of total body surface area (TBSA) burnt with first and second degree burns.
- Moderate burns:
  - 10 to 20 percent TBSA burnt and second degree burns.
  - 2 to 5 percent TBSA burnt and third degree burn, but not involving eyes, ears, face, genitals, hands, feet or circumferential burns (over chest or abdomen).
- Major burns
  - 20 percent or more TBSA burnt and second degree burns.
  - All third degree burns greater than 10 percent TBSA burnt.
  - All burns involving face, eyes, ears, feet, hands and/or genitals.
  - Complicated burns with trauma, fracture, head injury, cancer, diabetes mellitus, pulmonary diseases and all at-risk patients.

Table 20.1: "Rule of Five" of estimation of burns surface area

Area	Age 0–5 years	Age 5–10 years	Age 10 years onwards
• Head and Neck	20%	15%	10%
• Trunk - front	20%	20%	20%
• Trunk - back	20%	20%	20%
• Upper Limbs	10 × 2 = 20%	10 × 2 = 20%	10 × 2 = 20%
• Lower Limbs	10 × 2 = 20%	15 × 2 = 30%	15 × 2 = 30%
	100% (20 × 5)	105%* (20 × 5) = (105–5) = 100%	100% (20 × 5)

N.B. * 5% to be deducted from trunk

Estimation of Extent of Burns Surface Area

The extent of burns is expressed as the amount of surface area burnt in relation to total body surface area. Various methods are used to calculate the burnt area.

- The easiest way to calculate the extent of burns is the "rule of hand". One hand surface (child's own hand) with closed fingers, amounts to 1 percent of body surface area and this can be used for calculation the extent of burns.
- A convenient, easy and quick method of estimation of surface area in pediatric burns is "Rule of Five" (Lynch and Blocker, 1963) (Figs 20.1A and B and Table 20.1).
- The most accurate estimation of extent of burns surface area can be done by using Lund and Browder chart, which gives the exact percentage at different age groups in different parts of the body.
  It is time consuming and laborsome to calculate.
- The "Rule of Nine" is applicable for children above 10 years of age, same as like adults.

Clinical Manifestations

The clinical features of burn injury are manifested depending upon the degree of burns. The child may present with shock along with varied depth and extent of body surface area burnt.

Symptoms of shock usually appear soon after burns. The child presents with pallor, cyanosis, prostration, poor muscle tone (may become flaccid) and failure to recognize familiar people. There is rapid pulse, low blood pressure and subnormal temperature.

Inhalation injury causes inflammation of edema of the glottis, vocal cords and upper trachea leading to upper airway obstruction. The child usually presents with dyspnea, tachypnea, hoarseness, stridor, chest retractions, nasal flaring, restlessness, cough and drooling.

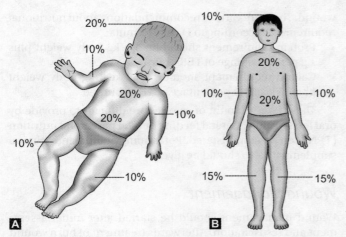

Figs 20.1A and B: Estimation of body surface area burnt by "Rule of Five". (A) Infant (B) Older children

Smoke inhalation initially may produce no symptoms or mild bronchial obstruction, but suddenly within 48 hours, may develop pulmonary edema, severe airway obstruction and bronchiolitis.

Symptoms of toxemia may develop after burns within one to two days. The patient usually manifested with fever, vomiting, edema, decreased urinary output, prostration, rapid pulse, glycosuria and unconsciousness.

Management

Management of burn injury includes first aid measures, assessment of extent of burns, fluid replacement, metabolic support, care of wound and use of topical antibiotics. Wound closure, prevention of infections and other complications, psychological support, nutritional support and rehabilitation are also major aspects of burn management. Best management can be provided in specialized burn unit with especially trained health personnel.

Minor burns can be managed at home with maintenance of aseptic techniques. Parents and family members need demonstration and specific instructions for home-care.

Moderate burns should be managed at general hospital/ district hospitals. But major burns, electrical burns and chemical burns should be managed initially with first aid measures and then must be transferred to specialized burn unit.

First Aid Measures

It is one of the important nurses responsibility to teach first aid measures along with prevention of burn injury to the general public. The first aid measures include:

- Immediate removal from heat source.
- In case of open flame, the child should help to lie flat on the ground and roll on the floor.
- Fire should be extinguished by pouring water.
- Avoiding pouring of water over the burnt area, once the fire has been extinguished, because it may be dangerous and lead to hypothermia, hyponatremia (due to water absorption), convulsions and brain edema.
- The child should be wrapped in clean sheet to prevent heat loss.
- Oral fluid or oral rehydration solution (ORS) should be given, if the child is thirsty and able to drink.
- Oro-pharyngeal secretion to be removed and airway to be kept patent. The child should be turned to one side and respiration to be checked. If necessary, mouth-to-mouth breathing may be given.
- Transfer to hospital to be arranged promptly.
- Avoiding use of pain killer and sedative. Not applying cotton or any household materials on the burnt area. Blister should not be peeled off and should be allowed to spontaneous collapse.

Assessment

Initial assessment should be done to determine the priority of care to protect the child from life-threatening complications.

- Assessment of airway, breathing and circulation (ABC) helps to initiate resuscitative measures on the basis of priority needs.
- Level of consciousness and vital signs to be evaluated quickly.
- Cause, duration and time of burn injury, first aid measures received and emergency care given should be find out.
- Extent and depth of burn injury to be assessed promptly to start fluid replacement, especially percentage of total body surface area (TBSA) burnt.
- Presence of additional injury and general health of the patient (especially body weight) to be examined quickly.

Obtaining history of the injury in details including complete medical history of illnesses, allergies, recent infections, immunization status, emotional deprivation, family history of illness and socioeconomic history.

Subsequent assessment includes fluid balance, urine output, vital signs, capillary filling, body weight, condition of wound, nutritional status, emotional status, signs of infections and other complications. Subsequent assessment is done after stabilization of child's condition with initial management and fluid replacement or as daily routine assessment. Laboratory testing of serum electrolytes, ABG, hematocrit, urine osmolality, etc. are also important.

Fluid Replacement

Fluid replacement is done promptly on the basis of TBSA burnt and body weight of the child. There are numbers of formula and there is different opinion regarding fluid resuscitation, about the types and amount of solutions to be used. The Parkland formula is most commonly used. The Brooks and Evans formulas may also be used.

Parkland formula
- In first 24 hours: The total amount of calculated fluid requirement is = 4 mL of Ringer's lactate X weight in kg X-percentage of TBSA burned.
- One-half amount of calculated fluid is given is the first 8 hours, calculated from the time of injury.
- The remaining half of the fluid is given over the next 16 hours.
- In next 24 hours: 2 mL of Ringer's lactate per kg per percent of burns.

The Parkland formula is commonly used to determine the fluid needed for resuscitation of burns greater than 15 to 20 percent TBSA. However, it must be kept in mind that the resuscitation formulas are only a rough guideline to the fluid therapy. Frequent clinical and laboratory assessment is necessary as a guide for hydration status. The best guide of tissue perfusion is urine output. Adequate renal perfusion is indicated by 0.5 mL per kg per hour.

Additional Measures

- Air way management is important to keep the clear airway and to prevent respiratory complications. Oxygen therapy and ventilator support and tracheostomy may be need in some patients.
- *Tetanus prophylaxis:* Tetanus toxoid and tetanus human immunoglobulins to be administered in gross contamination of the wound.
- Sedative and analgesics to be given as prescribed to relief pain and to reduce anxiety. Initially intramuscular injection should be avoided.
- Systemic antibiotics to be given as prescribed. It should be given depending upon the culture report. The patient should be protected from nosocomial infections. Wound should be protected by topical antibiotics.
- Urinary catheter may be needed for some patients.

Nutritional Support

Adequate nutrition is very important to assist in wound healing and to maintain growth of the child. Initially, the patient may be kept nothing by mouth. When bowel sound returns, oral fluid to be given and then gradually solid food should be offered as tolerated. Extra calories and protein are needed to combat the loss during injury and to heal the

wound. There are various recommendations about nutritional requirement. According to Davies formula:
- Protein requirement should be 3 g/kg body weight plus 1 g per percentage of TBSA burned.
- Calorie requirement should be 60 kcal/kg body weight plus 35 kcal per percentage of TBSA burned.

These large amount of calories are difficult to provide by oral feeding only. Enteral feeding or total parenteral nutrition (TPN) can be administered. Potassium, vitamin and mineral supplements also should be given.

Wound Management

Wound management should be started after initial assessment and resuscitation. Afterwards treatment of burn wound should be done daily or twice daily as cleansing of wound with debridement or hydrotherapy and/or change of dressing (if applied).

Initial wound dressing and debridement may be done after administration of sedative and analgesics. Environmental temperature should be higher (28°-30°C). Tight clothing and ornament should be removed and hair can be removed around the wound. Clean technique can be used, as sterile technique may not always be possible. Wound should be cleaned with normal saline or savlon-water solution. Dead and loose skin should be removed. Blisters may be managed by pricking and draining the fluid.

Burn wound management can be done by open method or closed method depending upon the nature of burn wound and available facilities. Wound should be covered with antibacterial cream/ointment, sterile Vaseline gauze and if needed sterile dressing to be applied to absorb the drainage and to protect the wound from dust, dirt and other environmental nuisances. The commonly used topical agent for burns wound are silver sulfadiazine, silver nitrate and mafenide acetate cream (sulfamylon).

Hydrotherapy is used to facilitate cleansing and debridement of the burned area. It is done by bathing of the burn patient in a tub of water or with a water shower (tubing, tanking or showering). Shower water should be about 32°C or 90°F, which flows over the child (same temperature for tubing). Debridement is then done along with showering,. Isotonic saline also can be used in spite of water.

Nonviable tissue or Eschar may be removed through natural, enzymatic, mechanical and/or surgical debridement. Eschar can be removed daily during wound dressing. In surgical excision of nonviable tissue, the wound should be covered by biological dressing, i.e. xenograft, allograft or auto graft. This may be temporary or permanent covering procedure.

Surgical excision (facial or tangential) of burn wound may be done in full thickness or deep dermal burns to apply split thickness graft after separation of Eschar. Grafting should be done to avoid formation of hyper tropic scars leading to contractures and deformities. Wound swab culture should be done before skin grafting and positive culture should be treated with appropriate antibiotics. General health of the child should be improved before skin grafting.

Electrical burns may require fasciotomies, serial wound debridements, reconstructive surgery and even amputation. Ventricular fibrillations and brain damage may develop as systemic effects of electrical burns, which should be managed appropriately.

Chemical burns should be managed with initial washing of burnt area thoroughly with water and buffer solution like monobasic or dibasic phosphate solution. Wound of chemical burns may also need management with surgical excision and skin grafting to prevent long-term complications.

Rehabilitation

Rehabilitation of burns patient is very essential and should include physical, social, psychological, occupational and economical rehabilitation.

Complications

Burn injury may cause several complications which depend upon severity of burns and available management facilities.

Early complications: Hypovolemic shock, respiratory failure, renal failure, paralytic ileus, GI bleeding due to curling's ulcer, wound sepsis, thrombophlebitis, urinary tract infections, hypostatic pneumonia, toxic shock syndrome, post-burn seizures, hypertension, depression, etc.

Late complications: Anemia, malnutrition, growth failure, Marjolin's ulcer (carcinoma in burn scar), contracture, psychological trauma and cosmetic problems.

Nursing Management

Nursing Assessment

It should be done to identify the priority need and to formulate nursing diagnosis on the basis of initial and subsequent assessment by detailed history, physical examination and laboratory investigations.

Nursing Diagnoses

The important nursing diagnoses for nursing interventions should include the followings:

- Decreased cardiac output related to hypovolemia and increased metabolism.
- Impaired oxygenation related to inhalation injury and pulmonary complications.
- Pain related to burn wound.
- Fear and anxiety related to pain and hospital procedures.
- Risk for infections related to alteration of skin integrity.
- Potential to injury of gastric mucosa related to stress response and decreased gastric motility.
- Impaired physical mobility related to pain and contracture.
- Altered nutrition, less than body requirements related to poor appetite and burn injury.
- Alteration of body image related to disfigurement in burn injury.
- Altered parenting related to crisis situation.

Nursing Interventions

- Promoting and supporting cardiac output by continuous monitoring of features of shock, vital signs, level of consciousness and electrolyte values. Administering IV fluid therapy, oxygen therapy and other medications, maintaining warmth, humid environment, strict recording of fluid intake, measuring output of urine (indwelling catheter if necessary) are important measures to promote cardiac function.
- Providing optimum respiratory functions by oxygen therapy, ventilator support and tracheostomy if needed, with monitoring of respiratory status, ABG analysis and pulmonary complications.
- Relieving pain and discomfort by comfort measures, use of bed cradle, administering analgesics and sedatives as prescribed, providing relaxation and diversion, emotional support and explanation, etc. Pain assessment should be done during nursing measures or by pain rating scales.
- Reduction of fear and anxiety by allowing parents to stay with child (if possible) and allowing child to verbalize feeling. Explanation of procedure, accepting regressive behaviors and encouraging self-care also help to relief anxiety.
- Preventing infections by aseptic wound care, administering prescribed antibiotics, change of position, maintaining general cleanliness and assessing signs of infections and following barrier nursing.
- Preventing GI problems by keeping the child NPO and with nasogastric aspiration until bowel sound returns. Encouraging small amount of tube feeding (as indicated), reinitiating oral feeding gradually when bowel sound resumes, administering H_2 blocker and assessing features of GI complications for early management.
- Promoting and preserving mobility by range of motion exercise, early ambulation, change of position, use of splint at joint and use of therapeutic play to prevent complications.
- Providing adequate nutrition by high-calorie, high-protein diet with vitamin and mineral supplementation and offering small-frequent feeding and enteral feeding

or TPN if required. Assessing weight gain, wound healing, serum albumin level and nutritional status.

- Preventing negative body image by reassurance, referring for skin grafting and cosmetic surgery, motivating to accept the changed image and use of special clothing, seeking advice from child psychologist and cosmetic specialist.
- Promoting effective parenting by involving them in child care with necessary teaching and demonstrations, supporting the parents to overcome guilt feeling and allowing opportunity to ask questions to help them to cope with the stress situation. Teaching the parents and family members about prevention and safety precautions for avoidance of burn injury and rehabilitative measures at home, school and community especially in the postburn period to assist them to promote their responsibility.

COMMON SKIN DISEASES IN CHILDREN

Scabies

Scabies is a skin disease commonly found among school children. Produced by the burrowing action of a parasite insect mite (sarcoptic scabies) in the epidermis. It results in irritation and formation of burrows, vesicles and pustules.

Scabies is transmitted by direct skin-to-skin contact with infected persons or indirect contact of clothing and bed linen. It occurs in all socioeconomic group regard less of standard of personal hygiene. Incubation period is 4 to 6 weeks.

Clinical Manifestations

The clinical features of scabies include itching as primary symptoms followed by skin lesions as papules and vesicles. The burrow, a gray or white tortuous threadlike line, is most commonly found in the older children between the fingers, in the wrist and in the axillary or buttock folds. The skin lesions may also found along the belt line, on the male genitalia and female breast, on the knees, elbows and ankles, or may occur in any part of the body, even face, neck and scalp. Vesicles on the palms and soles are characteristics. Warm and moist areas are generally affected. The skin lesions may found as reddish nodules on trunk and groins. Superadded infection of the lesions are common and may cause formation of pustules and crust. Acute nephritis may occur as a complication of scabies.

Diagnosis is confirmed by identification of mite, ova or its faces from skin scrapings.

Management

Managemet of scabies is done with application of scabicide agent. The commonly used scabicidal is 25 percent benzyl benzoate diluted in calamine or water. In case of small children, it is applied all over the body from neck to toes after preliminary bath and removed after 24 hours. The best scabicide is 5 percent permethrin cream used for infants over 2 months and children. Other scabicidals are lindane 1 percent, crotamiton, etc. Permethrin should be removed by bathing after 8 to 14 hours of application. Lindane to be removed by 8 to 12 hour and crotamiton after 48 hours.

Infected scabies should be treated with suitable antimicrobial agents. Second time application of scabicide may be necessary on next day or after one week. Antihistaminic drugs may be given, if itching continues 2 to 3 weeks after the therapy. Steroids may be needed for some children.

Protective gloves should be used during application of scabicide. All the household and close contacts should receive the prophylactic treatment with scabicide on the same time, even if they do not have any overt skin lesions. After the treatment, all clothing, linen and towel should be boiled, sun dried and ironed to kill all mites. Side-effects for the therapy should be assessed and necessary treatment to be given.

Superficial Fungal Infections

Fungal infections of skin may found in many forms. The common superficial fungal infections are candidiasis, dermatophytosis and pityriasis.

Candidiasis (Moniliasis)

Fungal infection caused by *Candida albicans* is common in early infancy. The most common site of infection is oral cavity and presents as oral thrush. Other sites of fungal infections are napkin areas (external genitalia, perianal region, inguinal region), axilla, nails and any other moist areas.

The lesions may found as scaly, papulovesicular or erythematous area with sharp border. Pain and discomfort may present in the affected area. Oral thrush is manifested by appearance of white plaques on the oral mucous membrane, gum and the tongue. The plaques look like milk card which cannot be removed easily and may bleed in forceful attempt. Swallowing difficulties and diarrhea may present along with oral thrush.

The fungal infections are commonly found in association with maternal vulvovaginitis, broad spectrum antibiotic therapy, malnutrition, prematurity, diabetes mellitus, immunodeficiency disorders and hypoparathyroidism.

Management: Treatment of fungal infections can be done with local application of nystatin, clotrimazole, amphotericin 'B', ketoconazole or with any antifungal agents suitable for children.

Parents should be explained about the importance of hygienic measures and continued treatment till complete cure of the condition. Application of local antifungal preparations should be demonstrated, especially oral suspension, which should be applied at the inner sides of the mouth after feeding and to retain the medication as long as possible in the mouth.

Dermatophytosis (Ringworm Infections)

Dermatophytes are aerobic fungi present in the soil. Dermatophytosis is also known as ringworm infections, a highly specialized fungal infections of skin and its appendages. It may be superficial or deep. Depending upon the involved part of the body different terms are used.

Types: The common ringworm (Tinea) infections are:

- *Tinea capitis:* Fungal infection of the scalp due to Trichophyton or Microsporum.
- *Tinea corporis:* Fungal infection of glabrous skin usually due to Trichophyton or Microsporum.
- *Tinea cruris:* Fungal infection in the crural or peritoneal folds, extending upto upper inside of the thigh and caused by epidermophyton.
- *Tinea pedis* (athlete's foot): A chronic superficial fungal infection of the skin of foot, especially between the toes and on the soles due to Trichophyton and Epidermophyton.
- *Tinea unguium* (onychomycosis): Fungal infection of nails caused by Trichophyton or Epidermophyton.
- *Tinea versicolor:* A chronic noninflammatory usually asymptomatic disorder due to Pityrosporum orbiculare, marked only by multiple macular patches on the skin.

These infections spread from one child to another child by direct contact or through common use of towels, pillows, combs, hair brush, etc. Household pets like cats and dogs also can be source of these infections.

Tinea capitis: It is usually found in children between 3 to 10 years of age. During puberty, keratin is able to resist the fungal infections. The lesions appear on the scalp as round seborrhea like scaly patches with loss of hair (alopecia) and breakage of hair. Pruritus usually occurs in the affected area. A kerion, an inflammation, that produces edema, pustules and granulomatous swelling may develop with oozing.

Diagnosis of fungal infection is confirmed by examining the scrapping of scalp or hair.

Treatment consists of oral administration of griseofulvin 15 to 20 mg/kg/day for 5 to 7 days. Topical application of antifungal cream may be effective. Selenium sulfide lotion can be used twice per weeks. Clotrimazole, tolnaftate, etc. can be used as cream or lotions.

Tinea corporis: It presents with multiple small red scaly round patches studded with minutes vesicles on any part of the body. Patches enlarge at the periphery and healing occurs at center giving a characteristic circular shape with pale center and raised edges. Itching usually present. Secondary bacterial infections and allergic reactions may occur. Diagnosis is made by presence of fungus in the skin scrapings.

Treatment of this condition is done with application of calamine lotion and mild fungicides. Griseofulvin is administer in severe generalized and resistant cases. Tolnaftate (Tinaderm) is used effectively for this infection.

Tinea cruris (Jock itch): Ringworm infection of genitocrural region is found in obese male children. The lesions are symmetrical, demarcated with well-defined border. Itching usually present in the scaly erythematous lesions. Treatment is done with griseofulvin or tolnaftate as topical applications.

Tinea pedis: Fungal infections of feet involving interdigital clefts of toes and soles found as fissures or macerations. It may found on the planter surface of the feet as vesicular patches. Secondary infection, marked itching and bad odor are commonly present.

The condition is treated with antifungal agent, aluminium chloride and gentian violet. Amorolfine spray can be used daily for 3 to 6 weeks to have good result. The web space between toes to be kept dry.

Tinea unguium: It is chronic and resistant type of fungal infection affecting nails. It requires treatment for long period. Griseofulvin or other antifungal agents can be applied for 3 to 4 months for finger nails and 6 to 12 months for toe nails. Newly available topical preparations (ciclopirox and natifine) can be used for better penetration in the nails.

Tinea versicolor (pityriasis): It is mild and common fungal infection found in moist and warm climates. It is superficial infection caused by Microsporum furfur. It presents as yellowish-brown macules. Later, hypopigmented lesions are found usually on face, neck, arms and trunk. Scrapping from the lesions helps to diagnose the infection. Local application of antifungal agent (Tolnaftate) and application of selenium sulfide shampoo over affected skin 15 to 20 minutes daily for 1 to 2 weeks are useful along with good skin hygiene. Repeated attacks are commonly found.

Superficial Bacterial Infections (Pyoderma)

Bacterial infections of the skin are usually caused by *Staphylococcus aureus* or group-A beta hemolytic *Streptococcus*. Common bacterial skin infections are impetigo, boils or furuncles, folliculitis, cellulitis, ecthyma, etc.

Impetigo

Impetigo is the most common bacterial skin infection characterized by formation of vesicles, pustules, crusts and bullae. The causative organisms are *Staphylococcus aureus* and *Streptococcus pyogenes*. It is common in children below 10 years of age with poor personal hygiene. It spreads by close contact. Skin abrasion may also act as portal of entry. Incubation period is about 10 days.

Clinical manifestations: Impetigo is characterized by appearance of pink-red macules which become vesicles and rupture to develop crusts and leave temporary superficial erythematous area. Bullous lesions may develop anywhere in the body but commonly found on the face, axilla and groin. They are large thin-roofed blisters and break to form thin light brown crusts. Crusted lesions appear with thick yellow crusts. Pruritus and lymph gland enlargement may present. Autoinoculation is major cause of spreading of infection.

Management: Management of impetigo is done by gentle washing of affected area with soap and water thrice a day and removal of crusts and debris by normal saline or candy's lotion. Application of topical antibacterial and systemic antibiotics (cephalosporins, erythromycin) are essential.

Close contact with other children should be avoided to prevent spread of infection. Autoinoculation should be prevented by frequent hand washing, short nails, daily soap-water bathing, regular laundering of contaminated towel, linen and clothing.

Complications: Impetigo can be complicated with cellulitis, osteomyelitis, septic arthritis, pneumonia and septicemia. Streptococcal infection can cause scarlet fever, lymphangitis and lymphadenitis. Poststreptococcal acute glomerulonephritis may occur due to infection by nephritogenic strains.

Psoriasis

Psoriasis is a chronic recurrent dermatisis marked by discrete vivid red macules, papules or plaques covered with silvery lamellated scales over scalp, knees, elbows, umbilicus and genitalia. Removal of scales leads to multiple small bleeding points (Auspitz sign). It is commonly found in girls and in the age group of 3 to 10 years. It has multifactorial etiology. It may be exacerbated by infection, trauma, stress and hormonal factors. Koebner response as the tendency to appear lesions at the site of trauma may also be seen.

Treatment is done with local application of steroids, coaltar preparations, natural sunlight, psoralens and ultraviolet light and with vitamin 'D' therapy.

Acne

Acne is an inflammatory skin disease manifested as pleomorphic eruptions usually seen over face, trunk and rarely on arms, legs and buttocks. It is most commonly found in adolescence and rarely in infancy and childhood.

The initial lesions are found as whiteheads or blackheads (comedones). Then after 2 to 3 years the classical signs of acne are seen. The blackheads may be infected with *Staphylococcus epidermidis* or *Propionibacterium acnes* which leads to formations of pupules and pustules. Deeper lesions may form nodular cysts and scaring.

Acne may be found in children with greasy scalp, dandruff, seborrhea and increased production of sebum due to hormonal response. Some lipids of sebum cause irritant dermatitis. Comedones are formed due to lack of essential fatty acid and linoleic acid in the skin surface lipids. Colonization of microorganisms leads to inflammation of comedones.

There are several varieties of acne, i.e. acne vulgaris, infantile acne, steroid acne, halogen acne, topical acne, acne conglobate, pomade acne, etc.

Management

Treatment of acne should be done with adequate explanation about the cause of the condition for psychological preparation of the child and adolescence. Information's should be given about harmful effects of use of cosmetics, hair preparations, facial manipulations and frequent cleansing. Instructions to be given regarding treatment compliance and discouraging use of commercially advertized medicine.

Topical application of clindamycin or erythromycin for several weeks gives better result. Benzyl peroxide gel or cream can be used to reduce the number of comedones. Other useful agents are azelaic acid, retinoic acid, sulfur, salicylic acid and resorcinol. Systemic antibiotic and vitamin 'A' may be helpful.

Physical therapy with ultraviolet light may be effective. CO_2 or snow or cold water will have good effect.

Surgical management may be done with round extractions of open and closed comedones, needle aspirations of nodulocystic lesions, steroid injections and cosmetic surgery for scaring.

Atopic Dermatitis

Atopic dermatitis is also known as infantile or childhood eczema. It is usually related with allergic reaction and characterized by erythema, edema, intense pruritus, exudation, lichenification, crusting and scaling. It may associated with allergic rhinitis (hay fever), asthma and immunodeficiency. There may be IgE mediated reaction due to immune system abnormalities as deficient suppressor T cell functions. This condition may also have relation with hereditary and psychogenic factors.

Clinical Manifestations

Atopic dermatitis has varied presentation. In early months of life, the infant may present with erythematous squamous patches over scalp, behind the ears, around nose, buttocks and genitalia. This is termed as seborrheic dermatitis. This condition usually resolves in 4 to 6 weeks. But in some infants, this condition may progress to infantile eczema.

Infantile eczema is characterized by rosy erythema over the cheeks with fissuring of skin fold behind the ears, saddening of the neck folds, dryness and scaling of the extensor surfaces of the arms, wrists and legs. There may be desquamation, papule formation and crusting. Generally perioral, peri orbital and nasal areas are spared. There is marked itching and scratching which lead to excoriation and superadded infection with bacteria or fungus. This condition recovers in majority of the cases within one or two years. But in few cases, it may continue with remissions and exacerbations.

Infantile eczema may continue after one to two years of age or found as late onset after one year of age. Then it is termed as late onset atopic eczema or *Flexural eczema*. It is characterized by the lesions over flexures of elbows and knees, anterior of neck and front part of ankles. The lesions are erythematous, scaling and with lichenification.

Atopic dermatitis may also present as coin-shaped vesicular lesions with severe pruritus and known as *nummular eczema*. Another form of atopic dermatitis is found as *pityriasis alba* with hypo pigmented patches over face.

Management

Management of atopic dermatitis is done with topical applications of steroids, antibiotics, sodium fusidate and antihistaminic drugs. Systemic antibiotic therapy for 7 to 10 days is useful in active disease.

Other supportive measures include gentle bathing with small amount of liquid antiseptic soap, short nails, avoidance of scratching and allergens (food, dust, nylon, irritating soap, cosmetics, feather, animal danders, etc). Dietary intake of fish oil containing omega-3 fatty acid shows favorable results.

Diseases of Central Nervous System

21

- Child in Coma
- Meningitis
- Encephalitis and Encephalopathies
- Guillain-Barré Syndrome (Infective Polyneuritis)
- Convulsive Disorders
- Cerebral Palsy
- Mental Retardation

- Down's Syndrome (Mongolism)
- Neural Tube Defects (Myelodysplasia, Dysraphism)
- Hydrocephalus
- Intracranial Space Occupying Lesions
- Brain Tumors
- Head Injury (Craniocerebral Trauma)

INTRODUCTION

Diseases of nervous system are fairly common in children. Almost 20 to 30 percent of children are victims of neurological illnesses. These are major contributors to childhood morbidity and disability. Neurological disorders of infancy and childhood are different than in adults. Neurological symptoms are also found in association with various systemic diseases. Common disease conditions in children involving central nervous system (CNS) include congenital malformations, perinatal problems (birth asphyxia, birth injury), developmental disabilities, CNS infections, craniocerebral trauma and brain tumor.

Newer diagnostic modalities such as CT scan, MRI, PET scan, SPECT scan, cerebral angiography, myelography, electromyography, neuropsychological testing, echoencephalography, magnetoencephalography, newer EEG techniques, ultrasonography, etc. are now available to help in accurate diagnosis and appropriate management. Specialized health care settings are now organizing intensive care for neurological disorders with specially trained health personnel. Nurses are key persons to provide need-based problem oriented care for those diseases and disorders.

CHILD IN COMA

Coma is a life-threatening emergency situation caused by various disease conditions affecting central nervous system directly or indirectly. Detection of the exact cause of coma and specific management are life saving measures.

Coma is a state of profound unconsciousness from which the patient cannot be aroused even by powerful stimuli. The word 'coma' derived from the Greek word '*Koma*' means deep sleep. It indicates prolonged state of unarousable sleep and alteration of consciousness, usually resulting from lesions involving reticular formation of the brainstem, the hypothalamus and connection with the cerebral hemispheres. There is decreased responsiveness to visual, auditory and tactile stimulations with no spontaneous movement.

Pathology

Consciousness in maintained by the interaction of reticular activating system (RAS) with the cerebral hemispheres. Coma occurs due to dysfunction of cerebral hemispheres, structural lesions or metabolic or toxic effects of CNS. Alteration in intracranial pressure and disturbances of cerebral blood flow are also associated with development of coma.

Stages of Altered Consciousness

- *Drowsy*—There is reduced awareness or wakefulness and presence of hyperexcitability with irritability, alternating with drowsiness or clouding.
- *Confusion*—There is inability to think clearly with presence of disorientation for time, place and person.
- *Delirium*—The patient is out of contact with the environment and having disorientation, hyperactivity, irritability, hallucinations and talkativeness.
- *Obtundation*—There is increased sleep, reduced alertness with mental blunting.
- *Stupor or semicoma*—The patient is unresponsive but arousable by vigorous, repeated stimuli, again goes back to unresponsiveness when the stimuli is withdrawn.
- *Coma*—Unresponsive and unarousable by any stimulus.

Grades of Coma

- *Stage 1 or stupor*—The patient can be aroused for short duration and shows verbal and motor response to stimuli.
- *Stage 2 or light coma*—The patient cannot be aroused easily except with painful stimuli.
- *Stage 3 or deep coma*—There is no response to painful stimuli. Due to loss of cortical control over the motor functions, the patient's limbs may be in primitive reflex posture. In case of intact brainstem, the comatose patient adopts decorticate posture, i.e. flexed arms on the chest with closed fists and legs are extended. In dysfunction of midbrain, the comatose patient adopts decerebrate posture with arms rigidly extended and pronated and legs are extended (Figs 21.1A and B).
- *Stage 4 or brain death*—All cerebral functions are lost and pupillary reflexes are absent in this stage. No spontaneous respiratory effort presents but local spinal reflexes may be preserved.

Causes of Coma

Common causes of coma can be listed as follows:

- *Infections*—Meningitis, encephalitis, brain abscess, subdural or epidural empyema, cerebral malaria, septicemia, enteric and shigella encephalopathy.

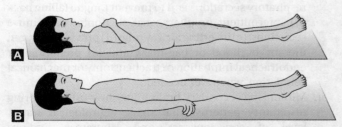

Figs 21.1A and B: Posturing in unconscious state: (A) Decorticate posture; (B) Decerebrate posture

- *Metabolic disorders*—Hypoglycemia, hyperglycemia, diabetic ketoacidosis, acid-base imbalance, dyselectrolytemia, uremia, hepatic failure, Reye's syndrome.
- *Drugs and poisons*—Opiates, barbiturates, sedatives, aspirin, organophosphates, snake bites, insect stings, lead poisoning.
- *Miscellaneous*—Head injury, intracranial hemorrhage, postictal coma, postcardiac arrest, demyelinating disorders of CNS, hypertensive encephalopathy, vascular malformations, brain tumors, hydrocephalus, hypoxia, hyperpyrexia, water intoxication and shock.

About 55 percent of nontraumatic cases of coma are due to CNS infections. Other most common causes include nontraumatic intracranial hemorrhage, hepatic encephalopathy, postictal coma, Reye's syndrome, etc.

Diagnostic Evaluation

A systematic approach of careful history of illness with thorough physical and neurological assessment are important to determine the provisional diagnosis. Specific laboratory investigations and imaging procedures are essential to detect the specific cause of coma.

History of illness should include detailed information related to the event, type of onset, associated symptoms, i.e. fever, vomiting, headache, convulsions, etc. History of ingestion of toxin or poisonous substances, any bites or stings, trauma, exposure to infections, chronic illness, malignancy, etc also provide useful guideline to diagnose the condition. Physical and neurological assessment should include head to foot examination, vital signs, blood pressure, pupillary signs, meningeal signs, features of increased intracranial pressure, neurological reflexes, etc. Other assessment include fundoscopy, level of unconsciousness with Glasgow coma scale (see Appendix–XII), presence of involuntary and abnormal movements (e.g. Doll's eye movement), abnormal posture, motor response, paralysis and paresis, skin color, peculiar odor, cardiac findings, bladder and bowel functions, presence of wound and infections, etc.

Laboratory investigations and diagnostic imaging should be planned according to provisional diagnosis. Examination of blood, urine, CSF, stomach aspirates, etc. are important diagnostic clues. Neuroimaging, like X-ray skull, CT scan, MRI, PET scan, SPECT scan can be arranged according to available facilities and suspected cause. EEG, EMG, ECG, etc. can help to confirm the diagnosis.

Management

Immediate Management

Emergency measures should be initiated as soon as the patient is hospitalized in comatose state. Before doing a complete physical examination and recording of detailed history, the patient should be resuscitated with clear airway and maintenance of breathing and circulation, after quick initial assessment.

The emergency management for a comatose child should include the followings:

1. Assess for patient airway and maintain clear airway by positioning (head extended), preventing fall back of tongue, or by suctioning. Mouth gag, oral airway tube, tracheostomy or endotracheal intubation may be needed for some patients.
2. Assess breathing patterns and maintain oxygenation by using 100 percent oxygen therapy with bag and mask or with ventilatory support, if needed.
3. Assess circulatory status (pulse, blood pressure) and administered intravenous fluid therapy with appropriate solutions (normal saline, ringer lactate, 10% dextrose) to restore hydration status, acid-base and electrolyte balance and to treat shock.
4. Administer medications to control seizures and high fever, if present and to give antidotes for poisoning or specific drug therapy for particular condition.
5. Assess for increased intracranial pressure (ICP) and provide measures to reduce ICP by the followings.
   - Head to be kept in neutral position with 15° to 30° elevation.
   - Ensure adequate oxygenation.
   - Maintain normal mean arterial blood pressure.
   - Restriction of fluid to 2/3rd of usual maintenance needs.
   - Provide hyperventilation with bag and mask or ventilator to maintain $PaCO_2$—25 to 30 mm Hg. It should be used for 1 to 2 days only.
   - Administer osmotic diuretics (mannitol, frusemide).
   - Use of dexamethasone in cytotoxic cerebral edema.
   - Administration of phenobarbital may be needed in refractory cases.
   - CSF drainage may be useful in obstructive hydrocephalus.
   - Provide supportive measures with reduction of fever and avoidance of pain, sudden movement, strong light, loud noise and noxious stimuli from environmental disturbances.
6. Intubate nasogastric tube to remove stomach contents to prevent aspiration and abdominal distension.
7. Monitor child's condition continuously and maintaining accurate records to provide specific management for the comatose child.

Specific Management

Specific management should be provided depending upon the exact cause of coma. Supportive measures should include maintenance of nutritional requirement and bladder-bowel functions, prevention of complications, continuous monitoring and expert nursing care.

Nursing Management

Nursing assessment: It should be done by details history, physical and neurological assessment along with review of diagnostic findings.

Nursing diagnoses: The important nursing diagnoses for a comatose child include:
- Ineffective airway clearance due to upper airway obstruction.
- High risk for secondary brain injury related to coma.
- Risk for fluid volume deficit due to inability to take oral feeding.
- Hyperthermia related to disturbance of brain functions.
- Impaired tissue integrity of cornea, related to diminished corneal reflex.
- Altered oral mucous membrane related to mouth breathing.
- Risk for impaired skin integrity related to immobility.
- Altered nutritional status less than body requirements related to inability of food intake.
- Altered urinary pattern (incontinence) related to unconsiousness.
- Bowel incontinence related to loss of neurological control in coma.
- Risk for injury related to convulsions and alteration of consciousness.
- Ineffective family coping related to life-threatening condition.

Nursing Interventions

A comatose child should be nursed in an intensive care unit (PICU, NICU) with specialized nursing techniques. The nursing interventions should be provided on the basis of priority nursing diagnoses. The important interventions are described below:

i. Maintaining an effective airway by—(a) positioning with extended head or head turned to one side to drain respiratory secretions and to prevent tongue falling back (b) intermittent oropharyngeal suctioning to remove secretions. (c) inserting airway tube (d) providing oxygen therapy by hood or bag-mask and (e) preparing for endotracheal intubation or tracheostomy or mechanical ventilation, whenever needed.
ii. Minimizing secondary brain injury by—(a) monitoring respiratory patterns, vital signs, neurological status, level of consciousness and laboratory findings (b) providing basic life support measures and measures

to reduce increased ICP and (c) administering prescribed medications.

iii. Maintaining fluid and electrolyte balance by—(a) administering fluid therapy, (b) monitoring hydration and electrolyte status and (c) administering antipyretics, antibiotics as prescribed, (d) monitoring vital signs and features of infections.

iv. Providing eye care with aseptic precautions and medications.

v. Maintaining healthy oral mucosa by special mouth care.

vi. Maintaining skin integrity by meticulous skin care to prevent pressure sore by back care, change of position, tidy clean bed, range of motion excercise and monitoring skin conditions.

vii. Providing adequate nutrition by NG tube feeding or TPN.

viii. Promoting urine elimination by indwelling urinary catheter or simple drainage with aseptic techniques and monitoring amount and nature of urine, features of infections or any other problems.

ix. Promoting normal bowel functions especially by preventing constipation or providing care in fecal incontinence. Monitoring features of GI obstructions or any other problems.

x. Preventing injury by placing on railcot bed, anti-convulsive drugs and allowing attendance (mother or any care giver), if possible. Constant observations for restlessness, involuntary movements and convulsions are important.

xi. Promoting family coping by emotional support, encouraging to ask questions and providing necessary information and instructions, regarding plan of care and prognosis.

MENINGITIS

Meningitis is the inflammation of the meninges, the covering membrane of the brain and spinal cord. It is a major cause of hospitalization of children with high mortality rate. The term meningitis to be considered as a misnomer, because it is virtually impossible that inflammation is limited to the meninges only. Meningoencephalitis is a better nomenclature, as brain tissue is also inflamed along with meninges.

Meningitis can be classified as:

a. Pyogenic or bacterial meningitis.

b. Tuberculous meningitis.

c. Aseptic meningitis caused by virus, fungus, or protozoa (toxoplasmosis, amebic).

Pyogenic Meningitis (Bacterial Meningitis)

Pyogenic meningitis is caused by bacterial infections. Acute bacterial meningitis is more common in neonates and infants due to immature immune mechanism and poor phagocytic functions.

Etiology

Inflammation of meninges may occur due to primary infections of meninges or due to metastatic spread from nearby or distant pyogenic focus. Infection may occur due to extension of local bacterial infections from sinusitis, mastoiditis or otitis media or from bacteremia through hematogeneous spread. It may also spread from pneumonia, empyema, pyoderma and osteomyelitis. It may develop following injury and penetrating wound. Diagnostic procedures and surgical interventions may cause the infection. Immunodeficiency state also can cause this infection. High-risk neonates are vulnerable to neonatal meningitis.

The causative organisms of meningitis in neonates are *E. coli, Streptococcus pneumoniae, Staphylococcus aureus, Streptococcus fecalis*, etc. In the infants and young children, the offending organisms are *H. influenzae, S. pneumoniae* and meningococci. *Pneumococci* is common beyond 3 years of age and *N. meningitidis* infection occurs in all ages. *Meningococcus* causes meningitis in epidemic.

Pathophysiology

Inflammatory cells infiltrate the leptomeninges. The cortex becomes edematous and exudative with proliferation of microglia. There is destruction of ependymal cells and collection of purulent exudate at the base of the brain. The subarachnoid space is filled with a cloudy and opaque fluid and exudates, which may block the foramina of luschka and Magnedie leading to internal hydrocephalus. Thrombophlebitis of the cerebral vessels may occur which results in infarction and neurological complications. Permanent neurological damage may develop due to tissue necrosis, infarction and hydrocephalus. Fatal endotoxic shock may occur in cases of meningococcal meningitis. Cerebral edema, change in composition of CSF, increased ICP and meningeal irritation due to inflammatory process produce the clinical manifestations.

Clinical Manifestations

The onset of the disease is usually sudden with high fever, headache, malaise, vomiting, restlessness, irritability and convulsions. The child may complain severe headache either diffuse or in the frontal region, spreading to neck and eyeballs. The neonates may present with insidious onset of refusal of feeds, high-pitched shrill cry, hypothermia, seizures, jaundice, lethargy and bulging fontanel.

The child may manifest mental confusion, with varying degree of alteration of level of consiousness, marked photophobia, generalized hypertonia and marked neck rigidity. Squint, ptosis and diplopia may found due to ocular palsies. Respiration may become periodic or cheyne-stokes type with features of shock.

On examination, meningeal signs are found as neck stiffness, positive Kernig's sign, positive Brudzinski's signs and papilledema. Neurological deficits like hemiparesis, cranial nerve palsies and hemianopia may present.

Special Features

In meningococcal meningitis, the patient is usually present with generalized purpuric rash, severe prostration, hypotension, shock and rapid coma. These occur due to hemorrhage and necrosis in the adrenal glands during meningococcal septicemia. This condition is known as Waterhouse-Friderichsen syndrome. Chronic meningococcemia may develop and presents with intermittent fever, chills, joint pains and maculopapular hemorrhagic rash.

Pneumococcal meningitis may develop in association with otitis media, sinusitis, pneumonia, or head injury. It can cause septic meningitis at all ages except neonates. This condition can be complicated with subdural effusion.

Staphylococcal meningitis is often found in neonates with umbilical sepsis, skin infections or septicemia. In older children, it is usually found following otitis media, mastoiditis, sinus thrombosis, arthritis and pneumonia.

Hemophilus influenzae type 'B' is responsible for meningitis in infants (3–12 months). They present with convulsions focal neurological signs and fever. These children may be complicated with subdural effusion and auditory deficit.

Complications

Pyogenic meningitis can be complicated with several neurological and systemic complications.

The complications include shock, myocarditis, status epilepticus, SIADH (Syndrome of inappropriate ADH secretions), subdural empyema or effusion, ventriculitis, arachnoditis, hydrocephalus, brain abscess, convulsive disorders, mental retardation, neurological deficits (like hemiplegia, ocular palsies, blindness, speech problem, deafness), obesity and precocious puberty.

Diagnostic Evaluation

Clinical manifestations are important diagnostic clue. The diagnosis is confirmed by lumbar puncture and CSF study.

The CSF examination shows turbid appearance, with increased cell count mainly polymorphonuclear leukocytes. There is increased protein level (more than 100 mg/dL) and decreased sugar (below 40 mg/dL) in CSF. Causative organism can be identified from CSF examination and culture. There is elevation of CSF pressure more than normal.

Other diagnostic approaches are CT scan, rapid diagnostic tests, (countercurrent immunoelectrophoresis, latex agglutination, etc.), nonspecific tests (C-reactive protein, CSF-lactic acid level) and polymerase chain reaction (PCR).

Routine examination of blood, urine analysis, X-ray skull and chest may help to exclude associated pathology.

Management

Pyogenic meningitis should be considered as medical emergency and following measures should be initiated promptly.

The specific antibiotic therapy is the important aspect of management. The commonly used drugs are—penicillin 4 to 5 lacs units/kg/day 4 hourly or cefotaxime 200 mg/kg/day 8 hourly IV or ceftriaxone 150 mg/kg/day BD. Ampicillin, gentamicin, amikacin, or chloramphenicol can also be used depending upon the causative organisms, combination of two antibiotics can be administered. Antibiotics can be given intrathecal in neonatal meningitis and in advanced cases.

Corticosteroids, dexamethasone, 0.15 mg/kg—every 6 hours IV is administered in severely ill patients with shock and to prevent neurological complications.

Osmotic diuretic therapy is given with mannitol (20%) 0.5 mg/kg every 4 to 6 hours IV, for maximum 6 doses to reduce the increased intracranial pressure.

Anticonvulsive drugs, diazepam 0.3 mg/kg is given to manage convulsions. Other anticonvulsives like phenobarbitone or phenytoin can also be used.

Vasopressors (dopamine) may be required in case of hypotension.

Other supportive management includes maintenance of fluid-electrolyte balance by IV fluid therapy, antipyretics, nasogastric tube feeding, vitamin supplementation, treatment of complications and good nursing care. Parents need emotional support and necessary information for continuation of care at home, follow-up and rehabilitation.

Prognosis

Prognosis depends upon initiation of treatment by early diagnosis. Generally patients with bacterial meningitis show distinct improvement in 10 days with appropriate antimicrobial agents. Some patients need treatment for more than 10 to 14 days. Delayed starting of management may lead to serious neurological complications. With the use of newer antibiotics, early diagnosis and treatment facilities, prognosis becomes favorable. Most of the mortality is found in neonatal meningitis.

Nursing Management

Nursing management should be performed based on subjective and objective data to formulate nursing diagnosis, to plan and implement nursing interventions. It should be provided same as the management of a comatose child.

In general, the nursing management should be provided with rest and comfortable position in rail cot bed with calm quiet dimlighted noise free environment. Important nursing measures include change of position, clearing of airway by removing oropharyngeal secretion, oxygen therapy, tepid sponge in case of fever for reduction of body temperature, maintenance of IV fluid therapy, nasogastric tube feeding, dietary support and administration of prescribed medications. Maintenance of personal hygiene (skin care, mouth care, eye care) and bladder-bowel functions are also significant. Prevention of injury, continuous monitoring of patient's conditions, care during convulsions, emotional support and teaching the parents about continuation of care after discharge are also important nursing responsibilities.

Tuberculous Meningitis

Tuberculous meningitis (TBM) is the inflammation of the meninges from tubercular infection caused by *Mycobacterium tuberculosis*. It is a serious complication of childhood tuberculosis. It may occur at any age, usually within a year of the primary infection of tuberculosis or may accompany with miliary tuberculosis. The numbers of TBM cases and mortality rate due to the condition had reduced but the survivors are usualy affected by various neurological complications.

Pathophysiology

The tubercular infection usually reaches the meninges by hematogenous route or through intracranial lymphatics or cervical lymph nodes. There is formation of submeningeal tubercular foci, which may discharge tubercle bacilli into the subarachnoid space. Proliferation of bacilli leads to perivascular exudation, caseation, gliosis and giant cell formation. The meningeal surface is then covered with exudates and tubercles. Small tubercles are scatterly develop over the convexity of the brain or periventricular area. Due to obliteration of subarachnoid space and arachnoid villi, CSF is poorly reabsorbed leading to increased amount of CSF and dilation of ventricles resulting hydrocephalus. Inflammatory changes result in diffuse edema of brain which leads to tubercular encephalopathy. Due to vascular occlusion, infarction of brain tissue may develop.

Clinical Manifestations

The onset of TBM is usually insidious. The clinical course of illness may be divided into three stages, i.e. prodromal, transitional and terminal.

The *prodromal stage* is the first stage of illness and the stage of invasion. It is presented with vague features like low grade fever, anorexia, drowsiness, apathy, headache, vomiting, irritability, disturbed sleep, restlessness, constipation, loss of weight, photophobia and sometimes with convulsions.

The *transitional stage* is the second stage of illness and also termed as stage of meningitis. In this stage, the child is manifested with features of increased ICP and meningeal irritation. The presenting features are positive Kernig's sign, neck rigidity along with fever, bradycardia, drowsiness, delirium, headache, vomiting, respiratory disturbances and even unconsciousness. Increased muscle tone and convulsions are usually present. Neurological deficits like monoplegia, hemiplegia, loss of sphincter control may develop. In infant, anterior fontanel may be found bulging. Cranial nerve involvement, ocular paralysis, strabismus, nystagmus and contracted pupils are common findings. Papilledema may present. Plantar reflexes may become extensor. Ankle and patellar clonus may be elicitable.

The *terminal or third stage* is the stage of coma. This stage is manifested with paralysis and coma. The child presents with fever, irregular respiration and bradycardia. Pupils are dilated and fixed, often unequal with nystagmus and squint. Ptosis and ophthalmoplegia are common. This condition may become fatal if left untreated for 4 weeks. Hydrocephalus develops in small children and infants, if the treatment is delayed or done inadequately.

There may be overlapping of the features of one stage into the other. Roughly duration of each stage is about one week. There may be prolongation of one stage or even absence of one stage, after the initiation of treatment.

Diagnostic Evaluation

History of illness in details along with family history of illness and history of contact with TB cases are important for diagnosis of TBM along with thorough physical examination.

The most important diagnostic procedure is CSF study by lumbar puncture. Increased CSF pressure, clear or slight turbid appearance of CSF, increased cell count with presence of lymphocytes and cobweb formation in CSF (when kept in test tube for 12 hours) are dependable information to diagnose TBM.

Identification of tuberculous bacilli in the CSF smear and culture helps to confirm the diagnosis. Biochemical study of CSF shows increased proteins but sugar and chlorides are reduced.

Other supportive investigations are chest X-ray to detect primary focus, X-ray skull, CT scan, Mantoux test, routine blood examination especially ESR and newer diagnostic approaches like biochemical markers, serodiagnosis and molecular diagnosis. Test for HIV infection should be performed in all suspected and at risk patients.

Management

Prompt management of TBM with adequate treatment for prolonged period should be provided. Antitubercular drugs should be given for 12 months. Initially four drugs are given with INH, rifampicin, pyrazinamide and ethambutol or streptomycin for two months. Then, in continuation phase, three drugs are given with INH, rifampicin and ethambutol for 10 months.

Adverse effects of the AT drugs should be monitored, specially auditory and vestibular nerve toxicity of streptomycin and ocular complications of ethambutol. Specific instructions for the AT drugs should be followed.

Parenteral corticosteroid therapy with dexamethasone for one to two weeks is useful to reduce cerebral edema and prevention of arachnoiditis with fibrosis. Afterwards, oral steroids should be continued with prednisolone for 6 to 8 weeks and then gradual tapered off.

Other symptomatic management includes mannitol (or glycerol or hypertonic glucose therapy) to reduce increased ICP, anticonvulsive drugs (diazepam, phenobarbitone) to control convulsions and IV fluid therapy to treat dyselectrolytemia and to maintain fluid-electrolyte balance. Pyridoxine (20 mg) orally once a day to be given to prevent side effects of INH.

Supportive nursing care, maintenance of nutritional requirements (NG tube feeding or oral feeding) and monitoring of features of complications, especially measurement of head circumference daily, to detect hydrocephalus are important measures. Ventriculoperitoneal shunt may be indicated in some cases with hydrocephalus.

Nursing Management

Nursing management of a child with TBM should be provided same as a case of bacterial meningitis and comatose child.

Complications

Hydrocephalus is the most common complication of TBM. Other complications include mental retardation, spasticity, cranial nerve paralysis, convulsive disorders, neurological deficits (hemiplegia, quadriplegia), endocrinal disturbances, precocious puberty, obesity, bladder-bowel dysfunction, optic atrophy and visual complications.

Prognosis

Early diagnosis, prompt and adequate treatment improve the prognosis. It depends upon age of the child, stage of illness, adequacy of treatment and presence of complications. Untreated cases may have fatal outcome within 4 to 8 weeks. The prognosis is poorer in younger children, malnourished children and advanced cases. About two-third of the TBM cases have long-term sequelae. Relapse may occur in incomplete antitubercular drug therapy.

ENCEPHALITIS AND ENCEPHALOPATHIES

Encephalitis is the inflammation of brain tissue. It may develop due to direct infection or via hematogenous route. It may occur across the olfactory mucosa or along the peripheral nerves. Immunological reaction also may cause encephalitis.

The term encephalopathy means the cerebral dysfunction occurs due to circulating toxic agents, abnormal metabolites, poisons or in case of intrinsic biochemical disorders. Encephalopathy can be static as in cases of cerebral palsy or may be progressive as in cases of galactosemia, leukodystrophy, etc.

Etiology

Encephalitis may found in epidemics. In India, some types of encephalitis occur in sporadic or endemic form.

The vast majority of cases of encephalitis are due to viral infections. The common viral agents are—DNA viruses (herpes simplex, cytomegalovirus, Epstein-Barr virus, chickenpox virus), RNA viruses (mumps, measles, rubella, enterovirus), rabies virus, dengue virus, arthropod-borne Japanese 'B' virus and HIV.

The other nonviral infectious agents are fungi (cryptococcus), protozoa (toxoplasmosis, malaria, amebiasis), bacteria (tuberculous, typhoid, shigella), helminths (cysticercosis, hydatid disease), etc.

The encephalopathies are caused by hypoxia, allergy, postvaccinal reaction, fluid electrolyte imbalance, metabolic disorders (hyperbilirubinemia in neonates, hepatic coma, uremia), insecticides, toxic (lead, mercury, carbon monoxide), malignancy, heat stroke, hyperpyrexia, diabetic ketoacidosis and Reye's syndrome.

Pathophysiology

Pathological changes in these conditions are nonspecific. Diffuse cerebral edema, congestion and hemorrhages may present. The neurons may show necrosis and degeneration. Meningeal congestion with mononuclear infiltration, perivascular tissue necrosis and myelin breakdown may found. The ground substance may show glial proliferation. Demyelination, vascular and perivascular destruction, cerebral cortical involvement may develop according to the type of infecting agent.

In case of rabies and herpes simplex infection, specific inclusions are identified. Characteristic pathological changes found in *Falciparum* malaria.

Acute disseminated encephalomyelopathy is more commonly found in children with scattered demyelination throughout the brain or spinal cord.

Clinical Manifestations

Clinical presentations of these conditions may vary depending upon severity of infections, host susceptibility, localization of infectious agent and presence of increased ICP.

The clinical features may show rapid variation from time-to-time with confusing neurological involvements. The features may be apparent or may found as mild abortive type of illness or severe encephalomyelitis.

The onset of the disease is usually sudden but may also be gradual. The patient may present initially with alteration of level of consciousness and convulsions along with high fever, headache, vomiting, mental confusion, irritability and lethargy. The child may present with peculiar behavior, hyperactivity, alteration of speech and ataxia.

Features of increased ICP, meningeal involvement and neurological deficits like ocular palsies, hemiplegia are usually present. Tense bulging fontanel, distended scalp veins, papilledema, hyperventilation, Cheyne-Stoke respiration and bradycardia may develop due to sudden and severe rise of intracranial pressure. Severe disturbances of vital centers resulting respiratory problems and cardiac arrest may found due to herniation of cerebellum through foramen magnum and compression of medulla oblongata. Focal paralysis and focal seizures with focal EEG changes usually found in herpes simplex encephalitis.

Diagnostic Evaluation

Careful history of illness and thorough physical examination are important diagnostic clue. CSF study helps to differentiate the condition from meningitis. Blood examination for sugar, urea, electrolytes and metabolic products are useful guideline for confirmation of diagnosis. Urine examination, toxicologic study, virological study, CT scan, etc. can be done to exclude the exact cause and pathology.

Management

Symptomatic and supportive management are important for better prognosis of these conditions. Initial management should be done promptly to save the life and prevent complications.

Airway clearance is the prime important by positioning and frequent suctioning. Oxygenation to be provided by nasal cannula or bag-mask technique. Mechanical ventilation may be necessary in cardiorespiratory insufficiency. Hydrotherapy and antipyretics is administered to relief from hyperpyrexia. IV fluid therapy and dopamine to be given to treat shock and fluid-electrolyte imbalance. Anticonvulsive drugs may be required to control convulsions. Mannitol or glycerol may be needed to reduce ICP. Steroid (dexamethasone) therapy may be given, though the role of the drug is not established.

Antiviral (acyclovir—30 mg/kg/day in 3 divided doses) is administered in herpes simplex encephalitis. Specific detoxification therapy is given in lead or insecticide poisoning. Cerebral malaria should be treated with antimalarial agent. Antibiotics to be prescribed to prevent secondary infections. Vitamin and mineral supplementation are usually given. Human immunoglobulin (IVIg) may be administered 200 to 500 mg/kg in early stage, which reduces the mortality rate.

Supportive nursing care is vital for the survival of these patients. Special attention to be given on skin care, continuous bladder drainage, care of eyes, change of position and monitoring of patient's condition with features of complications. Nasogastric tube feeding followed by gradual acceptance and intake of nutritional diet is very significant for promotion of better health in recovery period.

Nursing management of these patients should be done same as meningitis and comatose child.

Complications

The common complications following encephalitis or encephalopathy include, shock, cardiorespiratory disorders, epilepsy, paralysis, cerebellar ataxia, mental retardation, obesity and behavioral problems.

Prognosis

Prognosis may vary. The condition may be self-limiting. There may be complete recovery or may have severe neurological sequela. The mortality rate is usually high in complicated cases.

GUILLAIN-BARRÉ SYNDROME (INFECTIVE POLYNEURITIS)

Guillain-Barré (GB) syndrome or postinfectious polyneuritis is an autoimmune disorder following viral infections manifested with symmetric muscle weakness, diminished reflexes and paresthesia or other sensory disturbances resulting from demyelination.

These cases are found in the age group of 5 to 12 years. Neurological manifestations usually starts 2 to 4 weeks after the viral infections. The common offending virus for this condition are mumps, measles, chickenpox, rubella, infectious mononucleosis (EB virus infection), influenza, coxsackie or ECHO virus. Due to the infection, peripheral lymphocytes are sensitized to a protein component of the myelin, then there is alteration of myelin basic protein leading to demyelination.

Clinical Manifestations

Initial features are muscle pain followed by weakness of the proximal as well as distal group of muscle. Muscle involvement is symmetrical. It begins in the lower limbs, then spread to the trunk, upper limbs and face. Muscle tone is reduced resulting hypotonia. Respiratory difficulty occurs due to involvement of intercostal muscles. Respiratory failure may develop in some cases. Involvement of the autonomic nervous system leads to hypertension and urinary retention. Paresthesia, facial nerve involvement and ataxia are found in these patients.

Diagnostic Evaluation

History of illness and physical examination along with neurological assessment are the important basis of diagnosis.

CSF study shows a characteristic albumin-cytological dissociation in majority of the patients within 2 to 3 weeks of illness. There is increased protein level (more than 45 mg/dL), but cell count is usually normal or slightly raised.

This condition should be differentiated from other diseases, like poliomyelitis, transverse myelitis and traumatic neuritis, which are also important cause of acute flaccid paralysis (AFP). The GB syndrome should also be differentiated from cerebellar ataxia, polymyositis and postdiphtheric paralysis.

Electromyography in GB syndrome shows acute denervation of muscles. Motor nerve conduction velocities and sensory conduction times are found slow.

Management

In majority of the patients, the disease is self-limiting. In acute stage, symptomatic and supportive management are important and should be done same as poliomyelitis.

Assisted ventilation and tracheostomy may be needed in some patients with respiratory paralysis. Corticosteroid therapy, plasma exchange therapy and plasmapheresis can be provided.

Intravenous immunoglobin therapy with 200 to 300 mg/kg/day for 5 days gives good response, if it is given within 3 to 4 days of the disease.

Prevention of secondary infection and pressure sore, maintenance of nutrition and hydration, physiotherapy and good nursing care are important supportive measure. The patient may need specialized management is intensive care unit (ICU).

Prognosis

Full recovery is mostly achieved with restoration of full functions. But it may need 6 months to 2 years time. Fatal outcome may occur in case of respiratory paralysis. Many patients may develop chronic relapsing GB syndrome, which may have some residual disability and handicaps.

CONVULSIVE DISORDERS

Convulsion is the involuntary contraction or series of contractions of the voluntary muscles. It occurs due to disturbances of the brain functions resulting from abnormal excessive electrical discharge from the brain. It is manifested by involuntary, motor, sensory, autonomic or psychic phenomenon, alone or in combination. It may be associated with alteration of level of consciousness. Convulsion is also termed as seizure.

Convulsions are more commonly found in infants and children. It is a symptom found in various diseases. The overall incidence in childhood is about 8 percent. It is more commonly found along with cerebral palsy (35%) and in mental retardation (20%).

During convulsions motor movements are frequently observed, which may be associated with loss of consciousness. Generalized tonic-clonic convulsions, i.e. features of major fits are rarely found in neonates. Neonatal convulsions are seen as twitching of the limbs, fluttering of eyelids, conjugate deviations of eyes or as sucking movements. Convulsions should be differentiated from tremors, jitteriness, startle response to stimuli and sudden jerks.

Causes of Convulsive Disorders in Children

Neonatal Period

- Birth asphyxia, hypoxia, birth injury, intraventricular hemorrhage.
- Hypoglycemia, hypocalcemia, hypo- or hypernatremia hypomagnesemia.
- Narcotic drug withdrawal, accidental injection of local anesthetic drug into fetal scalp.
- Septicemia, kernicterus, meningitis, tetanus neonatorum.
- Congenital malformations—microcephaly, porencephaly, arteriovenous fistula.
- Pyridoxine deficiency, inborn errors of metabolism.
- Intrauterine infections such as STORCH infections.

In Infants and Young Children

- Febrile convulsions.
- CNS infections—meningitis, encephalitis, cerebral malaria, tetanus, Reye's syndrome and intrauterine infections.
- Postinfectious and postvaccinal encephalopathy-following acute viral infections (mumps encephalopathy, measles encephalopathy), pertussis vaccination.
- Metabolic disturbances—dyselectrolytemia, dehydration, alkalosis, hypocalcemia, hypoglycemia, inborn errors of metabolism, glycogen storage disease.
- Traumatic—accidental and nonaccidental injury.

- Space occupying lesions in the brain—brain tumor, brain abscess, tuberculoma, cysticercosis.
- Vascular—intracranial hemorrhage, DIC, arteriovenous malformations, hypertension.
- Drug and poisons—phenothiazine, diphenylhydantin salicylates, piperazine.
- Miscellaneous—heat stroke, cerebral anoxia, acute cerebral edema, poisoning, allergy, renal disease, breath holding spells, degenerative disorders.
- Idiopathic epilepsy.

Febrile Convulsions

Febrile convulsion refers to the seizures associated with fever but excluding those related to CNS infections. It is the most common cause of convulsions in early childhood. It is related to abrupt increase in body temperature rather than degree of temperature rise.

Type

The febrile convulsions can be simple benign typical type or atypical complex type.

Typical febrile convulsions: These are generalized rather than focal and last less than 10 minutes. It is usually found in children between 6 months and 5 years of age. The fits occur within 24 hours of the onset of fever and usually single per febrile episode. There is no recurrence before 12 to 18 hours of attack and no residual paralysis of limbs. CSF study and EEG are normal after the attack.

Family history of convulsions is frequently present. Higher incidence occurs in twins and children of consanguineous parents. The condition may have genetic predisposition or may be due to immature neuronal membrane response to rise of body temperature.

Atypical febrile convulsions: They predispose to idiopathic epilepsy. The children may have focal convulsions of more than 20 minutes duration even without significant fever. There may have abnormal EEG for two weeks after the attack.

Management

Management of febrile convulsions should be done to control convulsions, to reduce increased body temperature and to treat the cause of fever, usually ARI.

Anticonvulsive drugs are indicated in prolonged convulsions. Diazepam 0.3 mg/kg IV or 0.5 to 1 mg/kg per rectum or phenobarbital 5 mg/kg IM can be administered.

Antipyretics (paracetamol, mefenamic acid) and tepid sponge should be given to treat fever. Hydration and nutrition status to be maintained. Clearing of airway and oxygen therapy may be needed for some children. Rest, comfortable position and hygienic measures to be provided. Explanation and emotional support to the parent are important along with necessary health teaching.

Investigations to be done to ruled out other possible causes of convulsions and treatment to be planned accordingly.

Prevention of febrile convulsion may be needed. Antipyretics, hydrotherapy and temperature recording are essential for all febrile children. Intermittent prophylaxis with antiepileptic drug (diazepam) is indicated to prevent recurrence of convulsive episodes. Continuous prophylaxis can be given in case of failure of intermittent therapy, or in atypical convulsions, or in family history of epilepsy. Sodium valproate (10–20 mg/kg/day) or phenobarbital (3–5 mg/kg/day) are effective for febrile convulsion prophylaxis. The duration of therapy can be 1 to 2 years or up to 5 years of age.

Prognosis

In typical febrile convulsions prognosis is good. In atypical type, there is chance of development of complications like intellectual impairment, behavioral problems and epilepsy. Chance of recurrence is about 30 to 80 percent. Recurrence is more commonly found in younger age, females, presence of risk factors and in atypical prolonged episodes.

Epilepsy

Epilepsy is recurrent, episodic, paroxysmal transient disturbances of brain function due to abnormal electrical activity of the neurons. It is manifested as abnormal motor, sensory or psychomotor phenomena and often with impaired or loss of consciousness. It may be idiopathic or organic.

Almost one percent of all children have epilepsy with highest incidence in the preschool years. Family history is commonly present with probable genetic predisposition.

Pathophysiology

The basic mechanism of all convulsions appears to be prolonged depolarization, causing brain cells to become overactive and to discharge in a sudden violent disorderly manner. This paroxysmal burst of electrical energy spreads to adjacent areas of the brain and may jump to distant areas of CNS resulting in a seizure. The biochemical basis of seizures is not completely understood.

Classification of Epilepsy

Clinically epilepsy can be broadly classified into two groups, i.e. generalized or partial.

Generalized Seizures

a. Tonic-clonic seizures (Grand mal)
b. Absence seizures:
   i. Typical (petit mal)
   ii. Atypical
c. Atopic seizures (drop attacks)
d. Myoclonic seizures.

Partial Seizures

a. Simple partial seizures (with elementary symptoms and no impaired consciousness)
   i. With motor signs (Jacksonians or focal motor).
   ii. With somatosensory or special sensory, i.e. visual or auditory.
   iii. With autonomic manifestations (abdominal epilepsy)
b. Complex partial seizures—Manifested with impaired consciousness and with automatism. It includes psychomotor or temporal lobe seizures.

Clinical Manifestations

Generalized tonic-clonic seizures (Grand mal type): It is most frequent form of childhood epilepsy. Onset is abrupt. The classical form has four phases, i.e. an aura, tonic spasm, clonic phase and postictal phase.

An aura, a peculiar sensation with dizziness occurs in about one-third epileptic children before tonic-clonic seizure. It is a transitory premonitory symptom which the child may recognize as the impending convulsions and adopt measures for self-protection. Aura may be sensory, visceral, motor or autonomic.

In *tonic spasm phase* child's entire body becomes stiff, face may become pale and distorted, eyes fixed in one position, back may be arched, head turned to backward or in one side, arms are usually flexed and hands are clenched. The child usually falls on the ground from standing or sitting position and may utter a peculiar piercing cry. The child loses consciousness and having frothy discharge from mouth due to inability to swallow the saliva. Due to spasm of respiratory muscles, there is ineffective breathing and cyanosis. Pulse may become weak and irregular. Duration of this stage may be about 30 seconds. These features occur due to muscular spasm and rigidity.

The *clonic phase* is manifested with rhythmic jerky movements due to alternating contractions of muscle groups following the tonic state, which usually start in one part and become generalized including the facial muscles. The child may pass stool and urine involuntarily and may have tongue or cheek bite due to sudden forceful contraction of abdominal muscles and jaw. The duration of this stage may be few minutes to even a few hours (in status epilepticus).

In the *postictal or postconvulsive state*, the child is usually become sleepy, confused or exhausted or perform automatic actions and may complain headache. The child may not be able to recall the episode and rarely may develop a transient paresis.

Tonic-clonic fits may not occur in children and may be predominatly tonic or clonic phase.

Absence seizures (Petit mal): Absence seizures rarely appears before 5 years of age. It is manifested as the followings:
- The child may loss contact with the environment for a few seconds.
- The child may appear as staring or day dreaming.
- The child may discontinue the activity suddenly (e.g. reading, writing) and may resume the same activity when the seizure is over.
- Atypical absence seizure may present as rolling of the eyes, nodding of the head, slight hand movements and smacking of lips.

The child appears normal and not aware of having the episode in the postseizure state. The duration is usually 5 to 10 seconds and frequency varies from one to two per month to hundred times each day. The precipitating factors include hyperventilation, fatigue, hypoglycemia and stress situation.

Status Epilepticus

It is a state of continuing or recurrent seizures that prolonged for more than 30 minutes or occur in a series without regaining consciousness in between attacks. It is a medical emergency as cerebral damage may occur due to prolonged cerebral hypoxia or hypoglycemia. In postictal state, the child may have ataxia, aphasia and mental sluggishness. Mortality rate due to this condition is about 4 percent. The child may have cardiorespiratory arrest or aspiration of vomitus. Residual neurological deficits may develop in 9 percent cases. Todd's paresis or postictal paralysis may result due to metabolic exhaustion of epileptic neurons.

Partial Seizures

Partial seizures account for 60 percent of convulsive disorders in children. The common causes are inflammatory granulomas, atropic lesions, birth asphyxia, head injury, neoplasms and neurocysticercosis. Partial seizures can be classified as—(a) Simple partial seizures (20%) (b) Complex partial seizures (25%) and (c) Partial with secondary generalization seizures (15%). Partial seizures may be found as psychomotor or temporal lobe seizures and as focal motor (Jacksonian seizures) or focal sensory.

Myoclonic Seizures (Infantile Spasms)

This seizures occurs in infants usually between 3 to 8 months age and second in incidence only to generalized seizures in this age group. It is almost always associated with cerebral abnormalities and mental retardation. The child presents with sudden forceful myoclonic contractions involving the muscles of trunk, neck and extremities. The contractions can be flexor type or extensor type or mixed. The duration is usually less than one minute. Frequency may varies from a few to hundred attacks per day. Usually this type of seizure disappear spontaneously by the age of 4 years, but in some causes generalized or other type of seizures may develop.

Neonatal Seizures

Seizures are most common in neonatal period due to poor myelination and incomplete dendritic arborization. Neonatal seizures present as (a) subtle (b) multifocal clonic (c) focal clonic (d) generalized tonic and (e) myoclonic types.

Subtle seizures may present with eyeblinking, fluttering and buccolingual movements. There may be pedaling or automatic movements. The common causes of subtle seizures are perinatal asphyxia, sepsis and bacterial meningitis. Focal clonic seizures are caused by metabolic disorders like hypoglycemia, hypocalcemia and due to intracranial bleeding. Tonic and myoclonic types develop due to malformations and dysgenetic state. About one-third cases are multifactorial and idiopathic. It is important to detect the exact cause of neonatal seizures for appropriate management.

Diagnosis of Convulsive Disorders

Careful history with description of the convulsive episodes along with detailed physical and neurological examination help in clinical diagnosis of the disease and to differentiate it from hysterical attacks.

Confirm diagnosis can be done by examination of blood, urine and CSF, specially on the basis of suspected cause.

EEG is the most useful investigation in case of epilepsy. Cranial imaging like X-ray skull, CT scan, PET or SPECT scan and MRI are also very useful diagnostic approach. Metabolic or cytogenetic studies is indicated in case of suspected inborn error of metabolism.

Management of Epilepsy/Convulsive Disorders

Management of convulsive disorder depends upon the identified cause. The management mainly done with drug therapy, diet therapy and surgery, if indicated. Emotional support, psychosocial rehabilitation and vocational guidance are also important aspects of management. Long-term management may continue over 1 to 4 years and needs supervision and explanation for treatment compliance.

Drug Therapy

The selection of antiepileptic drugs depends upon age, type of seizure and economical status. The commonly used drugs are:

1. Phenobarbital—3 to 5 mg/kg/day in 1 or 2 divided doses and indicated in tonic-clonic, partial, akinetic and febrile convulsions.
2. Diphenylhydantoin—5 to 8 mg/kg/day in 2 divided doses, indicated in tonic-clonic, atonic, akinetic and partial seizures.
3. Carbamazepine—10 to 20 mg/kg/day in 2 to 3 divided doses and indicated in tonic-clonic, atonic, akinetic and partial seizures.
4. Diazepam—0.2 mg/kg/dose IV or per rectal is indicated in status epilepticus.
5. Sodium valproate—15 to 20 mg/kg/day in 3 to 4 divided doses is indicated as broadspectrum anticonvulsive agent.
6. Ethosuximide—10 to 20 mg/kg/day in 2 divided doses is indicated in absence seizure.

Usually single drug is used but if fails to relieve seizures than addition of a second drug is needed. Duration of treatment may vary, usually 2 to 4 years, but mentally retarded children may need longer duration. Side effects of the drugs should be observed and special precautions to be followed during administration and thereafter.

Success of treatment depends upon regularity in taking drugs. Duration will be decided and must be informed to the parent or caregiver.

Diet Therapy

Ketogenic diet may be given to raise the seizure threshold with calculated amount of proteins and fats without carbohydrates. This diet makes the child ketotic as fat is used for energy production rather than carbohydrate. It seems that ketones may inhibit the seizure.

The child should not be given IV fluid with dextrose and strict fluid restriction to be maintained.

Surgical Management

Neurosurgery is indicated in some cases of convulsive disorders, especially in anatomical lesions like brain tumor, hematoma and in medically intractable seizure disorders.

The possible surgical interventions include corpus callosotomy, focal resection of parts of cerebral cortex such as temporal lobe, extratemporal regions involved as epileptogenic foci.

Nursing management

A. *Nursing assessment:* Detailed subjective and objective data to be collected to formulate nursing diagnosis and to plan nursing interventions.

B. *Nursing diagnoses:* The important nursing diagnoses include the followings:
- Risk for injury related to convulsive episodes.
- Ineffective breathing related to spasms of respiratory muscles.
- Social isolations related to misconceptions.
- Altered self-esteem related to lack of control over seizures.

- Knowledge deficit related to long-term care of seizure disorder.

C. Nursing interventions
1. Ensuring safety during seizures:
   i. Provide preventive measures to protect the child from injury by removal of hard objects, sharp things or toys from the child and placing child on floor or bed.
   ii. Side rails of the bed or crib to be padded.
   iii. Removing oropharyngeal secretions by suctioning and turning head to one side (if possible). Suction machine to be kept ready beforehand.
   iv. Oxygen therapy to be given and all emergency equipment to be kept ready to manage cardiorespiratory problems.
   v. Close observation and frequent monitoring of child's condition for vital signs, airway, breathing patterns, preseizure events, presence of aura, types of movements during seizures, sites of contractions or twitching, eye movements, pupil size, bladder incontinence, pallor/cyanosis/flushing, teeth clenched, tongue bite, frothy discharge/vomitus aspirations, level of consciouness, neurological status and postictal events (memory, paralysis, speech alteration, restlessness, behavior change), etc.
   vi. Administering prescribed medications, IV/IM or per rectal or oral, as indicated.
   vii. Following special instructions about diet, rest and activities.
2. Preventing respiratory arrest and aspiration:
   i. Loosen the clothing around neck and placing the child flat.
   ii. Avoid restraining the child and not to give anything in between teeth or in the mouth, when the teeth are clenched during convulsions.
   iii. Clear airway, remove secretions, turn head to one side during seizures and on sidelying position in postictal stage.
   iv. Record the events in details.
3. *Promoting socialization:* Instructing the parent to allow the child to perform normal life as possible with some restricted activities like, not to climb high places, or to avoid swimming and exertional activities. An identity card should be kept with the child.
4. *Strengthening self-esteem:* Explanation, reassurance, encouraging to discuss about feeling, promoting independence in self-care and family counseling are important for child and parents to improve their self-esteem.
5. *Providing health teaching:* Necessary related health teaching to be given with special emphasis on continuation of medications, care during convulsions, diet therapy, restricted activities, misconception regarding the disease and follow-up.

CEREBRAL PALSY

Cerebral palsy (CP) is a group of nonprogressive disorders resulting from malfunctions of the motor centers and pathways of brain. It is a noncurable and nonfatal condition due to damage of the growing brain before or during birth. It is most common cause of crippling in children. It's severty is ranging from minor incapacitation to total handicap. Mental retardation is associated in about 25 to 50 percent of cases of CP. Other associated handicapped conditions are epilepsy, orthopedic deformities, partial or complete deafness, blindness and psychological disturbances. The prevalence rate is about 4 per 1000 live births. Mild cases are likely to be missed.

Etiology

The cerebral palsy occurs due to multiple risk factors. It is not a familial disease. Genetic factors may have influence in this condition. It may result from maldevelopment and disorganization of the brain. Perinatal hypoxia, intraventricular hemorrhages, birth trauma, acid-base imbalance, indirect hyperbilirubinemia, kernicterus, metabolic disturbances and intrauterine or acquired infections, Low birth weight and congenital malformations (especially of CNS and chromosomal) are considered as important etiological factors. These factors may operate prenatally, during delivery and in postnatal period. Birth asphyxia, previously believed to be a leading cause of CP, but at present, considered as uncommon etiology.

Pathology

In mild cerebral palsy, the brain appears normal, but may be under weight and has sparse subcortical white matter and sparse nerve fibers.

In severe cerebral palsy, there may be various pathological lesions like cerebral atrophy, cavity formation in subcortical white matter, atrophy of basal ganglia, leukomalacia, porencephaly, microcephaly, cerebellar lesions, vascular occlusions and gliosis.

Types/Classification of Cerebral Palsy

Based on Motor Deficit and Distribution of Handicaps

Cerebral palsy can be classified based on motor deficit and distribution of handicaps:
- Spastic cerebral palsy (pyramidal CP).
- Extrapyramidal cerebral palsy (Dyskinetic CP)
- Atonic cerebral palsy (cerebellar CP).
- Mixed type CP.

Classification According to Severity

Mild cerebral palsy (20%): Patients are ambulatory, fine movements are impaired only.

Moderate cerebral palsy (50%): These children achieve ambulation by self-help. There is impaired gross motor, fine motor and speech development.

Severe cerebral palsy (30%): The children present with multiple defects and unable to perform usual activities of daily living.

Clinical Manifestations

Early signs of cerebral palsy include one or more of the followings. These include asymmetric movements, listlessness, irritability, difficulty in feeding or swallowing or poor sucking with tongue thrust, excessive high pitched or feeble cry, poor head control and slow weight gain.

Late signs include one or more of the followings. These are delayed gross motor development, persistent infantile reflexes, weakness, abnormal postures, drooling, recurrent infections, constipation or incontinence of stool, malocclusion of teeth, caries teeth, delayed or defective speech and evidence of mental retardation.

Common associated problems are seizures, GER (Gastroesophageal reflux), visual defects (coloboma, squint, blindness, refractive errors), hearing impairment, perceptual disorders, mental retardation, speech disorder, growth failure and behavioral problems.

Special Features of Different Types of CP

Spastic Cerebral Palsy

It is most common type (65%). There is defect in the cortical motor area or pyramidal tract which causes abnormally strong tonus of certain muscle groups.

Depending upon the involvement of spasticity, the child may behave quadriplegia, paraplegia, hemiplegia, triplegia, diplegia or monoplegia. Early diagnostic features are persistent neonatal reflexes, feeding difficulties and scissoring of lower limbs due to spasms of adductor muscles. Other features are opisthotonic posture, pseudobulbar palsy, restricted voluntary movements, deep tendon reflexes become brisk, positive ankle clonus and convulsions. The child may have multiple handicaps and neurological deficits with behavioral problems. Permanent contractures may develop without muscle training.

Extrapyramidal Cerebral Palsy

It is found in about 30 percent of patients of all CP. The child presents with dyskinesia, like athetosis, choreiform movements, dystonia, tremor and rigidity. Arms, legs, neck and trunk may be involved. Mental retardation and deafness are commonly found as associated problems. The lesions of the extrapyramidal tract and basal ganglia are considered as the cause of involuntary, uncoordinated, uncontrolable movements of the muscle groups. Cerebral damage due to kernicterus is considered as the etiological factors.

Atonic Cerebral Palsy (Cerebellar Involvement)

This type occurs in less than 5 percent of the patients. Hypotonia and hyporeflexia are common features. Ataxia and tremors appear by the age of two years.

Mixed Type Cerebral Palsy

Some patients with CP have features of diffuse neurological involvement of mixed type.

Diagnostic Evaluation

Details history related to the condition is most important for diagnosis. These should include history of prenatal and perinatal period including apgar score, resuscitation, birth injury, etc. History of neonatal period with physical, neurological and developmental assessment are significant diagnostic evidence. Language development, personal-social behavior and learning disability should be examined along with gross motor and fine motor development.

Special diagnostic approach should includes CT scan, MRI, EEG, psychometry test, examination of blood and urine.

Prevention of Cerebral Palsy

Prevention of cerebral palsy can be done by adequate antenatal care with prevention of maternal infections, fetal problems and perinatal hazards. Prevention of birth injury, perinatal asphyxia, neonatal hyperbilirubinemia are important measures for prevention of CP. Early diagnosis and prompt initiation of appropriate management of etiological factors along with the condition, reduce the incidence of neurological, psychosocial and emotional handicaps of the child.

Management

Management should be planned in a team approach. Coordination among team members is needed between pediatricians, pediatric surgeons, pediatric nurse specialist, physical therapist, occupational therapist, speech therapist, pediatric social worker, child psychologist, teacher, special educator, family members and parents. The holistic approach is required to achieve fullest possible functional ability and skill in keeping the child with developmental age.

Management includes drug therapy, physiotherapy, surgical corrections of deformities, occupational therapy and rehabilitation.

Drug therapy: It is indicated in symptomatic management for the child with CP. The commonly used drugs are— diazepam for spasticity, strychnine for hypotonia, chlordiazepoxide or levodopa for athetosis, carbamazepine for dystonia, anticonvulsives for epilepsy, tranquilizers for behavioral problems and muscle relaxants to imporove muscular functions.

Surgical correction: It may be needed for bony deformities and stabilizing the joints or relieving the contractures. Selective dorsal rhizotomy can be done to decrease spasticity. Orthopedic support can be provided by splints or orthotic devices.

Physiotherapy: It is effective to prevent contractures, to promote relaxation of spastic muscles and for maintenance of posture. Occupational therapy can be arranged as some simple occupation (e.g. typing) so that when they grow up, they can earn something for their own. Positive application of certain repetitive movements of legs, hands and fingers can be used during occupational training which also help to relax spastic muscles. The child should be trained in self-care like feeding, dressing, bathing, brushing, etc. Family support and community support are vital for socioeconomic rehabilitation of these handicapped children.

Nursing Management

Nursing assessment: It should includes the detection of ability to perform activities of daily living (ADL), developmental milestones, neurological reflexes, feeding behavior, nutritional status, bladder and bowel habits, problem related to vision, hearing and language, associated health hazards or congenital anomalies, present problems, parent-child interactions, treatment compliance, etc. Nursing diagnoses should be formulated accordingly to plan and to provide nursing interventions.

Nursing interventions: The nursing care of a child with cerebral palsy should include specialized care in the following aspects along with routine care of a child.
1. *Increasing mobility and minimizing deformity:* These should be achieved by encouraging exercise as directed by physical therapist, use of splints or brace to facilitate muscle control, motivation for practicing self-care and arranging specially prepared self-care articles (long handed spoon, sponge handle toothbrush, etc.) Play materials to be provided for improvement of co-ordinated movement. Good body alignment to be maintained to prevent contractures. Adequate rest period, avoidance of exiting events, administration of prescribed drugs,

avoidance of stress and frustration and continuation of physical therapy are also important measures.
2. *Maximizing growth and development:* Planning daily care with special approach for feeding, sleeping, toileting, play, physical therapy, special interest of the child, safety measures and emotional needs according to the level of the child's disability.

Allowing independence and self-help with comfortable environment (both physical and emotional) and educational opportunities by special schooling or arranging special training. Strengthening family process by encouraging to express feelings, frustrations and need for help for continuation of care of the child.
3. *Protecting the child* from physical injury and providing security by good parent child relationship and family support.
4. *Teaching the parents* and family members about home based care and continuation of treatment with regular follow-up. Information to be given about the available facilities for specialized care of the children with CP, (e.g. spastic society, Institution for cerebral palsy or handicapped children, etc). Parents also need guidance from social workers or community health nurse regarding the continued care and management of these children.

MENTAL RETARDATION

Mental retardation refers to the most severe general lack of cognitive and problem solving skills. It is also known as cognitive developmental delay. It is significant subaverage general intellectual functioning existing concurrently with deficits in adaptive behaviors and manifested during the developmental periods. The child presents with low learning capacity, poor maturation and inadequate social adjustment.

In general population 2 to 3 percent children are mentally retarded. About 3/4th of total cases are only mild type and 5 percent are having severe to profound mental retardation.

Classification

Mental retardation is classified depending upon IQ level. IQ or intelligence quotient is calculated by the formula:

$$= \frac{\text{Assessed mental age}}{\text{Chronological age}} \times 100$$

The mental retardation can be classified as:
- Mild mental retardation with IQ level 51 to 70.
- Moderate mental retardation with IQ level 36 to 50.
- Severe mental retardation with IQ level 21 to 35.
- Profound mental retardation with IQ level below 20.

The children with IQ level between 71 to 90 is considered as borderline intelligence who are vulnerable to learning problems and usually sorted out. They need special help in regular classes in school. They are not included as mentally handicaps.

Mild mentally retarded children need some special class placement and can attain only up to 4th to 6th standards at school levels. They are designated as "educable".

Moderate mentally retarded children can able to attain up to 2nd class standards in academic skills. They are considered as "trainable". They can learn maximum up to self-care activities.

Severe mentally retarded children can learn only self-care and simple conversational skills. They need much supervision and considered as "custodial".

Profound mentally retarded children can able to learn very minimal self-care abilities and language. Total supervision is must for them and they are also considered as "custodial".

Some degrees of education and training are possible for all groups of mentally retarded children, even in severe and profound mental handicaps.

Etiology of Mental Retardation

The etiology of mental retardation are multifactorial and may be combination of medical, sociocultural and psychological factors. Approximately in 50 percent of mentally retarded children no identifiable organic or biological cause can be found. The predisposing factors of the condition include poor-socioeconomic status, low birth weight, preterm birth advanced maternal age and consanguineous marriage.

The potential contributory factors or the possible identifible causes of mental retardation can be as follows:

a. Genetic syndromes—For example, Down's syndrome, Fragile 'X' syndrome, galactosemia, Klinefelter syndrome, etc.
b. Congenital anomalies—For example, congenital hydrocephalus, microcephaly, cranial malformations, craniosynostosis.
c. Intrauterine influences—For example, maternal infections, and exposure to teratogens, placental insufficiency, pre-eclampsia, antepartum hemorrhages, etc.
d. Perinatal conditions—For example, birth trauma, perinatal asphyxia, intracranial hemorrhage, prematurity, low-birth weight, etc.
e. Postnatal conditions—For example, CNS infections, kernicterus, head injury, toxic or postvaccinal encephalopathy, thrombosis of cerebral vessels, iodine deficiency, hypothyroidism, severe PEM, metabolic disorders, PKU, galactosemia, etc.
f. Environmental and sociocultural factors—For example, poverty, broken family, faulty parenting, child abuse and neglect, parental psychopathology, and environmental deprivation.

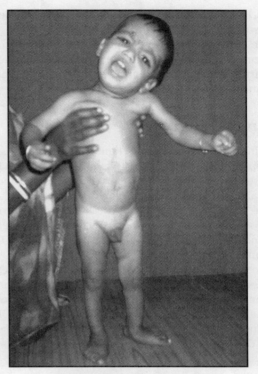

Fig. 21.2: Mental retardation

Clinical Manifestations

The child with mental retardation presents with failure to achieve age appropriate development to some degrees. The mental age is below the chronological age. There is poor maturation with learning difficulties and inappropriate family and social adjustment (Fig. 21.2).

In infancy, the child manifested with poor feeding, weak or uncoordinated sucking leading to poor weight gain, delayed or decreased visual atertness and auditory response, reduced spontaneous activity, delayed head and trunk control, hypotonia or spastic muscle tone and poor mother-child interaction.

In toddler, the presentations are delayed speech and language disabilities, delayed motor milestones (standing, walking), failure to achieve independence (like self-feeding, dressing and toilet training), short attention span and distractibility, clumsiness, hyperactivity, poor memory, poor concentration, emotional instability, sleep problems, impulsiveness and low frustration tolerance.

Convulsions are commonly found with mental retardation. Associated defects of musculoskeletal system, vision and hearing are commonly present. Congenital anomalies are often associated. Neurodegenerative disorders, psychiatric illness, emotional problems and cerebral palsy may be found along with mental retardation.

The presence of specific physical characteristics like microcephaly, Down's syndrome, cretinism, mucopolysaccharidosis helps to diagnosis the mental retardation at birth and infancy.

Diagnostic Evaluation

The clinical diagnosis can be done with detailed history of developmental period along with family history, birth history and history of past illnesses, supported by findings of thorough physical examination and neurological examination.

The important diagnostic measures to confirm the diagnosis of mental retardation are IQ test and detection of associated diseases or etiological factors like Down's syndrome, cretinism, etc.

The investigations may include urine test for metabolic diseases, urine chromatography, chromosomal studies, hormonal assay, enzyme estimation, serological test to detect intrauterine infections, CSF study, X-ray skull, EEG, CT scan, MRI, angiography, etc. In suspected cases prenatal diagnosis can be done by amniocentesis.

Management

Mentally retarded child needs management in multidisciplinary team approach. Adequate diagnostic facilities to detect associated problems and appropriate management of the specific condition should be arranged.

Family members and parents need counseling regarding various aspects of the condition and necessary management. Parents should be explained, informed and discussed about the long-term care at home situation according to the child's IQ level and associated problems. Importance to be given on promotion of self-care ability and independence of the child. Routine basic care, immunization, growth monitoring, nutritional requirements and tender loving care to be provided to the child. Necessary drug therapy should be discussed with the parents. Psychological and emotional support needed for parents and family members. The child needs love affection, appreciation, discipline and minimal criticism for tender loving care from parents and family members.

Special educational arrangement and available facilities should be discussed with the parents. The child may be send to day care center or special schools or vocational centers or workshop. The child needs support to develop potentials to the maximum and to become independent as possible for self-help.

Preventive Management

Prevention of mental retardation can be done with the following measures:

- Welfare of the girl child should be emphasized as they are the soil and seed of the future generation. Care of the girl child needs special attention from the young age with good nutrition and immunization especially for rubella. Iodine deficiency should be prevented. Early marriage and teenage pregnancy should be avoided. Consanguineous marriages to be prevented. 'Healthy mother can give birth of the healthy child'—this information should be propagated.
- Genetic counseling is the important measures to prevent genetic and chromosomal abnormalities. Advanced maternal age above 35 years is the risk condition for Down's syndrome and associated mental retardation. It should be prevented by health education.
- Good obstetrical care is important to prevent etiological factors related to mental retardation.
- Essential neonatal care to be provided to prevent neonatal complications like CNS infections, kernicterus, etc which can cause mental retardation.
- Prevention and management of low birth weight, preterm delivery, PEM and iodine deficiency during infancy and childhood should be emphasized.
- Whole cell pertussis vaccine should be avoided to the children with history of neurological disease.
- Neonatal assessment and screening of metabolic disorders, congenital hypothyroidism or other congenital anomalies should be done in suspected cases. Routine physical and neurological assessment should be done for all neonates and suspected infants before the screening procedures.

DOWN'S SYNDROME (MONGOLISM)

Down's syndrome is the most common chromosomal disorder and most common identifiable cause of mental retardation. It is a condition associated with a variety of congenital anomalies. The incidence of Down's syndrome in India is about 2.2 per 1000 live births which is higher than the average. Overall figure of 1 in 600 for all races.

Types

There are three known types of Down's syndrome
1. Trisomy-21 (95% of all cases). It is also called as Trisomy 'G'. There are total 47 chromosomes instead of 46. The extra chromosome presents in 21st pair. The origin of extra chromosome is either from mother or from father. In most cases, it is from mother especially of advanced age pregnancy. It occurs due to nondisjunction, i.e failure of chromosomal separation during meiosis. A mongol baby is generally first born or the last born in multigravida mother.
2. Translocation of chromosome 21 with 14 or may be with 13 or 15 (4% of all cases). In this type total number of

chromosome remains normal (46), though one is large and atypical.

3. Mosaicism (1%). It may occur rarely. The affected child has two number of chromosomes and other cell line trisomic for the number 21 chromosome. It occur due to postconception error in chromosomal division during mitosis.

Clinical Manifestations

The children with Down's syndrome have a characteristics look like mongolian races, i.e Chinese, Tibetans, Japanese, so they are called as "mongol" and the condition as mongolism.

The affected child is cheerful, affectionate, friendly, fond of music and has grossly delayed milestones with both physical and mental retardation. The maximum mental age is around 8 years and average IQ is about 40. So these children were previously termed as " Cheerful idiot".

The physical characteristics of a child with Down's syndrome are as follows:

- Head is small (microcephaly) with flat occiput.
- There is typical facial grimace on crying.
- Face is flat with upwards slanting of eyes and epicanthal folds at inner angles. Oblique palpebral fissure is obvious only when the eyes are open. Brushfields spots, i.e. small whitish spots near the periphery of the iris, and late onset cataract may present.
- Nose is short with flat nasal bridge. This gives an impression of increased distance between the eyes along with epicanthal folds and termed as pseudohypertelorism.
- Ears are small, low-set and may have deformed ear lobes, as small or absence.
- Mouth shows high arched palate, malocclusion of teeth or small teeth with protruded and furrowed tongue (Scrotal tongue) in the small oral cavity.
- Neck is short and broad with low hairline and may seems that head is almost resting on the trunk.
- Hands are short and broad, little fingers are short and incurved due to hypoplasia of middle fingers (clinodactyly). There is single transverse crease (simian crease) in the palm in spite of 3 major creases.
- In the feet, there is wide gap between the big and second toes (sandle gap). A deep crease is found on the sole starting between the big and second toes and extending towards heel.
- Typical dermatoglyphics are observed in these children.
- There is significant generalized hypotonia with hyperflexibility of joints. Skin is usually dry and rough.
- Associated congenital heart disease are commonly (40%) found. GI malformations and Hirschsprung's disease are also seen in these children.
- Other associated and potential problems are visual defects, hearing problems, speech and communication disorders, hypothyroidism, short stature, obesity, growth retardation and recurrent respiratory infections. The mydriatic effect of atropine instilled into the eye of a child with Down's syndrome is exaggerated.

Diagnostic Evaluation

Physical characteristics of the child with Down's syndrome are sufficient to diagnose the condition. The confirm diagnosis is done with the help of chromosomal study, dermatoglyphic findings and radiological findings of bony abnormalities.

Antenatal diagnosis can be done in suspected cases by amniocentesis, chromosomal study, estimation of alpha-fetoprotein, hCG and estriol assay. USG can be helpful to reveal the bony (femur, humerus) abnormalities and nuchal thickening.

Management

There is no specific management of Down's syndrome. Symptomatic treatment for infections, nutritional deficiencies and associated congenital malformations are important measures. Daily supportive care should be provided to prevent acquired health hazards. Physiotherapy, speech therapy, special educational facilities, occupational training can be helpful for some children. According to the IQ level, the child can be trained in self-care or parents should provide daily routine care for health maintenance.

Parental counseling is significant aspect of management, especially when they are planning to have another child. When parents are normal and the child has trisomy 21, the risk or recurrence in subsequent siblings are only one percent. If the mother is a carrier of the translocated chromosomes, there is 10 percent chance of recurrence in the future offspring. If the father is the carrier, there is only 5 percent risk or recurrence.

Prognosis

Prognosis of the child with Down's syndrome depends upon the presence of associated condition and management facilities. The major causes of early mortality is mainly congenital heart disease. Respiratory infections are another life-threatening condition. These children are prone to develop juvenile type of chronic myeloid leukemia.

NEURAL TUBE DEFECTS (MYELODYSPLASIA, DYSRAPHISM)

Neural tube defects are the congenital malformations of the CNS resulting from a defective closure of the neural tube during early embryogenesis between 3rd and 4th week of intrauterine life. It involves the defects in the skull, vertebral column, the spinal cord and other portion of CNS. It occurs in about 1 to 5 per 1000 live births. Risk in second sibling is high. The defect is usually obvious at birth and varies in severity from spina bifida occulta to anencephaly.

Etiology

The exact cause of neural tube defect is not known, but the triggering factors are maternal radiation exposures, drug (valproic acid), exposure to chemicals, malnutrition especially folic acid deficiency and genetic determinant. These factors alone or in one or the other combination, adversely affect the normal development of the neural tube, thereby causing the defect.

Types of Neural Tube Defects

Spina Bifida

Spina bifida is one of the most common anomaly of neural tube development seen in infants. It is the congenital defect of the spinal column due to failure of the fusion of vertebral arches with or without protrusion of the meninges and dysplasia of the spinal cord. It is the malformation of the spine in which the posterior portion of the lamina of the vertebra fails to close. It can be only a small deformed lamina separated by a midline gap or may be a complete absence of lamina.

Spina bifida can be broadly divided into two groups, spina bifida occulta and spina bifida cystica. Spina bifida cystica is commonly found as meningocele and meningomyelocele.

Spina Bifida Occulta

It is most frequent and most benign neural tube defect. There is defective closure of the posterior arch and laminae of the vertebrae, usually L5 and S1. There is no protrusion of the meninges. But the dysplasia of the spinal cord is a prominent feature. Most of the cases are asymptomatic.

Some children present with cutaneous lesions over the defect, as tuft of hairs, nevus, lipoma, hemangioma, dermal sinus or as dimple in the skin. There may be intraspinal lesions like dermoid cyst, intramedullary lipoma, etc. which produces neurological deficit.

The symptomatic children usually present after 6 to 8 years of age with any of the followings (a) progressive deformity of the foot, (b) changes in micturition pattern, (c) alteration in the gait and (d) trophic ulcers on the toes and feet. Other significant anomalies of the spinal cord (syringomyelia, diastematomyelia, tethered cord, etc.) may be found in association of the condition. Progressive neurological deficits require surgical correction of the defect. Laminectomy is done and the intraspinal lesion is excised. Operation can be

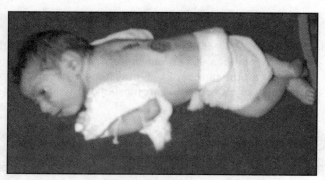

Fig. 21.3: Meningocele *(For color version, see Plate 6)*

done even before neurological deficit appears in selected cases. Myelo-CT scan and MRI help to confirm the diagnosis before operation.

Meningocele (Fig. 21.3)

It is hernial protrusion of the meninges through a midline defect in the posterior vertebral arch. It forms a fluctuating cystic swelling filled with CSF and covered by a thin transparent membrane or with skin. It transilluminates easily. It is generally found in the lower back, i.e. lumbosacral region. It may also be found in the thoracic region and in the skull (cranial meningocele). The spinal cord and nerve roots are usually normal. There is no dysplasia of the spinal cord and the child may found asymptomatic. It is relatively uncommon lesion (4–5%). The symptomatic child may present weakness of the legs or lack of sphincter control. Associated anomalies like hydrocephalus, tethered cord may be present. As the skin or membrane covering is thin, CSF leakage may present and there is chance of infections.

Head circumference of the child should be measured daily and anterior fontanel to be checked for bulging or widening. These help to detect the development of hydrocephalus. The meningocele sac should be protected from infection and injury. The infant should be positioned on the abdomen to avoid pressure on the sac. If the sac is not covered with skin, it should be protected with sterile moist dressing. X-ray spine and skull, CT scan can be done to determine the defect and associated anomalies.

Surgical closure of the sac should be done as early as possible to prevent infections. Prognosis is generally good unless hydrocephalus and neurological deficits are develop.

Meningomyelocele (Myelomeningocele) (Fig. 21.4)

It is a midline cystic sac of meninges with spinal tissue and CSF, which herniates through a defect in the posterior vertebral arch. It is one of the most common lesion (90 to

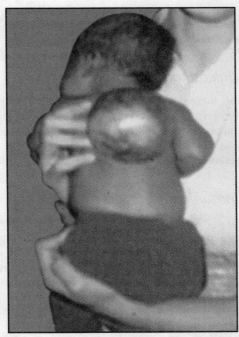

Fig. 21.4: Myelomeningocele *(For color version, see Plate 7)*

95%) and can be present anywhere on the midline in the back, but lumbosacral area is the most common site. There is dysplasia of the spinal cord and this is always accompanied by neurological deficit. These can be found as two types—(a) myelocele (open type) and (b) myelomeningocele (closed type), the most common cystic lesion containing neural tissue which may be dysplastic spinal cord or nerve fibers. Transillumination is not easy.

The child with myelomeningocele may present with flaccid paralysis, absence of sensation and drop reflex. Postural abnormalities like club foot, subluxation of hips may be present. Spasticity and hyperactive reflexes may present in thoracic or cervical myelomeningocele. Hydrocephalus is usually associated with this anomaly. Musculoskeletal deformity and hydrosyringomyelia may occur in neonates. Later, in older children, contractures of joints, scoliosis and kyphosis may develop. There is risk or infection of CNS and rupture of sac.

Primary diagnosis is done by clinical manifestations. Associated anomalies can be detected by X-ray, CT scan, MRI and complete neurological assessment. Routine blood and urine examination are also necessary. Prenatal diagnosis can be done by amniocentesis and estimation of alpha fetoprotein.

Management of this condition can be done by surgical correction of the defect and essential care of the infant. Afterwards correction of musculoskeletal deformities and regulation of bladder and bowel functions should

be performed. Additional supportive measures include prevention of injury and infection of the sac by appropriate positioning with protective covering (sterile wet dressing), prevention of skin breakdown and monitoring of signs of hydrocephalus (head circumference, fontanel, feeding behavior). Other measures are provision of adequate nutrition, promotion of urinary elimination and bowel regularity, prevention of leg or hip deformities and other complications. Perioperative care, promotion of growth and development, emotional and psychological support, health teaching regarding care of the child are also important aspect of management.

Anencephaly

Anencephaly is a congenital absence of cranial vault with the cerebral hemisphere completely missing or reduced to small masses. Various congenital anomalies can be associated with this condition, like congenital heart disease, cleft palate, etc. This condition is incompatible with life, death usually occurs with a week or two of birth.

Encephalocele

It is a sac like protrusion of meninges with brain substance (cerebral cortex, cerebellum, or part of brainstem) herniating through a congenital bony defect in the skull. It is commonly found in the midline and in the occipital or parietal area. It may also found on frontal bone, in the orbit or in the nose. The size may vary from small to as big as size of head. The survived child may develop hydrocephalus, visual problems, seizures, microcephaly and mental retardation. Associated congenital anomalies are usually present, i.e. cleft lip and palate, abnormal genitalia, congenital nephrosis, etc.

Prenatal diagnosis can be done by estimation of alpha fetoprotein and USG. In postnatal period, the condition is evident at birth. X-ray skull and CT scan help to detect the associated anomalies.

Surgical repair of the defect can be done unless there is gross malformation of the brain. Hydrocephalus can be treated with shunt. Gentle nursing care, prevention of infection and injury are important measures along with other supportive care. Outcome depends upon the extent and location of encephalocele with available treatment facilities.

Other neural tube defects include syringomyelia, diastematomyelia, tethered spinal cord, lissencephaly schizoencephaly, porencephaly, agenesis of corpus callosum, agenesis of cranial nerves, Acardi syndrome, etc.

HYDROCEPHALUS

Hydrocephalus is the abnormal accumulation of cerebrospinal fluid (CSF) in the intracranial spaces. It occurs due to imbalance between production or absorption of CSF or due to obstruction of the CSF pathways. It results in the dilatation of the cerebral ventricles and enlargement of head.

CSF Circulation and Pathways

Cerebrospinal fluid is secreted at the choroid plexus within the cerebral ventricles by ultrafiltration and active secretion. From the lateral ventricles CSF passes to the third ventricle through the foramina of Monro. From third ventricle, it passes through cerebral aqueduct (aqueduct of Sylvius) to the fourth ventricle. From fourth ventricle, CSF passes to the basal cisterns and subarachnoid spaces through the foramina Luschka and foramina Magendie. CSF is absorbed via the archnoid villi into the venous channel and sinuses. About 20 mL of CSF is secreted in an hour, and 500 mL/day. The total volume of CSF is about 100 to 150 mL. In the child, the quantity is proportionately less and gradually increasing with age to the adult figure.

Etiology of Hydrocephalus

Hydrocephalus may occur due to congenital or acquired causes.

Congenital Hydrocephalus

It occurs due to the followings conditions:
a. Intrauterine infections—mainly in rubella, toxoplasmosis, cytomegalovirus.
b. Congenital brain tumor obstructing the CSF flow.
c. Intracranial hemorrhage.
d. Congenital malformations like aqueduct stenosis, Arnold-Chiari malformation (displacement of the brainstem and cerebellum through formen magnum), Dandy-Walker anomaly (congenital septum or membrane blocking the outlet of 4th ventricle).
e. Malformations of arachnoid villi.

Acquired Hydrocephalus

It occurs usually following the conditions like:
a. Inflammation—Meningitis, encephalitis.
b. Trauma—Birth injury, head injury, intracranial hemorrhage.
c. Neoplasm—Space occupying lesions like tuberculoma, subdural hematoma or abscess, gliomas, ependymoma, astrocytoma, choroid plexus papilloma, pseudotumor cerebri.
d. Chemical—Hypervitaminosis 'A'.
e. Connective tissue disorder—Hurler syndrome, achondro-plasia.
f. Degenerative atrophy of brain—Hydrocephalus Ex-vacuo.
g. Arteriovenous malformations, ruptured aneurysm, cavernous sinus thrombosis, etc.

Types

Hydrocephalus can be divided into two types.

Communicating Hydrocephalus

In this type, there is no blockage between ventricular system, the basal cisterns and the spinal subarachnoid space. There may be failure in the absorption of CSF (cavernous sinus thrombosis) or excessive production of CSF as in choroid plexus papilloma, pseudotumor cerebri, etc.

Noncommunicating Hydrocephalus

In this type of hydrocephalus, there is obstruction at any level in the ventricular system, commonly at the level of aqueduct or at foramina Luschka and/or Magendie. The obstruction may be partial, intermittent or complete. It develops mainly due to inflammation and developmental obstructive lesions. It occurs in majority of cases.

Pathology

The ventricular system becomes greatly distended and dilated. Increased intraventricular pressure leads to thinning of cerebral cortex and cranial bones. Ependymal lining of ventricles is disrupted resulting in periventricular ooze. Subependymal edema occurs and white matter is compressed. Downward bulging of third ventricle compresses the optic nerves and hypophysis cerebri with dilation of sella turcica. Choroid plexus is usually atrophied to some degrees. Cortical atrophy may also occur.

Clinical Manifestations

Congenital hydrocephalus starts in fetal life and presents at birth or within first few months of life.

Acquired hydrocephalus develops in association with underlying cause or as its complications. Clinical manifestations depend upon age of the child, types and duration of hydrocephalus, closing of anterior fontanel or fusion of cranial sutures. The features may manifest rapidly, slowly, steadily advancing or remittent.

The features include excessive enlargement of head, delayed closure of anterior fontanel, tense and bulging fontanel with open sutures. Presence of signs of increased intracranial pressure and alteration of muscle tone (spasticity) of the extremities are common presenting features. There is delayed in head holding of the infant (Figs 21.5A and B).

Later, with gradual increase in size of the head, the child presents with protruding forehead, shiny scalp with prominent scalp veins. The eyebrows and eyelids may be drawn upwards exposing the sclera above the iris with impaired upward gaze resulting the 'sun-set' sign of eyes. The

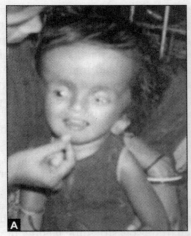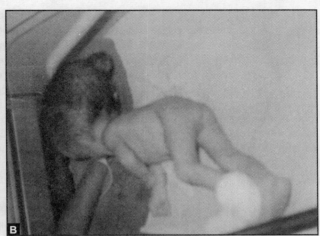

Figs 21.5A and B: Hydrocephalus *(For color version, see Plate 7)*

cracked-pot (Macewen's) sign may be elicited by percussion of head. Transillumination is positive. Mental functions and neurological manifestations are usually vary with the causative and associated factors. The children may have normal intelligence.

Hypocephalus occurring late in childhood, may not present with large head. The features may be found as increased intracranial pressure (ICP) with papilledema, spasticity, ataxia, urinary incontinence and progressive deterioration of mental activities.

Increased ICP presents with the signs and symptoms as nausea, vomiting, restlessness, irritability, high pitched shrill cry (in infants), irregular and decreased respiration, decreased pulse, increased temperature and systolic blood pressure. Pupillary changes, tense and bulging fontanel, separation of cranial sutures, increase of head circumference, papilledema, convulsions, lethargy, stupor and coma also usually present. In older children headache, lethargy, fatigue, apathy, personality changes and visual problems are manifested.

Diagnostic Evaluation

Physical examination and neurological assessment along with serial measuring of head circumference is helpful to diagnose the condition. Increase in head circumference in first 3 months of life, more than 1 cm every 15 days and persistent widening of squamoparietal sutures should arouse suspicion of hydrocephalus. Positive transillumination of infant head, typical cracked-pot sound (Macewen's sign) of the skull bone, ophthalmoscopy are important diagnostic measures.

MRI, CT scan, cranial ultrasonography and X-ray skull also can be performed to diagnose the underlying pathology and involvement of the intracranial structures.

Management

Management of hydrocephalus depends upon specific cause, associated malformations, clinical course and severity of the condition.

Surgery may not be indicated, if the hydrocephalus gets spontaneous arrest. When the surgical management is not necessary, then medical management is done to reduce increased ICP by carbonic anhydrase inhibitor, acetazolamide (Diamox) 50 mg/kg/day to reduce CSF production in slow progressive hydrocephalus. Oral glycerol and isosorbide can also be used for the same purpose.

Surgical management is indicated in obstructive hydrocephalus, in rapid enlargement of head, visual disturbances or in life-threatening increase ICP. Ventriculostomy and choroid plexectomy have been performed with variable results. Surgical shunts are the treatment of choice at the present time.

Intracranial or extracranial shunt is done to bypass the obstruction and to divert the CSF from the ventricular system to other compartment. The most commonly performed extracranial shunt is ventriculoperitoneal shunt (V-P shunt) (Fig. 21.6). Other approaches are ventriculoatrial shunt, ventriculopleural shunt or ventriculogallbladder shunt.

Intrauterine surgical intervention in fetal hydrocephalus has not yet given good results.

Nursing Management

Nursing Assessment

Along with routine nursing assessment, the most important is the measurement of head circumference. The measurement should be done at the occipitofrontal circumference at largest point and approximately at same time each day and in centimeter.

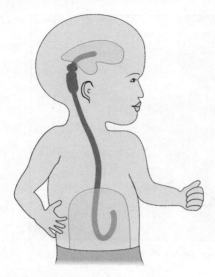

Fig. 21.6: Ventriculoperitoneal shunt

Other important aspects of assessment are status of fontanel, level of consciousness, pupillary response, vital signs, pattern of respiration, signs of increased ICP, condition of the scalp, presence of pressure sore or any skin breakdown, incontinence of bladder and bowel, neurological deficits, motor activity, change in feeding behavior and signs of complications.

Nursing Diagnoses

The important nursing diagnoses are:
a. Altered cerebral tissue perfusion related to increased ICP.
b. Altered nutrition, less than body requirement related to reduced oral intake and vomiting.
c. Risk for impaired skin integrity related to enlarged head.
d. Anxiety related to the abnormal condition and surgical interventions.
e. Risk for infection related to introduction of infecting organism through the shunt.
f. Risk for fluid volume deficit related to CSF drainage.
g. Ineffective family coping related to life-threatening problem of infant.

Nursing Interventions

1. Maintaining cerebral perfusion by assessment and management of increased ICP and assisting in diagnostic procedures to detect the exact pathology and administering treatment schedule as indicated. Taking care of shunt, if done.
2. Providing adequate nutrition by exclusive breastfeeding to the neonates and the infants up to 6 months of age. For older children, offering small frequent feeding and

placing the infant or child in semisitting position with elevation of head during and after the feeding.
3. Maintaining skin integrity by preventing pressure on the enlarged head with thinned skull and scalp. Firm or soft pillow under child's head, frequent change of position and keeping the area clean and dry are important measures. Good skin care and range of motion exercise are also essential to prevent skin breakdown.
4. Reducing parental anxiety by explanation reassurance and encouraging to express feeling.
5. Preventing infections by aseptic technique, frequent hand washing of caregivers, maintaining general cleanliness, giving eye care and mouth care and administering antibiotics as prescribed.
6. Maintaining fluid balance by IV fluid therapy, intake-output chart, nasogastric tube feeding or oral feeding as indicated.
7. Strengthening family coping by teaching daily care of V-P shunt, as needed for the particular shunt, like pumping the shunt, positioning the child as directed (initially flat to prevent excessive CSF drainage then gradual elevation of head of child's bed to 30–45 degree) and assessing for excessive drainage of CSF (sunken fontanel, agitation, decreased level of consciousness). Parents should also be informed about the signs of increased ICP, which indicate shunt malfunctions.

Other necessary health teaching to be given to help the parents to cope with the stress situation and to provide continued home-based care with regular medical help.

Complications

Hydrocephalus can be complicated with seizures, herniation of brain, persistent increased ICP, developmental delay, infections, neurological deficits, motor and intellectual handicaps, visual problems (squint, optic atrophy, field defect), aggressive and delinquent behavior, etc.

Shunt complications are found as shunt revision due to shunt occlusion, malfunction, infection and physical growth of the child. Ventriculoatrial (V-A) shunt may be complicated with endocarditis, bacteremia, thromboembolism, ventriculitis, corpulmonale, etc. Shunt dependency also may develop.

Prognosis

Prognosis of the children with hydrocephalus depends upon initiation of management and associated problems. Following appropriate medical and neurosurgical treatment, about 70 percent of these patients with infantile hydrocephalus live beyond first year of life. Without treatment, mortality is as high as 50 to 60 percent.

Two-third of the survived children have motor and intellectual handicapped conditions. A long-term follow-up in a specialized setting may improve the prognosis. Many children lead fairly normal life with normal motor and intellectual development.

INTRACRANIAL SPACE OCCUPYING LESIONS

Intracranial space occupying lesions (ICSOLs) are usually localized in nature and may be either neoplastic, inflammatory, parasitic or traumatic in origin. These lesions occupy space within the cranium and can cause increased intracranial pressure and pressure symptoms.

Some of the intracranial space occupying lesions are:
a. *Intracranial neoplasms:* Astrocytoma, glioma, medulloblastoma, ependymoma, choroid plexus papilloma, craniopharyngioma.
b. *Inflammatory granulomas:* Tuberculoma, brain abscess, subdural effusion, amebic granuloma.
c. *Parasitic:* Neurocysticercosis, hydatid disease of the brain.
d. *Traumatic:* Subdural hematoma.

These neurological lesions are requiring prompt recognition and early referral to the neurosurgeon.

Clinical features depend on the site and nature of the lesion, age of the child and the presence of complications. ICSOLs generally present with progressive focal neurological symptoms and signs like focal fits, cerebellar signs (like incoordination, nystagmus, ataxia), monoplegia hemiplegia, visual defects and respiratory problems. These children may present with hydrocephalus, endocrine abnormalities or generalized attacks depending upon the site of the lesion. Sometimes they may have life-threatening conditions like cardiorespiratory arrest.

Neurodiagnostic procedures to be followed to ruled out the exact pathology and appropriate management to be planned.

BRAIN TUMORS

Brain tumors are expanding lesions within the skull. About 20 percent of the childhood malignant tumors are brain tumors. These are the second most common group of neoplasms in children next to leukemia. Primary brain tumors may be benign or malignant. Benign tumors may become life-threatening, if located in the vital area of the brain.

Majority (two-third) of the brain tumors are infratentorial and close to midline which lead to hydrocephalus. About one-third to half of these are medulloblastomas and one-third are astrocytomas of cerebellum. Brain stem gliomas and ependymomas account for the rest.

Common supratentorial tumors are astrocytomas, ependymomas, craniopharyngioma and malignant gliomas.

Choroid plexus papilloma and pineal body tumors are less common.

Common Brain Tumors

Cerebellar Astrocytoma

It is slow growing malignant tumor commonly found as cystic tumor of cerebellum with unilateral cerebellar signs and slowly increasing ICP. It is seen in 3 to 8 years age group. It can be classified from grade I to grade IV. Management is done by surgical excision, chemotherapy and brachytherapy.

Medulloblastoma

It is highly malignant, rapidly growing invasive tumors and usually found in cerebellum. It is more common in male children (2:1) than females. The clinical features are truncal ataxia, early papilledema, unsteadiness in sitting position and signs of increased ICP. Prognosis is very poor, death occurs within few weeks to few years. Management is done with surgery, irradiation and chemotherapy.

Brainstem Glioma

It is composed of neuroglia, sometimes extended to include all intrinsic neoplasmas of the brain and spinal cord. There is progressive, bilateral cranial nerve palsies with pyramidal signs and ataxia. Brain stem gliomas carry the worst prognosis. Most children die within 18 months. Surgery is difficult. Chemotherapy does not have significant role. Radiotherapy is used for management by local irradiation.

Ependymoma

It is usually slow growing benign tumor derived from ependymal cells or lining of the central canal of the spinal cord and cerebral ventricles. It is commonly appears on the floor of the 4th ventricle, causing obstruction of flow of CSF. It can invade cardiorespiratory centers, cerebellum and spinal cord. These patients may present with subarachnoid hemorrhage and increased ICP.

Clinical Manifestations

Brain tumors are manifested with features of increased intracranial tension, and some common clinical features with localized signs for the particular tumor.

The common features include increased head size or papilledema, vomiting, headache, head tilting to the side of lesions, unsteady gait, ataxia, diplopia and nystagmus. The child may present with convulsions, visual disturbances, cranial nerve palsy, behavior problems, intellectual impairment and speech disturbances. Separation of cranial sutures, tense and nonpulsatile fontanel and delayed closure of fontanel with features of increased ICP are significant. Focal motor weakness and hemiparesis may be found.

Diagnostic Evaluation

Detailed history of illness, thorough physical and neurological examination give suspicion about the diagnosis. The diagnosis can be confirmed by CT scan, MRI, positron emission tomography (PET) scan, EEG, CSF cytology and angiography.

Management

The management of brain tumor is done mainly by neuro-surgery to excise the lesion as much as possible and to determine the type of tumor and extent of invasiveness.

Radiotherapy and chemotherapy are recommended in malignant tumors after confirmation of diagnosis.

Ventriculoperitoneal shunt may be done in case of hydro-cephalus. Symptomatic and supportive treatment should be provided in perioperative period. Immunotherapy or gene therapy are the newer treatment modalities.

Nursing Management

Important nursing management in the postoperative period should include positioning the head in unaffected side or as directed and monitoring the signs of increased ICP, CSF drainage, level of consciousness, edema of head and neck and vital signs at frequent interval. Ventilatory support and intensive care unit to be arranged. Routine care to be provided along with involvement of the parents.

Special precautions to be followed during radiotherapy, chemotherapy and in ventriculoperitoneal shunt. Emotional support to the parent and discussion about possible outcome to be emphasized.

HEAD INJURY (CRANIOCEREBRAL TRAUMA)

Head injury includes any injury involving scalp, skull, meninges or any portion of the brain caused by external forces. It is one of the most important cause of childhood mortality and morbidity. One-third of all head injury cases are children. They are by nature accident prone and injury of the head is common among accidental injury.

Causes of Head Injury

According to different age group the causes of head injury can be described as follows:
- *Neonates:* Birth injury, instrumental delivery.

- *Toddlers and preschoolers:* Fall from height, hard object falling on the head or hits on head by hard object.
- *Older children:* Automobile accidents, road traffic accidents, sports and recreation injury, fall from height, penitrating injury through eyes, crush injury, fall of heavy objects on head.

Pathology

Pathological changes due to head injury depends upon various factors like thickness of the skull, presence of open fontanels, type of suture and developing brain.

Pathological changes in brain may be primary or secondary. Primary injury includes all types of hematoma, cerebral contusion and laceration. Secondary changes mostly include cerebral edema, hypoxia and ischemic injury.

Common pathological changes in brain in neonates following head injury include cephalhematoma, skull fracture, subdural hematoma, intracerebral hematoma and brain swelling.

In toddlers the common pathological changes are found as depressed or comminuted fracture, extradural or subdural hematoma, concussion, contusion, laceration and brain swelling.

In older children the common pathological changes are extradural or subdural hematoma, cerebral contusion and laceration, intracerebral hemorrhage, ischemic-hypoxic injury and brain swelling.

The external force transmitted to the intracranial structure and produces acceleration of the skull with subsequent injury and distortion with movement of the brain. Injury of the brain can occur at the site of trauma, i.e. coup, or at some distance from the area of injury, i.e. contrecoup. The force of injury can cause tearing of small arteries and veins causing hemorrhage or can lacerate the brain tissue and meninges or can stretch and shear nerve fiber tracts.

Types of Head Injury

Fracture of the Skull

In neonates, a typical 'ping-pong' fracture may occur due to elasticity of the bone. The fracture may be fissured or depressed type. The linear fracture is the most common.

Older children may have comminuted fracture with dural tear and laceration with brain damage. There may be CSF rhinorrhea or CSF otorrhea. Fracture of anterior fossa may involve orbit and leads to orbital hematoma and black eyes.

Intracranial Hemorrhage

It is found in neonates due to excessive moulding of skull bones or forceps delivery. Rupture of delicate surface veins leads to acute subdural hemorrhage and intracerebral hematoma which may cause neonatal death. About 20 to 25 percent neonatal death are due to intracranial hemorrhage, which is usually nontraumatic and found in sick preterm babies.

Concussion of the Brain (Cerebral Concussion)

Concussion is the reversible neurologic dysfunction. Transient loss of consciousness and loss of memory are the part of concussion. The child may be stunned for a short time. The cause of concussion may be an injury at the occipital area and shearing strain at the brain stem level due to violent blow on head. The children recover promptly and completely from concussion.

Cerebral Contusion

It is bruishing or petechial hemorrhage in the brain tissue at the site of blow following direct trauma. It may occur due to angular head down motion producing high tensile strains throughout the brain. Cerebral contusion consists of hemorrhagic brain necrosis and infarction. Contusion at frontal and temporal lobes are common.

Extradural Hematoma

It may occur following head injury mostly in the temporal or frontal lobe or in posterior fossa. Hematoma may be arterial or venous depending upon the type of fracture and vessels involved by the fracture. Blood may be collected due to bleeding from fracture line and form a thin layer of clot.

Acute Subdural Hematoma

It results from severe injury but may occur due to minor injury with bleeding disorders in the patients. Subdural hematoma (SDH) is an accumulation of fluid, blood and its degradation products within the potential subdural space between dura and arachnoid. It can be acute or chronic depending on the time between injury and the onset of symptoms. Frequent fall and injury to the head accounts for higher incidence of SDH. When the sutures are not fused, the hematoma can grow slowly. The hematoma may remain silent for sometimes, because the skull can expand to accommodate the SDH.

Brain Swelling

It may found in association with head injury and may be due to vascular congestion. It can cause fatal outcome due to generalized brain swelling. Focal brain swelling occurs in contusion or intracerebral hematoma due to release of neurotransmitters. Cerebral edema may occur due to hypoxia. Brain swelling due to vasocongestion may be due to neurogenic vasoparalysis or vasodilation and increased blood flow.

Clinical Manifestations

The child with head injury may arrive at hospital with history of trauma, presence or absence of wound on the scalp, respiratory obstruction and loss of consciousness. The child may be drowsy, irritable or lethargic. Features of shock, alteration of vital signs and signs of increased ICP may present. Severe headache, vomiting, convulsions and loss of memory may found. There may be bladder and bowel dysfunction as incontinence. Fracture skull may be evident on examination.

The neurological features which may be noticed in case of head injury include the followings:

- Level of consciousness can be altered as depressed, stuporous or comatose.
- Hemiparesis, monoparesis or hemiplegia may found due to focal brain damage. There can be alteration of neurological reflexes and disturbances of vision, hearing or taste. Sensation to pain, touch or temperature may be altered. Cranial nerve palsy is common. Seventh cranial nerve involvement leads to facial palsy and change in facial expression.
- Bruises over ipsilateral ear, bleeding through ear, CSF otorrhea and hearing loss may present.
- Unilateral or bilateral dilated fixed pupils may found depending upon severity of injury. Optic nerve injury may present with fixed dilated pupil and positive consensual light reflex, as pinpoint pupil size with slow, unequal or absent pupillary reaction.
- Acute subdural hematoma is commonly develop with deterioration of level of consciousness, progressive hemiplegia, focal seizures, pupillary enlargement, changes in vital signs, decerebrate posture and respiratory failure.
- Chronic subdural hematoma can develop with gradual onset and variable symptoms according to age of the child. Early signs include anorexia, difficulty in feeding, vomiting, irritability, low grade fever and retinal hemorrhage. Late signs are enlargement of head, bulging and pulsating anterior fontanel, glossy scalp with prominent scalp veins. Ocular palsies (rare), strabismus, pupillary inequality, hyperactive reflexes and convulsions are common. In older children lethargy, anorexia, increased ICP, convulsions and unconsciousness are presenting features.

Additional systemic injuries are found in about 50 percent cases with severe head injury. Limb fracture is most common. Other associated injury like fracture long bone, spinal injury, chest injury with hemopneumothorax, abdominal injury and pelvic injury may present.

Complications

Head injury has numbers of complications. These include shock, persistent increased intracranial pressure, epidural hematoma, leptomeningeal cyst, visual disturbances, convulsive disorders or post-traumatic epilepsy, post-traumatic amnesia, hydrocephalus, behavioral disturbances (aggressiveness), mental retardation, learning disabilities, growth failure and psychiatric illness.

Diagnostic Evaluation

Detailed history about the injury with description of the event is very important. Thorough physical examination must be done to detect the severity of cerebral trauma and presence of additional injuries.

Assessment of level of consciousness by Modified Glasgow Coma Scale for children (see Appendix XII) and presence of focal neurological deficits are the most vital aspects of neurological examination in case of craniocerebral trauma.

Although adequate baseline clinical evaluation is major importance, but the investigations are also needed to detect the site, size, nature and extent of brain injury for better management.

The diagnostic evaluation should include CT scan and X-ray (skull, abdomen, pelvis, chest, spine). EEG may be done to determine focal destructive lesions or seizure activity. Echoencephalography and cerebral angiography also can be done. Blood for ABG analysis and other routine examination is important. Lumber puncture is not done generally in presence of increased ICP due to danger of herniation of brain.

Management

Emergency Management

Emergency management in first 5 to 6 hours after head injury is the most crucial aspect. First aids at the place of injury with basic life support measures promote better prognosis. First aids measures should include resuscitation (clear airway, breathing support and maintenance of circulation), prevention of further accidents, and safe transport to the hospital under optimum support. Immediate hospitalization is necessary for close observation (12–24 hours), continuous neurological assessment and subsequent management.

After hospitalization, initial management should be done with following steps:

- *Maintenance of airway:* It should be done by positioning and removal of secretions by oropharyngeal suctioning. Nasopharyngeal tube or simple oral airway tube may be needed for some children. Endotracheal intubation or tracheostomy may be required in children with respiratory obstruction.
- *Establishment of breathing:* It can be done by ventilatory support with simple bag and mask or by mechanical ventilators. Intensive care unit may be necessary for these children.
- *Maintenance of circulation:* Intravenous fluid therapy to be started to maintain blood pressure within normal change. Blood transfusion may be needed. CVP line should be made.
- Assessment of neurological status to be performed by modified Glasgow Coma Scale (GCS), neurological examination, pupillary reaction, etc. External and associated injury to be assessed. Necessary investigations to be performed after stabilization of patient's condition.
- Continuous urinary drainage by foley's catheterization.
- Nasogastric intubation to be done to prevent abdominal distension and aspiration of gastric content.
- Intensive care unit placement for further management and continuous monitoring, especially in case of severe head injury, whether managed medically or surgically.

Medical Management

- Continuous monitoring of neurological status, vital signs and intracranial pressure (ICP).
- Management of increased ICP by slight head up position, controlled hyperventilation, barbiturate, osmotic diuretic and corticosteroid therapy.
- Prevention and treatment of convulsion, fever and other problems.
- Prevention of infections.
- Supportive expert nursing care as unconscious patients.

Surgical Management

Surgical management is indicated in large intracranial hematoma, compound depressed fracture and penetrating injuries along with deterioration of level of consciousness, neurological deficits, generalized convulsions and abnormal pupillary reaction. In case of small subdural hematoma or contusion, surgical intervention is not indicated. The following surgical interventions are commonly performed:

- Craniotomy or Burr hole operation is required in acute subdural hematoma for evacuation of the clot.
- Subdural tap or V-P shunting is done to remove collecting fluid in case of chronic subdural hematoma.
- In penetrating wound, repair of CSF leakage may be necessary along with debridement of the wound.
- Elevation of fracture segment is done in depressed fracture skull.

Nursing Management

Nursing Assessment

a. Nursing history should include mode and time of injury, duration of unconsciousness, presence of vomiting, convulsions, headache, loss of memory, loss of vision, any discharge from ear, nose and bleeding. Routine history to be collected when the patient is stabilized.

b. Physical examination and assessment of neurological status are important to evaluate effectiveness of management, deterioration of child's condition and to plan further management. The following aspects should be assessed with special attention along with routine examination:

   i. Signs of increased ICP and alterations of vital signs.
   ii. Level of consciousness by GCS score.
   iii. General behavior—irritability, lethargy, change in personality, etc.
   iv. Pupillary and visual change—dilated or contracted pupil, no response to light, double vision, etc.
   v. Convulsions, tremor, twitching and neck rigidity.
   vi. Alteration of motor functions and abnormal movement.
   vii. Incontinence of bladder and bowel.
   viii. Cerebrospinal fluid leakage and presence of wound.
   ix. Neurological reflex and paralysis.

Nursing Diagnoses

Important nursing diagnoses related to head injury can be as follows:

- Ineffective breathing related to increased ICP.
- Altered cerebral tissue perfusion related to head injury.
- Impaired physical mobility related to alteration of consciousness.
- Altered hydration and nutrition related to unconsciousness.
- Risk for infection related to injury.
- Ineffective family coping related to life-threatening situation.
- Knowledge deficit related to care of injured child.

Nursing Interventions

Nursing interventions in a child with head injury can be same as the comatose child with the following strategies.

- Maintaining respiration and clearing airpassage.
- Maintaining adequate cerebral perfusion.
- Organizing emergency measures for life saving.
- Providing perioperative care related to neurosurgery with specific precautions for children.
- Monitoring neurological status and vital functions with appropriate recording.
- Preventing complications of immobility.
- Providing care for specific conditions like convulsion, fever, fluid-electrolyte imbalance, hemorrhage, wound, etc.
- Maintaining nutrition and hydration status.
- Preventing infections and related complications.
- Strengthening family coping and promoting crisis interventions.
- Teaching the parents about routine care, long-term care and prevention of accidental injury.

Prognosis

Prognosis in case of head injury depends upon type of injury, initiation of management and available facilities for specialized care.

- Maximum children with head injury recover within 24 to 48 hours.
- Approximately 70 to 75 percent of injured children will die, if the initial GCS score is 3 to 4 and about 20 percent may be severely disabled.
- Post-traumatic sequela may develop in some children with various complications. About 5 percent children may have post-traumatic epilepsy.

Endocrine Disorders in Children

22

- Short Stature
- Disorders of Pituitary Glands
- Diabetes Insipidus
- Disorders of Thyroid Glands
- Disorders of Parathyroid Glands
- Disorders of Adrenal Glands
- Congenital Adrenal Hyperplasia

- Ambiguous Genitalia
- Undescended Testes (Cryptorchidism)
- Precocious Puberty
- Delayed Sexual Development (Delayed Puberty)
- Menstrual Abnormalities
- Obesity
- Diabetes Mellitus

INTRODUCTION

Endocrine system and its metabolic and biochemical effects are more vital in infancy and childhood. Because, stimulation of physical and sexual growth is the unique feature of these age group. Growth and development are greatly influenced by the hormones with their over-secretions and undersecretions. Abnormal endocrine functions leads to altered growth and development and various disorders and diseases with life-threatening conditions or long-term complications.

Nurses, working in the hospitals or community, are responsible for early detection of hormonal influences on variations of growth and development and endocrine disorders and diseases. Appropriate referral, participation on diagnostic procedures and management of the children to prevent long-term sequelae and to promote growth and development are important nursing responsibility.

SHORT STATURE

Short stature is defined as length/height below 3rd percentile for age according to international standard, below 5th percentile according to ICMR standard or below 3 standard deviation of mean for age. It is a common pediatric problem with a large number of etiological factors.

Short stature may be primary or secondary and proportionate or disproportionate (with short limb and trunk).

Primary short stature is usually due to an intrinsic defect in the skeletal system related to some genetic or prenatal damage (e.g. IUGR). In this condition, potential for normal bone growth is impaired though skeletal age is unaffected. Main effect is found on diaphyseal growth.

Secondary short stature is characterized by impairment of bone age and height to the same extent. In this condition, the potential for reaching the adult height depends upon availability of proper treatment.

Causes of Short Stature

Genetic Cause

- Genetic disorders (chromosomal and metabolic disorders), e.g. Down's syndrome, Turner syndrome, chondrodysplasia, cystic fibrosis, osteogenesis imperfecta.
- Familial short stature.
- Constitutional delay—delayed skeletal growth, delayed puberty.

- Primordial—intrauterine growth retardation, low birth weight.

Endocrine Disorders

Growth hormone insufficiency, hypothyroidism, Cushing, syndrome, hypogonadism, precocious puberty, diabetes mellitus.

Nutritional Disorders

Prolonged malnutrition, rickets, nutritional dwarfism, anemia.

Chronic Organic Diseases

- Gastrointestinal—Malabsorption syndrome, intestinal parasitosis, cirrhosis of liver, cystic fibrosis of pancreas, congenital megacolon, etc.
- Cardiovascular—Congenital heart disease, rheumatic heart disease.
- Respiratory—Pulmonary tuberculosis, bronchial asthma, bronchiectasis.
- Skeletal—Caries spine, kyphosis.
- Chronic infections—Malaria, *H. pylori* infection, kala-azar.
- Chronic renal disease and renal ricket.

Drug Induced

Prolonged use of anabolic steroids or corticosteroids.

Psychosomatic

Emotional deprivation, child abuse and neglect (CAN).

About 5 percent cases causes are idiopathic. The term dwarfism is not used at present for short stature. Disorders of growth are now termed as dysplasia.

Diagnostic Evaluation

Diagnostic evaluation for a short stature child should be based on detailed history, physical examination, routine investigations, bone age and study of growth rate. Hormonal studies and karyotyping are needed in selected cases.

Management

Management depends on the underlying cause. The cause may be treatable to resolve the growth problem, be amenable to growth hormone supplementation or may be untreatable due to genetic cause. Parents need adequate explanation and support to cope with situation. Genetically engineered GH therapy is now possible but it is very expensive and should be started before 11 years of age for attaining the optimal height.

DISORDERS OF PITUITARY GLANDS

Pituitary gland lies in the sella turcica of the sphenoid bone. It consists of adenohypophysis (anterior lobe), neurohypophysis (posterior lobe) and in between the vestigial intermediate lobe.

The hormones produced by the anterior pituitary gland are growth hormone (GH), thyroid stimulating hormone (TSH), adrenocorticotropic hormone (ACTH), prolactin and gonadotropins, i.e. follicle stimulating hormone (FSH) and luteinizing hormone (LH).

The posterior pituitary hormones are oxytocin and antidiuretic hormone (ADH) or vasopressin.

The disorders of pituitary glands may affect all the respective target glands. Hypopituitarism is the deficiency of one, some or all the hormones secreted by the glands.

Growth hormone (GH) is the only hormone that does not have a target gland to induce further hormonal secretion. Deficiency of growth hormone causes pituitary dwarfism and rarely Frohlich's syndrome. Excess secretions of GH results in gigantism and acromegaly.

Growth Hormone Deficiency

Growth hormone (GH) insufficiency results from lack of pituitary production or lack of hypothalamic stimulation on the pituitary gland. The lack of GH impairs metabolism of proteins, fats and carbohydrates.

Infants with congenital GH deficiency may appear normal at birth. Growth impairment starts within a few months of life, but the features become obvious at about 1 to 2 years of age.

Etiology

The causes of GH insufficiency can be listed as follows —
- *Genetic cause:* In case of Turner syndrome (XO) and in GH gene deletion and development defects.
- *Organic cause:* CNS tumors, infections and irradiation, birth injury, head injury, vascular problems (infarction, aneurysm) and autoimmune disorders.

Clinical Manifestations

Neonates with GH deficiency may present with hypoglycemic convulsions. Children with GH insufficiency are short stature with normal body proportions. They have more weight according to their height and having high subcutaneous adiposity. Skeletal maturation, dentition and bone age are delayed. The height age is less than the skeletal age and chronological age. Other features are doll-like face, frontal bossing, depressed nasal bridge, prominent philtrum, single central incisor tooth, truncal obesity, hypoplastic penis and scrotum, increased skin fold thickness, high pitched voice, delayed sexual development and younger look than their actual age.

Diagnostic Criteria

- Height is less than 3rd percentile of chronological age.
- Bone age is less than chronological age.
- Growth velocity is less than 4 cm per year during pre-pubescent period.
- Abnormal GH secretory pattern.
- Maximum GH level is less than 10 ng/mL during provocative stimulation test.
- Reduced somatomedin-C or insulin like growth factors (IGF).
- Normal growth resumption following GH administration.

Management

A short stature children should be kept under regular check-up for assessment of growth for 6 months to one year before all the investigations are planned. If the child is gaining more than 4 cm height per year, then the child is not likely to have hypopituitarism. If GH level is low, the child should be treated with recombinant GH (0.07–0.1 IU/kg/day subcutaneously) till the adequate growth is achieved. Associated pituitary deficiency should be treated.

DIABETES INSIPIDUS

Diabetes insipidus (DI), is the disorders of the posterior pituitary gland due to a deficiency of antidiuretic hormone (ADH). It is characterized by failure of the body to conserve water due to a deficiency of ADH, decreased renal sensitivity to ADH or suppression of ADH secondary to excessive ingestion of fluid, i.e. primary polydipsia.

Pathophysiology

Intake and output of water are governed by the centers in the hypothalamus to control thirst and synthesis of ADH. Thirst ensures adequate intake of water and ADH prevents water loss through the kidney. The child with DI is unable to produce appropriate levels of ADH or it's action leading to polyuria, increased plasma osmolality and increased thirst.

Classification

- *Central or neurogenic diabetes insipidus:* It may be due to congenital and acquired causes leading to low level of ADH. The congenital causes are mainly hereditary and CNS defects. Acquired causes are due to CNS tumors, CNS infections, head injury and vascular disorders. In some cases it may be idiopathic.
- *Nephrogenic diabetes insipidus:* It occurs due to renal unresponsiveness to the ADH and caused by chronic renal disease.

Clinical Manifestations of Diabetes Insipidus

The child with DI manifests suddenly with the disease. The child presents with excessive thirst and polyuria. Some patients may present with nocturnal enuresis. There is pale dry skin with reduced sweating and weakness. Dehydration, hyperthermia and poor appetite may found. Polyuria produces disturbances in rest, sleep, play and schooling.

Infant with DI present with excessive crying, quieted with water more than milk feeding. They also have rapid weight loss due to water preference over feeding. Sunken fontanel with dehydration, constipation and growth failure are commonly seen.

Complications

The child with DI can be complicated with hypovolemic hypotension, hypernatremia, precocious puberty, visual disturbances and emotional disorders.

Diagnostic Evaluation

History of illness and physical examination and 24 hours intake and output help in clinical diagnosis. Laboratory investigations to be done to confirm the diagnosis. Urine examination shows decreased specific gravity, sodium and osmolality. Blood examination shows elevation of serum sodium and serum osmolality, with low ADH level. Water deprivation test can be done to confirm the diagnosis, though potentially dangerous. Definitive renal function test can also be done in nephrogenic DI. MRI or CT scan is indicated to detect underlying cause in hypothalamic pituitary region.

Management

Daily replacement of ADH using desmopressin (DDAVP), a synthetic analogue is necessary in IM or SC route. It can be given as nasal spray or in oral or sublingual route. Thiazide diuretics in nephrogenic DI can be administered.

Supportive care should include sufficient water intake, maintenance of intake and output, prevention of fluid and electrolyte imbalance, low sodium intake and recording of body weight. Care of dry skin, safety measures in weakness, adequate nutritional intake in poor appetite, prevention of constipation and hyperthermia, special mouth care with soft tooth brush and promoting good sleep are additional measures. Parents should be explained about the care after discharge. Psychogenic compulsive water drinking may requires psychotherapy.

The prognosis of the disease depends upon adequate treatment. The disease is a chronic condition and usually not life-threatening.

DISORDERS OF THYROID GLANDS

Thyroid gland secretes thyroxin (T_4), triiodothyronine (T_3) and calcitonin. These hormones promote cellular growth, metabolism and mental development. Disorders of thyroid gland are broadly classified as hypothyroidism and hyperthyroidism.

Hypothyroidism

Deficiency or low circulating level of thyroid hormones result in hypothyroidism. It can be congenital which is known as cretinism and can be acquired as juvenile hypothyroidism.

Low level of T_4 causes rise in TSH. Absence or deficiency of T_4 leads to abnormal development of CNS in the neonates. In older children deficiency of the hormone causes decreased metabolism, growth retardation and delayed physical maturation.

Causes of Hypothyroidism

The congenital causes of hypothyroidism are thyroid agenesis or dysgenesis, defect in thyroid hormone synthesis, inherited defects of thyroid hormone receptors, maternal thyroid antibodies acrossing placenta, iodine deficiency and antithyroid medications during pregnancy (Radioiodine, carbimazole).

Acquired postnatal causes of hypothyroidism are autoimmune thyroiditis (Hashimoto's disease), radiation exposure, antithyroid drugs, iodine deficiency, thyroidectomy and ingestion of goitrogens.

Secondary hypothyroidism occurs due to deficiency of TSH or TRH and hypopituitarism.

Clinical Manifestations

A neonate with congenital hypothyroidism are unusually large and heavy at birth with marked open posterior fontanel and wide sutures. The earliest clinical manifestations may be found as lethargy, sluggishness, hoarse cry, feeding difficulties, hypotonia and over sleeping. Other features are persistent constipation, prolonged physiological jaundice, abdominal distension and cold, dry, rough thick skin. Umbilical hernia and anemia are common.

The classical features of cretinism appear usually in 8 to 12 weeks. The characteristic coarse facial feature found with a large protruding tongue from large open mouth with thick lips, puffy eyelids, depressed nasal bridge, seemingly wide apart eyes (pseudohypertelorism) and wrinkle forehead with sparse eyebrows and low level of hairline.

The scalp hair is scanty, rough, dry and brittle. Anterior fontanel and coronal sutures are usually widely open. The neck is short with a pad of supraclavicular fat. Voice is hoarse. Dentition is delayed. Hypotonia is commonly found. Abdomen is distended with presence of an umbilical hernia. Hands are broad with short fingers. Poor feeding and constipation are commonly present. The child is having sluggish behavior, mental retardation, delayed physical growth with infantile skeletal proportion.

In acquired or late onset hypothyroidism, the child present with growth retardation, short stature, stocky appearance, large head, dull expression, puffy face, myxedematous skin (thick and pigmented), lethargic, cold intolerance, hypotonia, delayed dentition, delayed puberty, delayed skeletal maturation, goiter and poor school performance. Gross mental retardation may be absent.

Diagnostic Evaluation

Detailed family history with history of antenatal period and physical examination are important. Neonatal screening (in suspected cases) for T_4 and TSH showing elevation of TSH and low T_4, indicate congenital hypothyroidism.

In older children, free T_4, T_4 and T_3 resin uptake are reduced with TSH elevation. Elevation of thyroid antibodies indicates autoimmune thyroiditis. X-ray shows delayed bone age and abnormal growth rate. Thyroid nuclear scan shows reduced uptake. Serum cholesterol is usually elevated (beyond the age of 2 years). Serum carotene and prolactin level is raised. Alkaline phosphate is low. Low thyroglobulin level indicates inborn error of thyroid hormone synthesis. Low urinary iodine excretion indicates iodine deficiency. TSH estimation helps to detect secondary hypothroidism. FNAC of thyroid gland may be needed in case of continued thyroid enlargement.

Management

Replacement therapy with synthetic levothyroxine should be started as early as possible to maintain normal thyroid functions. Replacement therapy needs to be continued through out the life. Therapy should be monitored periodically by clinical symptoms and biochemical testings. Gain in height, normal activity and improvement of mental performance indicate good therapeutic response. Bone age should be checked once a year.

Parents need explanation about the life long treatment compliance, blood testing, follow-up and special instructions. Features of overdose of levothyroxine should be informed.

Prognosis

Prognosis depends upon the degree of hypofunction, age of onset of features, initiation and adequacy of treatment. In late onset hypothyroidism, with mild features, the mental development is better.

With adequate replacement therapy within 6 months of age, physical growth is fairly gratifying. About 50 percent of these children can have good mental development with an IQ level 90 or even more.

Hyperthyroidism

Hyperthyroidism is a disorder of the thyroid gland when a high level of circulating T_4 results in abnormally increased body metabolism.

It may be caused by autoimmune process in Graves disease, i.e. diffuse toxic goiter (most common). It may also occur in toxic nodular goiter, lymphocytic thyroiditis, thyroid adenoma, carcinoma thyroid, pituitary adenoma and iodine induced hyperthyroidism. The condition may also be found in neonates with history of maternal thyrotoxicosis. It may also be caused by ingestion or overdose of thyroid medication. Preadolescents and adolescents girls are commonly affected.

Clinical Manifestations

The clinical features of hyperthyroidism include thyromegaly (enlargement of the thyroid gland), polyphagia with weight loss and hyperactivity as restlessness, nervousness, hand tremors, sleep disturbances, emotional lability. Other features include hyperexcitability, excessive diaphoresis, and heat intolerance. The child may also present with exophthalmos, proptosis, lid retraction, tall stature (under weight for height) and poor school performance.

The patient may have palpitation, tachycardia, wide pulse pressure, progressive cardiomegaly and cardiac insufficiency.

Thyroid crisis is less common in children. It may occur with sudden onset, high temperature, restlessness, tachycardia, rapid progression to delirium, coma and eventually death.

Diagnostic Evaluation

History of illness, physical examination, along with laboratory investigations help in diagnosis. Serum thyroid function tests reveals elevated T_3 (total and free) and T_4 (total and free) with suppressed TSH. Radioactive iodine uptake is high and radionuclide scan shows the pathology (carcinoma). Microsomal antibodies are positive.

Management

Management of hyperthyroidism is done with antithyroid drugs (propylthiouracil, methimazole, neomercazole), radioactive iodine therapy, and surgical intervention as subtotal or total thyroidectomy. In severe thyrotoxicosis, potassium iodide solution or Lugol's iodine may be indicated to inhibit the release of thyroid hormone. Propranolol, beta-adrenergic blocking agents may be prescribed for cardiac effects.

Supportive care should include high caloric nutritious diet, avoiding overactivity, promoting rest, sleep and relaxation, special care during radioactive ablation therapy (disposal of stool and urine as directed by nuclear medicine department) and regular follow-up with continuation of treatment.

Goiter (Thyromegaly)

Goiter is the enlargement of the thyroid gland. When the lateral lobe of thyroid gland becomes larger than the terminal phalanx of child's thumb, then it is diagnosed as thyromegaly. It may be congenital or acquired, sporadic or endemic. Thyroid function may be normal, diminished or increased.

Goiter may develop due to high production of TSH in response to decreased thyroxine level, inflammatory or neoplastic infiltration or due to long acting thyroid stimulator. All goiters in childhood are not due to environmental iodine deficiency or due to increased physiological requirement of adolescence. The important causes of goiter are inflammatory, autoimmune, dysgenetic, neoplastic, compensatory (drug induced) and colloid goiter.

Endemic goiter is common in the region of Himalayan mountains due to poor intake of iodine in water. Sporadic goiter is due to failure to organify iodide due to autosomal recessive transmission. Congenital goiter may result from ingestion of goitrogenic agents (antithyroid) during pregnancy. Acquired goiter occurs due to Hashimoto's thyroiditis, the most common cause of childhood goiter in non endemic area. Nontoxic diffuse goiter also known as simple goiter, colloid or adolescent goiter. It is an acquired thyroid enlargement with normal thyroid function not due to inflammation or neoplastic process. It is found more in girls (95%) around puberty. The enlargement is due to increased TSH secretion because of iodine deficiency and thyroid growth stimulating immunoglobulin. Levothyroxine is given for 2 years, which leads to complete regression in about 30 percent of cases.

DISORDERS OF PARATHYROID GLANDS

Parathyroid glands produce parathormone which controls calcium and phosphate metabolism. It increases absorption of calcium from intestine, and reabsorption of calcium from bones. It enhances mobilization of calcium and phosphorus from bone. It inhibits renal tubular reabsorption of phosphate and promotes reabsorption of calcium.

Disorders of parathyroid glands leads to hypoparathyroidism and hyperparathyroidism.

Hypoparathyroidism

Hypoparathyroidism may occur due to congenital absence of parathyroids or in neonates born to mothers with parathyroid adenoma. Autoimmune hypoparathyroidism is usually seen along with Addison's disease, pernicious anemia and lymphocytic thyroiditis. It may found following surgery of subtotal thyroidectomy, in which parathyroids are also removed. It may also develop in neck irradiation and hemosiderosis in thalassemia.

Pseudohypoparathyroidism may occur due to failure of end-organ response in which hormone secretion is good but the patients are found mentally retarded with poor bony development and short fingers and toes.

Clinical Manifestations

Hypoparathyroidism is related to low calcium level. Mild cases may remain asymptomatic. Severe condition causes tetany which manifested with tingling sensations, numbness and stiffness of hands and forearms. Patients may have painful muscle spasms or cramps and hyperventilation. Skin may be coarse and dry. Nails are ridged and brittle. There is delayed and irregular dentition. Convulsions and unconsciousness may occur with evidence of increased intracranial pressure and papilledema. Extrapyramidal symptoms may develop due to calcification of basal ganglion.

Diagnostic Evaluation

Diagnosis is confirmed by the blood examination for presence of low calcium and parathyroid hormone with high phosphate level. Alkaline phosphate may be normal or low. Serum magnesium levels and renal functions are normal.

X-ray of bones show increased density of metaphyses. CT scan of brain shows calcification of basal ganglia. ECG may show prolongation of QT interval. EEG may reveal slow activity level.

Management

Management of the condition is done by correction of hypocalcemia and hyperphosphatemia by IV calcium gluconate. Vitamin 'D' should be administered. Oral intake of calcium should be increased. High phosphate containing food like milk and egg should be avoided. Blood and urine test should be done to monitor the calcium level.

Hyperparathyroidism

Primary hyperparathyroidism in children is usually due to single benign adenoma in which features are evident about 10 years of age. It may found in association with multiple endocrine neoplasia. Secondary hyperparathyroidism may develop due to low calcium level such as vitamin 'D' deficiency ricket, malabsorption syndrome and chronic renal failure. In certain instances parathyroids continue to be hyperactive even after the removal of primary cause and known as tertiary hyperparathyroidism.

Clinical Manifestations

This condition is characterized by hypercalcemia, hypophosphatemia and hypercalciuria. The clinical manifestations are muscular weakness, anorexia, vomiting, constipation, polydipsia, polyuria and weight loss. Renal function may be impaired due to calcium deposition in the renal parenchyma. Renal calculi may develop and hematuria may occur. Progressive oliguria, azotemia and coma may develop in high rise of calcium level. Bony changes manifested with backache, leg pain, abnormal gait, knocked knee, fracture and poor bone growth. The patient may present with acute abdominal pain due to acute pancreatitis.

Infants may present with poor feeding, hypotonia, failure to thrive, mental retardation, convulsion and blindness.

Diagnostic Evaluation

Physical examination and careful history of illness should be obtained. The diagnosis should be confirmed by blood examination, urine analysis and X-ray.

Blood examination shows high serum calcium, low serum phosphate, raised serum PTH and normal calcitonin.

Urine specific gravity is low. RBC may present in the urine. X-ray shows extensive demineralization of bones and presence of renal calculi. Radionuclide scan reveals the presence of adenoma.

Management

Management should include treatment of hypercalcemia with high fluid intake and administration of furosemide. Dietary calcium intake to be reduced. Calcitonin may be prescribed. Surgical removal of adenoma is required. Monitoring of sodium and calcium level to be done at regular interval.

DISORDERS OF ADRENAL GLANDS

Adrenal glands secrete a large number of hormones. Adrenal cortex produces approximate 30 steroid hormones which are responsible for maintenance of electrolyte balance, carbohydrate and protein metabolism, growth and development and sexual maturation.

Adrenal medulla produces catecholamines, i.e. adrenaline and noradrenaline. Adrenaline is responsible for increasing systolic blood pressure, heart rate and cardiac output, but for reducing coronary blood flow and peripheral resistance. Noradrenaline is responsible for increasing both systolic and diastolic blood pressure and for increasing coronary flow and peripheral resistance.

The disorders of adrenal glands present as adrenal insufficiency, adrenal hyperactivity and adrenal medullary disorders.

Adrenal insufficiency may develop due to suppression of gland activity in prolonged steroid therapy in case of nephrotic syndrome, rheumatic fever or ITP. It may also occur due to adrenal hemorrhage. This condition develops in adrenal necrosis in fulminant infections like septicemia or meningococcemia and known as Waterhouse-Friderichsen's syndrome. Chronic adrenal failure may found rarely in children, in case of tuberculosis or in autoimmune process and known as chronic idiopathic adrenocortical insufficiency or Addison disease.

Adrenal cortical hyperactivity or hyperadrenocorticism causes (a) Cushing's syndrome in case of cortisol secreting lesions, (b) adrenogenital syndrome from androgen producing lesions such as adrenal tumors or adrenal hyperplasia and (c) hyperaldosteronism are rare.

Adrenal medullary disorders are found as (a) ganglioneuroma, a benign tumor, (b) neuroblastoma, a malignant tumor and (c) pheochromocytoma, a rare adrenaline secreting tumor.

CONGENITAL ADRENAL HYPERPLASIA

Congenital adrenal hyperplasia (CAH) is a group of inherited disorders marked by congenital deficiency or absence of one or more enzymes essential for the production of adrenal cortical hormones. It is inherited as an autosomal recessive disorder.

The enzyme involved most commonly is 21 - hydroxylase (90–95%). Deficiency of 11-beta-hydroxylase (5–8%) and 3-beta-hydroxysteroid dehydrogenase also lead to CAH. The production of adrenal mineralocorticoids and glucocorticoids is blocked by the enzyme deficiency in the steroid pathway.

Commonly there is insufficiency of cortisol, aldosterone and androgen productions. Due to lack of feedback suppression, ACTH and renin are secreted to stimulate adrenal gland production causing hyperplasia of the gland.

Aldosterone insufficiency results in fluid-electrolyte imbalance. Cortisol insufficiency results in diminished hepatic glucogenesis. Overproduction of androgens will virilize female external genitalia and under production of androgens will block virilization of male external genitalia.

Clinical Manifestations

The most common form of the condition is life-threatening and requires diagnosis and treatment soon after birth.

The important presenting feature is ambiguous genitalia. In female, there is varying degree of virilization due to exposure of androgens during intrauterine development. The infant presents with clitoromegaly, labial fusion, rugated labia appearing scrotal shaped and incomplete vagina. The male infant presents with incomplete virilization as small penis, and incomplete scrotal fusion.

Neonates with salt-losing CAH due to associated aldosterone deficiencies may cause life-threatening emergencies and present with severe vomiting, fluid-electrolyte imbalance and vascular collapse with shock.

In other form of CAH, decreased secretions of adrenal steroids and increased production of ACTH may cause a variety of clinical symptoms like hyperpigmentation, virilization and hypertension. About seven variants of CAH may present with menstrual irregularities, hirsutism and acne in later life.

Diagnostic Evaluation

Neonatal assessment and detection of ambiguous genitalia followed by enzyme assay, serum electrolytes and glucose estimations, pelvic ultrasonography and karyotyping help to confirm the diagnosis.

Prenatal diagnosis can be done by assay of 17-ketosteroids, 17-OHP and pregnanetriol in amniotic fluid or by genotyping or HLA typing of amniotic cells by chorionic villus sampling in suspected cases.

Management

Management of CAH include replacement of glucocorticoids and mineralocorticoids, addition of salt and surgical reconstruction of ambiguous genitalia. In prenatal period, administration of dexamethasone at 5th week of gestation can prevent the sexual ambiguity. In postnatal period, the adequacy of treatment should be monitored with serial estimations of enzymes and adrenal steroid levels. Growth parameters should be checked, especially bone age indicate the adequacy of treatment. Emotional support is essential for family members with necessary guidance for future management.

AMBIGUOUS GENITALIA

"Ambiguous" means being difficult to classify. Ambiguous genitalia indicates having external genitalia that are not distinguishable as being of either sexual form. It is a condition with discrepancy between the external genitals and internal gonads. There are characteristics of neither a male nor a female. Hence, they are designated as intersex or hermaphrodite. The condition is termed as hermaphroditism. It is a congenital abnormality evident at birth.

Types of Hermaphroditism

True Hermaphroditism

In this condition the individual possesses both ovarian and testicular glands either in the same (ovotestis) or opposite gonads. Majority of them have 46XX karyotype. It is quite rare condition.

Pseudohermaphroditism

In this condition the individual possesses sex glands of one sex but genitalia of the opposite sex. Gonads are normal. The condition is relatively common and found as female pseudohermaphroditism and male pseudohermaphroditism.

Female pseudohermaphroditism (FPH): It is the most common type and is characterized by female phenotype with XX genotype. Gonads are ovaries but the external genitalia are virilized. It occurs due to exposure of female fetus to androgens in early gestation due to maternal medication with androgens or progestational agent like diethylstilbestrol. Female pseudohermaphroditism may also occur due to maternal virilizing tumors (arrhenoblastoma) or due to congenital adrenal hyperplasia. The condition is manifested by a large clitoris resembling the penis and hypertrophied labia majora resembling the scrotum, thus producing a resemblance of a male genitalia.

Male pseudohermaphroditism (MPH): It is generally characterized by male phenotype and XY genotype. The external genitalia are incompletely virilized or may be ambiguous or completely female. This condition is considered as MPH, marked by a small penis, perineal hypospadias and scrotum without testes, which resembling the vulva. It occurs due to disease of the adrenal gland or a feminizing tumor of the undescended testis.

Diagnostic Evaluation

Clinical suspicion regarding pseudohermaphroditism should be made in case of small penis, hypospadias and undescended testes in male child and presence of mass in the labia majora or groin in female child. These conditions require detailed history, through physical examination and laboratory investigations.

Detailed history should include family history of ambiguous genitalia, history of abortion or early neonatal death, history of consanguinity and intake of hormone or medication during pregnancy.

Thorough head to foot examination to be done with special attention about presence of renal and other congenital abnormalities, presence or absence of testis, degree of labioscrotal fusion, size of penis or clitoris, presence of hypospadias, etc. Rectal examination to be done to identify the presence of uterus, vaginal pouch and prostate. Growth assessment is important to detect abnormality.

Radiological studies help to diagnose the condition. Plain X-ray helps to detect the bone age which is advanced in congenital adrenal hyperplasia but delayed in gonadal dysgenesis and hypopituitarism. Retrograde genitourethrogram helps to detect abnormal internal genital structures. USG, CT scan and MRI are helpful for detection of status of internal genitalia, undescended gonads and anomalies of adrenal glands.

The following laboratory investigations can be done to confirm the diagnosis:

- Buccal smear or peripheral blood or bone marrow study are helpful to diagnose the real gonadal sex by the presence of nuclear sex chromatin study.
- Chromosomal study, gonadal biopsy, urethroscopy, vaginogram and laparotomy can be done to detect the abnormal characteristics.
- Urinary excretion of increased pregnanetriol, 17-keto-steroid and 17-OHP is diagnostic of CAH.
- Serum electrolyte variations especially high serum potassium level in ambiguous genitalia with positive buccal smear and advanced bone age help to confirm the diagnosis of CAH.
- Serum testosterone or estrogen estimation is often useful in the diagnosis of intersex.

Management

Management depends upon underlying cause and associated conditions. Early diagnosis with specific management by hormonal therapy and steroid therapy with surgical reconstruction of external genitalia may be effective. Support to the parent and family members are very essential to cope with the situation. Necessary instructions and health teaching to be given for continuation of management.

UNDESCENDED TESTES (CRYPTORCHIDISM)

Undescended testes is the failure of one or both testes to reach the normal position in the scrotum through the inguinal canal.

It is more common in preterm infant. The testes lie intra-abdominally upto 7th month of intrauterine life. It descends to the scrotum between 8th and 9th month of fetal life. Due to several factors it fails to descent.

It is found in 3 to 4 percent of full term infants and 20 to 30 percent of preterm infants. Two-third of them descend ultimately into normal scrotal position within first year of life.

Causes

The most probable cause is an impairment of the hypo-thalamic pituitary gonadal axis, i.e. block in the hormonal pathways to stimulate the testes to descend or the testes may fail to respond to stimulus due to some inherent deficit. There may be anatomical obstruction along the pathway of descent or failure of intra-abdominal pressure to rise (e.g. examphalos). Heredity and chromosomal abnormalities or absence of one or both testes (anorchia) can be the cause of undescent or maldescent. Short spermatic cord and artery mechanically prevent the descent of small and ill formed immobile testes, which may fail to descend below the external inguinal ring. There may be ectopic attachment of the testes which prevent the descend. The undescended testes may found in the abdominal cavity near the pubic tubercle, in the inguinal canal and retroperitoneal space.

Clinical Types

Retractile Testis or Pseudocryptorchidism

Because of cremasteric reflex, testis may be temporarily pulled-up from the scrotum into the inguinal canal or abdomen especially in cold environment and during examination. That can be coaxed back into the scrotum by sliding the fingers from the internal inguinal ring towards the scrotum. Ascent of the testis can be prevented by placing the fingers first across the upper portion of the inguinal canal. This condition is termed as retractile testis or pseudocryptorchidism.

True Cryptorchidism

It is termed when the testis is located in the abdomen or inguinal canal. Rarely it can be found in perineum, femoral area or in front of symphysis pubis at the base of the penis as ectopic testis. Scrotum of the affected side may be smaller or flat in bilateral type. It may be associated with inguinal hernia. This condition can be complicated with malignancy and poor spermatogenesis leading to infertility or sterility in later life. True cryptorchidism can be described as follows:

- *Arrested descent (30%, bilateral):* Descent may stop anywhere along the normal pathway. The subtypes are intra-abdominal, canalicular, emergent and high scrotal.

- *Deviated or ectopic testis (30% bilateral):* Testes are found away from the normal line of descent. The testis is usually firmer and bigger. The subtypes are superficial, inguinal, pubopenile, perineal and crural.
- *Absence of testis:* It can be associated with or without intersex and destruction of testis following infarction, torsion or mumps (vanishing testis syndrome). Absence of testis is termed as anorchia.

Clinical Manifestations

Undescended testis can be unilateral or bilateral. The child presents with absence of testis in the scrotum showing the scrotum empty. There may be signs of complications like torsion, tumor, trauma and hernia which is usually associated with 60 to 70 percent cases.

If the problem is not treated, it can be complicated with impaired testicular function leading to sterility, as the sperm forming cells are damaged when testes remain in higher temperature in abdominal cavity than the scrotal temperature. Dysgenesis of sperms may cause malignancy. Psychological problems may found in some children with this condition.

Diagnostic Evaluation

Physical examination, related history, USG, laparoscopy and hormonal assay help to diagnose the condition and its complications.

Management

Natural and spontaneous descent of undescended testes occur by one year of age. The best time for therapy is between 1 to 2 years of age to prevent complications.

Administration of hormonal therapy with human chorionic gonadotropin (HCG) may cause descent of the testis in some children. HCG also results in enlargement of the testes. It is administered as 250 units below one year, 500 units between one and five years and 1000 units above 5 years, twice a week for 5 to 6 weeks. Usually good response found within one month. Leuteinizing hormone releasing hormone (LHRH) can also be used alternatively as injection or nasal spray. Post-treatment retraction rate may be high with poor response to hormonal therapy. In such cases, surgery (orchidopexy) should be done early by 2 years of age for good result.

Orchidopexy is performed to fix the testes in the scrotum. If there is an associated hernia, then herniotomy along with orchidopexy is indicated on the same time. Operative complications may develop as atrophy of testes due to damage of testicular vessels.

In case of absence of testes, a silastic prosthesis can be inserted at 8 to 10 years of age to overcome emotional problem.

PRECOCIOUS PUBERTY

Precocious puberty or advanced sexual development is unusual early sexual maturation and development of secondary sexual characteristics before the age of 8 years in girls and 9 years in boys. It can be two types: (a) central or true precocious puberty and (b) peripheral or pseudoprecocious puberty.

Central or true precocious puberty (CPP) is caused by premature activation of hypothalamic-pituitary-gonadal (HPG) axis. It may occur due to congenital anomalies, cranial irradiation, hydrocephalus, CNS tumor, CNS trauma, and as complications of CNS infections. Hypothalamic hamartoma is a common cause of precocious puberty. The condition is manifested as premature spermatogenesis or ovulation along with complete physical and sexual maturation same as in normal puberty. It is 4 to 5 times more common in girls.

Peripheral or pseudoprecocious puberty (PPP) occurs due to increased secretions of sex steroid hormones (androgen or estrogen) from either the adrenal glands or the gonads (ovaries or testes). It is independent of the activation of HPG axis. The sexual development is incomplete or partial with no spermatogenesis or ovulation, but other signs of sexual maturation are present. There is rapid somatic growth.

Combined type of both central and peripheral precocious puberty may occur secondary to peripheral precocious puberty with activation HPG axis.

The *diagnosis* of the condition can be done with detailed history, thorough physical examination, X-ray, MRI, endocrine assay, gonadal biopsy and laparotomy to find out the exact cause and associated problems.

Management of precocious puberty can be done by the treatment of underlying cause and drug therapy.

Drug therapy for CPP is given with gonadotropin releasing hormone (GnRH) analogous (triptorelin, leuprolid) intramuscular (IM) for once a month. In case of PPP, drug therapy is given with medroxy-progesterone acetate (Depoprovera) 100 mg/m^2 every 2 to 3 week, IM or 10 mg twice daily orally. Cyproterone (antiandrogenic) is administered to stop menstrual bleeding and to regress secondary sexual characteristics. It is given 75 to 100 mg/m^2 in 2 to 3 divided doses. Ketoconazole is also used in treatment of PPP to suppress gonadal hormone secretions.

Precocious puberty may lead to psychosocial problem and sexual abuse. The child and parents need counseling and guidance for protection from psychosexual hazards.

Sex education is very important for the child that should be planned according to the chronological age.

DELAYED SEXUAL DEVELOPMENT (DELAYED PUBERTY)

Delayed puberty is the lack or delayed sexual development and progression. It occurs due to lack of production or secretion of gonadal steroids from the testes (i.e. testosterone) or from the ovaries (i.e. estrogen) leading to failure to achieve sexual maturity. It can be two types, primary or secondary delayed puberty.

Etiology

Primary Delayed Sexual Development

It occurs due to absence or dysfunction of the gonads. It is found in Turner's syndrome (45, X0), gonadal dysgenesis and in bilateral gonadal failure due to radiation, chemotherapy, infections, defect in gonadal steroid synthesis, trauma, etc.

Secondary Delayed Sexual Development

It occurs due to lack of hypothalamic pituitary stimulation to gonads. It is found in hypothalamic lesions due to infections, trauma, irradiation, or isolated deficiency of GnRH. It may also occur in pituitary lesions, in hypopituitarism or isolated LH and FSH deficiencies.

Failure of end organs to respond to circulating gonadal hormone, i.e. in androgen insensitivity also can cause this problem. Other causes are chronic illness, anorexia nervosa and autoimmune atrophy.

Clinical Manifestations

In female, lack of breasts development by the age of 13 to 13.5 years indicate the delayed puberty. In male, lack of testicular enlargement by the age of 14 years is indicative of the condition. Failure to progress through the puberty changes and emotional lability are commonly found. Sterility is common complication.

Diagnostic Evaluation

History and clinical examination to detect nutritional deficiencies, chronic illness and family history related to delayed puberty should be obtained. Diagnosis is confirmed by X-ray to detect bone age and laboratory investigations of estimation of sex steroids (testosterone, estrogen) and gonadotropins (LH or FSH). Abdominal and pelvic USG to view the internal organs help to diagnose the abnormalities.

Management

Management of delayed puberty is done by replacement of gonadal steroids. For boys, testosterone supplement to be administered 50 to 100 mg monthly by injection until final height is achieved, then 200 mg monthly. For girls, conjugated estrogen 0.3 to 0.625 mg daily by oral tablet to be given. Progestational agents can be added to the therapy. This hormonal therapy may be warranted to promote puberty and sustain sexual characteristics. The cause of the condition should be detect and appropriate management to be planned. Psychological support to the adolescent is important and should be emphasized through discussion for improvement of body image, hair style, clothing, make up, etc. Continuation of treatment and its side effects to be discussed.

MENSTRUAL ABNORMALITIES

Menstrual abnormalities are common concerns of adolescent girls which include premenstrual syndrome, dysmenorrhea, amenorrhea, menorrhagia, etc.

Premenstrual Syndrome

Premenstrual syndrome (PMS) is also known as premenstrual tension syndrome and recently known as premenstrual dysmorphic disorder. It is related to hormonal imbalance like prostaglandins, endorphins and with psychoenvironmental factors.

It is characterized by symptoms such as markedly depressed mood, marked anxiety, marked affective lability and decreased interest in activities. The symptoms occurs regularly during last week of luteal phase in most menstrual cycle about 7 to 10 days before onset of menstruation. It usually disappears within one or two days after beginning of the menstrual periods. For the diagnosis of PMS, history of five or more of the episodes must be present in previous 12 months.

The adolescent girls with PMS usually present with feeling of sad, hopeless, feeling of tense, anxious with marked lability of mood and frequent tearfulness. The girls may have persistent irritability, anger, increased interpersonal conflicts, decreased interest in usual activities and withdrawal behavior. Difficulty in concentration, feeling of fatigue, lethargic, lacking of energy, marked changed in appetite with craving of salty and sweet foods are also present. Hypersomnia and insomnia may found.

Physical symptoms include breast tenderness or swelling, headaches, dizziness, vertigo, palpitation, sensation of bloating, weight gain, swelling of fingers and legs, joint or muscle pain, acne, etc. Suicidal thoughts may be accompanied.

The condition is diagnosed on the basis of clinical manifestations. Usually no diagnostic evaluation is necessary.

Management depends upon severity of symptoms. Mild analgesics, progesterone therapy or oral pill may be helpful. Tranquilizers may be needed. Diuretic can be given to reduce edema of the extremities. Limiting salt intake, refined sugar, caffine, animal fats and increasing intake of leafy green vegetables, whole grain cereals and complex carbohydrate are beneficial. Calcium and vitamin B_6 supplementation to be given. Regular exercise may help to relief discomfort. Explanation, reassurance and emotional support with diversional activities are essential aspect of management. The condition is usually self limiting without any complications.

Dysmenorrhea

Dysmenorrhea is painful menstruation, most common gynecologic dysfunction. Primary dysmenorrhea is usually intrinsic to uterus and most common type. It may be due to increased prostaglandin production by the endometrium. It may also occur due to hormonal, obstructive and psychological factors. Secondary dysmenorrhea is caused by congenital anomalies, uterine fibroids, ovarian cyst, endometritis and pelvic infections.

The *clinical features* occur due to uterine contractility and uterine hypoxia. The adolescent girls with dysmenorrhea present with characteristics menstrual cramps (i.e. colic or dull pain), spasmodic or constant and generally located in the lower mid-abdominal or suprapubic area. Associated symptoms are nausea, vomiting, diarrhea, headache, chills, tiredness, nervousness, low backache, abdominal discomfort, pallor, sweating and syncope. Pain may be moderate to severe and may last for a few hours to one or two days causing short-term school absenteeism.

The underlying cause of dysmenorrhea should be ruled out by abdominal and pelvic examination along with abdominal USG and other necessary investigations.

Management of primary dysmenorrhea to be done with application of local heat on abdomen or lower back by heating pad to increase blood flow and decrease spasms. Excercise, good posture, sleep, good nutrition, hygienic measures and mild analgesics or sedative are useful aspect of management to decrease the discomfort. Aspirin or acetaminophen may also be used. Prostaglandin inhibitor drugs is recommended. Ibuprofen 400 mg three to four times a day can also be effective. Oral contraceptives may be indicated to decrease uterine contractility. Usually, the condition is self-limiting without complications. Emotional support to the girl is essential to reduce stress and anxiety. The management of secondary dysmenorrhea to be done depending upon the underlying pathology.

Amenorrhea

Amenorrhea is the absence of menstruation due to primary and secondary cause.

In primary amenorrhea, menarche does not occur by the age of 16 years. It is caused by chromosomal, hormonal, nutritional and psychogenic disorders. Primary amenorrhea is found in gonadal dysgenesis, triple - X syndrome, imperforate hymen, hematocolpos, hematometrium, agenesis of cervix, uterine agenesis or malformations, etc.

Secondary amenorrhea occurs when menstruation stops for more than 3 months after establishment of regular cycle. The underlying causes are psychogenic, hormonal, nutritional or exercise-related disorders, polycystic ovary disease, pituitary tumors and hyperthyroidism. Other causes are anorexia nervosa, cystic fibrosis, chronic illnesses, malnutrition, cyanotic congenital heart disease, diabetes mellitus, inflammatory bowel disease and medications like phenothiazines, oral contraceptives, etc. Pregnancy is the most frequent cause of secondary amenorrhea.

Diagnostic Evaluation

Detailed history should include menstrual history of mother, sister and aunts. Physical examination to be done to detect associated problems. Laboratory investigations should include hormonal study for estrogen, progesterone, LH, FSH, prolactin, TSH level to exclude the hormonal disorders. Genetic karyotyping to be done to detect chromosomal abnormalities. Abdominal USG and X-ray may be indicated to confirm the diagnosis. Pregnancy test to be done in suspected cases.

Management

Management of amenorrhea depends upon the exact cause. Nutritional support, exercise and counseling are general measures. Hormone replacement therapy may be indicated in some cases. Emotional support is essential for effective condition. Specific management to be planned with consultation of gynecologist, when indicated.

Menorrhagia

Menorrhagia is excessive bleeding during regular menstruation. It can be increased in duration or amount of blood or both. Other conditions related to abnormal menstruation are metrorrhagia and polymenorrhea. Metrorrhagia is the uterine bleeding between regular menstrual periods. It is significant because usually it is a symptom of disease. Polymenorrhea is the frequent menstruation occurring at intervals of less than 3 weeks.

Menorrhagia may be caused by endocrine disturbances, hypothyroidism, estrogen secreting ovarian tumor or due to many other conditions like hypertension, diabetes mellitus, blood dyscrasias, etc. Excessive menstrual bleeding may be the first symptom of thrombocytopenic purpura.

Diagnosis of the underlying pathological condition can be done by detailed history, (especially menstrual history) thorough physical examination, hormonal estimation, blood tests and USG.

Management of the condition should be done depending upon the specific cause. Iron therapy, emotional support, hormonal therapy may be needed. Gynecological consultation should be required for definitive management.

OBESITY

Obesity is the excessive accumulation of fat in the subcutaneous tissues and other body parts. Overweight is the term used when the body weight is increased more than 110 percent of the standard weight and the triceps skinfold thickness is more than 30 mm. The term obesity is used when the body weight is increased more than 120 percent of the standard weight.

Body mass index (BMI) is the most useful screening parameter for children and adolescent to assess obesity. BMI correlates significantly with subcutaneous and total body fat. High BMI correlates with blood pressure and serum lipid levels. It has significant predictive value for adult obesity related to morbidity and mortality. BMI is calculated with the following formula:

$$BMI = \frac{Weight\ in\ kg}{(Height\ in\ meter)^2}$$

BMI value more than 30 or more than 95th percentile indicates presence of obesity.

Causes of Obesity

Endogenous Obesity

- *Genetic cause:* Prader-Willi syndrome, Laurence-Moon-Biedl-Bardet syndrome.
- *Endocrinal cause:* Hypothyroidism, Cushing syndrome, hypogonadism, pseudohypoparathyroidism, polycystic ovary, hyperandrogenic ovary syndrome, growth hormone deficiency.
- *Hypothalamic obesity:* Froehlich syndrome, postencephalitic obesity, postmeningitic obesity.

Exogenous Obesity

Constitutional, excessive dietary consumption or overeating due to psychogenic factors, poor energy expenditure, fat cell hyperplasia, etc.

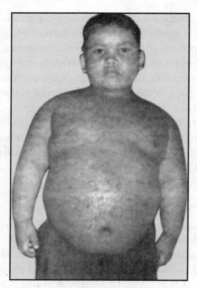

Fig. 22.1: Obesity in (65 kg body weight) the age of 7 years

Clinical Manifestations

The child is fatty with body weight more than 95th percentile for that age or in excess 20 percent of average weight for age or BMI above 30 kg/m² (Fig. 22.1).

There is fat deposition all over the body. Excessive fat deposition over the neck gives the look of double chin. Fat deposition found in gluteal region, thighs, abdomen and around breast. External genitalia, hands and feet appear small. Knocked knee, slipped femoral epiphysis may present. Emotional problem may also found in these children.

Management

Dietary restriction is important with avoidance of mid-meal snacks, chocolates, candies, sweets and icecream. Increasing physical exercise, sports and encouraging to loss weight gradually should be explained to the child and parents. Regular weight recording and follow-up are essential. Appetite can be reduced by drugs like amphetamines. Psychogenic overeating in children indicates need for counseling.

DIABETES MELLITUS

Diabetes mellitus (DM) is the most common endocrine metabolic disorder of childhood and adolescence with long-term effects on child's physical and psychological growth and development. It can lead to damage, dysfunction, or failure of various organs specially eyes, kidneys, nerves, heart, blood vessels, etc.

Diabetes mellitus is a disorder of glucose intolerance due to deficiency in insulin production and it's action leading to hyperglycemia and abnormalities in carbohydrate, protein and fat metabolism.

Approximately 5 percent of all diabetics are children. Peak incidence in children is found around 5 years and about 10 to 12 years. Insulin dependent diabetes mellitus (IDDM) occurs at younger age. About 25 to 50 percent patients are presenting before 15 years of age. Type I DM may be significantly altered by changes in geography and lifestyle.

Classification

Diabetes mellitus is now classified as two types: Type I and type II, as per Expert Committee of American Diabetes Association and WHO.

Type I Diabetes Mellitus

It results from autoimmune destruction of beta cells. It is characterized by gross deficiency of insulin (insulinopenia) and dependence on exogenous insulin for prevention of ketoacidosis. It occurs mainly in childhood, (juvenile-onset diabetes) though there is no age bar. Majority of type I cases are idiopathic.

Type II Diabetes Mellitus

It is rare in children and not associated with autoimmune process or disease. It is usually not insulin dependent and not complicated by ketoacidosis. Previously it was known as adult-onset diabetes or maturity onset diabetes or stable diabetes.

In pediatric age group, particularly in younger and school aged children, most cases are type 1 diabetes. The incidence of type II DM is now rapidly increasing due to morbid obesity, sedentary lifestyle, high caloric intake and family history of diabetes.

The terms insulin-dependent diabetes mellitus (IDDM), noninsulin dependent diabetes mellitus (NIDDM) and malnutrition related diabetes mellitus (MRDM) have been eliminated by the Expert Committee on the diagnosis and classification of diabetes mellitus sponsored by the American Diabetes Association and WHO.

Other Specific Types (Secondary DM)

- Genetic defects of betacell function.
- Genetic defects in insulin action.
- Diseases of exocrine pancreas, cystic fibrosis, pancreatitis, fibrocalculous pancreatopathy, surgery of the pancreas.
- Endocrinopathies—Cushing syndrome, hyperthyroidism.
- Drugs or chemical induced (steroids, pentamidine).
- Infections—Rubella virus, CMV.
- Immune mediated—anti-insulin receptor antibodies.

- Other genetic syndromes—Down's syndrome, Turner's syndrome, Klinefelter's syndrome.

Etiopathogenesis

Approximately 95 percent of childhood DM are idiopathic with absolute deficiency of insulin due to hereditary inborn error of metabolism. Etiology of type 1 DM are considered as genetic, environmental factors and autoimmune reactions. The environmental factors are necessary to trigger the onset of autoimmunity in genetically susceptible individuals. Infectious disease like mumps, coxsackie virus, CMV are associated with development of type I DM. Environmental toxins (rodenticides) and early introduction of cow's milk protein may be important factors for development of diabetes mellitus.

Due to autoimmune reaction, there is inflammation of the beta cells of pancreas. The inflammatory process seems to stimulate the beta cells to produce slightly abnormal class II human leukocyte antigens (HLAs). Lymphocytes recognize these antigen as nonself and destroy them, releasing more beta cell proteins that can make additional HLAs and stimulate an ongoing immune response that eventually destroys all the beta cells which secrete insulin. The HLAs in the pancreas are determined genetically. Because most patients with type I DM have HLA - DR_3, HLA - DR_4 or both for development of an autoimmune response.

Clinical Manifestations

Childhood diabetes is usually rapid in onset and may present with diabetic coma. It needs injectable insulin for treatment. Obesity plays no role in childhood DM. Dietetic control alone never helps the diabetic children to improve from the condition.

Clinical features of type I DM are evident, when 90 percent of pancreatic beta cell synthesis and release capacity is destroyed or effectively inactivated.

The onset of the disease is usually acute over a period of few weeks with classical triad features, i.e. polyuria, polyphagia and polydipsia. Other features include nocturia, enuresis (who was earlier dry), weight loss, general weakness, tiredness, and bodily pains. Fainting attack due to hypoglycemia, pain abdomen, nausea, vomiting, irritability, vulvovaginitis in girls, skin infection, dry skin, poor wound healing may also occur.

Diabetic coma may be the first presenting feature and the child may hospitalized with diabetic ketoacidosis (DKA).

The child with DKA may present in precomatosed state with drowsiness, dryness of skin, cherry red lips, increased respirations, nausea, vomiting and abdominal pain. In comatosed state, the child may have extreme hyperpnea (Kussmaul breathing), acetone breath, soft and sunken eyeballs, rigid abdomen, rapid weak pulse, decreased body temperature, dehydration and decreased BP. Circulatory collapse and renal failure may develop with fluid-electrolyte imbalance. There may be precipitating factors like infections, trauma and intercurrent infections. The diagnostic features of DKA are hyperglycemia (more than 250–300 mg/dL), ketonemia and acidosis (pH below 7.3 and bicarbonate level below 15–20 m Eq/L) with glucosuria and ketonuria.

Complications

Diabetes mellitus has wide range of complications and presented as acute, subacute or intermediate and chronic conditions.

Acute complications are usually reversible and found as diabetic coma, hypoglycemia, diabetic ketoacidosis (70%) and infections.

Subacute or intermediate complications are potentially reversible and presented as growth failure, delayed sexual maturation, impaired neurological development, poor school performance, poor psychological development, limited joint mobility and lipohypertrophy.

Chronic complications are usually irreversible. They occur due to macrovascular and microvascular pathological changes. Retinopathy, nephropathy and neuropathy are the most common complications usually manifested later in life. Retinopathy is the most common microvascular alteration. Metabolic cataract may also develop. Neuropathy is manifested as diminished motor nerve conduction velocity, changes in sensory nerve, decreased vibration perception along with peripheral and autonomic neuropathy. Nephropathy is found as Kimmelstiel-Wilson syndrome, renal failure and overt nephropathy. Other chronic complications are hepatomegaly, chronic infections like boils, styes, abscesses, fungal infections and tuberculosis. Hypertension, atherosclerosis, CCF, blindness may also develop in the children having diabetes mellitus.

Diagnostic Evaluation

History of classical triad symptoms, i.e. polyuria, polyphagia, polydipsia are very important diagnostic criteria. Physical examination along with other history of illness and laboratory investigations help to confirm the diagnosis. The following investigations and their findings are important.

- Blood sugar estimation reveals as follows:
  - Random blood sugar level 200 mg/dL or more on two separate occasions with clinical features of diabetes mellitus suggest the diagnosis.
  - Fasting blood sugar level 126 mg/dL or more or two occasions is suggestive and 100 to 126 mg/dL is highly suspicious and 160 mg/dL is diagnostic of the condition.
  - Oral glucose tolerance test is rarely required in children and may be done in doubtful cases with oral

glucose intake of 1.75 gm/kg of ideal body weight—(maximum 75 gm).
- Urine examination for the presence of sugar and ketones.

Management

Management of DM in children involves combination of insulin therapy, dietary management, physical exercise, prevention of complications, promotion of growth and emotional-social development. These children need care in team approach. Nursing personnel has a pivotal role in the management of the children and educating the parents, children and family members regarding different aspect of care.

The diabetic child can be managed at home but initially hospitalization is necessary for stabilization of child's condition and to educate the family members and the child about home care and follow-up.

Insulin Therapy

Initial requirement of insulin may be 1 to 1.75 units/kg/day. Then the dose may be less than 0.5 units per kg/day after 12 to 16 weeks. The total calculated dose is administered in divided amount, i.e. 2/3rd dose in morning and 1/3rd dose at night. Split mix regimen can be followed with 2/3rd lente (intermediate acting) and 1/3rd regular (short acting) insulin.

Adjustments of dosages may be required depending upon blood glucose level, urine sugar and ketone level, diet and exercise. Urine should be examined before each injection of insulin.

Exercise and Physical Activity

These should be emphasized to increase glucose utilization and sensitivity of muscles to insulin. Exercise should include walking, jogging, swimming, aerobic exercises and games.

Diet Therapy

Daily dietary planning for diabetic children is important for prevention of acute or long-term complications and promotion of growth and development. Diet should be recommended depending upon the blood sugar level, metabolic status, standard of living and requirements for growth and development.

Carbohydrates can be provided up to 55 to 60 percent of total calories. Increase in diet fiber is associated with lower glucose level in diabetics. It should be taken 20 to 35 gm/day from a varied diet. Concentrated carbohydrates like candies, sugar, sweets, chocolates and cakes to be avoided.

Protein intake should be 15 percent of total calories, though it depends upon renal function, glycemic status and

need for growth and development. In adolescents it can be lowered up to 8 percent of total calorie intake.

Fat should be allowed about 30 to 35 percent of total calorie and not more than 10 percent should be saturated or polyunsaturated fat.

Deficiency of micronutrients may occur in diabetic child so dietary intake should contain the essential micronutrients.

Diet should be planned for three major meals and three mid-meal snacks to avoid hypoglycemia.

Follow-up

The diabetic child should be reviewed every 3 to 4 months for follow-up. History of diet, exercise, activity and presence of any problems are essential for necessary modifications of treatment schedule. Physical examination should include assessment of growth (height, weight) blood pressure, condition of site of insulin injection, and presence of any infections. Ophthalmic check up with fundoscopy should be done once a year or as indicated. Blood examination to be done for glucose, glycosylated Hb, serum lipids (cholesterol, HDL, LDL, VLDL, triglycerides) and thyroid function tests (TSH, T4). Urine should be tested for sugar and protein. Self-monitoring of blood glucose, urine glucose and ketones are important aspects that should be explained and record book or diary to be maintained for follow-up.

Emotional Support and Diabetic Education

Emotional support and health teaching to the family members and children are essential to up-to-date their knowledge and skill in long-term care.

Demonstration should be given about urine testing, blood testing (self-monitoring), administration of insulin and diet therapy. Informations to be given regarding interpretation of signs and symptoms, need for follow-up, prevention of complications, etc. Instruction to be given to carry a "diabetic card" and to contact with diabetic association and other support facilities.

Management of Diabetic Ketoacidosis

Diabetic ketoacidosis (DKA) is a severe life-threatening complication of DM and serious manifestations of insulin deficiency as fluid electrolyte imbalance, metabolic acidosis, ketonemia and hypertriglyceridemia.

The child with DKA needs immediate management. Assessment should be done for level of consciousness, severity of dehydration, acidosis, BP, pulse, skin turger and body weight. Presence of infections or any precipitating factors to be assessed.

Laboratory investigations should be done to confirm the diagnosis of DKA. Blood examination for glucose, ketone, pH, bicarbonate, triglyceride, potassium, etc to be done. Urine examination is done for glucose acetone/acetoacetate.

Management of DKA should include fluid therapy, initially with normal saline (0.9%) or dextrose (5%) in normal saline (0.45%) and administration of insulin therapy, bolus dose (0.1 unit/kg) and then in continuous IV drip (0.1 unit/kg/hour), then S/C insulin therapy, when meals are tolerated. Potassium supplementation to be given (after urination). Bicarbonate replacement, antibiotic therapy and treatment of cerebral edema may be required. Monitoring of patients condition is vital and should be done with ECG, intake output chart, blood for glucose, eletrolytes, BUN, creatinine, pH, ketone, calcium, phosphorus, etc. Level of consciousness, vital signs and signs of deterioration or improvement should be monitored.

Nursing Management of Diabetes Mellitus

Nursing Assessment

- History of onset of signs and symptoms and associated problems like weight loss, pain abdomen, dehydration, etc. along with detailed history of illness.
- Physical examination to detect physical signs, slow healing sore, fruity smell to breath (acetone breath due to ketosis).
- Assessment of cardiac function—tachycardia, hypotension, arrhythmias, dehydration.
- Assessment of renal function—urine output, glycosuria, ketonuria, intake-output balance chart.
- Assessment of GI function—dietary intake, diarrhea, constipation, hunger, thirst, flatullence.
- Assessment of neurologic status—numbness, pain, change in gait, tingling sensation of the extremities.
- Assessment of growth and development, presence of complications, review of self-monitoring record, etc.

Nursing Diagnoses

Important nursing diagnoses should include the followings:
- Altered nutritional intake due to insulin deficiency and alteration of metabolism.
- Knowledge deficit related to insulin therapy.
- Knowledge deficit related to blood glucose monitoring.
- Risk of injury related to hypoglycemia.
- Fluid-volume deficit related to DKA.
- Fear and anxiety related to long-term illness.
- Risk for infection related to hyperglycemic state.

Nursing Interventions

- Providing nutritional requirement as planned to prevent complications and to promote growth.

- Increasing knowledge and skill about insulin therapy. Information and demonstration to be given to administer insulin before meal with prescribed dose and type of insulin. Using rotation of sites methods for injections at upper arms and thighs. Outer areas of abdomen and hips may also be used. Insulin syringe with measuring scale, (same as unit strength of insulin) is required for administration of insulin. Aseptic technique to be followed during SC injections. Urine testing to be done before insulin injection and meal to be kept ready. Record to be maintained for urine test findings and insulin dose. Observing for any complications and encouraging to express feeling.
- Providing instructions about self-monitoring of blood glucose level. Procedure of blood test by glucometer or reagent strip to be demonstrated. Explanation to be given about precautions and times of blood test and for maintenance of records for reference to health care provider.
- Identifying and controlling hypoglycemia—Informing about symptoms of hypoglycemia it's cause and prevention. Hypoglycemia may occur in overdose of insulin, reduction in diet and increased exercise. It is manifested with trembling, shaking, dizziness, sweating, apprehension, drowsiness, unusual behavior, mental confusion, convulsions, coma, etc.
- Restoring fluid balance by IV fluid therapy in DKA.
- Reducing fear and anxiety by emotional support and health teaching on home care, follow-up, ophthalmic checkup, blood testing, exercise, play, avoidance of stress and trauma, continuation of school activities, identity card as diabetic, signs of hypo- or hyperglycemia, etc.
- Preventing infections by aseptic measures of injection, routine immunization, general cleanliness, hygienic measures especially care of skin, feet, legs, hands and prevention of cuts and injuries.

Prognosis

Diabetes mellitus is a chronic incurable disease but symptoms can be improved, complications can be prevented and life can be prolonged by appropriate management. The introduction of insulin (by Banting and Best in 1922) made it possible to allow the patients to lead normal life with this disease. The diabetic children with adequate treatment usually have fairly reasonable growth and development with remarkable increase in average life span.

Prevention of diabetes is under trial. Detection of prediabetic stage by measurement of autoantibodies, genetic risk and beta cell functions, secondary prevention and immunosuppression are also in experimental phase.

Eye, ENT and Orodental Problems in Children

23

- Diseases of the Eye
- Ear Problems in Children
- Disorders of the Nose
- Disorders of Throat

- Dental Problems
- Problems of Oral Cavity
- Cleft Lip and Cleft Palate

DISEASES OF THE EYE

Diseases of the eye may be related to a variety of systemic disorders. Isolated problems like infections, congenital anomalies, trauma and vitamin deficiency are also commonly found in children. Prompt management is important for prevention of long-term complications. Detailed history related to eye problems, ophthalmological examination including test for visual acuity (using Snellen's chart) and color vision, (using Ishihara's chart), dark adaptation, pupillary reaction, external examination of eye ball, ophthalmoscopic examination, tonometry, refraction test, etc. should be performed to detect the abnormalities, their causes and complications.

Categorization of Common Ophthalmic Problems

Orbital Diseases and Disorders

Hypertelorism, hypotelorism, exophthalmos (proptosis), enophthalmos, microphthalmia, orbital cellulitis, periorbital cellulitis, orbital benign tumors (hemangioma, dermoid), orbital malignant tumors (rhabdomyosarcoma, lymphosarcoma, metastatic neuroblastoma, optic glioma, retinoblastoma), orbital injury.

Diseases of the Eyelids

Ptosis, lid retraction, lagophthalmos, blepharitis, entropion, ectropion, blepharospasm, hordeolum (stye), chalazion, coloboma, tumors, vascular anomalies.

Diseases of the Lacrimal System

Congenital nasolacrimal duct obstruction (dacryostenosis), dacryocystitis, alacrima (dry eye), chronic dacryoadenitis.

Diseases of Conjunctiva

Conjunctivitis, ophthalmia neonatorum, noninflammatory conditions like subconjunctival hemorrhage, conjunctival chemosis, pterygium, pingueculum, symblepharon, dermoid cyst, dermolipoma, conjunctival nevus, conjunctival xerosis, Bitot's spots, conjunctival discoloration, e.g. yellow in jaundice, deep red in polycythemia, neurofibromas, surface nodules over conjunctiva (in case of TB, leprosy, syphilis).

Corneal Diseases

Interstitial keratitis, dendritic keratitis, corneal ulcers, phlyctenules (phlyctenular keratoconjunctivitis), keratoconus, sclerocornea, microcornea, (anterior microphthalmia), megalocornea, congenital corneal opacity (leukoma), corneal pigmentation (in case of cystinosis), keratomalacia (in case of vitamin 'A' deficiency).

Abnormalities of Sclera

Blue sclera in Marfan's syndrome and osteogenesis imperfecta, blackish discoloration due to alcaptonuria, episcleritis and scleritis.

Pupillary and Uveal Tract Abnormalities

Aniridia, iris coloboma, congenital microcoria (miosis), congenital mydriasis, dyscoria, corectopia, anisocoria, leukocoria (cat's eye reflex, white pupil) persistent pupillary membrane, iridocyclitis, chorioretinitis, panophthalmitis, Brushfield spots, heterochronia (Horner's syndrome).

Disease of Lens

Cataracts, ectopia lentis.

Diseases of Eye Movement and Alignment

Strabismus (squint), nystagmus.

Refractive Errors

Hypermetropia (hyperopia), myopia, astigmatism, anisometropia.

Visual Disorders

Amblyopia, amaurosis, night blindness (nyctalopia), diplopia, dyslexia.

Diseases of Retina and Vitreous

Retinopathy of prematurity (Retrolental fibroplasia), retinopathy due to systemic disorders (hypertensive, diabetes, leukemia) retinal detachment, retinoblastoma, retinitis pigmentosa.

Optic Nerve Diseases

Papilledema (choked disk), optic neuritis, optic atrophy.

Increased Intraocular Pressure

Congenital increased intraocular pressure (also known as buphthalmos) and glaucoma (congenital, infantile juvenile).

Retinopathy of Prematurity (Retrolental Fibroplasia)

Retinopathy of prematurity (ROP) may develop in preterm infants (less than 33 weeks of gestational age) due to retinal immaturity and hyperoxia resulting from high concentration of oxygen therapy. The contributing factors are sick neonates with respiratory distress, apnea, bradycardia, infection, anemia, heart disease, hypoxia, hypercabia, acidosis, etc.

It is a bilateral complications of preterm infants. There is cessation of vasculogenesis with poor vascularization and myelination. Hyperoxia causes vasoconstriction of retinal arteries leading to retinal hypoxia, retinal edema and appearance of new blood vessels. A demarcated line developed between the vascularized and avascular retina. The line changes into a ridge with extraretinal fibrovascular tissue. This condition is followed by retinal hemorrhage, formation of retinovitreous fibrous tissue behind the lens and subtotal retinal detachment. ROP may be complicated with total retinal detachment followed by blindness.

Management of ROP can be done by early diagnosis, ROP screening and by laser therapy or by cryotherapy to the avascular retina, to prevent further progression of retinopathy. In case of total retinal detachment, vitreoretinal surgery may be perform to recover the condition.

ROP can be prevented by prevention of preterm delivery, appropriate use of oxygen therapy and vitamin 'E' supplementation as antioxidant in high risk neonates.

Congenital Nasolacrimal Duct Obstruction (Dacryostenosis)

The lacrimal gland is not well developed at birth. Approximately 2 to 5 percent neonates may have persistent watery discharge from eye and even conjunctivitis due to congenital obstruction of nasolacrimal duct. It occurs due to incomplete canalization of the nasolacrimal duct with a residual membrane at the lower end of the duct at the entrance of nasal cavity. It may be unilateral or bilateral.

The condition is manifested as continuous spilling of tear over onto the cheek. Excessive tearing may be found as 'wetness' of the eye or frank overflow of tears (epiphora). There may be mucoid or mucopurulent discharge, crusting of eyelids, erythema and maceration or excoriation of the cheek. In some children, reflux of fluid or discharge on massaging the nasolacrimal sac may be found. The condition may be complicated with secondary conjunctivitis and lacrimal duct infection.

The problem may resolve spontaneously by 1 to 3 months. Cleaning of eye with moist, sterile swab and gentle nasolacrimal massage to be done by downward and backward pressure, 15 to 20 times per day, over the tear passage to force the contents through the nasal orifice of the duct. Antibiotic eye drops may be required. Thorough hand washing before the cleaning and massaging is very important for prevention of infection.

If the problem persists beyond one year of age, 'probing' is performed to remove the obstruction. Probing may require to repeat once or twice. In some children, failure of repeated probing may need reconstructive surgery, i.e. dacrocystorhinostomy (DCR).

Childhood Cataract

Childhood cataract (opacity of lens) may be congenital or acquired. A wide number of conditions are responsible for pediatric cataracts.

The common causes of congenital cataract are prematurity, maternal infections (Toxoplasmosis, rubella, CMV, herpes simplex, measles, influenzae, etc.), chromosomal disorders (Trisomy-21, Turner's syndrome) and metabolic disorders (Galactosemia, PKU, cretinism mucopolysaccharidosis).

The acquired causes of cataract include eye trauma (contusion, foreign body, penetrating injury), child abuse, steroid induced, radiation, drug effects (tetracyclines, chlorpromazine), hypo- and hypervitaminosis 'D', juvenile onset diabetes mellitus, hypoglycemia, hypocalcemia, etc.

Congenital cataract is usually bilateral. The child presents with visible clouding of lens, varying impairment of vision and may found with amblyopia. The lamellar cataract is usually develop in children.

Management of cataract is performed with surgical removal of lens (early by 6 months of age) followed by correction of aphakia and amblyopia. Postoperative care should include sedation for first 24 hours to prevent crying (especially in infant), prevention of vomiting and prevention of increased intraocular pressure. Antibiotics and steroid eye ointments to prevent infections, aseptic eye care with eye patch and eye shield for several days to prevent injury are essential. Parental teaching and necessary information to be provided along with routine care.

Conjunctivitis

Conjunctivitis, the inflammation of conjunctiva, is most common eye problem in children. In neonates, it is termed as ophthalmia neonatorum.

Conjunctivitis may be infectious or noninfectious. The common causative organisms responsible for the infections are viruses (adenovirus, measles virus) or bacterias (*H. influenzae, N. gonorrheae, Chlamydia, Staphylococcus, Streptococcus*). The noninfectious conditions are due to allergy, irritants or toxins (chemicals, spray, cleansing agent, smoke, air pollutants) and systemic diseases (Stevens-Johnson syndrome). Endogenous allergic conjunctivitis may be found

in tuberculosis as phlyctenular conjunctivitis. Conjunctivitis may be a component of Reiter's disease (arthritis, urethritis and conjunctivitis).

The child with conjunctivitis presents with redness of the eye caused by dilatation of the blood vessels of the conjunctiva and excessive tearing with or without exudate. Sandy feeling, sticky eye lids, mucopurulent discharge and photophobia are commonly present. Vision is not usually affected and pupillary reaction to light is normal, unless in the presence of complications.

1. Bacterial conjunctivitis is managed with saline irrigation and application of antibiotic eye ointment (Bacitracin and Neomycin). The condition usually improves within 2 to 3 days.
2. Allergic conjunctivitis is characterized by itching of the eyes, increased lacrimation and mucoid discharge. Treatment is done with hydrocortisone ophthalmic ointment 3 to 4 times per day with antibiotic eye ointment. Antihistaminic is given orally. The condition may be complicated with corneal ulcer, if not treated appropriately. Cold compresses is helpful for allergic conjunctivitis.
3. Chronic follicular conjunctivitis may be seen commonly in children from orphanages, or schools. It is manifested by numerous follicles in the upper and lower conjunctiva. Response to treatment is usually poor. These children may suffer for 2 to 3 years.
4. Viral conjunctivitis commonly found in association with pharyngitis and characterized by watery discharge of eye. There is no specific treatment. Antibiotic eye ointment should be applied to prevent secondary infections.
5. Phlyctenular conjunctivitis may develop as allergic manifestations of tuberculosis or due to beta hemolytic streptococcal infections and in round worm infestations. The condition is manifested as painful erythema, irritation, lacrimation, soreness in one or both eyes. Other features are photophobia and blepharospasm with grey spot at the limbus in one or both eyes. The condition may be complicated with corneal ulcer. Management is done with hydrocortisone eyedrops, antibiotics eye ointment to prevent secondary infections and atropine eye ointment to keep the pupil dilated. Systemic diseases to be detected and necessary treatment should be done.

Strabismus (Squint)

Strabismus or squint means looking obliquely. It is an abnormality of ocular movements and an important cause of visual impairment. It is found in about 5 percents of infants. There are two types of strabismus, i.e. nonparalytic and paralytic.

1. Nonparalytic strabismus (concomitant) is commoner type. The movements of extraocular muscles are normal and diplopia never occurs. The condition may be

convergent or divergent. The deviation is secondary to visual or ocular defect of the affected eye.

2. Paralytic strabismus (nonconcomitant) occurs due to weakness or paralysis of extraocular muscles resulting limitation of eye movement and false orientation of eye muscles. Other features are dizziness and diplopia. Congenital paralytic strabismus may be due to neuromuscular anomalies and birth injury. Acquired paralytic squint may develop due to intracranial SOL, CNS infections, polioencephalitis, diphtheria toxins, vitamin B_1 deficiency, lead poisoning, fracture base of the skull, myasthenia gravis etc.

Diagnostic Evaluation

On examination, the squint eye deviates obliquely and the visual axis of the squinting eye in not directed at the object observed by other eye.

Slight deviation of the eye may present in the neonates which usually disappears by 3 to 6 months of age. It is known as transient strabismus. If this condition persists beyond 6 months of age and the infant does not develop eye-coordination and normal convergence then it should be considered as permanent strabismus.

Clinical examination, inspection, visual acuity test, corneal light reflex test, cover test, Krimsky test, Hirschberg's test, help to detect the degree of deviation and visual impairment.

Management

Management of strabismus should be done with early recognition of the problem. Correction of refractive errors and associated conditions like cataract are essential to develop best possible vision in both eyes. Occlusion therapy of normal eye for one to two weeks or longer helps the deviated eye to improve vision by continuous exercises.

Orthoptic training for special visual exercises is advised for improvement of vision. Surgical interventions may be needed in failure of above treatment. It involves shortening, lengthening and repositioning of the extraocular muscles. Delayed management beyond six to eight years of age can hardly succeed in reversing the problem, especially the acuity of vision and even the cosmetic cure.

Refractive Errors

The state of refractive error is termed as ametropia. It occurs when the images fail to come to a proper focus on the retina due to discrepancy between the size and refractive power of the eye. The ideal optical state is 'emmetropia', when the parallel light rays coming to a focus on the retina.

The refractive errors are presented as myopia (or near sightedness), hyperopia (or far sightedness), astigmatism and anisometropia (inequality in refractive power of the two eyes.)

Myopia (Near Sightedness or Short Sightedness)

It may occur in some children during the period of growth and development. The child usually complains blurred vision, for distant objects, as difficulty in reading blackboard writing in class room and pursuing the distant activities. Near vision is usually not impaired except in high myopia. Child tends to keep reading books close to the eyes.

Myopia occurs when parallel light rays come to focus in front of the retina, due to too long anteroposterior diameter of the eye, higher refractive power of the cornea or lens and anterior dislocation of the lens. The condition may be simple myopia as low degree and stationary problem. Progressive myopia with steady increase of problem throughout the life may develop as very high degree problem. Frawning and squint may result from child's inclination to improve the visual acuity. Myopia should be corrected with concave lenses.

Hyperopia (Far Sightedness or Hypermetropia)

In this condition, the child is able to see distant objects clearly but near vision is impaired. Usually, the children may complain eye strain, headache, redness of the eye, blurring of vision, fatigue, convergent strabismus and lid inflammation with eye rubbing. Some children report no symptoms.

Hyperopia occurs when the parallel light rays are focussed behind the retina, due to short anteroposterior diameter of the eye, poor refractive power of the cornea and lens or posterior dislocation of lens. The refractory error can be corrected by convex lenses.

Astigmatism

Astigmatism is a refractive error caused by the irregularity in the curvature of the cornea or lens. It causes light rays to converge unequally in different meridians causing distorted vision, a burning sensation in the eyes and headache. The parallel rays of light fail to focus sharply at a point on the retina. It may be complicated by amblyopia.

Astigmatism may occur following eye injury, or due to ptosis or hemangioma in eyelids or periorbital region. It is manifested as distortion of images, frowning, squinting, eye strain, headache, fatigue, eye rubbing due to sandy feeling in the eyes and lid hyperemia. The child may present with poor school performance and reading books too close. The error can be corrected by cylindrical or spherocylindrical lenses.

Visual Disorders

The important diseases recognized as responsible for visual impairment and blindness in India are cataract, refraction errors, corneal opacity, glaucoma, trachoma and associated infections. Malnutrition and systemic diseases are also important contributing factors. Other causes include eye injury, congenital disorders, retinal detachments, tumors, leprosy, etc.

The *visual disorders* can be found as the following problems:

- Amblyopia or dimness of vision or subnormal vision in one or both eyes inspite of correction of significant refractive errors.
- Amaurosis means partial or total loss of vision may be found in the form of profound impairment, near blindness or blindness.
- Night blindness (nyctalopia) is the inability to see well at night or in faint light. It may occur in retinitis, choroidoretinitis, vitamin 'A' deficiency, retinotoxic drugs (quinine) etc.
- *Double vision (diplopia):* It is found in squint, and ptosis. It may be a warning sign of increased intraocular pressure, a brain tumor, an orbital mass or myasthenia gravis.
- *Color blindness:* It is a genetically determined condition in which color perception is defective or absent. Red and green color deficiency is the usual form. It can be detected at the age of 5 to 6 years of age. It is found in about 4 to 8 percent of the male population and is inherited as sex linked recessive trait.

Color blindness may be total or partial and is tested with widely used *Ishihara chart.* There is no specific treatment of the condition.

Visual Impairment and Blindness

The WHO proposed a uniform criterion and defined blindness as "visual acuity of less than 3/60 (Snellen) or its equivalent". The WHO International Classification of Diseases (ICD) described the levels of visual impairment as shown in Table 23.1. In order to facilitate the screening of visual acuity by nonspecialized personnel, in the absence of appropriate vision charts, the WHO has now added the "inability to count fingers in daylight at a distance of 3 meters" to indicate as visual acuity of less than 3/60 or its equivalent.

The Table 23.1 shows differentiation between "low vision" (categories 1 and 2) and "blindness" (categories 3, 4 and 5). If the child reads 6/18 or better, he/she is coded "0", i.e. no visual impairment.

The important causes of blindness among children are trachoma, conjunctivitis, vitamin 'A' deficiency, eye injury, tuberculosis and STDS. Other causes are squint, glaucoma, refractive error (myopia), severe measles, leprosy, congenital anomalies (like cataract, optic atrophy), neurodegenerative diseases, malignancy, etc.

Blindness in children can be prevented by various simple measures. The measures include promotion of breast feeding, improvement of diet especially vitamin 'A' containing food, maintenance of ocular hygiene, avoiding harmful practices (kajal), good light, safety measures and immunization. Vitamin 'A' oil supplementation is an important measure to prevent related problems. Regular eye check-up especially for school children and health teaching about improvement of eye health and hygiene are also essential preventive measures. Avoidance of excessive watching of television and maintaining distance (at least 6 feet) away from the screen are good habit for eye health. Early detection of ocular diseases and disorders with appropriate treatment and healthy habits are helpful to prevent the visual impairment and blindness.

Retinoblastoma

Retinoblastoma is a malignant glioma of the retina. It may be unilateral (70%) or bilateral (30%). About 90 percent cases are found in less than 5 years of age. It is rare tumor, though the most common ocular neoplasm of childhood. It usually develops in the posterior portion of retina.

The disease have a genetic predisposition in majority of the cases. The retinoblastoma gene is located on chromosome 13. The gene carries risk of osteosarcoma and a secondary malignancy like a pineal tumor, the so called "trilateral retinoblastoma".

The *clinical features* of the condition include leukocoria, yellow white reflex in the pupil, loss of vision, pain in the eye, squint, pupillary irregularity and hyphema. In advanced cases frank proptosis, increased intracranial pressure and bony pain may be present. Metastasis may occur to bone, brain, liver, kidney etc.

Diagnosis is confirmed by fundoscopy to detect leukocoria and by CT scan to determine the extent of tumor. Other investigations should include X-ray to detect bone

Table 23.1: Categories of visual impairment

Categories of visual impairment	Visual acuity			
		Maximum less than		Minimum equal to or better than
Low vision	1.	6/18	*	6/60
	2.	6/60	*	3/60
Blindness	3.	3/60 (finger counting at 3 meters)	*	1/60 (finger counting at 1 meter)
	4.	1/60 (finger counting at 1 meter)	*	Light perception
	5.	No light perception		

involvement radionuclide bone scan, CSF study, bone marrow study, etc. to identify the metastasis.

Management of the condition includes radiotherapy, chemotherapy, scleral plaque irradiation, cryotherapy or photocoagulation. Enucleation may be done in unilateral cases. Prognosis depends upon the size and location of tumor.

Nursing Management of Childhood Eye Diseases

Nursing Assessment

History of illness, physical examination, ocular assessment with review of related laboratory and radiological investigations help to detect nursing diagnoses and to intervene nursing care.

Nursing Diagnoses

- Risk for infection related to exposure to environmental hazards.
- Pain related to inflammation or surgery or due to increased intraocular pressure.
- Risk for injury related to reduced visual acuity.
- Self-care deficit related to impaired vision and eye problems.
- Altered growth and development related to disturbances of visual stimulation.
- Fear and anxiety related to visual impairment.
- Knowledge deficit related to long-term care in eye diseases.

Nursing Interventions

- Preventing infections by caring and cleaning eyes with aseptic precautions following basic principles of eye care, handwashing, instillation of prescribed antibiotics and other medications, eye irrigation (if directed) and teaching instillation of eye drops/application of ointment, use of eye shield, etc.
- Minimizing pain by applying cold or warm compress to the affected part, allowing protection from bright light (sun glasses) in photophobia, provision of dimlight, administering analgesics and other therapy as directed, allowing interaction with others and diversional activities.
- Preventing injury by instructing about safety measures at hospital home, school and community. Proper use of eye glasses, keeping safety from falling off, dirt and damage, traffic rules and personal safety for preventing of eye injury and promotion of eye health to be explained. Orientation to be given to the visually impaired child about furniture, safety measures, food serving, toilets, use of side rails on bed, etc.

- Maintaining activity of daily living with assistance for eating, bathing, toileting, dressing and other hygienic care as needed.
- Promoting normal growth and development through various sensory stimulations, e.g. manipulating objects, hearing sound, noting smells, tasting eatables and providing other available opportunities of tender loving care.
- Reducing fear and anxiety by emotional support, explanation, reassurance, encouraging to express feeling and answering questions.
- Teaching the child and family members about the specific long-term care and giving instructions for restriction of activities, preparation for surgery, available medical help, follow-up, rehabilitation facilities (learning braille), schooling at special setting (blind school), etc.

EAR PROBLEMS IN CHILDREN

Ear problems are commonly found in children, especially the infections, which easily affect them due to immature immune system, structural difference from that of adult and due to lymphoid hypertrophy. Ear problems can be presented as congenital or acquired disorders.

Congenital malformations of ear may be found as small ear (microtia), total absent of ear (anotia), atresia or stenosis of external auditary canal, accessory skin tags, congenital cholesteotoma and congenital deafness.

Acquired conditions of ear are mainly otitis externa, otitis media, hearing impairment and diseases of internal ear, like labyrinthitis.

Problems of External Ear

Dermatitis

Dermatitis of the ear usually associated with seborrheic dermatitis of the scalp or middle ear discharge. It may be due to allergic reactions. Treatment should be done with antiseborrheic (selenium sulfide) application on scalp and steriod ointment on the inflamed area. Antiallergic and antibiotic therapy may be needed in case of allergic or bacterial infections. Hygienic measures to be emphasized.

Otitis Externa (Swimmer's Ear)

Otitis externa (Swimmer's ear) is common in children of warm and damp climate with excessive perspiration. It is usually associated with otitis media and chronic otorrhea. It may occur due to manipulation of pinna and pressure on the tragus. The condition is characterized by pain, redness, tenderness and swelling of external auditary canal. Infection usually spread to pinna and postauricular area. Treatment of the condition is done with hot packs, local antibiotics or antifungal and application of steriods (in most cases). Swimming should be avoided in acute stage. Irrigation with water and hydrogen peroxide should be avoided. Analgesics may be needed for short period to alleviate pain. Careful periodic cleaning of the external canal is necessary. The conditions may be complicated with hemorrhagic belbs and vesicles in case of viral infections along with similar lesions in soft palate. These features along with facial palsy constitute Ramsay-Hunt syndrome.

Furunculosis

Furunculosis is found at outer end of the external auditary canal with severe pain, difficulty in chewing, tenderness and even involvement of lymph glands over mastoid region. Treatment is done with hot fomentation and systemic antibiotics.

Foreign Body in the External Auditory Canal

Foreign body in the external auditory canal is a common problem. The child present with pain in the ear and discomfort. Careful removal of the foreign body should be done. Irrigation may be needed except in organic materials. Antibiotic ear drops may be applied to prevent infection.

Impacted Cerumen (Wax)

Impacted cerumen (wax) in the ear canal may found in the children causing discomfort and even hearing problems. Wax or cerumen is a product of glandular secretions and exfoliated keratin. It protects from entrance of dirt and insects. Wax can be accumulated which may become hard and black by drying up. Soft wax can be removed carefully by cotton-swab or smooth ring curette. Hard wax should be soften by olive oil or sodiumbicarbonate solution instillation 2 to 3 times a day for a few days, followed by syringing to remove the wax from the ear canal by irrigation or suction or by instrumentation for mechanical removal.

Otitis Media

Otitis media is the inflammation of middle ear. It is very common in infancy and early childhood. It is usually associated with upper respiratory tract infections. Infections from pharynx (nasopharynx) spread easily through the eustachian tube to the middle ear and the mastoid antrum causing otitis media and mastoiditis.

Children are more prone to otitis media due to: (a) Short, wide and horizontal eustachian tube which allow ascending infections from the nasopharynx, (b) upper respiratory infections which are more common and resulting obstruction by lymphoid tissue and (c) congestion of gum during eruption of teeth. These conditions promote spread of infection through the eustachian tube to the middle ear. The risk factors of the condition include exposure to cigarette smoke, overcrowding, bottle feeding, allergic rhinitis, cleft palate and in Down's syndrome.

Otitis media may be presented in three types, i.e. acute otitis media, (AOM), otitis media with effusion (OME) and chronic suppurative otitis media (CSOM). Most common complication of otitis media is mastoiditis.

Acute Otitis Media

Acute otitis media (AOM) is usually associated with upper respiratory infection (URI) and following measles, influenza or rubella. The most common causative organisms are *Streptococcus pneumonia* and *Haemophilus influenzae*.

Clinical manifestations: The child with AOM is commonly manifested with history or URI, pain in the affected ear, discomfort, irritability, restlessness, continuous crying and fever. Parenteral diarrhea and vomiting may occur. The child may present with pull or rubbing the affected ear, discharge and hearing impairment. On examination tympanic membrane looks lusterless, rough, red and bulging. Perforation of ear drum may occur leading to discharge from ear with reddish brown fluid, which may accumulate in the external ear canal. Culture and sensitivity test of ear discharge may be required for effective antibiotic therapy.

Complications: AOM can lead to extracranial and intracranial complications, if not treated effectively. Extracranial complications are acute mastoiditis, chronic and recurrent otitis media, facial palsy, hearing impairment, subperiosteal abscess and neck abscess. Intracranial complications are meningitis and cerebral abscess.

Management: Antibiotic therapy (amoxicillin, erythromycin, cephalosporins) for 10 to 15 days to be given to reduce the chance of complications. Dose may vary according to severity of infections. Other measures include symptomatic treatment with analgesics, antipyretics, decongestants and local heat application. Antihistaminics and local antibiotic ear drops have little value in the management of AOM. Aspiration of middle ear (tympanocentesis) or tympanotomy may be needed in severe pain to drain the middle area collection. Complications should be detected early for appropriate treatment. Discharge from the ear should be cleaned aseptically to keep the area dry.

Otitis Media with Effusion

Otitis media with effusion (OME) is commonly associated with AOM. Many children have no history of acute otitis media. The child with OME may present with middle ear effusion without pain in the ear and fever.

The effusion may be serous, mucoid or purulent. It may be infectious, allergic or immunological in origin. The presenting features are mild to moderate loss of hearing, feeling of ear blockage or pressure in the ear. The condition may be seen without any symptoms, on examination tympanic membrane is found dull with reduced mobility.

Majority of OME cases recover spontaneously within 3 months. If effusion persists more than 3 months, i.e. in chronic OME, management is done with antibiotic therapy followed by myringotomy and insertion of tympanostomy tube. Other indications of tube placement are pain and discomfort in the ear, altered behavior, delayed speech, recurrent attack of acute otitis media and significant loss of hearing. Adenoidectomy may be indicated in persistent symptomatic effusion above 4 years of age. Swimming should not be allowed to the children to prevent middle ear contamination.

Chronic Suppurative Otitis Media

Chronic otitis media (COM) is manifested as perforation of tympanic membrane with otorrhea and hearing loss, which is termed as active COM or chronic suppurative otitis media (CSOM). Inactive COM is presented with only hearing loss. These conditions are found as complication of AOM or recurrent otitis media.

The child with CSOM may present with cholesteatoma, a cyst like mass of squamous epithelium extending from the ear drum into the middle ear. The cholesteatoma may cause serious complications by slow expansions and destruction of ossicles with tympanosclerosis.

CSOM may be complicated with mastoiditis, abscess formation in mastoid and neck, inner ear infection with sensory hearing loss, facial palsy, meningitis and intracranial abscess.

Management of CSOM comprises antibiotic therapy (topical, oral or parenteral) and removal of cholesteatoma. Mastoidectomy may be necessary in some children. Tympanoplasty is performed in children older than 8 years age and having simple tympanic perforation without cholesteatoma. Reconstruction of ossicles (ossiculoplasty) may be indicated in some cases.

Mastoiditis

Mastoiditis is a common complication of otitis media with inappropriate treatment. It usually occurs one week after untreated and acute suppurative otitis media.

Mastoiditis is the inflammation of the air cells of the mastoid process characterized by fever, chills, retroauricular pain and swelling with tenderness over the mastoid. Swelling may be large enough to pull the pinna forwards. The tympanic membrane may be intact but dull and bulging. X-ray of the part helps in diagnosis in the later stage of the condition with bony destruction and absorption of mastoid air cells.

Complications of mastoiditis may be found as intracranial lesions, sinus thrombosis, otitic hydrocephalus, brain abscess and suppurative labyrinthitis, etc.

Management of mastoiditis is done with parenteral antibiotic therapy, myringotomy and mastoidectomy. Complications should be prevented by early treatment. Treatment of complications may require neurosurgical interventions.

Hearing Impairment (Deafness)

Hearing is important for the development of speech and verbal communication. Impairment of hearing may be congenital or acquired. It may be temporary or permanent, organic or inorganic and peripheral or central in origin. Hearing deficit can be mild, moderate, severe or profound. It is one of the common handicapped conditions in children. It is found about 9 to 15 percent among Indian school children.

Common Causes of Hearing Impairment

a. *Genetic:* Familial deafness, chromosomal abnormalities like trisomy 21, Pierre-Robin syndrome, Alport's syndrome, Hunter-Hurler syndrome and congenital craniofacial anomalies.
b. *Intrauterine infections:* Rubella, CMV, syphilis, toxoplasma, chickenpox,
c. *Teratogenic exposure during pregnancy:* Drug therapy with quinine, streptomycin, thalidomide and irradiation.
d. *Infection in postnatal period:* Meningitis, encephalitis, mumps, measles, chickenpox, recurrent and suppurative otitis media.
e. Mechanical obstruction of external auditory canal by wax and foreign body.
f. Brain damage, cerebral palsy, mental retardation, LBW baby (below 1500 g), severe respiratory depression, birth asphyxia, prolonged (more than 5 days) mechanical ventilation, birth injury.
g. *Toxic:* Neonatal hyperbilirubinemia.
h. *Ototoxic drug therapy:* Streptomycin, gentamicin, neomycin, chloroquine, loop diuretics.
i. *Endocrinal:* Cretinism.
j. *Injury:* Direct injury of ear, head injury, indirect injury by explosion (cracker, fireworks), constant exposure to loud noise.
k. *Nutritional:* Malnutrition, vitamin 'B' complex deficiency.

Classification of Hearing Impairment

In a quiet environment, the healthy child can hear tones between 0 to 25 decibel range. Hearing impairment is described as follows:

- Slight hearing impairment—15 to 25 decibels.
- Mild hearing impairment—25 to 40 decibels.
- Moderate hearing impairment—40 to 65 decibels.
- Severe hearing impairment—65 to 95 decibels.
- Profound hearing impairment—95 or more decibels.

Types

Hearing deficits can be classified as follows:

Conductive hearing deficit: It is dysfunction of sound transmission or conduction of sound wave through the external ear and middle ear. Any process interfering with sound transmission through ear canal, ear drum or ossicles may result in conductive hearing loss. It is common type of hearing deficit.

The most common cause of conductive deafness is otitis media with effusion. Other causes are impacted wax, foreign body, tympanic perforation, cholesteatoma, otosclerosis etc. Several congenital syndromes may also be associated with conductive hearing deficit, e.g. Apert's syndrome, Crouzon's syndrome etc.

Sensorineural hearing deficit: This condition is caused by damage or lesions of the cochlea (organ of Corti), auditory nerve or central auditory pathways. It is usually an acquired problem due to meningitis, perinatal CNS infection, birth asphyxia, neonatal hyperbilirubinemia, ototoxic drug effect and loud noise. This condition may be congenital due to genetic or nongenetic causes. Genetic causes are associated with Alport's syndrome, Jervell's syndrome, etc. Nongenetic causes are LBW baby, prematurity, neonatal sepsis, etc. These problems damage the auditory nerve and hair cells in the cochlea, thus prevent transmission of sound impulses to the brain for interpretation resulting in sensorineural hearing deficit.

Mixed type: It includes both conductive and sensorineural hearing deficit.
- Hearing deficit can also be classified as central or peripheral hearing deficit. It may also be due to psychogenic factor.
  - *Central hearing deficit:* It indicates auditory deficit originating along central auditory nervous system from the proximal 8th nerve to cortex due to convulsive disorders, tumors, demyelinating disease etc.
  - *Peripheral hearing deficit:* It indicates dysfunction in the sound transmission through the external or middle ear as also its conversion into neural activity at the inner ear and the 8th nerve. It may be conductive, sensorineural or mixed type.

Consequence of Hearing Impairment

Children with hearing impairment may not complain that they cannot hear well. Only about 6 percent of the hearing impaired children have profound hearing loss. The rest have some hearing ability. But even mild or unilateral hearing deficit has detrimental effect on development and performance of the child.

Consequences of hearing impairment may be found as poor or lack of response to sounds, delayed or poor speech development, poor attention span, poor academic performance, behavior problems in home and school, speaking loudly, listening radio and television at a loud volume, inadequate social and emotional development.

Diagnostic Evaluation

1. *Assessment of developmental milestones,* especially language development and personal social behavior along with response to sound help in suspicion of hearing impairment. Otoscopic examination to be done along with physical examination and history collection related to the condition for the suspected cases.
2. *Hearing tests*
   a. *Using tuning fork:* Weber test, Rinne test and Schwabach test are done in school children to detect the types of hearing deficit. These tests are not fully reliable. Before testing with these techniques, wax from ear canal to be removed.
   b. An ordinary test using wrist watch can be useful to detect the hearing deficit.
3. Audiometry to be done to confirm the diagnosis and the type of deficit. This test should be done through play and behavior assessment, when the child can co-operate and follow the instructions. The result is recorded in the form of audiogram. Pure tone audiometry is usually possible in children above 5 years of age.
4. Tympanometry may be performed to detect mobility of the tympanic membrane.
5. Labyrinthine test to be performed to detect vestibular functions in older children and adolescence. It is simple, inexpensive and accurate diagnostic test indicating presence or absence of labyrinthine response.
6. Auditory brainstem response (ABR) or otoacoustic emissions (OAE) test should be done to detect hearing impairment for all neonates with risk factors for hearing loss.

Management

Early detection and prompt treatment of ear diseases by medical and surgical interventions are important aspect of management. Treatment of infections by antibiotic therapy removal of cerumen or toxic agent and management the specific cause should be done effectively.

Surgical interventions may be required specially in conductive problems as myringotomy, tympanoplasty, tympanostomy tube insertion, stapedectomy and insertion of graft or prosthesis, adenotonsilectomy, cochlear implant etc.

Supportive and rehabilitative management are provided with hearing aids, speech therapy, lip reading, sign language, deaf education, etc. Cochlear implants are indicated in profound sensorineural deafness, which is unresponsive to 3 to 6 months trial with powerful hearing aids.

Parental involvement and counseling are important aspect of management. Necessary instructions to be given about maintenance and care of hearing aids with precautions. Improvement of communication ability of the child should be emphasized by visual cues, sign language, etc. Prevention of injury and accidents with environment modification, referral for rehabilitation and emotional support for facilitation of ventilation of feeling are also important.

DISORDERS OF THE NOSE

Congenital malformations involving nose are mainly cleft palate and choanal atresia. These conditions are detected at birth and their management depends upon the severity of condition.

Acquired problems of the nose include rhinitis, sinusitis, foreign body, nasal obstruction, trauma and epistaxis.

Rhinitis

Rhinitis is the inflammation of the nasal mucous membrane generally caused by viruses. Bacterial rhinitis may be severe and found complicated with sinusitis, otitis, laryngopharyngitis, etc. Allergic rhinitis may be found commonly due to inhalation of allergens like pollen, dust, mites or due to food allergy or seasonal changes, etc.

Acute rhinitis is manifested with fever, vomiting, nasal obstruction, sucking and breathing difficulty, mouth breathing, malaise and sleep disturbances. Mild diarrhea may present with the condition. This condition may be complicated with otitis media, bronchiolitis, bronchopneumonia, persistent sinusitis, spasmodic laryngitis, purulent rhinitis, etc. Management of acute rhinitis is done with antipyretics, decongestants, prevention of spread of infection and cleaning of nasal secretions. Antibiotic therapy is indicated only in presence of complications and with bacterial rhinitis.

Chronic rhinitis is characterized by chronic nasal discharge. It may be associated with adenoids, unhygienic environment, overcrowding, poor ventilation in housing, inadequate proteins and vitamins intake in diet and nasal allergy. Allergic rhinitis may present with sneezing, itching, nasal blockage, mucoid rhinorrhea, postnasal discharge, cough, redness of conjunctiva, etc. Management of chronic rhinitis is done with nose blowing exercises, breathing exercises, clearing nostril, avoidance of allergy and symptomatic relief by antihistaminics, decongestant and saline nasal spray.

Sinusitis

Inflammation of sinuses are common along with rhinitis. Maxillary and ethmoid sinuses are most commonly infected in infancy and early childhood. Frontal sinusitis may develop only after 4 to 5 years of age. The common etiological organisms are *S. pneumoniae, H. influenzae, B. catarrhalis* and *S. pyogenes*. Sinusitis can be acute or chronic.

Acute Sinusitis

It may develop following acute coryza or viral rhinitis. It is manifested with headache, facial pain, retro-orbital pain, fever, foul breath, postnasal discharge with persistent cough especially at night, tenderness, redness and swelling over the cheek or near the inner canthus of the eye, etc. The condition may be complicated with periorbital or orbital cellulitis, chronic sinusitis, cavernous sinus thrombosis, meningitis, optic neuritis, subdural abscess and osteomyelitis of maxila.

Nasal examination shows mucous or pus on the floor of the nasal cavity. Diagnosis is confirmed by X-ray of paranasal sinuses which shows air-fluid levels and complete opacification. CT Scan can be done to detect complications. Nasal swab culture helps to determine the causative organisms.

Management of acute sinusitis include effective antibiotic therapy, decongestants, mucolytic agents, nasal drops (ephedrine in normal saline), analgesics, steam inhalation (in older children), more fluid intake, application of local heat and avoiding contact with URI.

Chronic Sinusitis

Chronic sinusitis involved mainly the maxillary antrum and found as complication of acute sinusitis which develops from acute coryza. Other contributing factors of this condition are nasal polyps, infected tonsils and adenoids, septic tooth, nasal allergic reaction, deviated nasal septum (DNS), cystic fibrosis, etc. The common causative organisms are *Staph. aureus, Pneumococcus* and *Strep. viridans*.

Clinical features of chronic sinusitis include recurrent attack of nasal and postnatal discharge with cough. Nasal obstruction, sniffing, nose-twitching, mouth breathing, epistaxis and discharge from ear may present. General symptoms may found as low-grade fever, malaise, anorexia, easy fatigability, irritability and headache. Nasal examination reveals some enlargement and congestion of the inferior turbinates and mucopus or pus on the nasal floor. X-ray of the maxillary and ethmoid sinuses helps in diagnosis. It shows opacification of the sinuses due to pus or due to thickening of the lining membrane. Culture and sensitivity test of nasal discharge may be done to detect the causative agent.

Management of chronic sinusitis should be done with prolonged antibiotic therapy. Supportive measures should include breathing exercise, nose blowing, vitamin 'A' supplementation, lavage of the antrum (maxillary) followed by instillation of antibiotic, topical nasal corticosteroid and analgesics. Surgical intervention may be necessary when conservative management is unsuccessful. Endoscopic sinus surgery to remove the diseased tissue and nasal antrostomy (surgical placement of an opening under inferior turbinate) to provide aeration of the antrum and to permit exit for purulent material may be indicated in some children. Correction of deviated nasal septum or removal of nasal polyp may be needed.

Nursing responsibilities include early detection of the condition, motivating for appropriate treatment, encouraging for completion of therapy, follow-up, discouraging for swimming and diving in children with URI. Teaching about prevention of the condition and its complications, moving to dry climate, increasing humidity and fluid intake and local heat should be emphasized.

Epistaxis

Epistaxis or nose bleeding is common in children. Bleeding occurs usually from anteroinferior portion of the cartilaginous nasal septum due to rich capillary vasculature in this zone known as little's area or Kiesselbach's plexus.

The *common causes* of epistaxis in children are major trauma, nose-picking and vigorous nose blowing or rubbing. Other local causes of epistaxis are foreign body in nose, nasal injury, nasal polyp, rhinitis (allergic, acute, chronic), nasal diphtheria, nasopharyngeal tumors or vascular malformations (hemangioma, telangiectasia), etc. There are systemic causes which may result in epistaxis. These include leukemia, hemophilia, thrombocytopenia, DIC, rheumatic fever, typhoid fever, acute infections, ingestion of aspirin, hypertension, tuberculosis, leprosy, solar radiation, cirrhosis, nephritis, vitamin 'K' deficiency, scurvy, etc. Epistaxis may occur on adolescent girls during puberty. It may also occur in hot summer months and due to excessive emotional stress and strain.

Management of epistaxis should include first aid measures like digital pressure for 10 to 15 minutes by pinching the nose to stop bleeding and bending forwards, in comfortable position, loosing cloths and giving reassurance. The child should be instructed to avoid nose picking, forceful blowing and sneezing. Splashing cold water and cold compress over the nose bridge are helpful. Persistent nose bleed may require local application of vasoconstricting agent (epinephrine) and nasal packing with gauze or gelfoam pack, as it may be anterior, posterior, or combined (anterior and posterior) nasal bleeding.

Recurrent epistaxis can be managed by chemical (silver nitrate) or electrocautery. Application of antibiotic ointment for lubrication and for prevention of infection may be needed. Control of allergic reactions, detection and management of systemic causes and bleeding disorders to be done appropriately. Details family history and history of illness to be obtained and necessary investigations to be performed. Blood transfusion may be necessary in some children with epistaxis.

Nursing measures should include continuous monitoring of vital signs, bleeding, hypoxia, respiratory difficulty and nasal packing. Teaching the parents and family members about measures to stop epistaxis and immediate medical help are also important. Instructions to be given to the parents to apply lubricant to nasal septum twice daily to reduce dryness and to avoid nasal blowing or picking nose after nose bleed. Preventive measures of foreign body in the nose, nasal injury and solar radiation to be explained. Need for management of local and systemic cause of epistaxis should be informed and emphasized.

DISORDERS OF THROAT

The disorders and diseases of throat can be found as congenital or acquired problems. Congenital anomalies of throat include cleft palate, laryngomalacia, laryngeal webs, cysts and hemangiomas. Acquired problems are mainly inflammatory, i.e. pharyngitis, tonsillitis, adenoids, laryngitis and epiglotitis. Throat injury may occur accidentally with stick, pen, sharp objects or may found as external cut injury especially during kite-flying with sharp thread as laryngotracheal cut.

Pharyngitis

Pharyngitis is commonly termed as sore throat which involves inflammation of pharynx and tonsils. Inflammation of soft palate and lymphoid follicles of palate also may present with the condition. Laryngitis may occur in extension of this inflammation. Pharyngitis commonly occur after one year of age. Common causative organisms are viruses (adenovirus, enterovirus, parainfluenzae virus, EB virus, etc.) in about 80 to 90 percent. Bacterial infection may occur especially with group 'A' beta hemolytic streptococci, *S. aureus, H. influenzae,* etc.

Viral pharyngitis is characterized by nonexudative erythema of pharynx, tenderness of cervical lymph glands, fever, malaise, anorexia, hoarseness of voice, cough, nasal discharge and nasal obstruction. It is usually self-limiting. Lymphadenopathy and laryngeal involvement are common.

Bacterial (streptococcal) pharyngitis is manifested with bilateral tonsillar hypertrophy, erythema, whitish exudate, headache, vomiting, abdominal discomfort, fever and dysphagia due to sore throat. Throat examination shows diffuse congestion of the tonsils and its pillars with petechiae over the soft palate. Anterior cervical lymphadenopathy is commonly present. Diagnosis is confirmed by throat swab culture.

Pharyngitis may be complicated with otitis media, mastoiditis, chronic ulcer in the throat, peritonsillar abscess (quinsy), sinusitis, meningitis, mesenteric adenitis, rheumatic fever and acute glomerulonephritis.

Management of pharyngitis includes warm saline gargles (in older children), analgesics, antitussive, antipyretics, steam inhalation, extra fluid intake, liquid or soft diet and oral hygiene. Streptococcal pharyngitis should be treated with antibiotics (penicillin, amoxicillin, erythromycin, cephalosporin) for 10 to 15 days, and bed rest. Nasal decongestant and antiallergic may be needed for some children.

Tonsillitis

Inflammation of tonsils are common in children and may be found as acute tonsillitis and less frequently as chronic cases. The most important organism is group—A beta *Streptococcus* hemolyticus. Other organisms are *H. influenzae*. Spread of infection may occur in nursery, school and dormitories.

Acute Tonsillitis

Acute tonsillitis may be classified as follows:
1. *Catarrhal tonsillitis:* It is usually present with URI and measles. It is least severe form and manifested as redness and sore throat.
2. *Follicular tonsillitis:* There is involvement of crypts with discrete yellow patches of exudate on tonsils and enlargement of regional glands.
3. *Parenchymatous tonsillitis:* There is congestion and swelling of the entire organ.
4. *Peritonsillar abscess (quinsy):* It may develop in bacterial tonsillitis. The child may present with trismus and muffled voice with poor oral intake, severe pain on swallowing and opening of the mouth, high fever, offensive breath, enlarged cervical lymph glands and otalgia. On examination of throat, unilateral bulge in the soft palate and peritonsillar region with uvular deviation to the opposite side are seen.

The *clinical features* of acute tonsillitis usually present with abrupt onset of pain in the throat which may radiate to the ears. Painful swallowing with fever, shivering and convulsions may occur especially in younger children. Tonsils look markedly red and congested. Anterior cervical glands may enlarged and become tender. False membrane may develop in follicular tonsillitis. This condition should be differentiated from diphtheria, infectious mononucleosis (EB virus), vincent angina and oral thrush.

Management of acute tonsillitis should be done with bedrest, isolation from other children to prevent spread of infection, soft or liquid diet, analgesics and antipyretics. Systemic antibiotics (penicillin) should be administered parenterally for 7 days. Other antibiotics (erythromycin, cephalexin) can be given. Hot saline gargle or gargles with aspirin in solution may be useful. Analgesic lozenges in the early stage is helpful.

Chronic Tonsillitis

Repeated attack of tonsillitis may be frequently found in children. It results in scaring over the crypts leading to retention of infected materials within the tonsils. The clinical manifestations are more generalized than local features. The child may present with recurrent sore throat, tiredness.

Poor food intake, vomiting, bad smell in breath (halitosis), abdominal pain, swallowing and breathing difficulties, dryness and irritation in throat. Respiratory difficulties and chronic hypoxemia with pulmonary hypertension may develop.

This condition may be complicated with peritonsillar abscess (quinsy), retrotonsillar abscess and failure to thrive.

On examination, the child looks sick and throat is congested. Crypts of tonsils appear spongy and purulent material may found on pressure on crypts. Tonsils may become smaller in size due to fibrosis. Enlargement of cervical lymph glands may be seen.

Management of chronic tonsillitis is done with tonsillectomy. It is indicated, if medical treatment is unsuccessful and there is severe hypertrophy of tonsils. It should be advised in more than six significant attacks of tonsillitis in a year for two consecutive years and presence of peritonsillar or retrotonsillar abscess. Other indications of tonsillectomy are obstructive sleep apnea, contributing focus of suppurative otitis media and carrier of diphtheria. Controversy exists over indications for and benefits of surgery in tonsillitis.

Adenoidal Hypertrophy

Adenoids are diffuse lymphoid tissue and follicles in the roof and posterior wall of the nasopharynx. It is called as pharyngeal tonsils. Adenoids cause more problem than tonsils in the first four years of life. Hypertrophy of adenoids mass may almost fill the vault of the nasopharynx and block the air passage, (through nose) and obstruct the eustachian tube.

Recurrent throat infection, poor nasal and oral hygiene, allergy and poor ventilation at house are the etiological factors of chronic adenoiditis and hyperplasia of adenoids. It may be associated with tonsillitis.

The *clinical features* of adenoidal hypertrophy are found as nasal block, mouth breathing and even open-mouth during daytime. Other manifestations are dry mouth and lips, persistent rhinitis, chronic nasal discharge, pharyngitis, snoring at night, nasal speech, offensive breath, impaired taste, bad smell from mouth, harassing cough, hearing deficit, etc. Chronic otitis media, growth failure, dull looking, malocclusion of teeth and poor school performance usually found in these children. The condition may be complicated with apneic spells, arterial hypertension and cor-pulmonale.

Diagnosis of adenoidal hypertrophy is confirmed by digital palpation, indirect visualization with pharyngeal mirror or fiberoptic bronchoscope and pharyngeal X-ray along with careful history of illness and physical examination.

Management of the condition is done with adenoidectomy to relief the symptoms and improve the child's health. This surgical intervention is contraindicated in URI and presence of cleft palate. Tonsillectomy and adenoidectomy may be performed together or separately.

Postoperative care following tonsillectomy and adenoidectomy should provide special attention for assessment of bleeding from the site of operation. Indications of hemorrhage include increase pulse, frequent swallowing, pallor, restlessness, clearing throat, vomiting of blood and oozing of blood in back of throat. The child should be placed in comfortable and prone position, head turned to one side to allow drainage from mouth and pharynx. Airway clearance, adequate fluid intake, application of ice collor, analgesics, alkaline mouth wash and liquid or semi-liquid diet should be provided. Spicy, hot, cold and rough foods are avoided. Milk and milk products (ice cream) should be restricted, because they tend to increase mucous secretion and may be a good source of infections. Reducing fear of the child, relieving parental anxiety and teaching the parents about home based care with necessary precautions for prevention of complications are important aspect of nursing interventions.

Discharge advice following tonsillectomy and adenoidectomy should include the followings:

- Rest up to one week.
- Soft nonirritating foods with more amount of water intake.
- Allowing normal diet and normal activities after 2 weeks of operation.
- Discouraging frequent coughing and throat clearing.
- Avoid contact with infected persons.
- Maintain oral hygiene and general cleanliness.
- Avoid gargling, only rinsing mouth or mouth wash will be allowed.
- Avoid straw to drink any liquid which may injured the operated site.
- Practice nose breathing rather than mouth breathing.
- Avoid overcrowding and dusty place for few weeks.
- Take prescribed medications.
- Contact medical help in bleeding and pain in throat or ear and attend regular follow-up.

Croup's Syndrome

Croup refers to inflammation of the larynx characterized by croaking cough, stridor, hoarseness, cold and fever. Dyspnea, cyanosis and restlessness may also develop. Laryngitis usually present with infection of surrounding tissue. Croup is the common term used for those infection.

Croup's syndromes are the infections of supraglottis, glottis, subglottis and trachea. It includes the followings:

- Acute laryngotracheobronchitis (subglottic croup).
- Acute spasmodic laryngitis (spasmodic croup): Spasmodic croup is found in children that typically occurs in midnight. It presents with barky cough and noisy breathing, but no other features of viral illness are found. This symptom may repeat in next 2 or 3 nights. The child remains fine in the morning. Etiology is suspected as allergy. Hospitalization is rarely required. Humidification of the room is important only.
- Bacterial tracheitis (pseudomembranous croup): Bacterial tracheitis is found in young children following upper respiratory tract viral infection. The child presents with brassy cough and stridor with toxic look. Bronchoscopy helps as both diagnostic and therapeutic procedure. Removal of purulent tracheal secretions as emergency management must be performed to remove life-threatening obstructions along with others routine management
- Acute epiglottitis (supraglottic croup).

Acute Laryngotracheobronchitis

It is found in children between 3 months to 5 years of age. Peak age is 1 to 2 years. Usually found in male child during late autumn or early winter. This condition is manifested with history of URI and mild brassy or barking cough, hoarseness, stridor, nasal flaring, chest retraction, labored breathing, air hunger, cyanosis, elevated temperature, tachycardia, crying, restlessness and agitation. The child feels comfort in upright or sit up position. Dehydration, hypercapnia, hypoxemia, and airway obstructions are found as complication.

Diagnosis is confirmed with history of illness, physical examination and X-ray which shows subglottic edema and normal supraglottic structure.

Management of the condition is done with oxygen therapy, antibiotics, (ampicillin, chloramphenical, ceftriaxone), humidification of environment and racemic epinephrine (0.5 mL of 2 percent solution diluted with sterile water to a total volume of 3.5 mL) through nebulizer. Single dose of dexamethasone (0.6 mg/kg) IM, reduces severity of the condition. Inhalation of budesonide in doses of 1 to 2 mg gives significant effect. Nasotracheal intubation or tracheostomy may be indicated in cases of severe obstruction.

Supportive nursing care should include maintenance of upright position, rest, oxygen therapy, humidified environment, monitoring of vital signs, respiratory status, pulse oximetry, ABG analysis, nebulization of racemic epinephrine, intravenous fluid therapy, administration of medication and hygienic measures. Special care to be provided in case of tracheal intubation or tracheostomy. Avoiding examination of throat with tongue depressor should be followed strictly, because it may lead to sudden cardiopulmonary arrest.

Necessary health teaching regarding continuation of care and emotional support to be provided.

Acute Epiglottitis

It is a supraglottic inflammation with edema of arytenoepiglottic folds. Peak incidence is 3 to 5 years of age and may be found in 2 to 7 years old children during autumn and winter.

Clinical features of acute epiglottitis are sudden fulminating course of high fever, toxic appearance, sore throat, drooling, dysphagia, aphonia, cough, stridor, air hunger, tachycardia, hoarseness, restlessness, respiratory distress with fatal airway obstruction, increasing cyanosis, coma and even death. In survived child pulmonary edema and pneumothorax may be developed.

Diagnosis is done on the basis of history of illness, clinical assessment, monitoring oxygen saturation level, X-ray neck, throat swab culture and complete blood count.

Management of this condition includes emergency measures like airway clearance by removal of secretions, positioning, tracheal intubation or tracheostomy. Care in intensive unit may be necessary. Intravenous antibiotic therapy (cefotaxime, ceftriaxone), antipyretic, humidified oxygen therapy and maintenance of fluid electrolyte balance are important measures. Mechanical ventilation may be indicated in severe respiratory distress. Examination of throat, especially with tongue blade is contraindicated to prevent reflex laryngospasm, acute airway obstruction and cardiopulmonary arrest. The child should never be placed in supine position. Emotional support to parents and explanation about ICU care should be provided. Health teaching to be given to the parent regarding continuation of care, hygienic measures and follow-up.

DENTAL PROBLEMS

Eruption of teeth usually begins at about six months with wide variation in timing. All the twenty temporary teeth erupt by the age of 2.5 to 3 years. First permanent teeth erupt at 6 years of age.

Problems related to eruption of teeth are seen as delayed eruption and malocclusion. Baby may born with natal tooth. It is usually harmless. Absolute noneruption of teeth or anodontia may be found as a classical feature of ectodermal dysplasia. Partial anodontia may affect third molars. Supernumerary teeth may develop in the areas of incisors. Twining of teeth or joined teeth may found in maxillary incisors.

Infant may have discoloration of temporary teeth which may be due to maternal drug therapy with tetracyclines during 3rd trimester of pregnancy. Disturbed enamel formation may be found as mottled enamel due to excessive fluoride in water and vitamin 'D' resistant ricket. Thin enamel may result in abnormal yellow colored teeth as the color of dentin.

Delayed Eruption of Teeth

Delayed eruption of first teeth may be found in normal children as later as 15 months of age. The possible causes are familial or racial tendency, poor nutrition, ricket, hypothyroidism, hypopituitarism, osteogenesis imperfecta, etc.

Malocclusion of Teeth

Dental malocclusion is the malposition and faulty contact of the mandibular and maxillary teeth due to improper relationship between upper and lower dental arches. It results in incorrect mastication, cosmetic disfigurement of face and early loss of teeth. Malocclusion of the teeth of upper jaw and lower jaw leads to cross bite or open bite or closed bite. There may be dental crowding in permanent incisors due to lack of adequate spacing between teeth.

Genetic factors are responsible for congenital malocclusion. Thumb sucking and tongue thrusting habits can cause dental malocclusion. Dental injuries and teeth extraction may also result to this condition.

Early detection and management with orthodontic interventions including bracing are effective. Management depends upon degree of malocclusion and difficulty of the child.

Dental Caries

Dental caries is a progressive and destructive process causing decalcification of the tooth enamel, destruction of dentin and cavitation of the teeth. It can spread into the tooth pulp and may cause inflammation and abscess.

Etiology

Many microorganisms can cause dental caries. Streptococci is the main cariogenic organism which produces an extracellular polysaccharide and forms a plaque over the teeth. Gradually tooth decay begins following demineralization of enamel. Destruction of dentin with cavity formation occurs causing inflammation and abscess formation. Biting surface and contact surfaces between teeth are most common site of caries.

The factors responsible for dental caries are carbohydrate-rich foods, especially chocolate which stick to the teeth and poor oral hygiene with inadequate dental care. Sleeping with feeding bottle in mouth, use of dummy or pacifiers with honey or some other sweetening agents are also responsible factors of dental caries. Long time retention of carbohydrate foods in the mouth is more important as cariogenic factors. Faulty salivary gland functions also considered as risk factors of dental caries. Deficiency and excess of fluoride are both harmful.

Clinical Features

Dental caries is found as pits and fissures of biting surfaces of teeth, commonly in molars as initial features. Cavity formation, involvement of pulp, periapical abscess, dental abscess or sepsis may develop. Dental caries may spread to involve the pulp and contagious tissue which is manifested with significant toothache. Pulpitis may be complicated with dental or periapical abscess which is very painful. Dental caries affecting neck of the teeth may found with nursing bottle caries and termed as baby bottle tooth decay. Serious complication of dental caries may be seen as endocarditis.

Management

Dental caries should be treated with analgesics to relief pain and tooth extraction or pulpectomy. Involvement of tissue outside the dentoalveolar unit requires antibiotics mainly in infection of submandibular space, periorbital space and facial triangle. Oral antibiotics are not effective, parenteral administration should be given to prevent complication.

Preventive Measures

a. Dietary modification by reducing carbohydrate-rich food intake and avoiding oral retaining.
b. Use of fluoride toothpaste.
c. Avoidance of chewing gum, chocolates, bottle feeding, use of pacifiers, etc.
d. Good oral and dental hygiene with correct technique of tooth brushing.
e. Dental sealants and plastics to be applied to seal the pits and fissures on occlusal surfaces of teeth.
f. Mechanical removal of plaque and debris of the teeth are essential.
g. Regular dental check-up for early detection of problems and necessary advice.

Dental Fluorosis

Dental fluorosis usually develops due to high concentration of fluorine in drinking water supply or high content of fluoride in tooth paste. A mottled discoloration of teeth enamel is found due to this fluorosis as white flecking or linear opacity of enamel. In chronic cases, the condition may be complicated with osteosclerosis, osteomalacia and involvement of vertebral column and spinal cord with paraplegia.

PROBLEMS OF ORAL CAVITY

Congenital problems involving the oral cavity include cleft lip, cleft palate, microglossia, tongue tie, macroglossia, hemangioma on the oral mucosal surface, etc.

Inflammatory disorders are found as stomatitis, aphthous ulcer, oral thrush, glossitis, gingivitis, noma or cancrum oris etc. Vitamin deficiency may be found as angular stomatitis, glossitis and gum bleeding.

Stomatitis: It is inflammation of oral mucosa. It can be due to various etiological factors. The most common cause of stomatitis in young infants is oral thrush caused by *Candida albicans*. In older children, it may develop due to prolonged antibiotic therapy and poor orodental hygiene. Antifungal drugs and improved oral hygiene are effective to treat the condition.

Aphthous ulcer or aphthous stomatitis: It is characterized by small whitish painful lesions surrounded by a red border, usually associated with local trauma or irritation by tooth. It may be due to allergy, endocrine disturbances or emotional stress. The exact cause is not known. The lesions may be found as small ulcer with reddish spots inside the mouth. It is usually self-limiting. Good oral hygiene and detection of possible underlying cause with its treatment are important.

Herpetic stomatitis: It may be found in children due to acute infection by herpes simplex virus as vesicle formation in oral mucosa. It is usually associated with inflammation of gum (gingivitis) and tongue (glossitis). It is self-limiting, but infected condition requires special attention.

Other forms of stomatitis may found in children as necrotizing ulcerative stomatitis or gingivostomatitis which is known as *Vincent's stomatitis. Angular stomatitis* may be seen in vitamin B_2 deficiency. Diffuse purulent inflammation of the floor of the mouth may be found due to streptococcal infection, which is termed as *Ludwig's angina*.

Noma or *cancrum oris* may be seen as gangrenous ulcer of the mouth in the malnourished children. It begins as a small gingival ulcer and results in gangrenous necrosis of surrounding facial tissues and cheeks.

Glossitis: It is inflammation of the tongue and characterized by red, raw tongue with pain and burning sensation. It is followed by atrophy of the papillae with thin smooth tongue. Vitamin B complex deficiency is the main cause. It may be associated with cough and cold. Tongue bite, burns with hot foods or corrosives also may cause painful glossitis.

Glossitis should be managed with good oral hygiene, antiseptic mouth wash or gargling and correction of nutritional deficiency conditions. Ice packs can be used in trauma and hematoma. Oral ulcer can be treated with application of boroglycerine. Antibiotic therapy may be needed in infected cases. Health teaching for improvement of oral hygiene and intake of vitamin 'B' containing food items is important measure for prevention of the condition.

CLEFT LIP AND CLEFT PALATE (FIG. 23.1)

Cleft lip and cleft palate are congenital malformations of face resulting from the failure of fusion of first branchial arch during intrauterine development. The complete formation of lip often occurs by 5 to 12 weeks, whereas the formation of palate may occur only by 12 to 14 weeks of gestational age. These conditions are usually detected at birth and may

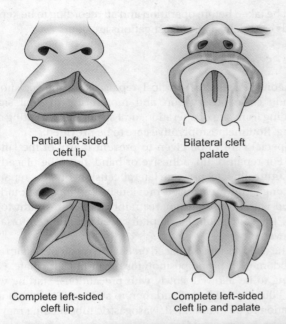

Partial left-sided cleft lip

Bilateral cleft palate

Complete left-sided cleft lip

Complete left-sided cleft lip and palate

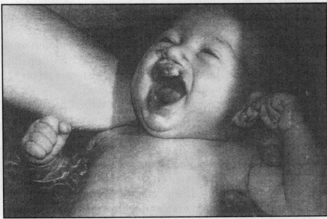

Fig. 23.1: Cleft of the lip and palate

be associated with other congenital anomalies in about 20 percent of cases. These may involve the CNS anomalies or cardiovascular and skeletal malformations.

Cleft lip and cleft palate may occur as single or in combination. It may be unilateral or bilateral.

Cleft Lip (Hare Lip)

It results from failure of the maxillary process to fuse with nasal elevations on frontal prominence. The extent of cleft lip is varying from a notch in the vermilion border to a large cleft reaching the floor of the nose. It is apparent at birth as incomplete formation of lip. It may be associated with cleft palate and supernumerary, deformed or absent teeth. Cleft lip may be found unilateral or bilateral.

Cleft Palate

It results from failure of masses of lateral palatine processes to meet and fuse together. It may be unilateral or bilateral or may occur in isolation or with cleft lip. Cleft palate in isolation may found in the midline involving only uvula or reaches the incisive foramen through soft palate. In association with cleft lip, it involves soft palate and exposes the nasal cavity on one or both side depending upon the defect. Cleft palate is found as an opening or elongated opening or fissure in the roof of the mouth, which should be detected during routine neonatal examination.

Causes

The causes of cleft lip and cleft palate may be genetic or due to unfavorable maternal factors. Maternal factors may be viral infections during 5th to 12th weeks of gestation or ingestion of drugs, exposure to X-ray, anemia and hypoproteinemia.

Types of Cleft Lip and Cleft Palate

- *Group I (Prealveolar):* It includes only cleft lip in right or left side or bilateral and rarely in midline. It can have subtypes, i.e. Group I-A, which indicates cleft lip and alveolus and Group I-B, indicating sub-surface cleft visible with smiling.
- *Group II (Postalveolar):* It includes only cleft palate. Submucous cleft may found as fistula or bifid uvula.
- *Group III (Combined):* It includes both cleft lip and palate in midline or may be unilateral or bilateral.

Combined types are found more frequently (50%) than the isolated cleft lip (25%) and cleft palate (25%).

Complications

Immediate Problems

1. Feeding problem due to ineffective sucking resulting in undernutrition.
2. Aspiration of feeds resulting respiratory infections.
3. Parental anxiety due to defective appearance of the infant.

Long-term Problems

1. Recurrent infections especially otitis media.
2. Disturbed parent-child relationship and maladjustment with nonacceptance of the infant.
3. Impairment of speech.
4. Malocclusion and malplacement of teeth.
5. Hearing problems due to oral malformation especially in cleft palate.
6. Impaired body image due to altered shape of face and oral cavity.

Surgical Management

In cleft-lip: Surgical repair of the defect of the lip is done, preferably at 2 to 3 months of age, when the infant is having good health (At 10 weeks age, 10 lb weight and 10 g Hb%). The operation is termed as cheiloplasty.

In cleft palate: Palatoplasty, the surgical reconstruction of the palate is done with repair of the cleft, at about age of 1 to 2 years of age. It should be done before the child develops defective speech.

Nursing Management

At Birth

Cleft lip and cleft palate should be detected at birth during initial neonatal assessment. Associated congenital anomalies and life threatening problems to be identified for prompt management. Mother needs adequate explanation and emotional support for the stressful event. Parents and family members should be encouraged to accept the infant and to provide tender loving care with love and affection.

Demonstration to be given to the mother and family members regarding feeding of the baby to prevent aspiration and to provide adequate nutrition for growth and development. Breastfeeding is possible in the baby with cleft lip and cleft palate. Cleft palate baby may require palatal obturator which can make feeding easier. If the baby is unable to suck the breast, then expressed breast milk or artificial feeding to be given with long handled spoon and bowl. Dropper or soft large hole nipple or soft feeder or syringe can also be used. Hygienic measures to be followed strictly to prevent diarrhea and other GI disturbances. Small quantity feeds to be given slowly at the side of the mouth. Precautions to be taken to prevent choking. The infant to be placed in upright position during feeding. Burping to be done in between feeds.

Essential care of the neonates to be provided with warmth, immunization, prevention of infections, hygienic care and follow-up. Explanation to be given to the parents about details of surgical correction of the birth defect.

Before Surgery

Basic preoperative preparation and care are important. Parents need emotional support. The child should be prepared with specific directions of the surgeon. Consent must be taken before operation and all recording to be kept in hands especially if any investigations are done.

After Surgery

Immediate care after surgical repair of the defect should include close observation and monitoring of vital signs, bleeding from site of operation, oral secretions, vomiting and crying. Routine postoperative care to be provided.

Special care to be given to prevent injury of the suture line. For repair of lip, adhesive or band aid to be placed on the suture line to prevent lateral tension on the repaired lip. Longan bow, was used previously. The infant should be placed within the mummy restraint or hand restraint to be used. The child should be kept dry, well fed and comfortable to prevent crying.

The child should be placed on back in repair of cleft lip and on abdomen in prone position for repair of cleft palate. Oral feeding to be allowed slowly with precautions, starting with clear liquid to full liquid and then to soft food. Nutrition and hydration to be maintained. Nasogastric tube feeding may be necessary in some children.

Care of suture line to prevent infection is very important. Mouth care and cleaning of suture line after each feed with normal saline or H_2O_2 or sterile water or antiseptic mouth wash to be done. Antibiotic ointment can be applied on suture line in case of lip repair. Removable suture can be removed on 5 to 14 days depending on the condition of wound.

Antibiotics, analgesics and other prescribed medications to be administered with specific precautions. Do not allow finger or straw inside mouth. Avoid sucking or talking loudly in repair of palate. Play and other diversions can be allowed to the child. Parents need continued emotional support and specific instructions to participate in child care. Discharge advice to be explained especially about prevention of infections of the operated area and follow-up. Information to be given about necessary rehabilitational facilities available for the better social adjustment of the child. Speech therapy may be needed.

Prognosis

Residual speech defect may result even after successful repair of palate which requires help from speech therapist. Cosmetic problem of scar on the lip may need cosmetic surgery and counseling.

Musculoskeletal Disorders in Children

24

- Disorders of Muscles
- Disorders of Bones

- Diseases of Joints

DISORDERS OF MUSCLES

Problems that interfere with locomotion are associated with disorders of muscle, bones and joints. Locomotor problems in children may be congenital or acquired during growth and development.

Disorders of muscles include numbers of diseases with progressive weakness of certain groups of muscles. Muscular dystrophies result from primary disease of the muscle, whereas muscular atrophies are secondary to neurological problems. Alongwith clinical manifestations, various investigations are useful to diagnose the muscular diseases. Electromyography (EMG), muscle biopsy, radiography, serum enzymes, blood test (for ESR, TLC, DLC) and examination of synovial fluids are important diagnostic measures.

The muscular disorders in children may be manifested as muscular dystrophies, muscular hypotonia (floppy infant), polymyositis, myositis ossifications, congenital myopathy, endocranial myopathy, torticollis, periodic paralysis (due to hypokalemia or hyperkalemia) and paroxysmal myoglobinuria. The disease of neuromuscular junction is found as myasthenia gravis.

Muscular Dystrophies

Muscular dystrophies are group of hereditary disorders with gradual atrophy of various skeletal muscle groups. It is characterized by gradual onset in early life with involvement of proximal muscles, loss of deep tendon reflexes and pseudohypertrophy of muscle. Initially, the muscle fibers swell, followed by hyaline degeneration and increased connective tissue formation. Infiltration of fat between the fibers may give the muscle an appearance of hypertrophy. Degenerative changes and central location of nucleus in the muscle fibers are often present.

Clinical Types

1. *Pseudohypertrophic muscular dystrophy (Duchenne and Becker type):* It is most common type of muscular dystrophy in children. Commonly found in 3 to 5 years of age. It is genetic disorder with X-linked recessive inheritance and primarily affects the males.

   The pelvic girdle is affected first and gradually weakness spreads to shoulder girdle. Pseudohypertrophy of calf muscles occurs in 80 percent of cases. Other features include symmetrical weakness of pelvic girdle muscles, a waddling gait, exaggerated lumbar lordosis and difficulty in getting-up from the supine position and climbing stairs. Mild mental retardation may present in some children. Cardiac involvement, respiratory infection and heart failure may complicate the condition. Prognosis is generally poor.

2. *Limb girdle type (Erb's type):* It involves the shoulder and pelvic girdles without affecting the face. Both sexes are affected. The prognosis is slightly better than Duchenne type.

3. *Pelvifemoral type (Leyden-Möbius type):* In this type, the quadriceps and the hamstring muscles show extreme weakness. The course is slowly progressive.
4. *Facioscapulohumeral type:* The face and shoulder girdle muscles affected first then spread to the pelvic girdle.
5. *Ocular myopathy:* It is presented as ptosis, weakness of orbicularis oculi muscles, external ophthalmoplegia and dysphagia.
6. *Distal myopathy:* It includes two distinct types (a) early onset with wasting of facial muscles and (b) late onset in adolescence involving hands and feet.

Diagnosis

Careful history of illness, physical examination, laboratory investigations of serum enzymes (CPK, SGOT, LDH, etc.), EMG and muscle biopsy are useful to confirm the diagnosis.

Management

There is no effective management of muscular dystrophy. Prolonged immobilization should be avoided. Physiotherapy, exercises, walking and use of tricycle help to maintain ambulation and to prevent deterioration of muscular functions and contracture. Complications to be prevented by symptomatic treatment. Orthopedic appliances and surgical interventions (tenotomy) are useful. Emotional support to the parents should be provided with explanation and reassurance.

Newer therapeutic approaches are steroids, gene replacement therapy, dystrophin replacement therapy, myoblast transfer therapy, etc.

Prognosis is very poor, majority of the cases may have fatal outcome due to cardiomyopathy and pulmonary complications.

Floppy Baby Syndrome

Floppy baby syndrome or floppy infant syndrome also termed as amyotonia congenita. It is a congenital disease marked by generalized hypotonia of the muscles.

Causes

The causes of floppy baby syndrome can be listed as follows:
1. *Neurological disorders:* Hypoxic-ischemic-encephalopathy, kernicterus, chromosomal anomalies (Down's syndrome), atonic cerebral palsy, intracranial hemorrhage, inborn error of metabolism (mucopolysaccharidosis), poliomyelitis, acute polyneuropathy, neonatal myasthenia gravis, Werdnig-Hoffman disease.
2. *Muscle disorders:* Muscular dystrophies, congenital myopathies, polymyositis, glycogen storage disease.
3. *Miscellaneous:* Advanced PEM, rickets, scurvy, cretinism, malabsorption syndrome.

Clinical Manifestations

The older children may present with delay in walking, running or climbing stairs. The infants are manifested with frog-legged position and assumes the position of a rag doll. There is diminished resistance to passive movements of the extremities. The range of movement of the peripheral joints is increased. When pulling up the baby from supine position to sitting position, there is head lag. Convulsions and mental retardation may present.

Diagnosis of floppy infant needs detailed investigations to find out the exact cause. History of illness, physical examination, EMG, presence or absence of deep tendon reflex help to confirm the diagnosis.

Management of the condition should be done according to specific cause. Symptomatic and supportive measures should be provided to prevent complications and promote prognosis.

Limping

Limping or defective walking in the child is a serious problem to the parents and health care providers. It may occur due to problem of any part of weight bearing structures including spine, hips, knees, ankles and feet. The diseases, which cause tenderness, weakness or asymmetry of the weight bearing apparatus, cause a limping gait. Most cases of limping are transient, which may recover with time and without any specific management.

Causes of Limping

1. *Neuromuscular disorders:* Postpolio residual paralysis (PPRP), hemiplegia, muscular dystrophies, hemihypertrophy of muscles.
2. *Disorders of bones and joints:* Rickets, bony injury, congenital dislocation of hip, suppurative arthritis, rheumatoid arthritis, transient synovitis, tuberculosis, osteochondritis (Perthes' disease), slipped epiphysis, scoliosis, congenital vertebral defect.
3. *Problems of foot:* Club foot, painful lesions of the nails, toes and soles (corns), paronychia, fracture, ill fitting shoes, etc.

The diagnosis is based on the history of the illness, age of the child, time of onset, duration, course of illness and associated clinical features. Thorough clinical examination, neurological examination and necessary investigations (X-ray, EMG) are necessary to determine the exact cause of limping. Management should be done according to the specific cause.

DISORDERS OF BONES

Bony abnormalities can be found as congenital malformations, infections, trauma and tumor. The congenital bone disorders includes congenital deficiency of long bones (like phocomelia, hemimelia or amelia), polydactyly, syndactyly, trigger thumb, congenital dislocation of hip, congenital dislocation of patella, osteogenesis imperfecta, osteopetrosis (Marble bone disease), club foot, Marfan's syndrome, achondroplasia, etc. Acquired bony problems are mainly trauma (accidents, sports injury) tumor, and inflammations (osteomyelitis, osteochondritis, tuberculosis, etc.)

Osteogenesis Imperfecta (Fragilitas Ossium)

It is a hereditary osteoporotic syndrome, characterized by multiple fractures due to osteoporosis and excessive bone fragility. Other features include skeletal deformities, blue sclera, congenital deafness and lax ligaments. It is an autosomal dominant disorder. The defect is in the quality of bone matrix with metabolic disorder of collagen and its derivatives.

Types

There are two clinical types, (a) Osteogenesis imperfecta congenita and (b) Osteogenesis imperfecta tarda. A third group with slightly increased fragility as dental changes alone may occur in some children and known as dentinogenesis imperfecta.

Osteogenesis imperfecta congenita is a severe form or fatal type. About 50 percent of these type of disorders are found as stillbirth and remaining infants usually die soon after birth due to respiratory complications as a result of multiple fracture and defective thorax. This baby is born with multiple deformities.

Osteogenesis imperfecta tarda usually manifested with symptoms in middle or late childhood or even in puberty.

According to severity, osteogenesis imperfecta can be classified as type I, type II, type III and type IV.

Type I osteogenesis imperfecta: It is autosomal dominant disorder and manifested with osteoporosis, excessive bone fragility with fracture, blue scera and conductive deafness. It may found in adolescence (Fig. 24.1).

Type II: It is a lethal syndrome and presented with low birth weight and length, hypotelorism, fracture of nasal bone, extremely short and deformed bent extremities, broad thighs fixed at right angles to the trunk, crumpled long bones, fracture and beaded ribs as shown in X-ray. Prenatal diagnosis is possible by USG, X-ray and biochemical studies. With this type of defect 50 percent baby born dead and 50 percent die soon after birth.

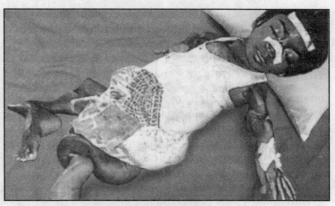

Fig. 24.1: Osteogenesis imperfecta, an adolescent of 5 feets height become one feet

Type III: It is an autosomal recessive disorder and manifested with multiple fractures, blue sclera which tend to become less blue with increase of age.

Type IV: It is an autosomal dominant disorder and may manifest any time from birth to adult life with fracture and deformities. The sclera becomes less blue with age and deafness is less frequent. In some cases opalescent dentin may be found.

Management

There is no specific management of the condition. Adequate nutrition or vitamin D supplementation, magnesium oxide (orally), and calcitonin may be effective to reduce the incidence of fracture. Careful nursing care on firm mattress and pillows, supervision of activities of daily living and prompt immobilization of fractures are essential measures. Surgical correction of deformities may be postponed till adolescence. Healing of fractures is always satisfactory and callus formation occur rapidly.

Developmental Dysplasia of the Hip

Developmental dysplasia of the hip (DDH) describes those conditions involving the abnormal development of the proximal femur and/or acetabulum. It may be associated with other congenital anomalies. Left hip is more commonly affected, but bilateral involvement occurs in more than 50 percent of cases. Girls are affected 8 times more than boys. The DDH was previously known as congenital dislocation of hip (CDH).

Etiology

Developmental dysplasia of the hip (DDH) is caused by genetic and environmental factors. It may develop following breech delivery or other difficult deliveries, when head of the femur may get dislocated upward and backward which may cause development of a false acetabulum.

Pathophysiology

The structures of hip joint, i.e. acetabulum, femoral head and capsule may not be developed properly. These lead to partial or complete dislocation of femoral head from the shallow acetabular cavity. Partial dislocation or subluxation is more common. Ossification centers are delayed in appearance. The degrees of DDH may include as follows:

- *Dysplasia:* This condition is found as shallow acetabulum with upward slant of acetabular roof.
- *Subluxation:* In this condition acetabular surface of the femoral head is in contact with shallow dysplastic acetabular surface but the head slides laterally and superiorly.
- *Dislocation:* Here articular cartilage of completely displaced femoral head does not contact with acetabular articular cartilage.

Clinical Manifestations

The physical findings of DDH may be detected during neonatal assessment. These findings may change as the child grown up.

The physical findings during neonatal examination or afterward include asymmetry of the thigh, presence of gluteal and knee folds, diminished spontaneous movements, shortening of the affected leg, inability to abduct the hip fully and posterior bulging of femoral head. The affected leg appears short and externally rotated.

Positive Ortolani sign (forced abduction of hip causes a clicking sound), positive Trendelenburg's sign (downward felt of pelvis on affected side) and positive Barlow's test including hip instability are important. If not treated, the child starts walking delayed with presence of pain in the joint, waddling gait and lordosis. Subluxation of the hip joint may be detected at birth or may manifest several months later.

Diagnostic Evaluation

Routine neonatal examination and physical examination during development assessment at regular interval are helpful to diagnose the condition.

The Barlow's text is the most important maneuver to detect hip instability. Holding the hips and knees at 90° angle of flexion, a backward pressure is applied while adducting hips. The femur head is felt slipping out of the acetabulum posterolaterally with a click sound indicating the test is positive.

The diagnosis of DDH is confirmed by X-ray, ultrasonography, CT scan, MRI or arthrograms.

Management

Management of DDH depends on the age of the child and the degree of the problem. The management should be started as early as possible to restore as closely as possible the anatomic alignment of the hip.

Subluxation of hip can be managed by Pavlik harness or abduction brace for maintenance of flexion abduction position till the hip becomes normal, usually by the 3rd months of age.

Dislocation of hip may require traction and closed reduction followed by application of hip spica cast for 3 months to maintain reduction. These are indicated when harness treatment is unsuccessful. Open reduction and innominate osteotomy followed by application of hip spica cast and abduction bracing are indicated when closed reduction and casting are unsuccessful. In acetabular dysplasia, use the NSAIDS, ambulation devices (crutches) and surgical correction are required. Follow-up should be continued until age of skeletal maturity.

Emotional support to the parents, maintenance of skin integrity and prevention of complications of immobility should be the important nursing responsibility along with the health teaching and instructions for participation in child care. Follow-up and rehabilitation should be emphasized.

Complications

Complications of DDH may be found as avascular necrosis, loss of range of motion of the affected hip, leg-length discrepancy, early osteoarthritis, femoral nerve palsy, recurrent dislocation or unstable hip and iatrogenic complication.

Congenital Club Foot (Fig. 24.2)

Congenital club foot or talipes is a nontraumatic deformity of the foot. The foot is twisted out of shape or position. The deviations may found in the direction of one or the other of the four lines of movement or of two of these combinations.

The foot may be deformed in plantar flexion (talipes equinus) or dorsiflexion (talipes calcaneus). The foot may be abducted and inverted (talipes varus) or abducted everted (talipes valgus) or various combination of these, i.e. talipes equinovarus, talipes calcaneovarus, talipes equinovalgus and talipes calcaneovalgus.

The most common type of club foot is *talipes equinovarus* (95%), in which the foot is in plantar flexion and deviated medially. Heel is elevated and foot is twisted inward.

In *talipes calcaneovalgus* type, the deformity is found as dorsiflexion and lateral deviation of the foot.

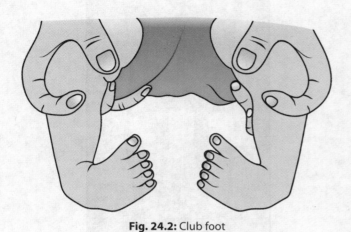

Fig. 24.2: Club foot

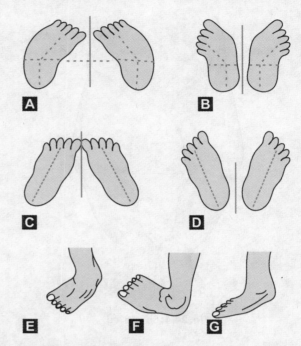

Figs 24.3A to G: Abnormal position of foot: (A) Metatarsus varus; (B) Metatarsus valgus; (C) Pes varus; (D) Pes valgus; (E) Talipes equinovarus; (F) Talipes calcaneovalgus; (G) Talipes equinovalgus

In *talipes equinus*, the toes are lower than heal, foot is extended and the child walks on toes. In *talipes calcaneus*, the toes are higher than heel, foot is flexed, heel alone touches the ground causing the child to walk on the inner side of the heel, which often follows infantile paralysis of the muscle of Achilles tendon.

In *talipes varus*, heel and foot turned inward. In *talipes valgus*, heel and foot are turned outward.

Talipes pes cavus is termed when there is excessive plantar curvature of the foot. *Talipes arcuates* or cavus indicates exaggerated normal arch of the foot. Flat foot indicates the arch of the foot is less or flat and it is a calcaneovalgus deformity (Figs 24.3A to G).

Incidence

Club foot is found in 1 to 3 per 1000 live birth. Half of these cases are bilateral. Boys are two times more affected than girls. Among all forms of talipes, about 95 percent cases are talipes equinovarus. Club foot may be associated with spina bifida, meningocele and myelodystrophy.

Etiology

The exact etiology of club foot is not known. The suggested contributing factors are familial tendency (about 10% of cases) and primary arrest or anomalous development of the foot in fetal life. Intrauterine malposition of fetal foot due to less amniotic fluid and defective neuromuscular development of fetus may also found as important contributing factors of club foot.

There may be bony defects or abnormalities in joints (subtalar joint) or contractures of the Achilles tendon. Usually the ligaments on the medial side of the foot are contracted, underdeveloped and short, whereas on the lateral aspect they are stretched and relaxed.

Diagnostic Evaluation

The defect is obvious at birth and detected during first neonatal examination. Family history about the presence of the condition should be obtained. X-ray of the affected foot helps to detect bony abnormality and to assess treatment efficiency.

Management

Management should be started as early as possible with the standard foot wear, may be in the first week of life.

Initial nonoperative management is done by serial manipulation followed by immobilization in a plaster cast or adhesive tape or strapping or splinting. It should be done at the time of diagnosis. Parents should be taught with adequate explanation and demonstration about the manipulation that can be done at home. These initial management may be continued for 2 to 6 months of age. Then assessment is necessary about the progress and to plan for further management.

Dennis Browne bar/splint may be used along with corrective shoes after initial period of management. Recently, Wheaton brace or Bebax shoe is used.

Surgical management is usually performed at 4 to 9 months of age with postoperative immobilization before the child begins to walk. Correction of bony deformities

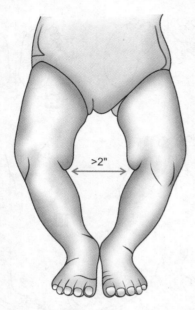

Fig. 24.4: Bowed leg

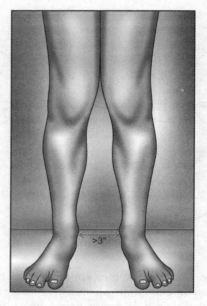

Fig. 24.5: Knocked knee

and to balance the muscle and tendons by a combination of fusion, release, lengthening and transfer are performed during surgical procedures. Tenotomy (of Achilles tendon) is indicated in some cases. Preoperative and postoperative care with prevention of infection is important.

Postoperative immobilization is done by cast for 12 weeks followed by use of brace (ankle-foot-orthosis) or corrective shoes for a period of 2 to 4 years. Parents need adequate explanations and instructions about correct use of shoes, brace, care of cast, skin care and regular follow-up till the completion of the total schedule of management.

Complications

In untreated cases, awkward gait, callosities and bursae may develop on weight bearing part. Overaggressive manipulation may produce disturbances in epiphyseal plate. Residual deformity may be found in long-term management schedule. Postoperative complications and problems related to plaster cast or inappropriate use of splint or brace or corrective shoes may develop in some children.

Genu Varus (Bowleg) (Fig. 24.4)

Genu varus or bowleg is termed when knees are abnormally divergent and ankles are abnormally convergent like a bent bow. It occurs due to lateral angulation of knee joints because of inward deviation of longitudinal axis of tibia fibula.

Physiological bowlegs are found when the child begins to walk but it recovers spontaneously within a short period. The pathological causes of bowlegs are rickets, trauma,

defective posture, developmental problems and endocrinal disturbances.

The condition needs to be identified early to correct the underlying cause and to prevent long-term complications. Persistent deformity may require orthotic devices or corrective osteotomy.

Genu Valgum (Knock Knee) (Fig. 24.5)

Genu valgum or knock knee indicates abnormal convergent of knees with divergent ankles. It is due to outward deviation of the longitudinal axis of both tibia and femur resulting medial angulation of knees. The intermalleolar distance becomes more than 8 cm.

Physiological knock knee are common in toddlers but it usually recovers within 7 years of age. The pathological causes of knock knee can be secondary to softening of the bone in case of rickets, juvenile rheumatic arthritis and bony dysplasia. Postpolio residual paralysis (PPRP), cerebral palsy, fractures, neoplastic disease of bone and postinfective bony lesions may also cause knock knee. The most common variety is idiopathic.

Early identification of the problem and orthopedic interventions like stapling or osteotomy and orthotic devices may be effective for the correction of deformity.

Kyphosis (Humpback or Hunchback)

Kyphosis is a deformity of the spine as an increased roundness of the thoracic curve. It occurs due to exaggeration or angulation of the normal posterior curve with convexity backward and forward curvature of the shoulders.

It may develop due to defective posture, rickets, congenital anomaly, diseased spine (syphilis, tuberculosis), malignancy, juvenile rheumatic arthritis, compression fracture or due to idiopathic cause as in Scheuermann disease.

Management is performed by orthotic devices or orthopedic surgery after clinical and radiological evaluation.

Scoliosis

Scoliosis is the lateral or side-to-side curvature of the spine due to alteration of normal spinal alignment occurring in the anteroposterior or frontal plane. It usually consist of two curves, the original abnormal curve and a compensatory curve in the opposite direction.

Etiology

In majority of the cases, the condition is due to idiopathic origin. Possible causes are congenital defects due to defective embryonic development of the spine as hemivertebra and wedge vertebra. Scoliosis may occur due to neuromuscular problems in muscular paralysis, cerebral palsy, intervertebral disk herniation, postpolio complications and myopathies. It may also occur due to rickets, sciatica, leg-length discrepancy, fracture, diseases of hip and spine, visual defects, defective posture and position, empyema and retraction of one side of chest.

In all types of scoliosis, the vertebral column develops lateral curvature. The vertebrae rotate to the convex side of the curve, which rotates the spinous processes toward the concavity. Vertebrae become wedge shaped. Disk shape is altered, as are the neural canal and posterior arch of the vertebral body. As the deformity progresses, changes in the thoracic cage increase leading to respiratory and cardiovascular problems.

Clinical Manifestations

Scoliosis may be presented with physical deformity like poor posture, increased or decreased thoracic kyphosis or lumbar lordosis and leg-length discrepancy. Shoulder asymmetry, scapular prominence, truncal imbalance, lump on back, uneven waistline and uneven breast size may be found. There may be visual deformity and bone pain.

Diagnostic Evaluation

Careful history, thorough physical and neurological examination and Adam's forward bending test are useful for diagnosis. X-ray spine, MRI, CT scan, myelograms and clinical photographs for appearance are effective to confirm the diagnosis.

Management

Management of scoliosis can be done with orthotic devices (Brace) and exercise therapy, to prevent progression of curve and to promote the flexibility in the spine. Surgical correction (Posterior spinal fusion) is indicated for stabilization of the spinal column and cosmetic purpose, when bracing is not possible or unsuccessful.

Preoperative traction or casting may be used to help to gain correction and increase flexibility. Postoperative casting also may be required to protect the fusion mass. Surgical intervention may be done in anterior or posterior approach with various instrumentation methods.

Parents and family members need emotional support and health teaching about care of cast, traction and brace, skin care, electrical stimulation, exercise and permitted activities, nutritious diet, breathing exercises, prevention of complications, etc. Continuation of school activities, social support and rehabilitation should be discussed with parents and family members.

Fracture

Fracture in children differ than those of adults in anatomy, physiology and biomechanics. The incidence of musculoskeletal injuries are increasing due to various reasons and environmental changes leading to long-term sufferings and fatal outcome in children. Prevention of musculoskeletal injuries and prompt initiation of management following the event are vital approach for better outcome.

Fracture is a break or disruption in the continuity of bone. In children, fracture usually occurs due to fall or direct trauma. It may found due to pathological cause or due to severe muscular contraction. Child abuse may result bony injury in children.

A bone gets fracture when the force applied to it exceeds the amount, the bone can absorb. The mechanism and effects of fracture in children differ in various aspect from that of adult.

In children, bones are having thick periosteum. Long bones are more resilient than those of adults, so they are able to withstand greater deflection without fracturing. Fracture involves the growth plate of the bone, which is weaker than surrounding ligaments, tendons and joint capsules and disrupted before these tissues are injured. Damage of growth plate may result in cessation of or disturbance in bone growth. There is often acceleration in bone growth after fracture in the long bones in children. Fracture bone heals more rapidly in young children and remodel more completely and actively with less disability and deformity.

Common Sites of Fracture in Children

1. Forearm fractures are most common site (50%). About 3/4th of the forearm fractures involve the distal third of radius and ulna.

2. Epiphyseal fractures involve the physis (growth plate) and accounts for about 15 to 30 percent of all fracture cases in children. The mechanism of injury is usually fall on an outstretched hand involving physeal injury of the distal radius and ulna.

3. *Fracture humerus:* It occurs due to fall onto an out-stretched arm or hand involving proximal part of the shaft of the humerus. Direct trauma may cause this fracture. Supracondylar fracture accounts for 60 percent of all elbow fracture in children. Lateral condylar fracture is second most common in distal humeral injuries. Medial epicondylar fractures are third most common of elbow fracture in children.

4. *Femur fractures:* It is common in children involving mid shaft of the femur and usually found following motor vehicle accidents.

5. *Tibial fracture and ankle fracture:* The most common lower extremity fracture in children occurs in the tibial and fibular shaft due to motor vehicle accidents and sports injury. Ankle fracture may occur in adolescents due to direct trauma.

Other sites of fractures include spinal injury due to fall from height (roof, trees) and automobile accidents. Pelvis and hip fracture may occur in high energy trauma such as motor vehicle accidents, bicycle accidents and fall from height. Foot fracture may occur following direct trauma, jumping or twisting injury involving metatarsals. Clavicular fracture may occur due to fall or direct trauma.

Common Types of Fracture in Children (Figs 24.6A to D)

a. *Open fracture:* It is a type of fracture in which a wound through the adjacent or overlying soft tissues communicates with the site of the break. It is also termed as compound fracture.

b. *Closed fracture:* The fracture that does not produce on open wound in the skin.

c. *Plastic deformation (bending):* A bending of the bone occurs in such a manner as to cause a microscopic fracture line that does not cross the bone. It is unique to children and commonly found in the ulna.

d. *Buckle (torus) fracture:* A fracture occurring on the tension side of the bone near the softer metaphyseal bone. It crosses the bone and buckles the harder diaphyseal bone on the opposite site causing a bulge. The bone cortex is not broken but is buckled.

e. *Greenstick fracture:* A fracture in which the bone is partially bent and partially broken, as a green stick breaks. The bone is bent and the fracture begins but does not entirely cross through the bone.

f. *Complete fracture:* A fracture in which the bone is completely broken, neither fragment is connected to the other. This fracture can be spiral, oblique, transverse and epiphyseal.

- Spiral fracture occurs from a rotational force that follows a helical line.
- Oblique fracture occurs diagonally across the diaphysis.
- Transverse fracture occurs when the fracture line is at right angles to the long axis of the bone and usually diaphyseal.
- Epiphyseal fracture occurs as a separation of the epiphysis from the bone between the shaft of the bone and its growing end.

Other types of fractures which may found in children are *pathological fracture* due to weakening of the bone structure by pathological processes such as neoplasm, osteomyelitis, etc.

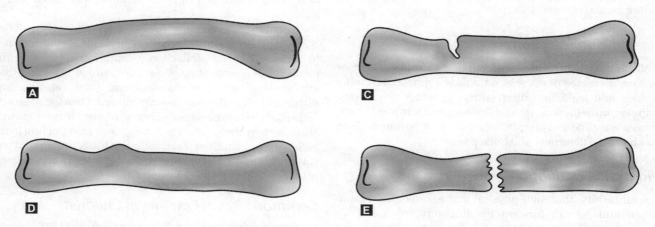

Figs 24.6A to D: Common fractures in children: (A) Plastic deformations (bend); (B) Buckle (torus); (C) Greenstick; (D) Complete

Depressed fracture: It may found in the neonates due to fracture of the skull, in which a fragment of fractured bone is depressed.

Clinical Manifestations

The clinical manifestations of fracture include inability to use the injured part (standing, walking, moving) and presence of deformity (visible or palpable). Other features are pain, tenderness, local swelling and brushing. Unusual mobility, shortening of the part, crepitus or grating sound due to movement between fractured bone fragments and muscular spasm may also present. History of trauma or injury is usually found. In pathological fracture, history of pathological conditions is present.

Diagnostic Evaluation

History of injury or trauma or chronic diseases (osteomyelitis, carcinoma) should be obtained. Clinical examination, radiologic studies (X-ray, CT scan, MRI, bone scan, fluoroscopy) and vascular assessment to be done to confirm the diagnosis.

Management

Management of children with fracture depends upon the age of the child, type of fracture and its location. The different management procedures are as follows:

- Immobilization of the fractured part by plaster cast, splint or brace.
- Closed reduction followed by a period of immobilization in the cast or splint.
- Closed reduction and percutaneous pining followed by immobilization.
- Closed or open reduction and application of external fixators.
- Open reduction with or without internal fixation followed by immobilization in a cast or splint.
- Traction (surface, skeletal) for slow reduction of fracture followed by a period of immobilization.

Specific traction: It used in children can be listed as the following:

1. *Bryant's traction:* It is indicated in fractures of femur and congenital dislocation of hip.
2. *Russell's traction:* It is applied to reduce the fractures of the femur or hip or specific types of knee injuries or contractures.
3. *Buck's extension:* It is used to prevent or to correct knee and hip contractures, to rest the limb, to prevent spasm of injured muscles or joints or to immobilize the fractured limb temporarily.
4. *Balanced suspension with Thomas splint and Pearson attachment:* It is used in older children and adolescents

for fractured femur to rest the injured lower extremity or joint.
5. *90-degree-90 degree traction:* It is indicated in fractured femur when skin traction is inadequate.
6. *Dunlop's traction:* It is used to treat fractures of the humerus and injures in or around the shoulder girdle.
7. *Cervical traction:* It is applied for stabilization of spinal fractures or injuries or in muscle spasms and muscle contractures.

Most childhood fractures usually heal within 12 weeks or less. Presence of wound needs special attention with aseptic precautions. Care of the child with plaster cast and tractions are the most important nursing responsibility. Preoperative preparation and postoperative care in case of open reduction should emphasize prevention of infections and other complications. Symptomatic treatment (analgesic, antibiotic) should be administered as prescribed.

Restoration of complete function of the fractured part can be achieved by physical therapy and exercise. Parents need adequate explanation and instructions to continue the management. Special instructions to be given regarding external fixators and internal fixation devices. Emotional support to the child and parents is essential. The child needs diversional therapy and continuation of school activities during the illness.

Complications

The complications of fracture in children are found as infections, avascular necrosis, vascular injuries, nerve injuries and palsies, visceral injuries, tendon and joint injuries, fat embolism, delayed union, nonunion or malunion, compartment syndrome, osteoarthritis, shortening due to the epiphyseal arrest and deformity.

Nursing Management

Nursing assessment: Initial assessment should be done for life-threatening problems (airway, breathing and circulation), same as a trauma victim. Hemorrhage, level of consciousness, vital signs, neurological signs and head to foot examination to be done to detect problems related to fracture and the associated injuries. Accident or trauma details should be included in the routine history. Presence of pain, ecchymosis, swelling and deformity or other features to be ruled out.

Nursing diagnoses: The important diagnoses are:
- Pain related to tissue injury and muscle spasms due to fracture.
- Altered tissue perfusion related to swelling and immobilization.
- Impaired skin integrity related to cast/traction/other orthopedic devices.
- Impaired physical mobility related to fracture and immobilization.

- Self-care deficit related to injury/fracture or surgery or immobilization by external orthopedic devices.
- Risk for infections related to trauma or wound or surgical interventions.
- Risk for peripheral neurovascular dysfunction related to cast, splint and orthopedic appliances.
- Ineffective coping related to hospitalization and long term illness with its possible complications.

Nursing interventions: Relieving pain by analgesics and nontraditional methods like diversion, relaxation, etc.

Promoting comfort by rest, position, alignments and support of the injured part.

Maintaining tissue perfusion by removing compressive and constricting bandage, elevating extremity above the heart level, encouraging movements and assessing the limb by checking temperature, color, sensation and pulses.

Promoting skin integrity by frequent change of position, care of pressure points, high protein and carbohydrate diet with rich in vitamins and minerals, massaging the healthy skin around the affected area and preventing skin infection and further injury. Skin should be assessed for any breakdown or pressure of cast, splint or bandage.

Promoting mobility by exercise of uninvolved limbs, appropriate ambulation and use of ambulatory aids (walker, cratch) with precautions.

Preventing infections by would care, antibiotic therapy, general hygienic measures, aseptic precautions, hand washing practices, universal precautions and dietary support.

Attaining independence and promoting self-care by the child, as possible.

Preventing neurovascular dysfunction by frequent assessment of affected limb (movement, sensation, numbness, tingling, excessive pain, etc.). Encouraging range of motion exercises.

Promoting effective coping by frequent interaction, assessment of problems, prompt interventions, explanation, emotional support, etc.

Teaching the parent about continuation of care at home after discharge (specially with cast, splint, traction, external fixators), immobilization and its importance, safety measures for prevention of infections and further injury, dietary support, assessment of problems, need for medical help, follow-up and rehabilitation.

Osteomyelitis

Osteomyelitis is the inflammation of bone, localized or generalized, and/or surrounding soft tissues caused by pyogenic infection. It may occur at any age, but mainly found as a disease of growing bone. Long bones are commonly affected at the metaphyseal region.

Etiology

The most common causative organism is *Staphylococcus aureus* (90%), which is responsible for acute hematogenous osteomyelitis. Other causative agents are group-B *Streptococcus* (common in infants and young children), *E. coli* (in neonates and young children) and *Pseudomonas aeruginosa*, *Aspergillus*, etc.

Osteomyelities can occur following trauma, surgical wound, penetrating wound, decubitus ulcer, septicemia, infections of skin and respiratory tract and in immunosuppression. Risk factors include external fixation devices, Foley's catheterization for urinary drainage, central or peripheral IV lines, IV drug users, etc.

Pathophysiology

Infections spread by three method, i.e. hematogenous, contiguous and direct inoculation. Hematogenous spread occurs through the bloodstream and found in children following blunt trauma to long bones. Contiguous infection occurs after surgery or from a primary infection directly from adjacent tissue. Direct inoculation occurs in open fracture or surgery through the puncture or stab wound.

There is inflammatory and immunological response at site of inoculation as pus formation, edema and vascular congestion. Infection spreads through Volkmann's and Haversian canal causing further vascular obstruction. Ischemia and necrosis develop following vascular obstruction, which allow separation of living bone from necrotic bone and formation of 'sequestrum'. Sequestra enlarge, spread and breach the cortex and form subperiosteal abscess and further interfere with blood supply.

If blood supply remains sufficient to maintain the life of bone tissue, new bone is originated and bone healing occurs. If blood supply is insufficient to maintain life of bone tissue, then the bone dies and becomes inert. Chronic sinuses may develop which leads to chronic osteomyelitis. Complete healing takes place only when the dead bone has been destroyed, discharged and excised.

Types

1. *Acute osteomyelitis:* It occurs as a result of hematogenous spread from a distant focus such as umbilicus, skin or throat or direct spread from a nearby specific focus. Metaphysis is the most susceptible site due to sluggish blood circulation and lack of phagocytic cells.
2. *Chronic osteomyelitis:* It develops due to inadequate treatment of acute osteomyelitis.

Clinical Manifestations

Acute osteomyelitis is manifested with fever, localized severe progressive pain, swelling, tenderness, erythema and warmth of the affected part. Limitation of range of motion, involvement of nearby joint, malaise, irritability with generalized signs of sepsis are usually present. History of local injury or trauma commonly found in about 50 percent of these cases. Previous history of upper respiratory or skin infection may present.

Chronic osteomyelitis is manifested as presence of sinus tract at the affected part. Discharging sinus is fixed with underlying bone. Nearby joint may become stiff due to secondary arthritis.

Complications

The complications of osteomyelitis may be found as septic arthritis, joint destruction and contracture, pathological fracture, skeletal deformity as leg-length discrepancy, immobility, abscess formation and systemic infection.

Diagnostic Evaluation

History of trauma or infection, physical examination, laboratory and radiological investigations are important to diagnose the condition.

Blood culture and culture of the material obtained by bone aspiration or biopsy help to identify the causative organism. Complete blood examination shows leukocytosis, low hemoglobin level and elevated ESR. X-ray of the affected part, bone scan and MRI help to determine the bony and soft tissue involvement.

Management

Acute osteomyelitis is managed with intravenous broad-spectrum antibiotic therapy (Cloxacillin, Gentamicin). Antibiotic therapy may be continued (orally) for 4 to 8 weeks. Selection of antibiotics depends upon culture and sensitivity report. Tuberculous etiology to be treated with antitubercular drugs. Symptomatic management with analgesics and antipyretics to be given. Supportive care should include adequate rest, nutritious diet, wound care, maintenance of hydration, immobilization of the part, exercise and ambulation as possible.

Surgical management may be needed in abscess formation as incision and drainage. Sequestrectomy and bone grafting may be required in chronic cases. Rehabilitation with orthotic devices may be needed in case of long-term complications and deformity.

Bone Tumor

Bone tumor may be classified as benign tumor and malignant tumor. Malignant bone tumors are common in adolescent age group. Approximately 90 percent of these tumors are osteosarcoma and Ewing's tumor.

A. *Benign bone tumors:* Bony growths which are not spreading by metastases or infiltration of tissue. Due to lack of invasive power and metastasis, there is less degree of anaplasia than malignant tumors. The benign bony abnormal mass include the followings.
   - *Reactive:* Benign osteoblastoma, osteoid osteoma, nonosteogenic fibroma
   - *Cystic:* Solitary cyst, aneurysmal cyst
   - *Hamartoma:* Osteoma, osteochondroma, enchond-roma.

   These benign tumors need surgical removal and supportive management.
B. *Malignant bone tumors:* These bony growth are able to infiltrate tissue, and spread by metastasis. These tumors frequently recur after attempts of surgical removal. These growth show high degree of anaplasia. The malignant bone tumors are found as follows:
   - *Primary:* Osteosarcoma, chondrosarcoma, fibro-sarcoma, multiple myeloma, Ewing's tumor, etc.
   - *Secondary:* From primary malignancy of any other site.

Osteosarcoma

Sarcoma is a malignant tumor of mesenchymal derivation. Osteogenic sarcoma is the malignant primary tumor of bone composed of a malignant connective tissue stroma with evidence of osteoid, bone and/or cartilage formation. Depending upon the dominant component, it can be classified as osteoblastic, fibroblastic, and chondroblastic.

Common sites of occurrence are distal femur, proximal tibia and proximal humerus. It may occur in pelvis, phalanges and jaw.

The clinical features are pain in the affected site with frequently causing limp or limitation of motion. Palpable, tender, fixed bony mass detected during examination. Diagnosis is confirmed by X-ray, CT scan, MRI, bone scan, angiogram and biopsy.

Management include surgery for amputation or limb saving procedure and chemotherapy.

Ewing's Tumor

It is a malignant tumor of bone arising in medullary tissue and more often in cylindrical bones. It occurs in femur but may involves flat bone such as pelvis, ribs and sternum. Pain, swelling in the affected part and constitutional symptoms are common features. Biopsy is done to confirm the diagnosis. Radiotherapy, chemotherapy and surgery are indicated for management of the condition.

DISEASES OF JOINTS

The common conditions affecting the joints in children are traumatic joint dislocation and inflammations like arthritis, osteochondritis, tuberculosis, synovitis and sports injury.

Traumatic joint dislocation occurs when the surface of the bones which form joint are no longer in anatomic contact. Shoulder, fingers and elbow are the common joints, which may be dislocated. This condition should be managed as emergency, because of associated disruption of surrounding blood and nerve supplies. There may be partial disruption of the articulating surface as subluxation.

Inflammation of joints (arthritis) are frequently found in children and associated with various etiology. The common inflammation of joints in children are juvenile rheumatoid arthritis and pyogenic arthritis. Nonrheumatic arthritis in children are related to hemophilia (hemarthrosis), scurvy (subperiosteal hemorrhage), tuberculosis and transient synovitis of hip.

Juvenile Rheumatoid Arthritis

Juvenile rheumatoid arthritis (JRA) is a chronic inflammatory, generalized systemic disease involving one or more joints and causing connective tissue damage and visceral lesions throughout the body. The JRA is termed when the onset is prior to 16 years of age and persisting for at least 6 weeks. It is common in girls than in boys.

Etiology

The cause of this collagen disorder is not known. The current hypotheses about the causes are infection from an unidentified organism or autoimmune process or hypersensitivity to unknown stimuli. Some subtypes have genetic predisposition.

Pathophysiology

In early stages, one or more joints become inflamed which localized in the joint capsule and primarily in the synovium. The tissue becomes thickened due to congestion and edema. The inflammatory response occurs in the interior of the joint leading to adherence and destruction of the articular cartilage. Inflamed and overgrown synovial tissue fills the joint space resulting in fibrous ankylosis and bony fusion. There may be premature epiphyseal closure or accelerated epiphyseal growth. Tendon and its sheath may also be affected by inflammatory changes. These conditions result in deformity, subluxation and fibrous or bony ankylosis of joints.

Clinical Manifestations

The clinical features of JRA is found as exacerbations and remissions. Precipitating factors are injections, injury or surgical procedures. The lesions may be widespread. The most dominant manifestations are the symmetrical involvements of both small and large joints including fingers and toes (proximal interphalangeal joints), wrists, ankles, knees, hips, cervical spine and temporomandibular joints. Joints become painful, swollen tender and warm. Reduced mobility and flexion position results in contractures and crippling. Fingers may become spindle shaped with shiny and smooth overlying skin within 1 to 3 months. The condition leads to joint destruction, dislocation and deformity which may occur gradually and sometimes suddenly.

Other manifestations of the disease are prolonged, remittent and irregular type fever with chills and rigors. Transitory rash over trunk, muscle aches, weight loss, subcutaneus nodules, iridocyclitis, hepatosplenomegaly, lymphadenopathy, pericarditis, myocarditis, pneumonia and pleurisy may present.

A clinical variant of JRA is Still's disease with Still's triad features as arthritis or arthralgia, lymphadenopathy and splenomegaly. It has acute febrile or systemic onset in single joint, gradually involving almost all the joints.

Types

Clinical manifestations of JRA can be grouped as follows according to presentation during the first 6 months of onset.
1. *Pauci articular type:* It is presented with four or fewer joints involvement. It is most frequent type (approximately 60 percent). It has two subtypes.
   Type I: It is more common in female children (80%) with the onset in about 5 years of age. But less than 10 years. Commonly nonsymmetrical and large joints, i.e. knees, ankles and elbows are involved. Antinuclear antibodies (ANA) are positive in 90 percent cases with rheumatoid factor (RF) negative. HLA-DR$_5$ and DRW$_8$ are positive (including genetic predisposition)
   Type II: It is more common in male children (90%) with the onset in about 8 to 10 years of age or more. Usually hip joints are involved nonsymmetrically with presence of sacroiliitis in some cases. The ANA and RF are negative with positive HLA B$_{27}$ (haplotype).
2. *Polyarticular type:* It is seen in about 30 percent of cases with involvement of 5 or more joints. Usually small joints are affected. Two subtypes are known with the presence or absence of rheumatoid factor with this type. The subtypes

are polyarticular RF (+)ve and polyarticular RF(–)ve. Serum ANA level is positive in about 25 percent cases of RF (–)ve and in about 75 percent cases of RF(+)ve.

3. *Systemic type:* It is more common in boys (60%) having acute febrile or systemic onset. It is seen in about 10 percent of all cases of JRA. The ANA may be positive or negative but RF is negative.

Diagnostic Evaluation

Details history of illness, physical examination and following findings of laboratory investigations help to diagnose JRA.

- Blood examination shows high TLC, high ESR, high serum proteins and positive C-reactive proteins.
- Antinuclear antibody (ANA) and rheumatoid factor (RF) may be positive or negative which help to detect the subtype of JRA.
- X-ray of the affected joint demonstrates bony changes.
- Synovial fluid examination and synovial biopsy show inflammatory reactions.
- Slit-lamp examination of eye helps to diagnose irido-cyclitis.
- ECG and echocardiography may be done to detect cardiac involvement.
- Other causes of joint disease should be ruled out by specific diagnostic tests, e.g. LE cells, bone marrow aspirations, etc.

Management

There is no specific management of this condition but supportive treatment is important aspect of management to reduce inflammation, relieve pain, prevent deformity of joints and ocular problems. The supportive management include:

- Rest during acute illness and comfortable position of affected part with assistance in self care.
- Relief of pain by NSAIDs (aspirin, ibuprofen, indo-methacin, etc.) along with H_2 receptor antagonist (cimetidine) and hot bath are important.
- Treatment of fever with tepid sponge and antipyretics.
- Physiotherapy and exercise (initially passive then active) to preserve joint mobility and to prevent contracture and deformity.
- Emotional support to reduce anxiety.
- Disease modifying antirheumatic drugs (DMARDs) like gold salts, d-penicillamine, hydroxychloroquine, may be administered when NSAIDs therapy is ineffective.
- Immunosuppressant cytotoxic drugs like methrotrexate (5 to 10 mg/m^2/week) orally can be given under medical supervision in NSAIDs and DMARDs failure cases.
- Other cytotoxic drugs such as cyclophosphamide, azathi-oprine, chlorambucil may be used for children with

severe debilitating disease and poor response to NSAIDs and DMARDs.

- Corticosteroid therapy is used as anti-inflammatory agents in life-threatening conditions with systemic and ocular manifestations.
- Gamma globuin therapy is useful in some children.
- Surgical management like synovectomy and joint replacement may be needed for extensive synovitis and destructive arthritis.
- Health teaching to the parents and the child is important for continuation of long-term treatment, promotion of self-care ability, growth and development monitoring, rehabilitation facilities and regular medical supervision.

Complications

Complications of JRA are mainly bony deformities including crippling and joint contracture, anemia, growth retardation, failure to thrive, short stature, problems of cervical spine (ankylosis, spondylitis) and problems of temporomandibular areas (microagnatha). Other complications include leg-length discrepancy, eye problems (like cataract, glaucoma, uveitis, blindness), cardiac problems and psychosocial problems.

Prognosis

Early detection and appropriate management of large majority of JRA cases have complete functional recovery with 75 percent complete remission.

Pyogenic (Septic) Arthritis

Pyogenic arthritis or acute bacterial inflammation of the joints usually occur in malnourished children or in association with acute infectious diseases such as septicemia, enteric fever, pneumonia or influenza. The common infecting organisms are *Staphylococcus aureus*, *Streptococcus*, *Pneumococcus*, *Gonococcus*, *Meningococcus*, *E. coli*, tubercle bacilli and *H. influenzae*. Infections usually occur by hematogenous route, but may spread from adjacent soft tissue inflammation. Commonly affected joints are hip, knee, elbow and shoulder, but any joints may be affected by the pyogenic arthritis.

Clinical Manifestations

Pyogenic arthritis is manifested as inflamed joint with severe pain, swelling, tenderness, warmth and marked restriction of movement of the limb, which is kept in flexed position. Usually, there is joint effusion which rapidly becomes purulent. The child looks very ill with fever, malaise and vomiting. As the disease progress, destruction of cartilage, septic necrosis of the heads of long bones and pathological dislocation may occur.

Diagnostic Evaluation

Diagnosis is confirmed by X-ray which shows reduction of joint space, destruction of cartilages, new bone formation and full bony ankylosis at later stage.

Aspiration of fluid from the infected joint and its culture helps to confirm the presence of pyogenic organism. It also helps to differentiate the condition from acute osteoarthritis, acute rheumatic fever and acute rheumatoid arthritis or tubeculous arthritis. History of illness and findings of physical examination also help in diagnostic evaluation.

Management

Management of pyogenic arthritis is performed with appropriate broad-spectrum antibiotics for 2 to 4 weeks parenterally. Other measures are joint aspiration or arthrotomy for drainage of affected joint and immobilization of the limb by POP cast or traction. Analgesics and other symptomatic treatment are provided. Supportive care is given including rest, support of the affected limb with comfortable position, nutritious diet, extra fluid intake, hygienic care, emotional support and necessary health teaching.

Prognosis

Early diagnosis and treatment lead to good prognosis. In neglected cases, sinus formation and pathological dislocation are common complications.

Handicapped Children and Child Welfare

25

- Handicapped Children
- Welfare of Children

HANDICAPPED CHILDREN

A handicapped condition makes the normal functions of the individual very difficult and leads to dependency. These conditions are increasing day by day due to changing lifestyle and complicated environment. It is a social problem. Numbers are increasing but estimation of exact numbers is difficult.

Handicapped child is one who deviates from normal health status either physically, mentally or socially and requires special care, treatment and education.

Concept of Disability

According to WHO, the sequence of events leading to disability and handicapped conditions are as follows:

Injury or Disease → Impairment → Disability → Handicap.

Impairment

It is defined as any loss or abnormality of psychological, physiological or anatomical structure or function, e.g. loss of vision, loss of hearing, etc. Primary impairment may lead to secondary impairment, e.g. defective hearing results in learning difficulties and poor school performance. Impairment can be temporary or permanent, progressive or regressive, visible or invisible and extrinsic or intrinsic. Impairment develops as consequence of disease or disorders, e.g. accidents leading to loss of lower limbs (amputation), is an impairment. Impairment leads to disability.

Disability

It develops as the consequence of impairment, e.g. loss of limbs result in inability to walk, i.e. an objectified event. Disability is the inability to carry out certain activities which are considered as normal for the age and sex. Disability has been defined as any restriction or lack of ability to perform an activity in the manner or within the range considered as normal for a human being.

Handicap

It develops as a consequence of the disability. It is a socialized event leading to disadvantages of individual's life and disturbances in the achievement of full potential. It results in social isolation.

Handicap is defined as a disadvantage for a given individual resulting from an impairment or a disability, that limits and prevents the fulfilment of a role which is normal for that individual, depending on age, sex, social and cultural factors.

Handicapped children refers to those with presence of an impairment or other circumstances, that are likely to interfere with normal growth and development or with the capacity to learn. Primary handicap condition leads to secondary handicap condition, e.g. blindness leads to economical handicapped situation, i.e. poverty. The child may have single or multiple handicap condition.

Classification

Handicapped children can be classified broadly into three groups:

Physically Handicapped Children

These groups include the children with blindness, deaf and dumb, congenital malformations like cleft lip, cleft palate, club foot, congenital heart disease, etc. Postpolio residual paralysis, leprosy, accidents, burns injury, etc. also lead to physical handicapped conditions. The most important causes of physical handicaps are birth defect, malnutrition, infections and accidents. These can be prevented by adequate support services.

Physically handicapped children can be grouped according to the affected part of the body. These include orthopedically handicapped, sensory handicapped, neurologically handicapped and handicapped due to chronic systemic diseases.

Orthopedically handicapped children are those having congenital bony defect (club foot), amputation due to accidental injury, bony defects following ricket, fracture, arthritis, leprosy, etc.

Sensory handicapped children present with following problems:
- *Visual problems:* Partial or complete blindness, refractory errors, etc.
- *Auditory problems:* Partial hearing loss, deaf and dumb.
- *Speech problems:* Stammering, dysphonia.

Neurologically handicapped children include cerebral palsy, mental retardation, convulsive disorders, hydrocephalus, spina bifida, postmeningitic, or postencephalitic sequelae, postpolio-residual paralysis, degenerative diseases of CNS, learning disabilities, etc.

Handicapped condition due to chronic systemic disease, e.g. heart disease, bronchial asthma, diabetes mellitus, muscular dystropy, etc.

Multiple physically handicapped children having combination of orthopedically, sensory and neurological handicaps.

Mentally Handicapped Children

The term 'mental handicap' is now used for the condition 'mental retardation'. At least 2 to 3 percent of Indian population are mentally handicap in any one form.

Mental retardation is the significantly subaverage general intellectual functioning existing concurrently with deficits in adaptive behavior manifested during the developmental period. It includes low learning abilities, poor maturation and social maladjustment in combination.

The malfunctioning of the brain is poorly understood in most cases, but the physiological alteration may be identified in some children. The cognitive and functional ability are affected with limitation in adaptive ability and communication. Self care, home-living, social interaction skill, community relationship, self directions, health behavior, safety measure, academic achievement, leisure time utilization and working capacity are altered in mentally handicapped children.

Mental handicaps are caused by multiple factors. In majority of the cases (75%) causes are not precisely understood. The causative factors can be genetic, social and physiological.

(Details of mental retardation are described in Chapter 21).

Socially Handicapped Children

Socially handicapped children are those having disturbed opportunities for healthy personality development due to social factors leading to nonachievement of full potentialities. Social disturbances are found in the form of broken family, parental inadequacy, loss of parents, poverty, lack of educational opportunities, environmental deprivation and emotional disturbances as lack of tender loving care.

These children include orphan child, abused child, addicted child, street children, child labor, maternal deprivation, emotional deprivation, neglected or destitute child, exploited or victimized and delinquent child. They are unable to adjust with their living environment.

Causes

Major causes of handicapped conditions in children are congenital anomalies, genetic disorders, poliomyelitis and other communicable diseases, perinatal conditions, malnutrition, accidental injury and sociocultural factors.

Prevention of Handicapped Conditions in Children

Handicapped conditions of children can be prevented by improvement of maternal health and adequate care during periconceptional, prenatal and intranatal period alongwith preventive measures during infancy, childhood and adolescents.

The *primary prevention* can be achieved by the following measures:

- *Genetic counseling:* Optimum maternal age for producing normal babies is between 20 to 30 years, this information should be explained to the couples along with prevention and different aspects of genetic and chromosomal problems.
- *Genetic screening* of 'at-risk' people to prevent inherited diseases like chromosomal or sex linked congenital anomalies (e.g. Down's syndrome, hemophilia, etc.)
- Reduction of consanguineous marriages by creating health awareness.
- Universal immunization coverage especially for poliomyelitis and MMR (mumps, measles, rubella).
- Improvement of nutritional status of mother and children especially for girl child, the future mother.
- Prevention of iodine deficiency and folic-acid deficiency conditions in periconceptional period.
- Essential care in antenatal, intranatal and neonatal periods. Prevention of maternal and neonatal infections, birth injuries, asphyxia, hyperbilirubinemia, etc.
- Avoidance of teratogenic agents in antenatal periods and special care of high-risk mothers and children.
- Medical termination of pregnancy of malformed fetus
- Improvement of health awareness about the preventive measures of handicapped conditions in children by elimination of causes like malnutrition, accidental injuries, etc.

Management of Handicapped Children

Management of handicapped children requires multidisciplinary approach. Early diagnosis and treatment of the particular cause of handicapping condition alongwith disability limitation and rehabilitation should be promoted. The aim of management is to safeguard against or halt the progression of the disease process from impairment to disability and handicap. The approaches of management should include the following aspects:

- Careful history, thorough physical examination and necessary investigations for early detection of handicapped conditions are important.
- Regular medical supervision and developmental assessment help to identify the abnormal condition early in initial stage by MCH or school health services.
- Treatment of particular handicapped condition by medical or surgical management, e.g. cataract, otitis media, leprosy, accidental injury, rickets, congenital anomalies, etc.
- Correction of deformity, e.g. visual or hearing problems by spectacles or hearing aids.
- Physiotherapy and exercise to improve physical conditions.
- Occupational therapy according to the child's ability and that should be provided with music, painting, weaving, wood-work, pottery, etc.

- Speech therapy to improve communication ability.
- Prosthetics, e.g. provision of artificial limb in a child with amputed leg.
- Special care for mentally handicapped children with love, warmth, patience, tolerance, discipline and avoidance of criticism.
- Counseling and guidance to the parents and family members for continuation of care of the children with emotional, educational and social support.
- Referral for welfare services (Govt., NGOs) for assistance of aids and appliances, for special training and education, rehabilitation and support services like pension, scholarship, special allowances, etc.

Rehabilitation of Handicapped Children

Rehabilitation of handicapped children should be approached by combined and coordinated use of medical, social, educational, psychological and vocational measures for training and retraining the children to the highest possible level of functional ability. It includes all measures to reduce the impact of disabled and handicapped conditions and to achieve social integration by active participation of the individual in the community.

The *process of rehabilitation* should involve the following aspects:

- Medical rehabilitation includes restoration of functions by prosthesis, artificial limbs, etc.
- Social rehabilitation includes restoration of family and social relationship by replacement in the family.
- Educational rehabilitation includes specialized training and educational facilities, e.g. braille for blind, sign language for deaf and dumb.
- Psychological rehabilitation includes restoration of personal dignity and confidence during the period of growth and development and in adult life.
- Vocational rehabilitation includes restoration of the capacity to earn a livelihood. This can be achieved by community participation and social legislation for the handicapped individual. The community needs to offer employment opportunities in shops, factories and other business establishment to the handicaps.

The handicapped child needs to be trained for an independent living with special training and education. In India, there are more than 150 schools and institution for the handicapped. These include day care centers, special school, (for blind, deaf and dumb) vocational training centers, special hospitals for crippled children, etc. These available welfare services of Government of India provide support services to the handicapped individuals and enabling the families to assume a large share of rehabilitation within the family cycle. Nongovernment organizations are also working along with government institutions for training, vocational guidance, counseling, manpower development, research, assistance for supply of aids and appliances to the handicapped and dissemination of informations.

The Ministry of Welfare, Government of India has introduced a comprehensive bill in the parliament known as "Persons with disabilities" (equal opportunities, protection of right and full participation) Bill, 1995. It deals with preventive and promotional aspects of rehabilitation.

The Children Act, 1960, provides for the care, protection, maintenance, welfare, education and rehabilitation of socially handicapped children.

The following National Institutes are working for the specific disabilities to provide care and welfare services in various aspects of the handicapped:

- National Institute for Orthopedically Handicapped, Bonhooghly, Kolkata.
- National Institute for Mentally Handicapped, Secunderabad.
- National Institute for the visually Handicapped, New Delhi and Dehradun.
- Ali Yavar Jung National Institute for the Hearing Handicapped, Mumbai.
- National Institute for Rehabilitation, Training and Research, Cuttack.

Nursing Management of Handicapped Children

Nursing personnel play a vital role to assist the family members to cope with the crisis situation for the handicapped condition. Planning and providing care to the handicapped children (especially physically and mentally handicapped) in health care institutions and community are important nursing responsibilities including parental involvement and community participation. Assisting the family to strengthen effective relationship and bondage to prevent children from becoming socially handicapped. Nurses are responsible for creation of awareness in the society about the prevention of handicaps, the abilities of the child with a handicap condition and the potentialities present in him/her. Nursing management should emphasize on three levels of prevention of handicapped individual.

Nursing care for the physically and mentally handicapped children in hospital and home should emphasize on the following aspects other than the specific problems present in them.

Nursing Assessment

Complete assessment of a handicapped child include detailed history of the condition, thorough physical and neurological examination, specific investigations, review of developmental screening, assessment of parent-child interaction and family coping, socioeconomic status, available support facilities, etc.

Nursing Diagnoses

The important nursing diagnosis related to handicapped conditions may include the following:

- Ineffective family coping and altered parenting related to handicapped condition.
- Anxiety of the parents and family members.
- Altered nutrition, less than body requirements.
- Potential for infection.
- Injury, risk for self-care deficit, bathing, feeding, dressing, toileting, hygienic care, etc.
- Communication impaired
- Physical mobility impaired.
- Elimination pattern
- Altered activity intolerance
- Altered sleep pattern
- Sensory alteration, visual/auditory
- Growth and development
- Altered diversional activity deficit
- Knowledge deficit related to continued care of handicapped children.

Nursing diagnosis should be made based on subjective data and objective data.

Nursing interventions should be planned on the basis of priority problems according to short-term and long-term goal. Handicapped children can be cared in the general hospitals, special health care setting, community health care centers in primary level and at home. Day-care centers, special schools, rehabilitation centers, occupational therapy and vocational training centers also can provide various services to these children. Nurses are key person for home based or hospital based care to guide and assist the parents and family members to promote optimum health of the handicapped children. Nurses are also contributing in the special care settings for the handicapped children to bring them as close to normality as possible, physically, mentally and socially.

WELFARE OF CHILDREN

Child welfare encompasses caring and attending to the entire spectrum of needs, i.e. physical, emotional, social and economical needs of the children through comprehensive child welfare services. Child welfare programs seek to provide supportive services to the families of the children, because one of the important responsibility of the society and state is to assist the family in its natural obligations for the welfare of the children. Welfare of the underprivileged children like street children, orphans, handicaps, etc. also needs special attention.

Child Welfare Services

Child welfare services involve preventive, promotive, curative, developmental, palliative and rehabilitative aspects of child care. The child health problems are gigantic and the available resources are only supplementary in nature and are designed to meet certain needs of the most deprived and vulnerable children. Attention is generally focused on three categories of children in the poor socioeconomic groups, i.e. children of working mothers, destitute children and handicapped children.

Comprehensive child welfare services are provided broadly of two types:
a. Services for the basic needs of normal children where the family and the community participate.
b. Services for the needs of physically, mentally or socially handicapped children.

Government of India adopted National Policy for Children in August 1974, keeping in view the constitutional provisions and United Nations Declaration of the Rights of the Child. Following the enunciation of National policy for Children, a number of programs were introduced by the Government of India viz ICDS scheme, programs for supplementary feeding, nutrition education, production of nutritious food, constitution of the National Children Fund' under the Charitable Endowments Acts, 1980, Institution of National Awards for child welfare, welfare of the Handicapped children, CSSM/RCH program, etc.

Details of National policy for Children, United Nation's Declaration of the Rights of the child and the Children Act are discussed in Chapter 1. Health programs for children, and child health services are described is Chapter 3. National Programs on Nutrition and Nutritional Policy are discussed in Chapter 5.

Child Welfare Agencies

The important child welfare agencies in India are:
1. Indian Council for Child Welfare (ICCW)
2. Central Social Welfare Board
3. Kasturba Gandhi Memorial Trust
4. The Indian Red Cross Society.

These voluntary health agencies get financial aid from the government to organize child welfare services in the country. The important activities of these agencies include the followings:
i. Day care services for children of working mothers through nursery schools, Balwadis, creches and day-care centers for infants and toddlers.
ii. Holding homes for children in the age group 12 to 16 years at hill stations and sea-side resorts.
iii. Recreation facilities by organization of play centers, public parks, children's libraries, Bal bhavans, children's films, national museums, hobby classes, etc.

Besides these national agencies, there are numerous other nongovernment organizations working for the child welfare in the country like Save-the-Children Fund, Child-In-Need-Institute (CINI), SOS village, etc.

International agencies are also interested and contributing in child welfare services in our country. Some of those are UNICEF, WHO, International Union for Child Welfare, CARE, FAO of the United Nations, USAID, International Red Cross, UNESCO and so on.

Welfare of Delinquent Children

The Children Act, 1960, in India defines delinquent as 'a child who has committed an offence'. Juvenile means a boy who has not attained the age of 16 years and a girls who has not attained the age of 18 years.

Delinquency is not merely "juvenile crime". It embraces all deviations from normal youthful behavior and includes the incorrigible, ungovernable, habitually disobedient and those who desert their homes and mix with immoral people, those with behavioral problems and indulge in antisocial practices.

Juvenile delinquency is increasing in India due to change in the cultural pattern of the people, urbanization and industrialization. The highest incidence is found in children aged 15 and above. The incidence among boys is 4 to 5 times more than the girls.

Causes

Biological causes: Biological factors like hereditary defects, feeble mindedness, physical defects, glandular disturbances and chromosomal anomaly may contribute for the delinquent behavior.

Social causes: Broken homes due to death of parents, separation of parents, step-mothers, disturbed home conditions, e.g. poverty, alcoholism, parental neglect, child abuse, battered baby, ignorance about child care, too many children, etc. may be responsible for delinquency.

Miscellaneous: Absence of recreation facilities, cheap recreations, sex-thrillers, violence in cinemas and television, slum dwelling, urbanization, industrialization, social disintegration, change in moral standards and value system, etc. also may cause delinquency.

Preventive Measures

• Improvement of family life and tender loving care of children.
• Appropriate schooling and healthy teacher taught relationship.
• Social welfare services by recreation facilities, parent counseling, child guidance, educational facilities, etc.

- Adequate general health services for early detection and management. [Details of juvenile delinquency is discussed in Chapter 10].

Child Guidance Clinic

Child guidance clinic (CGC) was started in 1909 in Chicago to deal with problems of juvenile delinquency. At present, it deals with all children or adolescents who for one reason or other are not fully adjusted to their environment. The objective of CGC is to prevent children from the possibility of becoming neurotics and psychotics in later life.

The most important aspects of child guidance is psychotherapy to restore positive feelings of security in the child. Physical health also need to be cared and maintained. Mental health improvement is done through play therapy, counseling and guidance, suggestions, change in the physical environment, easing of parental tensions, modification of parental attitude, etc.

Child guidance needs a team approach for correct diagnosis and management. The psychiatrist is the central figure and helped by clinical psychologist, educational psychologist, psychiatric social workers, community health nurses, speech therapist, occupational therapist, neurologist and pediatrician.

Juvenile Justice Act, 1986

With the implementation of the Juvenile Justice Act, 1986, all Children's Acts applicable in different parts of India have been canceled. The new act, provides a comprehensive scheme for care, protection, treatment, development and rehabilitation of delinquent juveniles. The new act has come into force from 2nd October, 1987.

Some of the special features of the Juvenile Justice Act are the followings:
- It provides a uniform legal framework for juvenile justice in the country, so as to ensure that no child under any circumstances is put in jail or police lock-up.
- It envisages specialized approach towards prevention and treatment of juvenile delinquency in keeping with the developmental needs of children.
- It establishes norms and standards for administration of juvenile justice in terms of investigation, care, treatment and rehabilitation.
- It lays down appropriate linkage and coordination between the formal system of juvenile justice and voluntary organizations. It specifically defines the roles and responsibilities of both.

By the year 1992, there were 609 institutions under Juvenile Justice Act, out of these 269 were observation homes, 249 juvenile homes, 40 special homes and 51 after care institutions.

This act was amended in the year 2000 and is applicable for those children who have not attained the age of 18 years.

Welfare of Destitute Children

Destitute children are in great need, especially of food and shelter. They may be deprived of parents. The children who have no home or who for some reason could not be cared for by their parents are placed in orphanage, an institution for orphans.

Psychosocially handicapped children who are orphans or delinquents or pavement dwellers or sufferer of parental/maternal deprivation, need for placement in special setting for rearing or bringing up and to promote growth and development.

Child Placement

Orphanages: A house of orphans. It may be government organization or voluntary organization. Small institutions are preferred to provide opportunity for the child to experience the warmth and intimacy of family life, to develop emotional security and to participate in activities that would help him or her to become an adequate citizen.

Foster Homes: It is concerned with the care of the orphans or destitute children. This is an institution where many facilities are available for rearing children other than their natural families. Foster care is given by the persons not related by blood. A good foster home can provide necessary love affection and security to meet the needs of the child.

Borstal Homes: It is an institution to which young offenders may be sent for reformative training. Boys over 16 years of age and who are too difficult to handle in a certified school or have misbehaved there, are sent to a borstal homes. This institution falls in a category between certified school and an adult prison. Boys are placed in borstal sentence usually for three years for training and reformation. There are about six borstal homes for boys in India, but none for girls. Borstals are not governed by the Children Act, but by the State Inspector General of Prisons.

Remand Homes: It is a place of detention for juvenile offenders. The child is placed under the care of physician, psychiatrist, and other trained personnel to improve the mental and physical well-being. Elementary schooling, various arts and crafts, games and other recreational activities are arranged for healthy development of the child.

Adoption: It is the assumption of the responsibility of caring for a child by a person (or persons) who is not the natural parents. This requires a legal procedure. The laws of adoption vary from country to country. The relevant law in India is the Hindu Adoptions and Maintenance Act, 1956." Legal adoptions confers upon the child and adoptive parents, rights and responsibilities similar to that of natural parents. Non-Hindus can only be appointed as legal guardians of the child. A child below 15 years of age can be adopted through the legal process.

Legal guidance should be provided to the person (persons) who wishes to adopt a child. They should be prepared for parenthood and child-care with adequate information and support. In agency adoption, the natural parents and adoptive parents are unknown to each other. The process of legal adoption depends on the policy of the agency.

Child Adoption

The Juvenile Justice (Care and Protection of Children) Act 2000 enables citizen of all religions, the freedom to adopt a minor child, irrespective whether he/she is a single parent and/or such adoptive parent/parents adopt a child of the same sex, irrespective of the number of living biological sons or daughters. Prior to 2000, adoption was allowed to Hindus only. Other religious groups were governed by Guardianship and Wards Act.

In India, only government recognized agencies can deal with adoption placement. Direct adoption placement by hospitals, maternity homes and nursing homes are not permitted. Private adoption is illegal and should be discouraged.

Adoption is an important alternative for the rehabilitation of children who are destitute and abandoned or for any social reasons cannot be brought up by their parents.

Procedures

Abandoned or destitute child must be first presented to the Child Welfare Committee, who will declare the child free for adoption. In case the biological parents want to give up a child, they have to execute a document in favor of adoption agency, duly witnessed by any authority of the hospital and a relative. A waiting period of two months is allowed to the biological parents to reconsider the decision, following which the child is free for adoption.

Registered agency which is licensed to process adoption by both State Government and the Central Adoption Resource Authority (an autonomous body under the Ministry of Women and Child Development, Government of India) can process the application for In-country and Inter-country adoptions of Indian children.

A social worker from the adoption agency provides guidelines and support to parents and help them to make informed decisions by preadoption counseling. Professional social worker conducted home visit to study the family before adoption is permitted. Parents are asked to submit documents regarding their health, financial status, social status, etc. All essential diagnostic tests (HIV, hepatitis-B, blood disorders, etc.) and screening for congenital anomalies of the child should be done prior to adoption.

A suitable child is shown to the parents, when everything is appropriate and the application is approved. After the acceptance of the child by the adoptive parents, the placement is legalized. The placement in the family is followed up for three years until the legal adoption is complete. Confidentiality is maintained for the total procedure. Necessary support is provided to the adoptive parents whenever needed.

Doctors and nursing personnel can help the family members during adoption process by counseling and providing necessary information regarding health status and home care of the child. They can help to increase public awareness about the process of adoption and its legal aspect.

Welfare of Working Children

In 1973, the International Labor Organization (ILO) passed a convention establishing 15 years as the minimum work age for the most sectors, while permitting light work from age of 13 years, provided that such work was unlikely to harm child's health, morals and safety or prejudice his/her school attendance.

Child labor is rooted in poverty, unemployment and lack of education. Labor at very young ages can have serious consequences on the child's development, both physical and mental. Working children always had lower growth and health status compared to their nonworking counter parts. (Details of child labor is described in Chapter 3).

The Declaration of the Rights of the Child and Indian Constitution has laid down that childhood and youth should be protected against exploitation. In our country various health and social legislation have been enacted to protect the health, safety and welfare of working children below the age of 15 years. The Child Labor (Protection and Regulation) Act, 1986 is the most important one. The Factories Act, 1948, (Amendment in 1987) also described about the employment of young persons.

The Factories Act prohibits employment of children below the age of 14 years and declares persons between the age 15 and 18 years to be adolescents. Adolescents should be duly certified by the certifying doctors regarding their fitness for work. Adolescent employee is allowed to work only between 6 am to 7 pm in the factories.

The Child Labor (Prohibition and Regulation Act, 1986)

Main features of the act are as follows:
1. No child who has completed his 12th year and no adolescent shall be required or allowed to work in any plantation unless (a) a certificate of fitness granted with

reference to him under section 27 is in the custody of the employer and (b) such child or adolescent carries with him, while he is at work, a token giving a reference to such certificate.

2. No child shall be required or permitted to work in any establishment in excess of such numbers of hours as may be prescribed for establishment.

3. The period of work on each day shall be fixed in a way that no period shall exceed three hours before he has had an interval of rest for at least one hour.

4. No child shall be required or permitted to work overtime.

5. Children are not permitted to work in occupations concerned with passenger and goods mail transport by railway, carpet weaving, cement manufacturing, cleaning ash pits, building construction operation, cloth printing, dyeing, manufacturing of matches, explosives and fireworks, beedi making, wool cleaning, etc.

Inspite of various health and social legislation, the numbers of child labor is increasing. It is felt that in the present context, it is not feasible to abolish child labor, but importance should be given on elimination of child labor from exploitative and hazardous works and to bring health services where they work through a strategy involving parents, employers, community, NGOs, voluntary agencies and government agencies.

The Supreme Court of India on 8th December, 1996 has directed all State Governments and Union Territories to take concrete steps to abolish child labor. It identified nine industries for priority action and directed setting up of Child Labor Rehabilitation Welfare Fund. The offending employers are supposed to pay for each child a compensation of ₹20,000 to be deposited in the fund.

A great deal of effort is needed to eliminate this evil and to protect such children against abuse, exploitation and health hazards, thus to regulate the conditions of work in occupations where child labor is permitted.

Prohibition of Child Marriage

The child marriage was forbidden by the Sarda Act, in British India in 1929. Inspite of spread of literacy and legislations prohibiting early marriages, child marriages are still in practice in many states of India (Rajasthan, MP, UP) and in rural populations.

The Child Marriage Restraint Act (Amendment), 1978 fixed the legal minimum age of marriage 21 years for boys and 18 years for girls. Improvement of public awareness about the age of marriage is very important.

Early marriage has a great impact on the various aspect of child health and regulation of fertility. Females who marry before the age of 18 years, give birth to a large number of children than those who married later. The offsprings of adolescents may have various health hazards. Teenage mother can be considered as child mother having a child to look after and cared. Early marriage results in school drop out, sexual hazards, obstetrical problems, poor physical and mental health, marital disharmony, inadequate parenting, etc.

Early marriage is a long standing custom in India. However, there is a gradual rise in the age at marriage in our country towards the positive approach for welfare of the children and their fullest growth and development. Nurses are responsible to inform and educate the people about the ill effects of child marriage and to motivate them to eliminate this problem from our country.

Children in Difficult Circumstances

As per the report of Ministry of Women and Child Development Government of India, by the working group on development of children for 11th Five-year Plan (2007–2012), the following children are sufferers and victims of difficult circumstances in our society. These children need support and welfare services.

Over the years some children have been struggling for survival and categorized as children in difficult circumstances. They include:

- Homeless children-pavement dwellers, displaced children, etc.
- Orphaned or abandoned children.
- Children whose parents cannot or not able to take care of them.
- Children separated from parents.
- Migrant and refugee children.
- Street children.
- Working children.
- Children in bondage.
- Children in prostitution.
- Children of sex worker/prostitutes/sexual minorities.
- Children of prisoners.
- Children affected by conflict.
- Children affected by natural disasters.
- Children affected by HIV/AIDS.
- Children suffering from terminal diseases.
- The girl child.
- Children with disabilities and related special needs.
- Children belonging to the ethnic and religious minorities and other minority communities and those belonging to scheduled castes and scheduled tribes.
- Children in institutional care-in state-run institutions or religious and other charitable institutions.
- Children in conflict with law (who commit crimes).
- Children who are victims of crimes.

These children are victims of their socioeconomic and geopolitical circumstances and demand for more focused attention.

National Plan of Action for Children 2005, mandate that state must take responsibilities for children both before and after birth and the child's interest are to receive paramount attention. This national plan sets the frame for future planning and interventions to secure the well-being of all children of the country and provide them a caring and protective environment.

There are various social welfare programs for women and children in India, which can be broadly, categorized under six heads.

1. Programs for welfare of women.
2. Programs for welfare of children.
3. Composite programs for both women and children.
4. Schemes for maladjusted groups.
5. Schemes for physically handicapped persons.
6. Programs for welfare of backward classes.

The children are the future citizen of the nation. So the child health problems need to be managed and prevented carefully with prime importance. Thus, child welfare should be the vital responsibility of the country in all levels to have healthy children and healthy nation.

Appendices

Appendix I

Basic Care of the Baby at Birth
Plea of a Baby at Birth

- I have come from an extremely warm, clean, quiet and comfortable abode.
- Protect me at birth from microbes and cold.
- I am wet and naked, dry me, cover me and place me under a heater.
- I do not know how to smile, let me announce my arrival by a cry.
- Do not hurt me but gently clean my windpipe to let me cry.
- Do not give me injections but give me a breath to save my life.
- I have been swimming all through in the womb, do not be in a hurry to bathe me in the labor room.

Meharban Singh

Appendix II

Children Learn what they Live

If a child lives with criticism,
  he learns to condemn.
If a child lives with hostility,
  he learns to fight.
If a child lives with ridicule,
  he learns to be shy.
If a child lives with shame,
  he learns to feel guilty.
If a child lives with tolerance,
  he learns to be patient.
If a child lives with encouragement,
  he learns confidence.
If a child lives with praise,
  he learns to appreciate.
If a child lives with fairness,
  he learns justice.
If a child lives with security,
  he learns to have faith.
If a child lives with approval,
  he learns to like himself.
If a child lives with acceptance and friendship,
  he learns to find love in the world.

Source Unknown

Appendix III

Prelude

Your children are not your children
They are the sons and daughters of life's longing for itself.

They come through you but not from you.
And though they are with you yet they belong not to you.

You may give them your love but not your thoughts.
For they have their own thoughts.

You may house their bodies but not their souls.
For their souls dwell in the house of tomorrow,
which you cannot visit,
not even in your dreams.

You may strive to be like them, but seek not to make them like you.
For life goes not backward nor tarries with yesterday.

You are the bows from which your children as living arrows are sent forth.

Kahlil Gibran from "The Prophet"

His Name is 'Today'

We are guilty of many errors
     and many faults,
But our worst crime is abandoning
     the children,
Neglecting the fountain of life.
Many of the things we need can wait,
     The child cannot.
Right now is the time his bones are
     being formed,
His blood is being made,
And his senses are being developed.
To him we cannot answer
     'Tomorrow'
His name is 'Today'

Gabriela Mistral
Nobel Prize Owner Chilean Poet

Appendix IV

Height and Weight of Indian Boys and Girls from 1 to 18 Years

Age in years	Height in centimeters		Weight in Kilograms	
	Boys	Girls	Boys	Girls
1	72.5	72.5	8.5	7.5
2	87.5	86.6	12.6	12.3
3	96.2	95.7	14.6	14.4
4	103.4	103.2	16.5	16.4
5	108.7	108.1	18.5	18.4
6	118.9	117.3	22.1	21.4
7	123.9	122.7	24.5	24.8
8	127.9	126.8	26.4	26.1
9	133.6	132.3	30.0	29.7
10	138.5	138.5	32.4	33.5
11	143.4	144.1	35.3	36.5
12	148.9	150.3	38.8	42.6
13	154.9	153.0	42.9	44.4
14	161.7	155.1	48.3	46.7
15	165.3	155.3	52.2	47.2
16	168.4	155.4	55.5	49.8
17	169.9	156.4	59.0	49.9
18	169.9	156.8	61.1	50.1

Source: ICMR—Growth and development of Indian infants and children

Appendix V

Normal Blood Pressure Values at Various Ages

Age	Mean systolic ± 2SD (mm Hg)	Mean diastolic ± 2SD (mm Hg)
Newborn	80 ± 16	46 ± 16
6–12 months	89 ± 29	60 ± 16
1 Year	96 ± 30	66 ± 25
2 Years	99 ± 25	64 ± 25
3 Years	100 ± 25	67 ± 23
4 Years	99 ± 20	65 ± 20
5–6 Years	94 ± 14	55 ± 9
6–7 Years	100 ± 15	56 ± 9
7–8 Years	102 ± 15	56 ± 8
8–9 Years	105 ± 16	57 ± 9
9–10 Years	107 ± 16	57 ± 9
10–11 Years	111 ± 17	58 ± 10
11–12 Years	113 ± 18	59 ± 10
12–13 Years	115 ± 19	59 ± 10
13–14 Years	118 ± 19	60 ± 10

Note: Blood pressure measurement should be done using an appropriate cuff covering two-thirds of the upper arm

Appendix VI

Calculation of Approximate Surface Area from Weight in Children with Normal Physique

Weight range (kg)	Approximate surface area (m²)
1–5	(0.05 × weight) + 0.05
6–10	(0.04 × weight) + 0.10
11–20	(0.03 × weight) + 0.20
21–40	(0.02 × weight) + 0.40

1. Lowe's formula: Surface area (m²) = $\sqrt[3]{\text{weight}^2(\text{kg}) \times 0.1}$

2. Costeff's formula: Surface area (m²) = $\dfrac{4W+7}{W+90}$

   Where 'W' is weight in Kg.

Appendix VII

Mean Urine Output at Different Ages

Age	Normal urine output		Oliguria (mL/Kg/hr)
	(mL/ 24 hr)	mL/Kg/hr	
Newborn	250	2.5	< 1.0
2 months	450	3.5	< 1.25
1 year	500	2.0	< 0.60
2 years	550	1.7	< 0.50
4 years	650	1.7	< 0.50
7 years	750	1.7	< 0.45
11 years	1100	1.4	< 0.40
14 years	1200	1.4	< 0.40
Adult	1500	0.8	< 0.30

Appendix VIII

Normal Biochemical Values

Determination	Specimen	Age/Sex	Normal value

• Alanine aminotransferase (SGPT) (U/L)	• Serum	• Infant
		• Thereafter
		  – Male
		  – Female
			• 5–28
			
			• 6–12
			• 4–17

• Albumin (g/L)	• Serum	• Newborn	• 25–35
		• Child	• 40–50
• ASLO (Antistreptolysin-O) titer or ASO	• Serum	• Child	• 170–330 Todd units

• Asparate aminotransferase (SGOT) (U/L)	• Serum	• Infant
		• Thereafter
		  – Male
		  – Female
			• 5–40
			
			• 7–21
			• 6–18

• Bilirubin (mg/dL) – Total – Direct (conjugated)	• Serum	• Cord • 0–2 weeks • Infant and child	• < 3 • < 15 • < 2 • < 0.2
• Cholesterol (mg/dL)	• Serum	• Children	• 119–263
• Glucose (fasting) mg/dL	• Serum	• Neonate • Premature • Child • Thereafter	• 30–60 • 20–60 • 60–100 • 70–105
• Lactate dehydrogenase (LDH–U/L)	• Serum	• Newborn • Neonate • Infant • Child • Thereafter	• 290–500 • 300–1500 • 100–250 • 60–170 • 40–90
• Phosphatase, alkaline	• Serum	• Newborn • Child • Thereafter	• 50–165 • 20–150 • 20–70
• Potassium (mEq/L)	• Serum	• Newborn • Infant • Child • Thereafter	• 3.7–5 • 4.1–5.3 • 3.4–4.7 • 3.5–5.3
• Protein, total (gm/dL)	• Serum	• Premature • Newborn • Child • Thereafter	• 4.3–7.6 • 4.6–7.6 • 6.2–8.0 • 6.0–8.0
• Sodium (mEq/L)	• Serum	• Newborn • Infant • Child • Thereafter	• 134–144 • 139–146 • 138–145 • 135–148

Contd...

Contd...

Determination	Specimen	Age/Sex	Normal value
• Thyroxin (T4) (mcg/dL)	• Serum	• Child	• 5.4–14.8
• Triiodothyronine (T3) (ng/dL)	• Serum	• Newborn • Thereafter	• 50–400 • 100–250
• TSH (mU/L)	• Serum	• Child	• 2–10

• Triglycerides (mg/dL)	• Serum	• Infant
		• Adolescent
		• Thereafter
		  – Male
		  – Female
			• 5–40
			• 30–150
			
			• 40–160
			• 35–135

• Uric acid (mg/dL)	• Serum	• Child
		• Thereafter
		  – Male
		  – Female
			• 2–5.5
			
			• 3.5–7.2
			• 2.6–6.0

• Urea nitrogen (mg/dL)	• Serum	• Newborn • Infant/child • Thereafter	• 4–18 • 5–18 • 7–8

Appendix IX

Acid-base Status (Arterial)

	Newborn	Infant	Child	Adult
• pH	7.26–7.49	7.30–7.46	7.35–7.45	7.35–7.45
• pCO_2 (torr)	30–40	27–40	30–45	32–48
• HCO_3 (mEq/L)	17.2–23.6	19.0–23.9	16.3–23.9	18–23
• pO_2 (torr)	55–95	85–110	85–110	85–110
• O_2 saturation	40–90	95–98	95–98	95–98
• Base excess	(–10)– (–2)	(–7)– (–1)	(–4)–(+2)	(–2)–(+3)

Appendix X

Normal Hematological Values

Determination	Reference range
• Bleeding time	• 1–9 min
• Clotting time	• 1.50–2.30 min
• Factor VIII assay (Antihemophilic factor)	• 50–200%
• Fibrinogen	• 200–400 mg/dL
• Partial thromboplastin time (PTT) (activated)	• 20–45 sec
• Prothrombin time	• 9.5–12 sec
• Platelets (per cu mm)	• Neonate — 1,00,000–3,00,000 • Thereafter — 1,50,000–4,50,000
• Erythrocyte count (per cu mm)	• Newborn — 5–6×10^6 • 3 months to 6 years — 3.5–5.6×10^6 • Adult female — 3.9–5.6×10^6 Male — 4.5–6.5×10^6
• Erythrocyte sedimentation Rate (ESR)—(Westergren method)	• Male — less than 15–20 mm/h • Female — less than 20–30 mm/h
• Reticulocytes (%)	• Newborn — 3–7 • 3 months to 6 years — 0–2 • Adult — 0.2
• Hemoglobin (gm%)	• Newborn — 14–20 (17) • 3 months to 6 years — 10.5–14 (12) • Adult female —12–16 (14) Male —14–18 (16)
• Hematocrit (%)	• Newborn — 45–65 (55) • 3 months to 6 years — 33–42 (38) • Adult female — 37–47 (42) Male — 42–52 (46)
• WBC (per cu mm)	• Newborn — 9,000–30,000 (18,000) • 3 months to 6 years — 6,000–15,000 (10,000) • Adult — 5,000–10,000 (7500)
• Neutrophils (%)	• Newborn — 40–80 (60) • 3 months to 6 years — 32–52 (42) • Adult — 40–75 (60)
• Eosinophils (%)	• Newborn — 2 • Up to 6 years — 2–3 • Adult —1–6
• Basophils (%)	• 0–0.5
• Lymphocytes (%)	• Newborn — 32 • 3 months to 6 years — 51 • Adult — 20–45 (30)
• Monocytes (%)	• Newborn — 7–14 • 3 months to 6 years — 4–8 • Adult — 2–10

Appendix XI

Cerebrospinal Fluid Constituents

Determination	Reference range
• Albumin	• 15–30 mg/dL
• Protein (Lumbar) (mg/dL)	• Premature — 32–240 (63)
	• Term newborn — 40–148 (73)
	• Infant and child — 15–40
• Sugar (mg/dL)	• Premature — 32–78 (51)
	• Term newborn — 35–64 (48)
	• Infant — 60–80
	• Child — 40–70
• Chloride (mEq/L)	• Term newborn — 109–123
	• Infant — 111–130
	• Child — 118–132
• Polymorphs (Per cu mm)	• Premature — 0–70 (3)
	• Term newborn — 0–26 (23)
	• Infant/child — 0
• Lymphocytes	• Premature — 0–20 (2)
	• Term newborn — 0–16 (5)
	• Infant/Child — 0–5
• Pressure (mm CSF)	• Term newborn — 50–80
	• Infant — 40–50
	• Child — 70–200
• Volume	• Child — 60–100 mL
	• Adult — 100–160 mL

Appendix XII

Modified Glasgow Coma Scoring System

Eye opening		
Score	Over 1 year	Under 1 year
4	• Spontaneous	• Spontaneous
3	• To verbal command	• To shout
2	• To pain	• To pain
1	• No response	• No response
Best motor response		
Score	Over 1 year	Under 1 year
6	• Obeys	• Spontaneous
5	• Localizes pain	• Localizes pain
4	• Flexion withdrawal	• Flexion withdrawal
3	• Flexion abnormal (Decorticate rigidity)	• Flexion abnormal (Decerebrate rigidity)
2	• Extension	• Extension
1	• No response	• No response

Best verbal response			
Score	Over 5 years	2 to 5 years	0 to 23 months
5	• Oriented and converses	• Appropriate words and phrases	• Smiles, coos, appropriately
4	• Disoriented and converses	• Inappropriate words	• Cries, consolable
3	• Inappropriate words	• Persistent cries or screams	• Persistent inappropriate crying or screaming
2	• Incomprehensible sounds	• Grunts	• Grunts, agitated or restless
1	• No response	• No response	• No response

Note: A score of 9 or more rules out coma, whereas a score of less than 7 confirms coma. Most subjects scoring 8 are too having coma.

Appendix XIII

Oxygen Therapy and Delivery Devices

Device	Flow rate	Oxygen%
A. Low flow systems		
• Nasal cannula*	• 1–6 L/min	• Maximum 45%
• Nasal catheter	• 1–6 L/min	• Maximum 45%
• Face mask	• 5–10 L/min	• 35–60%
• Venturi type mask	• 5–10 L/min	• 25–60%
B. High flow systems		
• Oxygen hood*	• 10–15 L/min	• 80–90%
• Partial rebreathing mask	• 10–12 L/min	• 50–60%
• Nonrebreathing mask	• 10–12 L/min	• Up to 90%
• Anesthesia bag with	• 10–12 L/min	• Up to 95%
• Nonrebreathing mask		
*In newborn baby, flow rate of oxygen therapy should be 1–2 L/min by nasal cannula and 5–8 L/min by oxygen hood		

Appendix XIV

Basic Life Support (BLS) Maneuvers of Cardiopulmonary Resuscitation (CPR)

Maneuver	Infant	Child (1–8 years)	Child and adult (Above 8 years)
• Airway	• Head tilt-chin lift • If trauma is present, use Jaw-thrust	• Same as infant	• Head tilt-chin lift or jaw thrust in trauma
• Breathing			
– Initial	• Two breaths at 1–1$^1/_2$ sec. per breath	• Same as infant	• Two breaths at 1.5–2 sec. per breath
– Subsequent	• 20 breaths/min	• 20 breaths/min	• 10–12 breaths per minute
• Circulation			

– Pulse check
  – Compression area
  – Compression width
  – Compression depth
 	
  – Rate
	• Brachial/Femoral
	• Lower half of sternum
	• 2 or 3 fingers together
	• 0.5″ – 1″
	Approximately $^1/_3$ – $^1/_2$ the depth of the chest
	• At least 100/min
		• Carotid
		• Lower half of sternum
		• Heel of one hand
		• 1″ – 1.5″
		Approximately $^1/_3$ – $^1/_2$ the depth of the chest
		• 100 per min
			• Carotid
			• Lower half sternum
			• Two hand stacked
			• 1.5″ – 2″
			
			• 80–100/min

• Compression – Ventilation ratio	• 5 : 1 (Pause for ventialtion)	• 5 : 1 (Pause for ventilation)	• 15 : 2 (one rescuer) • 5 : 1 (two rescuer)
• Foreign body airway obstruction	• Back blows or chest thrusts	• Heimlich maneuver	• Heimlich maneuver

Adapted from M Singh. Medical Emergencies in Children, 3rd edition. Sagar Publications, New Delhi, 2000.

Appendix XV

Optimal Timing for Surgical Correction

A. *Common neonatal emergencies requiring immediate surgical correction* as soon as they are diagnosed to prevent serious life-threatening complications:

- Diaphragmatic hernia
- Esophageal atresia
- Lobar emphysema
- Tension pneumothorax
- Neonatal intestinal obstruction
- Leaking meningomyelocele
- Gastroschisis
- Ruptured omphalocele
- Supralevator anorectal malformations
- Acute abscess

B. *Nonemergency conditions requiring urgent* surgical correction as early as possible to avoid complications. Common conditions and timing of surgery are mentioned below:

Condition	Timing of surgery
• Inguinal hernia	• As soon as diagnosed
• Talipes equinovarus	• In first week after birth
• Congenital dislocation of hip	• In first week after birth
• Hypertrophic pyloric stenosis	• 4–5 weeks of age
• Meningomyelocele with thin sac and exposed neural plaque	• As early as possible
• Congenital hydrocephalus	• As early as possible
• Sacrococcygeal teratoma	• Within 2 weeks after birth
• Masses suspected to be malignant	• As early as possible
• Patent ductus arteriosus causing complications	• As soon as possible

C. *Elective surgical correction*

Condition	Optimal age for surgery
• Cleft lip	• 2–3 months
• Cleft palate	• 12–15 months
• Tongue tie	• 12 months
• Sternomastoid tumor	• Tenotomy before hypoplasia of face
• Congenital biliary atresia	• Before 6–8 weeks
• Umbilical hernia	• After 3–4 years
• Undescended testis	• 2 years
• Hydrocele	• After 6 months
• Phimosis: a. Circumcision b. Preputial separation	• After 2–3 years • After 1 year of age

Contd...

Contd...

• Hypospadias:			
a. Meatotomy	• Any time after birth		
b. Chordee correction	• 2 years		
c. Urethroplasty	• 3 years (before child goes to school)		
• Epispadias:			
a. Chordee correction	• 2 years		
b. Urethroplasty	• 4 years		
• Exstrophy of bladder:			
a. 'Turn in' of bladder	• 2–3 weeks		
b. Chordee correction of epispadias, bladder neck repair and antireflux surgery	• 3–4 years		
c. Urethroplasty	• After achieving continence or after 2 years of chordee correction and rerepair of bladder neck		
d. Augmentation colocystoplasty	• 8–10 years		
• Supralevator anorectal malformations (PSARP)	• 10–12 months		
• Hirschsprung's disease (definitive surgery)	• 12–15 months or 6–8 months after colostomy.		
• Syndactyly	• 1–2 years		
• Ventricular or atrial septal defect	• 5– 6 years		
• Coarctation of aorta	• 5–6 years		

NB: Adapted from Clinical Hand Book of Surgical Pediatrics by R Kulshrestha.

Appendix XVI

Neutral Thermal Environmental Temperatures

Age and weight	Starting temperature (°C)	Range of temperature (°C)
0–6 hours		
Under 1200 gm	35.0	34.0–35.4
1200–1500 gm	34.1	33.9–34.4
1501–2500 gm	33.4	32.8–33.8
Over 2500 (and > 36 weeks)	32.0–33.8	
6–12 hours		
Under 1200 gm	35.0	34.0–35.4
1200–1500 gm	34.0	33.5–34.4
1501–2500 gm	33.1	32.2–33.8
Over 2500 (and > 36 weeks)	32.8	31.4–33.8
12–24 hours		
Under 1200 gm	34.0	34.0–35.4
1200–1500 gm	33.8	33.3–34.3
1501–2500 gm	32.8	31.8–33.8
Over 2500 (and > 36 weeks)	32.4	31.1–33.7
24–36 hours		
Under 1200 gm	34.0	34.0–35.0
1200–1500 gm	33.6	33.1–34.2
1501–2500 gm	32.6	31.6–33.6
Over 2500 (and > 36 weeks)	32.1	30.7–33.5
36–48 hours		
Under 1200 gm	34.0	34.0–35.0
1200–1500 gm	33.5	33.0–34.1
1501–2500 gm	32.5	31.4–33.5
Over 2500 (and > 36 weeks)	31.9	30.5–33.3
48–72 hours		
Under 1200 gm	34.0	34.0–35.0
1200–1500 gm	33.5	33.0–34.0
1501–2500 gm	32.3	31.2–33.4
Over 2500 (and > 36 weeks)	31.7	30.1–33.2

Age and weight	Starting temperature (°C)	Range of temperature (°C)
72–96 hours		
Under 1200 gm	34.0	34.0–35.0
1200–1500 gm	33.5	33.0–34.0
1501–2500 gm	32.2	31.1–33.2
Over 2500 (and > 36 weeks)	31.3	29.8–32.8
4–12 days		
Under 1500 gm	33.5	33.0–34.0
1501–2500 gm	32.1	31.0–33.2
Over 2500 (and > 36 weeks)		
4–5 days	31.0	29.5–32.6
5–6 days	30.9	29.4–32.3
6–8 days	30.6	29.0–32.2
8–10 days	30.3	29.0–31.8
10–12 days	30.1	29.0–31.4
12–14 days		
Under 1500 gm	33.5	32.6–34.0
1501–2500 gm	32.1	31.0–33.2
Over 2500 (and > 36 weeks)	29.8	29.0–30.8
2–3 weeks		
Under 1500 gm	33.1	32.2–34.0
1501–2500 gm	31.7	30.5–33.0
3–4 weeks		
Under 1500 gm	32.6	31.6–33.6
1501–2500 gm	31.4	30.0–32.7
4–5 weeks		
Under 1500 gm	32.0	31.2–33.0
1501–2500 gm	30.9	29.5–32.2
5–6 weeks		
Under 1500 gm	31.4	30.6–32.3
1501–2500 gm	30.4	29.0–31.8

Data from Scopes JW, Ahmed 1: Minimal rates of oxygen consumption in sick and premature infants. *Arch Dis Child* 1966;41:407-16 and range of critical temperatures in sick and premature newborn babies. *Arch Dis Child* 1996;41:417-19.

Appendix XVII

Neonatal Resuscitation Program Guideline-2005

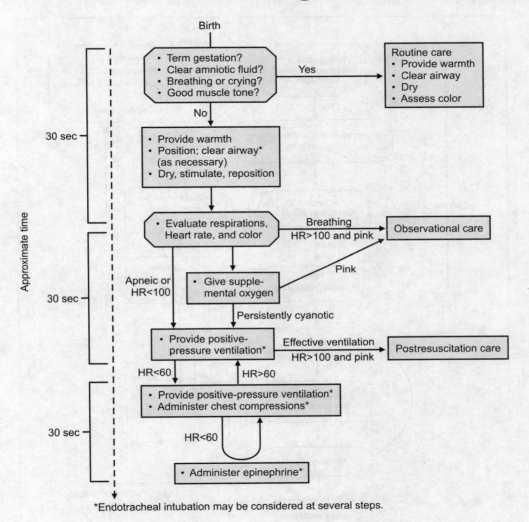

*Endotracheal intubation may be considered at several steps.

Appendix XVIIA

Newborn Resuscitation Algorithm: 2010 (AAP)

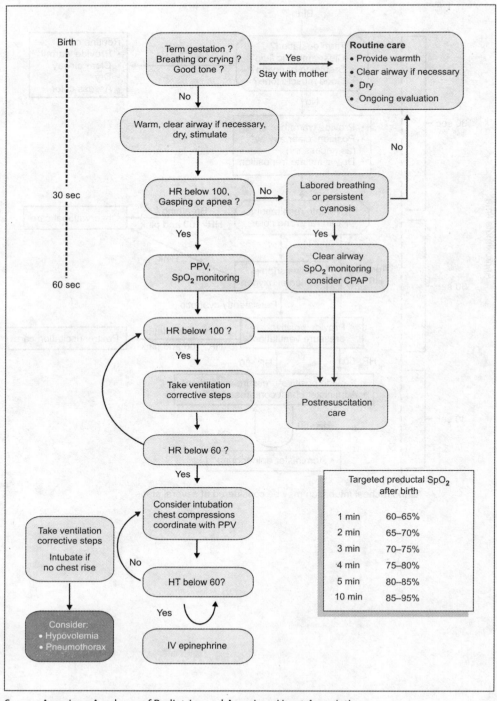

Source: American Academy of Pediatrics and American Heart Association.

Appendix XVIIB

Neonatal Resuscitation Program™: Reference Chart

! The most important and effective action in neonatal resuscitation is ventilation of the baby's lungs.

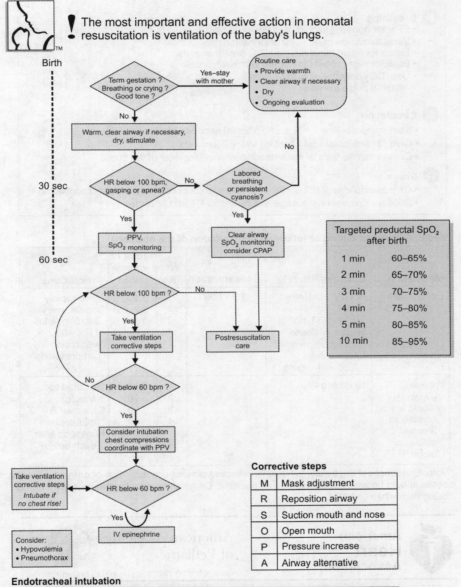

Corrective steps

M	Mask adjustment
R	Reposition airway
S	Suction mouth and nose
O	Open mouth
P	Pressure increase
A	Airway alternative

Endotracheal intubation

Gestational age (weeks)	Weight (Kg)	ET Tube size (ID, mm)	Depth of insertion* (cm from upper lip)
<28	<1.0	2.5	6–7
28–34	1.0–2.0	3.0	7–8
34–48	2.0–3.0	3.5	8–9
>38	>3.0	3.5–4.0	9–10

*Depth of insertion (cm) = 6+ weight (in Kg)

Contd...

Contd...

A **Airway**
- Put baby's head in "sniffing" position
- Suction mouth, then nose
- Suction trachea if meconium-stained and NOT vigorous

B **Breathing**
- PPV for apnea, gasping or pulse <100 bpm
- Ventilate at rate of 40 to 60 breaths/minute
- Listen for rising heart rate, audible breath sounds
- Look for slight chest movement with each breath
- Use CO_2 detector after intubation
- Attach a pulse oximeter

C **Circulation**
- Start compressions if HR is <60 after 30 seconds of effective PPV
- Give (3 compressions: 1 breath) every 2 seconds
- Compress one-third of the anterior-posterior diameter of the chest

D **Drugs**
- Give epinephrine if HR is <60 after 30 seconds of compressions and ventilation
- Caution: Epinephrine dosage is different for ET and IV routes

Medications used during or following resuscitation of the newborn

Medication	Dosages/Route*	Concentration	Wt (Kg)	Total IV volume (mL)	Precautions
Epinephrine	IV (UVC preferred route) 0.01–0.03 mg/Kg Higher IV doses not recommended Endotracheal 0.05–0.1 mg/Kg	1:10,000	1 2 3 4	0.1–0.3 0.2–0.6 0.3–0.9 0.4–1.2	Give rapidly repeat every 3 to 5 minutes if HR <60 with chest compressions
Volume expanders Isotonic crystalloid (normal saline) or blood	10 mL/Kg IV		1 2 3 4	10 20 30 40	Indicated for shock. Give over 5–10 minutes. Reassess after each bolus.

*Note: Endotracheal dose may not result in effective plasma concentration of drug, so vascular access should be established as soon as possible. Drugs given endotracheally require higher dosing than when given IV

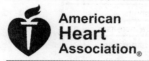

American **Heart** Association®

American Academy of Pediatrics

DEDICATED TO THE HEALTH OF ALL CHILDREN™

© 2011 American Academy of Pediatrics and American Heart Association
Supported in part by Fisher & Paykel Healthcare

NRP 307

ISBN 978-1-58110-505-6

90000>

9 781581 105056

Appendix XVIII

Identifying Intrauterine Growth Retardation in a Newborn

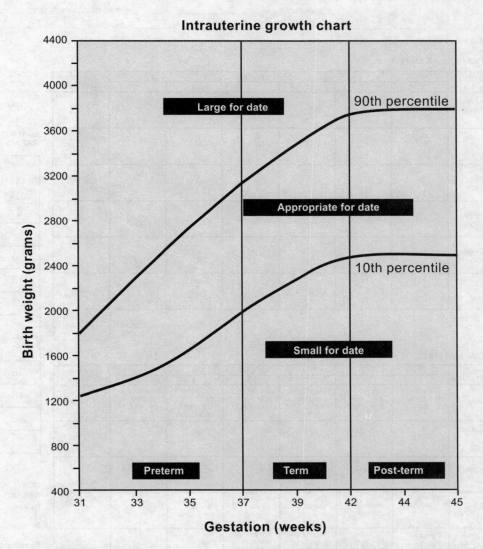

Intrauterine growth chart

Source: Facility based newborn care operational guide (Guidelines for planning and implementation)

Appendix XIX A

Gestational Age Assessment (Ballard)

NAME _____ DATE/TIME OF BIRTH _____ BIRTH WEIGHT_____

HOSPITAL NO. _____ DATE/TIME OF EXAM _____ LENGTH _____

                                 AGE WHEN EXAMINED _____ HEAD CIRCUMFERENCE_____

RACE _____ SEX _____ EXAMINER _____

APGAR SCORE : 1 MINUTE _____ 5 MINUTES _____

NEUROMUSCULAR MATURITY

NEUROMUSCULAR MATURITY SIGN	SCORE						RECORD SCORE HERE
	0	1	2	3	4	5	
POSTURE							
SQUARE WINDOW (WRIST)	90	60	45	30	0		
ARM RECOIL	180			<90–100	90		
POPLITEAL ANGLE	180	160	130	110	90	90	
SCARF SIGN							
HEEL TO EAR							

TOTAL NEUROMUSCULAR MATURITY SCORE

SCORE
Neuromuscular
physical
 Total

MATURITY RATING

TOTAL MATURITY SCORE	GESTATIONAL AGE (WEEKS)
5	26
10	28
15	30
20	32
25	34
30	36
35	38
40	40
45	42
50	44

PHYSICAL MATURITY

PHYSICAL MATURITY SIGN	SCORE						RECORD SCORE HERE
	0	1	2	3	4	5	
SKIN	Gelatinous red transparent	Smooth pink, visible veins	Superficial peeling, and/or rash few veins	Cracking pale area rare veins	Parchment deep cracking no vessels	Leathery cracked wrinkled	
LANUGO	None	Abundant	Thinning	Bald areas	Mostly bald		
PLANTAR CREASES	No crease	Faint red marks	Anterior transverse crease only	Creases ant. 2–3	Creases cover entire sole		
BREAST	Barely percept.	Flat areola no bud	Stippled areola. 1–2 mm bud	Raised areola. 3–4 mm bud	Full areola 5–10 mm bud		
EAR	Pinna flat, stays folded	Sl. curved pinna; soft with slow recoil	Well-curv. pinna; soft but ready recoil	Formed and firm with instant recoil	Thick cartilage ear sift		
GENITALS (Male)	Scrotum empty no rugae		Testes descending few rugae	Testes down good rugae	Testes pendulous deep rugae		
GENITALS (Female)	Prominent clitoris and labia minora		Majora and minora equality prominent	Majora large, minora small	clitoris and minora completely covered		

TOTAL PHYSICAL MATURITY SCORE

GESTATIONAL AGE (WEEKS)

By dates _____

By ultrasound _____

By score _____

Reference
Ballard JL. Novak KK. Driver M./A. Simplified score for assessment of fetal maturation of newly born infants. J Pediatr 1979;95;769-74, Reprinted by permission of Dr Ballard and Journal of Pediatrics

Appendix XIX B

Maturational Assessment of Gestational Age (New Ballard Score)

MATURATIONAL ASSESSMENT OF GESTATIONAL AGE (New Ballard Score)

NAME _____   SEX _____

HOSPITAL NO. _____   BIRTH WEIGHT _____

RACE _____   LENGTH _____

DATE/TIME OF BIRTH _____   HEAD CIRCUMFERENCE _____

DATE/TIME OF EXAM _____   EXAMINER _____

AGE WHEN EXAMINED _____

APGAR SCORE: 1 MINUTE _____ 5 MINUTES _____ 10 MINUTES _____

NEUROMUSCULAR MATURITY

Neuromuscular maturity sign	SCORE							Record score here
	−1	0	1	2	3	4	5	
Posture								
Square window (Wrist)	>90°	90°	60°	45°	30°	0°		
Arm recoil		180°	140–180°	110–140°	90–110°	<90°		
Popliteal angle	180°	160°	140°	120°	100°	90°	<90°	
Scarf sign								
Heel to ear								

Total neuromuscular maturity score

SCORE

Neuromuscular _____
Physical _____
Total _____

MATURITY RATING

Score	Weeks
−10	20
−5	22
0	24
5	26
10	28
15	30
20	32
25	34
30	36
35	38
40	40
45	42
50	44

PHYSICAL MATURITY

Physical maturity sign	SCORE							Record score here
	−1	0	1	2	3	4	5	
Skin	Sticky friable transparent	Gelatinous red translucent	Smooth pink visible veins	Superficial peeling and/or rash few veins	Cracking pale areas rare veins	Parchment deep cracking no vessels	Leathery cracked wrinkled	
Lanugo	None	Sparse	Abundant	Thinning	Bald areas	Mostly bald		
Plantar surface	Heel-toe 40-50 mm:-1 <40:-2	>50 mm no crease	Faint red marks	Anterior transverse crease only	Creases ant. 2/3	Creases over entire sole		
Breast	Imperceptible	Barely perceptible	Flat areola no bud	Stippled areola 1–2 mm bud	Raised areola 3–4 mm bud	Full areola 5–10 mm bud		
Eye/Ear	Lids fused loosely:-1 tightly:- 2	Lids open pinna flat stays folded	Sl. curved pinna; soft; slow recoil	Well-curved pinna; soft but ready recoil	Formed and firm instant recoil	Thick cartilage ear stiff		
Genitals (Male)	Scrotum flat, smooth	Scrotum empty faint rugae	Testes in upper canal rare rugae	Testes descending few rugae	Testes down good rugae	Testes pendulous deep rugae		
Genitals (Female)	Clitoris prominent and labia flat	Prominent clitoris and small labia minora	Prominent clitoris and enlarging minora	Majora and minora equally prominent	Majora large minora small	Majora cover clitoris and minora		

Total physical maturity score

Gestational age (weeks)

By dates _____
By ultrasound _____
By exam _____

Reference
Ballard JL, khoury JC, Wedig K, et al. New Ballard score, expanded to include extremely premature infants. *J Pediatr* 1991; 119; 119:417-423. Reprinted by permission of Dr Ballard and Mosby-Year Book, Inc.

Appendix XX

Routine Examination of Newborn Infants

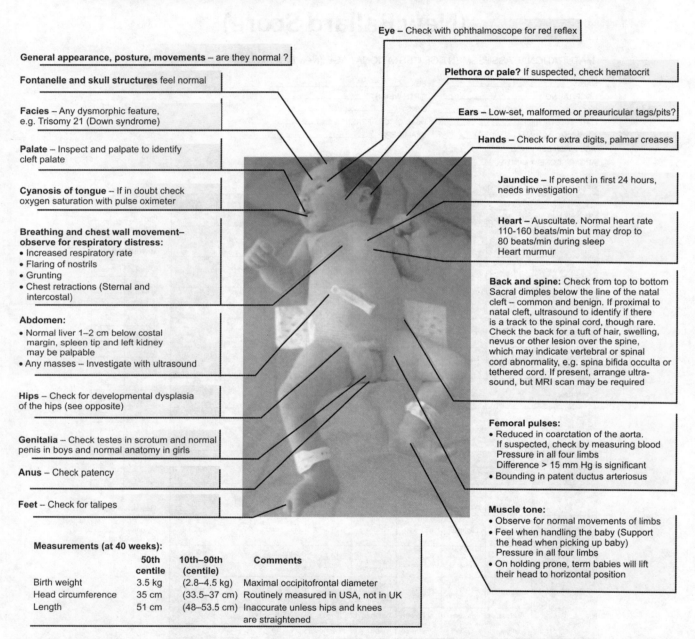

General appearance, posture, movements – are they normal ?

Fontanelle and skull structures feel normal

Facies – Any dysmorphic feature,
e.g. Trisomy 21 (Down syndrome)

Palate – Inspect and palpate to identify
cleft palate

Cyanosis of tongue – If in doubt check
oxygen saturation with pulse oximeter

**Breathing and chest wall movement–
observe for respiratory distress:**
• Increased respiratory rate
• Flaring of nostrils
• Grunting
• Chest retractions (Sternal and
  intercostal)

Abdomen:
• Normal liver 1–2 cm below costal
  margin, spleen tip and left kidney
  may be palpable
• Any masses – Investigate with ultrasound

Hips – Check for developmental dysplasia
of the hips (see opposite)

Genitalia – Check testes in scrotum and normal
penis in boys and normal anatomy in girls

Anus – Check patency

Feet – Check for talipes

Eye – Check with ophthalmoscope for red reflex

Plethora or pale? If suspected, check hematocrit

Ears – Low-set, malformed or preauricular tags/pits?

Hands – Check for extra digits, palmar creases

Jaundice – If present in first 24 hours,
needs investigation

Heart – Auscultate. Normal heart rate
110-160 beats/min but may drop to
80 beats/min during sleep
Heart murmur

Back and spine: Check from top to bottom
Sacral dimples below the line of the natal
cleft – common and benign. If proximal to
natal cleft, ultrasound to identify if there
is a track to the spinal cord, though rare.
Check the back for a tuft of hair, swelling,
nevus or other lesion over the spine,
which may indicate vertebral or spinal
cord abnormality, e.g. spina bifida occulta or
tethered cord. If present, arrange ultrasound, but MRI scan may be required

Femoral pulses:
• Reduced in coarctation of the aorta.
  If suspected, check by measuring blood
  Pressure in all four limbs
  Difference > 15 mm Hg is significant
• Bounding in patent ductus arteriosus

Muscle tone:
• Observe for normal movements of limbs
• Feel when handling the baby (Support
  the head when picking up baby)
  Pressure in all four limbs
• On holding prone, term babies will lift
  their head to horizontal position

Measurements (at 40 weeks):

	50th centile	10th–90th (centile)	Comments
Birth weight	3.5 kg	(2.8–4.5 kg)	Maximal occipitofrontal diameter
Head circumference	35 cm	(33.5–37 cm)	Routinely measured in USA, not in UK
Length	51 cm	(48–53.5 cm)	Inaccurate unless hips and knees are straightened

Source: "Neonatology at a glance" by Tom Lissauer and Avroy Fanaroff by Blackwell Publishing and Jaypee Brothers Medical Publishers

Appendix XXI

Transient Abnormalities in the First Few Days of Life

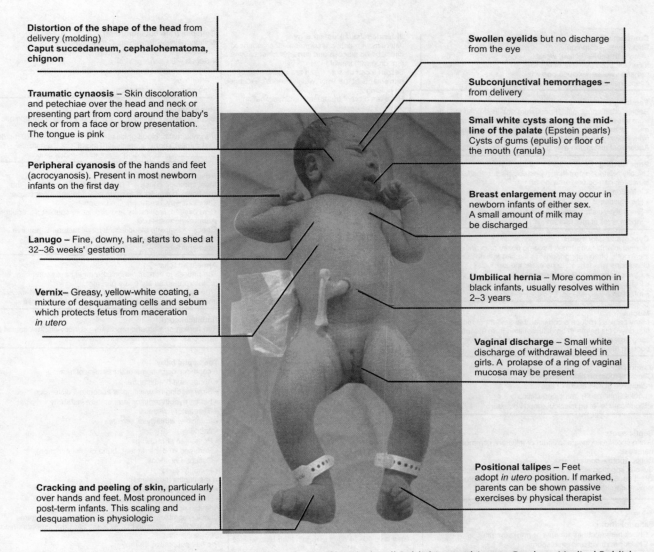

Distortion of the shape of the head from delivery (molding)
Caput succedaneum, cephalohematoma, chignon

Traumatic cynaosis – Skin discoloration and petechiae over the head and neck or presenting part from cord around the baby's neck or from a face or brow presentation. The tongue is pink

Peripheral cyanosis of the hands and feet (acrocyanosis). Present in most newborn infants on the first day

Lanugo – Fine, downy, hair, starts to shed at 32–36 weeks' gestation

Vernix– Greasy, yellow-white coating, a mixture of desquamating cells and sebum which protects fetus from maceration *in utero*

Cracking and peeling of skin, particularly over hands and feet. Most pronounced in post-term infants. This scaling and desquamation is physiologic

Swollen eyelids but no discharge from the eye

Subconjunctival hemorrhages – from delivery

Small white cysts along the mid-line of the palate (Epstein pearls) Cysts of gums (epulis) or floor of the mouth (ranula)

Breast enlargement may occur in newborn infants of either sex. A small amount of milk may be discharged

Umbilical hernia – More common in black infants, usually resolves within 2–3 years

Vaginal discharge – Small white discharge of withdrawal bleed in girls. A prolapse of a ring of vaginal mucosa may be present

Positional talipes – Feet adopt *in utero* position. If marked, parents can be shown passive exercises by physical therapist

Source: "Neonatology at a glance" by Tom Lissauer and Avroy Fanaroff by Blackwell Publishing and Jaypee Brothers Medical Publishers.

Appendix XXII

Overview of Common Neonatal Medical Problems

Conjunctivitis
Sticky eyes – common
clean with sterile (boiled) water
If conjunctivitis purulent or eyelids
red and swollen, exclude bacterial
cause including *Gonococcus* and *Chlamydia*

Vomiting
Babies often vomit milk. If persistent or bile stained may be
from intestinal obstruction. If it contains blood, malrotation
must be excluded, but is usually swallowed maternal blood
from delivery or maternal breast
Abdominal distension may be from lower intestinal obstruction

Poor feeding
Usually related to problems in establishing breastfeeding
However, can be presentation of:
• Infection
• Hypoglycemia
• Electrolyte disturbance
• Inborn error of metabolism

Cyanotic/dusky spells
Normal infants sometimes become dusky or cyanosed around
the mouth, often during feeds, in the first few days.
Conditions which need to be excluded are:
• Cyanotic congenital heart disease
• Polycythemia
• Infection

Mucus
Many babies produce a considerable amount of mucus on the
first day. This needs to be differentiated from the infant with
esophageal atresia who is unable to swallow saliva, which
pools in the mouth

Jaundice
Check bilirubin on blood sample if:
• Jaundice at <24 hours of age
• Looks significantly jaundiced clinically
• Significant level on transcutaneous monitor

Septic spots
White spots – erythema toxicum or milia are common and
harmless
Septic spots – contain pus
Bullous impetigo – Serious (Staphylococcal or streptococcal)
infection. Sacs of serous fluid; their roof is easily broken
leaving denuded skin

Pallor/plethora
• Check hematocrit for anemia or polycythemia
• Check breathing and circulation

Jitteriness/seizures/lethargy
Jittery movements are common – if pronounced
check blood glucose and consider other causes,
e.g. drug withdrawal
Seizures can be subtle, but are rhythmic jerky
movements of the limbs which cannot be stopped
on holding
Requires prompt treatment and investigation –
admit to the neonatal unit
Lethargy may be a sign of sepsis,hypoglycemia
or inborn error of metabolism

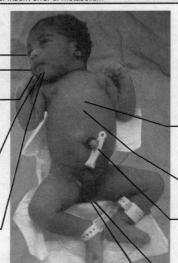

Delay in passing meconium (>24 hours)
check for intestinal obstruction

Delay in voiding urine (> 24 hours)
Voiding may be unobserved – often void
immediately after birth
Consider urinary outflow obstruction
(palpable bladder, ultrasound)
or renal failure (serum creatinine, ultrasound)

Weight loss
Babies initially lose weight (1–2% of birth
weight per day up to 7–10% of birth weight).
They take 10–14 days to regain their birth weight

Collapse (rare but important)
Maintain Airway, Breathing, Circulation
Causes:
• Sepsis – Bacterial or viral
• Duct-dependent heart disease – closure of ductus
  arteriosus
• Inborn error of metabolism

Hypoglycemia
Blood glucose <40 mg/dL (<2.6 mmol/L) and asymptomatic
– feed infant and recheck
If symptomatic, blood glucose levels are very low <20 mg/dL
(1.1 mmol/L) or persistently <40 mg/dL (<2.6 mml/L)
despite adequate feeding – give intravenous glucose

Respiratory distress
Most common cause – TTNB (transient tachypnea of the
newborn), but need to exclude infection and other causes
Check Airway, Breathing, Circulation
Give oxygen, respiratory and circulatory support as required
Admit to neonatal unit
Check – complete blood count, blood culture, C-reactive
protein and chest X-ray
Start antibiotics

Apneic attacks
The pauses in normal periodic breathing are sometimes
misinterpreted as apnea by parents
True apnea with desaturation is uncommon in term infants
and is a serious symptom; infection must be excluded

Umbilical cord
Red flare in skin around umbilicus – usually staphylococcal or
streptococcal. Give intravenous antibiotics

The septic baby
A combination of some of these clinical features:
• Apnea and bradycardia
• Slow feeding or vomiting or abdominal distension
• Fever, hypothermia or temperature instability
• Respiratory distress
• Irritability, lethargy or seizures
• Jaundice
• Petechiae or bruising
• Reduced limb movement (bone of joint infection)
• Collapse or shock
• Hypoglycemia
in meningitis (late signs):
• Tense or bulging fontanelle
• Head retraction (opisthotonus)
Admit to neonatal unit
Check – complete blood count, blood and other cultures,
C – reactive protein and chest X-ray consider lumbar puncture
Start antibiotics
Provide supportive therapy

Source: "Neonatology at a glance" by Tom Lissauer and Avroy Fanaroff by Blackwell Publishing and Jaypee Brothers Medical Publishers

Appendix XXIII

Fetal-Infant Growth Chart for Preterm Infants

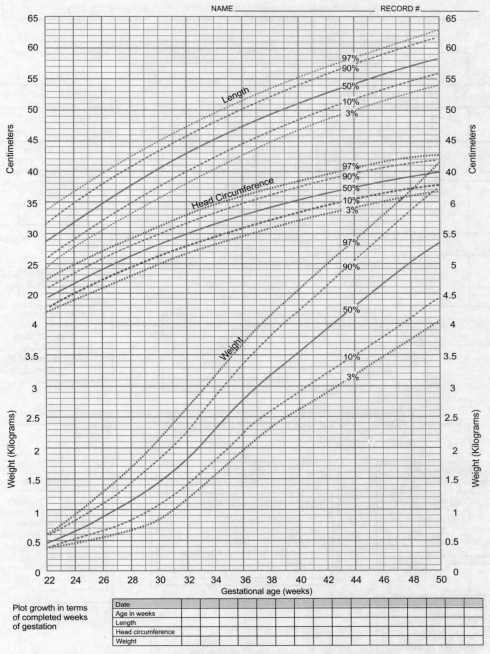

Plot growth in terms
of completed weeks
of gestation

Date													
Age in weeks													
Length													
Head circumference													
Weight													

http://www.biomedcentral.com/1471-2431/3/13

Appendix XXIV

IMNCI Case Management Process

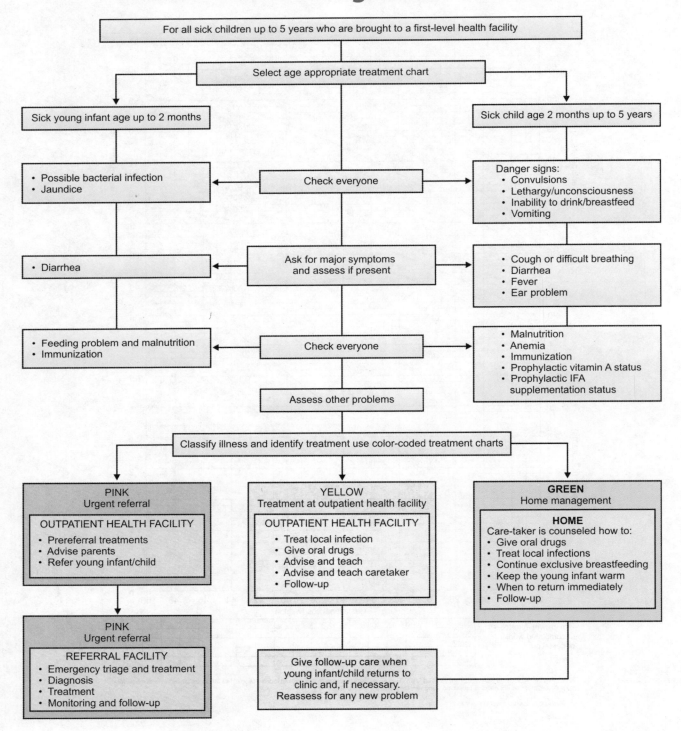

Appendix XXV

Emergency Triage Assessment and Treatment (ETAT)

Chart 1: Proforma for Assessment of Sick Child

Case Recording Form   Date_____

Name _____   Age _____   Sex _____   Wt _____   Temp _____

ASK: What are the infant's problems?

ASSESS (Circle all signs present)	Emergency treatments
	• Check for head/neck trauma before treating child—do not move neck if cervical spine injury possible. • EMERGENCY SIGNS: If any sign positive: give treatment(s), call for help, draw blood for emergency laboratory investigations (glucose, malaria smear, Hb)
AIRWAY AND BREATHING • Not breathing or gasping or • Central cyanosis or • Severe respiratory distress (Respiratory rate $\geq$ 70/min, Severe lower chest in-drawing, Grunting, Head nodding, Apneic spells, Unable to feed due to respiratory distress, Stridor in a calm child)	
CIRCULATION Cold hands with: • Capillary refill longer than 3 seconds, and • Weak and fast pulse IF POSITIVE Check for severe acute malnutrition	
COMA CONVULSING • Coma (AVPU) or • Convulsing (now)	
SEVERE DEHYDRATION (ONLY IN CHILD WITH DIARRHEA) Diarrhea plus any two of these: • Lethargy • Sunken eyes • Very slow skin pinch If two signs positive check for severe acute malnutrition	
PRIORITY SIGNS • Tiny baby (< 2 months) • Respiratory distress (RR >60/min) • Temperature < 36.5°C or >38.5°C • Bleeding • Restless, continuously irritable, or lethargy • Trauma or other urgent surgical condition • Referral (urgent) • Pallor (severe) • *Malnutrition:* Visible severe wasting • Edema of both feet • Poisoning • Burns (major)	
Check temperature if baby is cold to touch, rewarm *Source:* F-IMNCI Protocol by Govt. of India.	

Contd...

Contd...

Chart 2: Triage

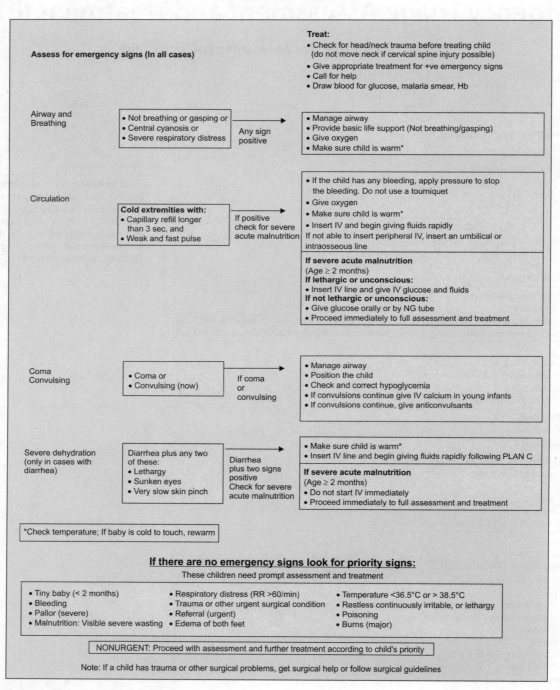

Treat:
- Check for head/neck trauma before treating child (do not move neck if cervical spine injury possible)
- Give appropriate treatment for +ve emergency signs
- Call for help
- Draw blood for glucose, malaria smear, Hb

Assess for emergency signs (In all cases)

Airway and Breathing
- Not breathing or gasping or
- Central cyanosis or
- Severe respiratory distress

Any sign positive →
- Manage airway
- Provide basic life support (Not breathing/gasping)
- Give oxygen
- Make sure child is warm*

Circulation

Cold extremities with:
- Capillary refill longer than 3 sec, and
- Weak and fast pulse

If positive check for severe acute malnutrition →
- If the child has any bleeding, apply pressure to stop the bleeding. Do not use a tourniquet
- Give oxygen
- Make sure child is warm*
- Insert IV and begin giving fluids rapidly
  If not able to insert peripheral IV, insert an umbilical or intraosseous line

If severe acute malnutrition
(Age ≥ 2 months)
If lethargic or unconscious:
- Insert IV line and give IV glucose and fluids
If not lethargic or unconscious:
- Give glucose orally or by NG tube
- Proceed immediately to full assessment and treatment

Coma Convulsing
- Coma or
- Convulsing (now)

If coma or convulsing →
- Manage airway
- Position the child
- Check and correct hypoglycemia
- If convulsions continue give IV calcium in young infants
- If convulsions continue, give anticonvulsants

Severe dehydration (only in cases with diarrhea)

Diarrhea plus any two of these:
- Lethargy
- Sunken eyes
- Very slow skin pinch

Diarrhea plus two signs positive Check for severe acute malnutrition →
- Make sure child is warm*
- Insert IV line and begin giving fluids rapidly following PLAN C

If severe acute malnutrition
(Age ≥ 2 months)
- Do not start IV immediately
- Proceed immediately to full assessment and treatment

*Check temperature; If baby is cold to touch, rewarm

If there are no emergency signs look for priority signs:
These children need prompt assessment and treatment

- Tiny baby (< 2 months)
- Bleeding
- Pallor (severe)
- Malnutrition: Visible severe wasting
- Respiratory distress (RR >60/min)
- Trauma or other urgent surgical condition
- Referral (urgent)
- Edema of both feet
- Temperature <36.5°C or > 38.5°C
- Restless continuously irritable, or lethargy
- Poisoning
- Burns (major)

NONURGENT: Proceed with assessment and further treatment according to child's priority

Note: If a child has trauma or other surgical problems, get surgical help or follow surgical guidelines

Source: F-IMNCI Protocol by Govt. of India.

Appendix XXVI

Neonatal Drug Chart

Drug	Dose	Route
Ampicillin	< 7 days 50 mg/kg dose, q 12 hr	IV
	> 7 days 50 mg/kg/dose, 1 8 hr	
Gentamicin	Sepsis/pneumonia 2.5 mg/kg/dose, q 12 hr or 5 mg/kg/dose, q 24 hr Meningitis: < 7 days 2.5 mg/kg/dose, q 12 hr > 7 days 2.5 mg/kg/dose, q 8 hr	IV IV
Amikacin	< 7 days 7.5 mL/kg/dose, q 12 hr	IV
Cefotaxime	< 7 days 50 mg/kg/dose, q 12 hr > 7 days 50 mg/kg/dose, q 8 hr	IV
Chaloramphenicol	12 mg/kg/dose q 12 hr	IV
Aminophylline	5 mg/kg loading, then 2 mg/kg/dose, q 8–12 hr	IV
Vitamin K	1 mg	IM
Phenobarbitone	20 mg/kg loading over 10–15 min then 3–4 mg/kg q 24 hr	Loading IV then IV, IM or oral
Phenytoin	15–20 mg/kg loading over 10–15 min then 5 mg/kg q 24 hr	IV
Dopamine/Dobutamine	5–20 micro g/kg/min	IV continuous

Source: Facility based newborn care (FBNC) Protocol by Govt. of India

Appendix XXVII

Pediatrics Drug Dosages/Regimens

Drug	Dose	Route
Aminophylline	For asthma *Loading dose:* 5–6 mg/kg (max. 300 mg) slowly over 20–60 minutes *Maintenance dose:* 5 mg/kg up to every 6 hours or By continuous infusion 0.9 mg/kg/hour	IV IV
Amoxicillin	15 mg/kg three times per day For pneumonia 25 mg/kg two times a day	Oral
Ampicillin	25 mg/kg four times a day 50 mg/kg every 6 hours	Oral IM/IV
Cefotaxime	50 mg/kg every 6 hours	IM/IV
Ceftriaxone	80 mg/kg/day as a single dose give over 30 minutes For meningitis 50 mg/kg every 12 hours (maximum single dose 4 g) Or 100 mg/kg once daily	IM/IV IM/IV IM/IV
Chloramphenicol	Calculate exact dose based on body weight. Only use these doses if this is not possible. *For meningitis:* 25 mg/kg every 6 hours (maximum 1 g per dose) For other conditions: 25 mg/kg every 8 hours (maximum 1 g per dose)	IV IM Oral
Chlorphenamine	0.25 mg/kg once (can be repeated up to 4 times in 24 hours)	IM/IV or SC
Ciprofloxacin	10–15 mg/kg per dose given twice per day (maximum 500 mg per dose)	Oral
Cloxacillin	25–50 mg/kg every 6 hours	IV
Cotrimoxazole (trimethoprim-sulfamethoxazole, TMP-SMX)	4 mg trimethoprim/kg and 20 mg sulfamethoxazole/kg two times per day	Oral
Dexamethasone	For several viral croup 0.6 mg/kg singe dose	Oral
Diazepam	For convulsions 0.5 mg/kg 0.2–0.3 mg/kg	Rectal: IV
Epinephrine (adrenaline)	*For wheeze:* 0.01 mL/kg (up to a maximum of 0.3 mL) of 1:1000 solution (or mL/kg of 1:10000 solution) *For several viral croup:* A trial of 0.3 mL/kg of 1:1000 nebulized solution	SC
Furosemide (frusemide)	For cardiac failure 1–2 mg/kg every 12 hours	Oral or IV
Gentamicin	7.5 mg/kg once per day	IM/IV
Nalidixic acid	15 mg/kg 4 times a day	Oral
Paracetamol	10–15 mg/kg, up to 4 times a day	Oral
Benzylpenicillin (penicillin G)	*General dosage:* 50000 units/kg every 6 hours *For meningitis:* 100000 units/kg every 6 hours	IM/IV
Phenobarbital	Loading dose 15 mg/kg Maintenance dose 2.5–5 mg/kg	Oral/IM/IV
Potassium	2–4 mEq/kg/dose/kg/day	Oral
Prednisolone	1 mg/kg twice a day	Oral
Salbutamol	1 mg per dose < 1 year; 2 mg per dose 1–4 years; Acute episode 6–8 hourly *Inhaler with spacer:* 2 doses contains 200 µg *Nebulizer:* 2.5 mg/dose	Oral

Contd...

Contd...

Anti-tuberculosis antibiotics

Calculate exact dose based on body weight			
Essential anti-TB drug (abbreviation)	Mode of action	Daily dose mg/kg (range)	Intermittent dose: 3 times/week/mg/kg (range)
Ethambutol (E)	Bacteriostatic	20 (15–25)	30 (25–35)
Rifampicin (R)	Bactericidal	10 (8–12)	10 (8–12)
Isoniazid (H)	Bactericidal	5 (4–6)	10 (8–12)
Pyrazinamide (Z)	Bactericidal	25 (20–30)	35 (30–40)
Streptomycin (S)	Bactericidal	15 (12–18)	15 (30–40)
Thioacetazone (T)	Bacteriostatic	3	Not applicable

Note: Avoid thioacetazone in a child who is known to be HIV-infected or when the likelihood of HIV infection is high, because severe (sometimes fatal) skin reactions can occur.

Source: F-IMNCI Protocol by Govt. of India

Management of Pediatric Tuberculosis under the Revised National Tuberculosis Control Program (RNTCP)

1. Diagnosis

Suspect cases of pulmonary tuberculosis: Children presenting with fever and/or cough for more than 2 weeks, with or without weight loss of no weight gain; and history with a suspected or diagnosed case of active TB disease within the last 2 years.

Diagnosis to be based on a combination of:
- Clinical presentation
- Sputum examination wherever possible
- Chest X-ray (PA view)
- Mantoux test (positive if induration > 10 mm after 48–72 hours)
- History of contact.

2. Treatment of Pediatric Tuberculosis

DOTS is the recommended strategy for treatment of TB and all pediatric tuberculosis patient should be registered under RNTCP.

Category of treatment	Type of patient	Intensive phase	Continuation phase
Category I	- New sputum smear positive pulmonary tuberculosis - Seriously ill* sputum smear negative pulmonary tuberculosis - Seriously ill extrapulmonary tuberculosis	2 H3 R3 Z3 E_3***	4H3R3
Category II	- Sputum smear positive relapse - Sputum smear positive treatmet failure	2 S3 H3 R3 Z3 E_3/IH3R3Z3E_3	5H3R3E_3 4H3R3
Category III	- Sputum smear negative - Extrapulmonary tuberculosis, not seriously ill**	2 H3 R3 Z3	4H3R3

*Seriously ill sputum smear negative pulmonary tuberculosis includes all forms of pulmonary tuberculosis other than primary complex, seriously ill extrapulmonary tuberculosis includes TBM, disseminated TB/miliary TB, TB pericarditis, TB peritonitis and intestinal TB, bilateral or extensive pleurisy, spinal TB with or without neurological complications, genitourinary tract TB, bone and joint TB.
**Not seriously ill extrapulmonary tuberculosis includes lymph node TB and unilateral pleural effusion
***Prefix indicates month and subscript indicates thrice weekly.

- In patients with TBM on category I treatment, the 4 drugs used during intensive phase should be HRZS or HRZE. Continuation phase in TBM or spinal TB with neurological complications should be given for 6–7 months, extending the total duration of treatment to 8–9 months
- Steroids should be used initially in cases of TBM and TB pericarditis and reduced gradually over 6–8 weeks.
- Before starting category II treatment, patient should be examined by a pediatrician or a TB expert. Ethambutol is to be used for all age groups.

Chemoprophylaxis

Asymptomatic children under 6 years of age, exposed to an adult with infectious (smear positive) tuberculosis, from the same household, will be given 6 months of isoniazid (5 mg/kg daily) chemoprophylaxis.

Management algorithm for treating acute asthma in a hospital

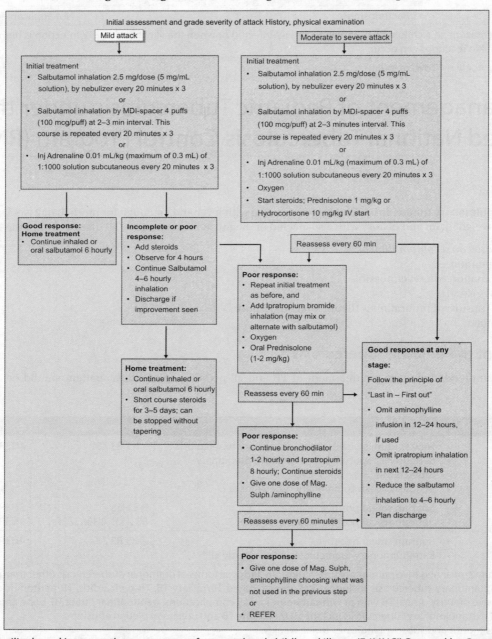

Source: Facility based integrated management of neonatal and childhood illness (F-IMNCI) Protocol by Govt. of India.

Appendix XXVIII

Safe Disposal of Hospital Waste

Proper disposal of hospital waste is important to keep the environment clean. To keep the environment clean, in each unit of ward, the waste should be disposed off in a proper way.

The following are different color drums with different color polythene for different type of waste, to be disposed off in a different way.

Black Drums/Bags

Left over food, fruits feeds, vegetables, waste paper, packing material, empty box, bags, etc. This waste is disposed off by routine municipal council committee machinery.

Yellow Drums/Bags: Infected Nonplastic Waste

Human anatomical waste, blood, body fluids, placenta, etc. This type of waste requires incineration.

Blue Drums/Bags: Infected Plastic Waste

Used disposable syringes, needles (first destroy the needle in the needle destroyer).

Used sharps, blade and broken glass, etc. Patients IV set, BT set, ET tube, catheter, urine bag, etc. should be cut into pieces and disposed in blue bag. This waste will be autoclaved to make it noninfectious. This is then shredded and disposed off.

Source: Facility based integrated management of neonatal and childhood illness (F-IMNCI) Protocol by Govt. of India.

Appendix XXIX

IMNCI Protocol

ASSESS AND CLASSIFY THE SICK YOUNG INFANT AGE UP TO 2 MONTHS

ASSESS	CLASSIFY	IDENTIFY TREATMENT

ASSESS

ASK THE MOTHER WHAT THE YOUNG INFANT'S PROBLEMS ARE
- Determine if this is an initial or follow-up visit for this problem.
- if follow-up visit, use the follow-up instructions on the bottom of this chart.

USE ALL BOXES THAT MATCH INFANT'S SYMPTOMS

A child with a pink classification needs URGENT attention, complete the assessment and pre-referral treatment immediately so referral is not delayed

CHECK FOR POSSIBLE BACTERIAL INFECTION / JAUNDICE

ASK:
- Has the infant had convulsions?

LOOK, LISTEN, FEEL:
- Count the breaths in one minute. Repeat the count if elevated.
- Look for severe chest indrawing.
- Look for nasal flaring.
- Look and listen for grunting.
- Look and feel for bulging fontanelle.
- Look for pus draining from the ear.
- Look at the umbilicus. Is it red or draining pus?
- Look for skin pustules. Are there 10 or more skin pustules or a big boil?
- Measure axillary temperature (if not possible, feel for fever or low body temperature).
- See if the young infant is lethargic or unconscious.
- Look at the young infant's movements. Are they less than normal?
- Look for jaundice?
- Are the palms and soles yellow?

YOUNG INFANT MUST BE CALM

SIGNS	CLASSIFY AS	IDENTIFY TREATMENT (Urgent pre-referral treatments are in bold print.)
Classify ALL YOUNG INFANTS: • Convulsions or • Fast breathing (60 breaths per minute or more) or • Severe chest indrawing or • Nasal flaring or • Grunting or • Bulging fontanelle or • 10 or more skin pustules or a big boil or • If axillary temperature 37.5°C or above (or feels hot to touch) or temperature less than 35.5°C. (or feels cold to touch) or • Lethargic or unconscious or • Less than normal movements	POSSIBLE SERIOUS BACTERIAL INFECTION	➤ *Give first dose of intramuscular ampicillin and gentamicin.* ➤ *Treat to prevent low blood sugar.* ➤ *Warm the young infant by Skin to Skin contact if temperature less than 36.5°C (or feels cold to touch) while arranging referral.* ➤ *Advise mother how to keep the young infant warm on the way to the hospital.* ➤ *Refer URGENTLY to hospital#*
• Umbilicus red or draining pus or • Pus discharge from ear or • <10 skin pustules.	LOCAL BACTERIAL INFECTION	➤ *Give oral co-trimoxazole or amoxicillin for 5 days.* ➤ Teach mother to treat local infections at home. ➤ Follow-up in 2 days.
And if the infant has jaundice: • Palms and soles yellow or • Age < 24 hours or • Age 14 days or more	SEVERE JAUNDICE	➤ *Treat to prevent low blood sugar.* ➤ *Warm the young infant by Skin to Skin contact if temperature less than 36.5°C (or feels cold to touch) while arranging referral.* ➤ *Advise mother how to keep the young infant warm on the way to the hospital.* ➤ *Refer URGENTLY to hospital*
• Palms and soles not yellow	JAUNDICE	➤ Advise mother to give home care for the young infant. ➤ Advise mother when to return immediately. ➤ Follow-up in 2 days.
And if the temp. is between 35.5–36.4°C: • Temperature between 35.5 - 36.4°C	LOW BODY TEMPERATURE	➤ Warm the young infant using Skin to Skin contact for one hour and REASSESS. ➤ Treat to prevent low blood sugar.

\# *If referral is not possible, see the section **Where Referral is Not Possible** in the module **Treat the Young Infant and Counsel the Mother.***

Contd...

Contd...

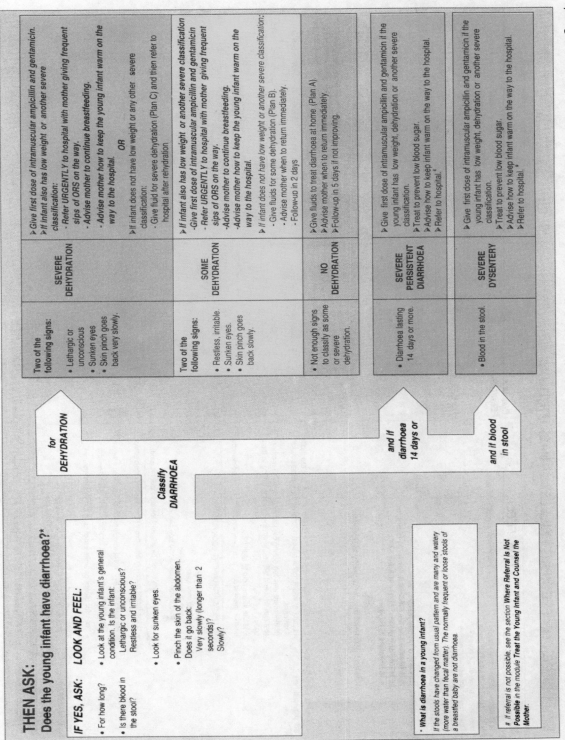

THEN ASK:
Does the young infant have diarrhoea? *

IF YES, ASK: **LOOK AND FEEL:**

- For how long?
- Is there blood in the stool?

- Look at the young infant's general condition. Is the infant:
  Lethargic or unconscious?
  Restless and irritable?

- Look for sunken eyes.

- Pinch the skin of the abdomen. Does it go back:
  Very slowly (longer than 2 seconds)?
  Slowly?

Classify
DIARRHOEA

for
DEHYDRATION

Two of the following signs: • Lethargic or unconscious • Sunken eyes • Skin pinch goes back very slowly.	**SEVERE DEHYDRATION**	➤ Give first dose of intramuscular ampicillin and gentamicin. ➤ If infant also has low weight or another severe classification: - Refer URGENTLY to hospital with mother giving frequent sips of ORS on the way. - *Advise mother to continue breastfeeding.* - *Advise mother how to keep the young infant warm on the way to the hospital.* **OR** ➤ If infant does not have low weight or any other severe classification: - Give fluid for severe dehydration (Plan C) and then refer to hospital after rehydration
Two of the following signs: • Restless, irritable. • Sunken eyes. • Skin pinch goes back slowly.	**SOME DEHYDRATION**	➤ *If infant also has low weight or another severe classification* -Give first dose of intramuscular ampicillin and gentamicin - Refer URGENTLY to hospital with mother giving frequent sips of ORS on the way. -Advise mother to continue breastfeeding. -Advise mother how to keep the young infant warm on the way to the hospital. ➤ If infant does not have low weight or another severe classification: - Give fluids for some dehydration (Plan B). - Advise mother when to return immediately. - Follow-up in 2 days
• Not enough signs to classify as some or severe dehydration.	**NO DEHYDRATION**	➤ Give fluids to treat diarrhoea at home (Plan A) ➤ Advise mother when to return immediately ➤ Follow-up in 5 days if not improving.

and if diarrhoea 14 days or

• Diarrhoea lasting 14 days or more.	**SEVERE PERSISTENT DIARRHOEA**	➤ Give first dose of intramuscular ampicillin and gentamicin if the young infant has low weight, dehydration or another severe classification. ➤ Treat to prevent low blood sugar. ➤ Advise how to keep infant warm on the way to the hospital.# ➤ Refer to hospital.#

and if blood in stool

• Blood in the stool.	**SEVERE DYSENTERY**	➤ Give first dose of intramuscular ampicillin and gentamicin if the young infant has low weight, dehydration or another severe classification. ➤ Treat to prevent low blood sugar. ➤ Advise how to keep infant warm on the way to the hospital.# ➤ Refer to hospital.#

* **What is diarrhoea in a young infant?**

If the stools have changed from usual pattern and are many and watery (more water than fecal matter). The normally frequent or loose stools of a breastfed baby are not diarrhoea.

If referral is not possible, see the section *Where Referral Is Not Possible* in the module *Treat the Young Infant and Counsel the Mother.*

Contd...

Contd...

THEN CHECK FOR FEEDING PROBLEM & MALNUTRITION:

ASK:

- Is there any difficulty feeding?
- Is the infant breastfed? If yes, how many times in 24 hours?
- Does the infant usually receive any other foods or drinks? If yes, how often?
- What do you use to feed the infant?

IF AN INFANT: Has any difficulty feeding, or
Is breastfeeding less than 8 times in 24 hours, or
Is taking any other foods or drinks, or
Is low weight for age,
AND
Has no Indications to refer urgently to hospital:

ASSESS BREASTFEEDING:

- Has the infant breastfed in the previous hour?

  If the infant has not fed in the previous hour, ask the mother to put her infant to the breast. Observe the breastfeed for 4 minutes.
  (If the infant was fed during the last hour, ask the mother if she can wait and tell you when the infant is willing to feed again.)

  - Is the infant able to attach?
    no attachment at all   not well attached   good attachment

    TO CHECK ATTACHMENT, LOOK FOR:
    - Chin touching breast
    - Mouth wide open
    - Lower lip turned outward
    - More areola visible above than below the mouth

    (All of these signs should be present if the attachment is good)

  - Is the infant suckling effectively (that is, slow deep sucks, not suckling at all   not suckling effectively   suckling effectively

    Clear a blocked nose if it interferes with breastfeeding.

  - Look for ulcers or white patches in the mouth (thrush).

- Does the mother have pain while breastfeeding? If yes, look and feel for:
  - Flat or inverted nipples, or sore nipples
  - Engorged breasts or breast abscess

LOOK, FEEL:

- Determine weight for age.

Classify FEEDING

Signs	Classify as	Treatment
• Not able to feed or • No attachment at all or • Not suckling at all or • Very low weight for age.	NOT ABLE TO FEED - POSSIBLE SERIOUS BACTERIAL INFECTION OR SEVERE MALNUTRITION	➤ Give first dose of intramuscular ampicillin and gentamicin. ➤ Treat to prevent low blood sugar. ➤ *Warm the young infant by skin to skin contact if temperature less than 36.5°C (or feels cold to touch) while arranging referral.* ➤ *Advise mother how to keep the young infant warm on the way to the hospital.* ➤ *Refer URGENTLY to hospital"*
• Not well attached to breast or • Not suckling effectively or • Less than 8 breastfeeds in 24 hours or • Receives other foods or drinks or • Thrush (ulcers or white patches in mouth) or • Low weight for age or	FEEDING PROBLEM OR LOW WEIGHT	➤ If not well attached or not suckling effectively, teach correct positioning and attachment. ➤ If breastfeeding less than 8 times in 24 hours, advise to increase frequency of feeding. ➤ If receiving other foods or drinks, counsel mother about breastfeeding more, reducing other foods or drinks, and using a cup and spoon. • If not breastfeeding at all, advise mother about giving locally appropriate animal milk and teach the mother to feed with a cup and spoon. ➤If thrush, teach the mother to treat thrush at home. ➤ If low weight for age, teach the mother how to keep the young infant with low weight warm at home. ➤If breast or nipple problem, teach the mother to treat breast or nipple problems. ➤Advise mother to give home care for the young infant. ➤ Advise mother when to return immediately. ➤Follow-up any feeding problem or thrush in 2 days. ➤Follow-up low weight for age in 14 days.
• Not low weight for age and no other signs of inadequate feeding.	NO FEEDING PROBLEM	➤Advise mother to give home care for the young infant. ➤Advise mother when to return immediately. ➤Praise the mother for feeding the infant well.

If referral is not possible, see the section *Where Referral Is Not Possible in the module Treat the Young Infant and Counsel the Mother.*

Contd...

Contd...

Contd...

ASSESS AND CLASSIFY THE SICK CHILD
AGE 2 MONTHS UP TO 5 YEARS

ASSESS   CLASSIFY   IDENTIFY TREATMENT

ASSESS

ASK THE MOTHER WHAT THE CHILD'S PROBLEMS ARE

- Determine if this is an initial or follow-up visit for this problem.
  - if follow-up visit, use the follow-up instructions on *TREAT THE CHILD* chart.
  - if initial visit, assess the child as follows:

CHECK FOR GENERAL DANGER SIGNS

ASK:
- Is the child able to drink or breastfeed?
- Does the child vomit everything?
- Has the child had convulsions?

LOOK:
- See if the child is lethargic or unconscious

A child with any general danger sign needs *URGENT* attention; complete the assessment and any pre-referral treatment immediately so referral is not delayed.

THEN ASK ABOUT MAIN SYMPTOMS:
Does the child have cough or difficult breathing?

IF YES, ASK:
- For how long?

LOOK, LISTEN:
- Count the breaths in one minute.
- Look for chest indrawing
- Look and listen for stridor

} CHILD MUST BE CALM

Classify COUGH or DIFFICULT BREATHING

If the child is:	Fast breathing is:
2 months up to 12 months	50 breaths per minute or more
12 months up to 5 years	40 breaths per minute or more

USE ALL BOXES THAT MATCH THE CHILD'S SYMPTOMS AND PROBLEMS TO CLASSIFY THE ILLNESS.

SIGNS	CLASSIFY AS	IDENTIFY TREATMENT (Urgent pre-referral treatments are in bold print.)
• Any general danger sign or • Chest indrawing or • Stridor in calm child.	SEVERE PNEUMONIA OR VERY SEVERE DISEASE	➤ **Give first dose of injectable chloramphenicol** *(If not possible give oral amoxycillin).* ➤ **Refer *URGENTLY* to hospital.#**
• Fast breathing.	PNEUMONIA	➤ Give *Cotrimoxazole for 5 days.* ➤ Soothe the throat and relieve the cough with a safe remedy if child is 6 months or older. ➤ Advise mother when to return immediately. ➤ Follow-up in 2 days.
• No signs of pneumonia or very severe disease.	NO PNEUMONIA: COUGH OR COLD	➤ If coughing more than 30 days, refer for assessment. ➤ Soothe the throat and relieve the cough with a safe home remedy if child is 6 months or older. ➤ Advise mother when to return immediately. ➤ Follow-up in 5 days if not improving.

If referral is not possible, *see the section Where Referral is Not Possible in the module Treat the Child.*

Contd...

Does the child have diarrhoea?

IF YES, ASK: LOOK AND FEEL:

- For how long?
- Is there blood in the stool?

- Look at the child's general condition. Is the child:
  - Lethargic or unconscious?
- Look for sunken eyes.
- Offer the child fluid.
  - Not able to drink or drinking poorly?
  - Drinking eagerly, thirsty?
- Pinch the skin of the abdomen.
  - Very slowly (longer than 2 seconds)?
  - Slowly?

Classify DIARRHOEA

	Signs	Classify as	Treatment
for DEHYDRATION	Two of the following signs: • Lethargic or unconscious • Sunken eyes • Not able to drink or drinking poorly • Skin pinch goes back	**SEVERE DEHYDRATION**	➤ If child has no other severe classification: - Give fluid for severe dehydration (Plan C). ➤ *If child also has another severe classification : Refer URGENTLY to hospital.# With mother giving frequent sips of ORS on the way. Advise the mother to continue breastfeeding.* ➤ *If child is 2 years or older and there is cholera in your area, give doxycycline for cholera.*
	Two of the following signs: • Restless, irritable • Sunken eyes • Drinks eagerly, thirsty • Skin pinch goes back	**SOME DEHYDRATION**	➤ Give fluid and food for some dehydration (Plan B). ➤ *If child also has a severe classification: Refer URGENTLY to hospital# with mother giving frequent sips of ORS on the way. Advise the mother to continue breastfeeding.* ➤ Advise mother when to return immediately. ➤ Follow-up in 5 days if not improving.
	Not enough signs to classify as some or severe dehydration.	**NO DEHYDRATION**	➤ Give fluid and food to treat diarrhoea at home (Plan A). ➤ Advise mother when to return immediately. ➤ Follow-up in 5 days if not improving.
and if diarrhoea 14 days or more	• Dehydration present.	**SEVERE PERSISTENT DIARRHOEA**	➤ Treat dehydration before referral unless the child has another severe classification. ➤ Refer to hospital.#
	• No dehydration.	**PERSISTENT DIARRHOEA**	➤ Advise the mother on feeding a child who has PERSISTENT DIARRHOEA. ➤ Give single dose of vitamin A. ➤ Give zinc sulphate 20 mg daily for 14 days. ➤ Follow-up in 5 days.
and if blood in stool	• Blood in the stool.	**DYSENTERY**	➤ *Treat for 5 days with cotrimoxazole.* ➤ Follow-up in 2 days.

If referral is not possible, see the section *Where Referral Is Not Possible* in the module *Treat the Child.*

Contd...

Contd...

Does the child have fever?
(by history or feels hot or temperature 37.5°C or above)

IF YES:
Decide Malaria Risk: High Low

THEN ASK:	LOOK AND FEEL:
• Fever for how long?	• Look or feel for stiff neck.
• If more than 7 days, has fever been present every day?	• Look and feel for bulging fontanelle.
• Has the child had measles within the last 3 months?	• Look for runny nose.
	Look for signs of MEASLES
	• Generalized rash and
	• One of these: cough, runny nose, or red eyes.

If the child has measles now or within the last 3 months:

• Look for mouth ulcers. Are they deep and extensive?

• Look for pus draining from the eye.

• Look for clouding of the cornea.

Classify FEVER

→ **High Malaria Risk**

HIGH MALARIA RISK

• Any general danger sign or • Stiff neck or • Bulging fontanelle.	**VERY SEVERE FEBRILE DISEASE**	➤ Give first dose of IM quinine after making a blood smear. ➤ Give first dose of IV or IM chloramphenicol (If not possible, give oral amoxycillin). ➤ Treat the child to prevent low blood sugar. ➤ Give one dose of paracetamol in clinic for high fever (temp. 38.5°C or above). ➤ Refer URGENTLY to hospital.#
• Fever (by history or feels hot or temperature 37.5°C or above).	**MALARIAL**	➤ Give oral antimalarials for HIGH malaria risk area after making a blood smear. ➤ Give one dose of paracetamol in clinic for high fever (temp. 38.5°C or above). ➤ Advise mother when to return immediately. ➤ Follow-up in 2 days if fever persists. ➤ If fever is present every day for more than 7 days, refer for assessment.

→ **Low Malaria Risk**

LOW MALARIA RISK

• Any general danger sign or • Stiff neck or • Bulging fontanelle.	**VERY SEVERE FEBRILE DISEASE**	➤ Give first dose of IM quinine after making a blood smear. ➤ Give first dose of IV or IM chloramphenicol (If not possible, give oral amoxycillin). ➤ Treat the child to prevent low blood sugar. ➤ Give one dose of paracetamol in clinic for high fever (temp. 38.5°C or above). ➤ Refer URGENTLY to hospital.#
• NO runny nose and NO measles and NO other cause of fever.	**MALARIA**	➤ Give oral antimalarials for LOW malaria risk area after making a blood smear. ➤ Give one dose of paracetamol in clinic for high fever (temp. 38.5°C or above). ➤ Advise mother when to return immediately. ➤ Follow-up in 2 days if fever persists. ➤ If fever is present every day for more than 7 days, refer for assessment.
• Runny nose PRESENT or • Measles PRESENT or • Other cause of fever PRESENT**	**FEVER - MALARIA UNLIKELY**	➤ Give one dose of paracetamol in clinic for high fever (temp.38.5°C or above). ➤ Advise mother when to return immediately. ➤ Follow-up in 2 days if fever persists. ➤ If fever is present every day for more than 7 days, refer for assessment.

→ **If MEASLES Now or within last 3 months, Classify**

• Any general danger sign or • Clouding of cornea or • Deep or extensive mouth ulcers.	**SEVERE COMPLICATED MEASLES#**	➤ Give first dose of Vitamin A. ➤ Give first dose of injectable chloramphenicol (If not possible give oral amoxycillin). ➤ If clouding of the cornea or pus draining from the eye, apply tetracycline eye ointment.## ➤ Refer URGENTLY to hospital.##
• Pus draining from the eye or • Mouth ulcers.	**MEASLES WITH EYE OR MOUTH COMPLICATIONS**	➤ Give first dose of Vitamin A. ➤ If pus draining from the eye, treat eye infection with tetracycline eye ointment. ➤ If mouth ulcers, treat with gentian violet. ➤ Follow-up in 2 days.
• Measles now or within the last 3 months.	**MEASLES**	➤ Give first dose of Vitamin A.

If referral is not possible, see the section **Where Referral is Not Possible** in the module

* This cutoff is for axillary temperatures; rectal temperature cutoff is approximately, 0.5°C higher.
** Other causes of fever include cough or cold, pneumonia, diarrhoea, dysentery and skin infections.
# Other important complications of measles - pneumonia, stridor, diarrhoea, ear infection, and malnutrition - are classified in other tables.

If referral is not possible, see the section **Where Referral is Not Possible** in the module **Treat the Child.**

Contd...

Contd...

Does the child have an ear problem?

IF YES, ASK: **LOOK AND FEEL:**

- Is there ear pain?
- Is there ear discharge?   • Look for pus draining from the ear.
- If yes, for how long?   • Feel for tender swelling behind the ear.

Classify EAR PROBLEM

Signs	Classification	Treatment
• Tender swelling behind the ear.	MASTOIDITIS	➢ Give first dose of injectable chloramphenicol (if not possible give oral amoxycillin). ➢ Give first dose of paracetamol for pain. ➢ Refer URGENTLY to hospital[#].
• Pus is seen draining from the ear and discharge is reported for less than 14 days, or • Ear pain.	ACUTE EAR INFECTION	➢ Give cotrimoxazole for 5 days. ➢ Give paracetamol for pain. ➢ Dry the ear by wicking. ➢ Follow-up in 5 days.
• Pus is seen draining from the ear and discharge is reported for 14 days or more.	CHRONIC EAR INFECTION	➢ Dry the ear by wicking. ➢ Follow-up in 5 days.
• No ear pain, and • No pus seen draining from the ear.	NO EAR INFECTION	No additional treatment.

*If referral is not possible, see the section **Where Referral Is Not Possible** in the module **Treat the Child**.*

Contd...

Contd...

THEN CHECK FOR MALNUTRITION

LOOK AND FEEL:

- Look for visible severe wasting.
- Look for oedema of both feet.

Classify NUTRITIONAL STATUS

• Visible severe wasting or • Oedema of both feet.	**SEVERE MALNUTRITION**	➤ Give single dose of Vitamin A. ➤ Prevent low blood sugar. ➤ Refer URGENTLY to hospital.# ➤ While referral is being organized, warm the child. ➤ Keep the child warm on the way to hospital.
• Very low weight for age.	**VERY LOW WEIGHT**	➤ Assess and counsel for feeding (If feeding problem, follow-up in 5 days) ➤ Advise mother when to return immediately ➤ Follow-up in 30 days.
• Not very low weight for age and no other signs of malnutrition.	**NOT VERY LOW WEIGHT**	➤ If child is less than 2 years old, assess the child's feeding and counsel the mother on feeding according to the FOOD box on the COUNSEL THE MOTHER chart. - If feeding problem, follow-up in 5 days. ➤ Advise mother when to return immediately.

THEN CHECK FOR ANAEMIA

LOOK:

- Look for palmar pallor. Is it:
Severe palmar pallor?

Classify ANAEMIA

• Severe palmar pallor	**SEVERE ANAEMIA**	➤ Refer URGENTLY to hospital.#
• Some palmar pallor	**ANAEMIA**	➤ Give iron folic acid therapy for 14 days. ➤ Assess the child's feeding and counsel the mother on feeding according to the FOOD box on the COUNSEL THE MOTHER chart. - If feeding problem, follow-up in 5 days. ➤ Advise mother when to return immediately. ➤ Follow-up in 14 days.
• No palmar pallor	**NO ANAEMIA**	➤ Give prophylactic iron folic acid if child 6 months or older.

THEN CHECK THE CHILD'S IMMUNIZATION *, PROPHYLACTIC VITAMIN A & IRON-FOLIC ACID SUPPLEMENTATION STATUS

IMMUNIZATION SCHEDULE:

AGE	VACCINE
Birth	BCG + OPV-0
6 weeks	DPT-1+ OPV-1(+ HepB-1**)
10 weeks	DPT-2+ OPV-2(+ HepB-2**)
14 weeks	DPT-3+ OPV-3(+ HepB-3**)
9 months	Measles + Vitamin A
16-18 months	DPT Booster + OPV + Vitamin A
60 months	DT

PROPHYLACTIC VITAMIN A
Give a single dose of vitamin A:
100,000 IU at 9 months with measles immunization
200,000 IU at 16-18 months with DPT Booster
200,000 IU at 24 months
200,000 IU at 30 months
200,000 IU at 36 months

PROPHYLACTIC IFA

Give 20 mg elemental iron +100 mcg folic acid (one tablet of pediatric IFA or 5 ml of IFA syrup or 1 ml of IFA drops) for a total of 100 days in a year after the child has recovered from acute illness if:
➤ The child 6 months of age or older, and
➤Has not received Pediatric IFA tablet/syrup/drops for 100 days in last one year

* A child who needs to be immunized should be advised to go for immunization the day vaccines are available at AW/SC/PHC
** Hepatitis B to be given wherever included in the immunization schedule

ASSESS OTHER PROBLEMS

MAKE SURE CHILD WITH ANY GENERAL DANGER SIGN IS REFERRED after first dose of an appropriate antibiotic and other urgent treatments.
Exception: Rehydration of the child according to Plan C may resolve danger signs so that referral is no longer needed.

If referral is not possible, see the section *Where Referral Is Not Possible in the module Treat the Child.*

Suggested Reading

1. American Academy of Pediatrics, Neonate Resuscitation Guidelines 2005, 2010.
2. Banerjee SR. Community and Social Pediatrics, Jaypee Brothers Medical Publishers (P) Ltd, New Delhi, 2008.
3. Basavanthappa BT. Community Health Nursing, Jaypee Brothers Medical Publishers (P) Ltd, New Delhi, 2008.
4. Behrman RE, et al. Nelson's Essentials of Pediatrics, 18th edition, WB Saunders Company: Philadelphia, 2008.
5. Birpuri SS. Principles and Practice of Nursing, Jaypee Brothers Medical Publishers (P) Ltd, New Delhi.
6. Cloherty JP, et al. Manual of Neonatal Care, 6th edition, 2010. Wolters Kluwer Lippincott Williams and Wilkins, New Delhi, Philadelphia, 2010.
7. Das Gupta S. Nursing Interventions for the Critically Ill. Jaypee Brothers Medical Publishers (P) Ltd, New Delhi, 2005.
8. Das PC. Textbook of Medicine, Current Books International, Kolkata, 2005.
9. Datta S. Principles and Practice of Nursing, West Bengal Nursing Council and TNAI, (West Bengal), Academic Publishers, Kolkata, 2003.
10. Dawn CS. Textbook of Obstetrics and Neonatology. Dawn Books. Kolkata, 2005.
11. Deorari AK, Paul VK. Neonatal Equipment: Everything that you would like to know, Sagar Publications, New Delhi, 2010.
12. Desai AB. Achar's Textbook of Pediatrics. Orient Longman: Hyderabad.
13. Drug Today Lorina Publications (India) INC. Delhi, 2013.
14. Dutta DC. Textbook of Obstetrics Including Perinatology and Contraception. New Central Book Agency (P) Ltd; Kolkata, 2009.
15. Facility Based IMNCI (F-IMNCI) Participants Manual Ministry of Health and Family Welfare, Govt. of India, 2009.
16. Facility based Newborn Care. Operational guide Ministry of Health and Family Welfare, Govt. of India, 2011.
17. Ghai OP. Essential Pediatrics. CBS Publishers and Distributors: New Delhi, 2009.
18. Glomella TL. Neonatology, 6th edition, McGraw Hill Companies, New York, 2009.
19. Golwalla AF. Handbook of Emergencies, Kothari Medical Publishing House: Mumbai.
20. Govt of India, Ministry of Health and Family Welfare, National Child Survival and Safe Motherhood Program, Modules for Health Workers, New Delhi.
21. Govt. of India, Ministry of Health and Family Welfare, HIV/AIDS, Prevention, Care and Control, Self Instructional Module, National AIDS Control Organization: New Delhi.
22. Government of India, National Institute of Health and Family Welfare, Reproductive and Child Health, Module for Health Worker (female) and Health Assistant (female).
23. Govt. of West Bengal, Dept. of Health and Family Welfare, Module for Clinical Training-Pediatric Nursing: Kolkata.
24. Govt. of West Bengal, Ministry of Health and Family Welfare, Swasthya Kalyan: Kolkata.
25. Great JW. Manual of Pediatric Therapeutics, Little Brown Company, Boston.
26. Guha DK. Neonatology: Principles and Practices. Jaypee Brothers Medical Publishers (P) Ltd, New Delhi, 2005.
27. Guha DK. Manual of Newborn Critical Care Medicine, Jaypee Brothers Medical Publishers (P) Ltd, New Delhi, 2006.
28. Guha DK. Practical Newborn Critical Care Nursing. Jaypee Brothers Medical Publishers (P) Ltd, New Delhi, 2006.
29. Gulani KK. Community Health Nursing. Principles and Practices. Kumar Publishing House, Delhi, 2005.

30. Gupta MC, Mahajan BK. Textbook of Preventive and Social Medicine. Jaypee Brothers Medical Publishers (P) Ltd, New Delhi, 2013.
31. Gupta Piyush. Essential Pediatric Nursing, 2nd edition, New Delhi, CBS Publishers and Distributors, 2007.
32. Gupta Suraj. The Short Textbook of Pediatrics. Jaypee Brothers Medical Publishers (P) Ltd, New Delhi.
33. Indian Public Health Association, Indian Journal of Public Health, IPHA, Kolkata.
34. Jogi Renu. Basic Pediatrics, Ajit Publications: New Delhi.
35. Kliegman RM, et al. Nelson's Textbook of Pediatrics, 18th edition, New Delhi, Saunders Elsevier, Philadelphia, Indian edition, 2008.
36. Kulshrestha R, Chellani H. Clinical Handbook of Surgical Pediatrics. Book from Child Care Series: New Delhi.
37. Kulshrestha R. Common Problems in Pediatric Surgery. Book from Child Care Series: New Delhi.
38. Marlow DR, Redding BA. Textbook of Pediatric Nursing. WB Saunder Company: Philadelphia.
39. National Institute of Cholera and Enteric Diseases, Module for Training of Diarrheal Diseases and Program Implementation: Kolkata.
40. National Neonatology Forum, Chronicle - NNF: New Delhi.
41. National Neonatology Forum, Resource Book 1 and 2, Care of the Normal and Sick Neonate.
42. Neonatal Resuscitation, Textbook of American Heart Association, American Academy of Pediatric, Jaypee Brothers Medical Publishers, New Delhi, 6th edition, 2012.
43. Nettina SM. The Lippincott Manual of Nursing Practice, (South Asia Edition), Lippincott: Philadelphia, 2010.
44. Park K. Community Health Nursing, 20th edition, M/S Banarsidas Bhanot Publishers, Jabalpur, 2009.
45. Park K. Park's Textbook of Preventive and Social Medicine, M/S Banarsidas Bhanot Publishers, Jabalpur.
46. Prakasamma M. The Indian Journal of Nursing and Midwifery: Hyderabad.
47. Singh Meharban. Care of the Newborn. Sagar Publications: New Delhi, 2010.
48. Singh Meharban. Drug Dosages in Children. Sagar Publications: New Delhi, 2008.
49. Singh Meharban. Essential Pediatrics for Nurses. Sagar Publications: New Delhi, 2006.
50. Singh Meharban. Medical Emergencies in Children. Sagar Publications: New Delhi, 2004.
51. Singh Meharban. The Art and Science of Baby and Child Care. Sagar Publications, New Delhi.
52. Singh Meharban. Pediatric Clinical Method Sagar Publications: New Delhi.
53. Smeltzer SC, Bare BG. Brunner's Textbook of Medical and Surgical Nursing, Lippincott: Philadelphia.
54. Taber's Cyclopedic Medical Dictionary, Jaypee Brothers Medical Publishers (P) Ltd, New Delhi, 2010.
55. Tambulwadkar RS. Pediatric Nursing, Vora Medical Publications: Mumbai.
56. Tom Lissauer, Avroy Fanaroff. Neonatology at a glance. Blackwell Publishing, Ist edition, 2006, Massachusetts.
57. Trained Nurses Association of India, Nursing Journals of India, TNAI: New Delhi.
58. Udani PM. Textbook of Pediatrics. Jaypee Brothers Medical Publishers (P) Ltd, New Delhi.
59. Waechter EH, et al. Nursing Care of Children. JB Lippincott Company: Philadelphia.
60. Wagle CS. Principles and Practice of Clinical Pediatrics. Vora Book Centre: Mumbai.
61. Watson J. Nurses Manual of Laboratory and Diagnostic Tests. Jaypee Brothers Medical Publishers (P) Ltd, New Delhi.
62. West Bengal Nursing Council, Nursing Theories and practices, volume - I and II, WBNC: Kolkata, 2000.
63. WHO Mother-Baby package, Implementing Safe Motherhood in countries.
64. WHO Safe Motherhood, Newsletter of worldwide activity.
65. Wong DL, et al,. Nursing Care of Infants and Children, 8th edition, Mosby, St Louise, ASZ, 2009.
66. Wong DL, et al,. Wong's Essential of Pediatric Nursing, 8th edition, Mosby: St. Louise, 2009.
67. Wong, Whaley's. Clinical Manual of Pediatric Nursing, Mosby; St. Louise, 2008.
68. www.nebi.nlm.nih.gov.pubmed
69. www.newbornwhocc.org
70. www.savethechildren.org

Index

Page numbers followed by *f* refer to figure and *t* refer to table.

A

Abdominal
  colic 178
  distension 166
    management 167
  pain 166
    causes of 166
    management 166
    with uncertain mechanism 287
Accidents and safety precautions, prevention of 132
Acid-base
  balance 209
  disturbances 208
  imbalance 213
  status 454
Acquired
  hydrocephalus 382
  intestinal obstruction 285
Actual hepatomegaly 297
Acute
  abdomen 287
    causes of 287
    diagnosis 287
    management 288
  glomerulonephritis 342
    complications 342
    etiology 342
    management 342
  lymphocytic leukemia 329
    chemotherapy 330
    complications 330
    management 330, 331
  nonlymphocytic leukemia 331
  otitis media 412
  renal failure 346
    diuretic phase 348
    etiology 346
    management 348
    oliguric phase 348
    phases of 346
    recovery phase 348
  respiratory infections 259, 262
    classification 260
    complications 261
    definition 259
    diagnostic measures 261

    management 261
  nursing
    assessment 261
    diagnosis 261
    interventions 261
    management 261
    preventive measures 262
    prognosis 261
  rheumatic fever 311
    complications 313
    prognosis 313
  sinusitis 415
  subdural hematoma 387
Adaptation in nursing care, strategies for 141
Adequacy of breastfeeding, indicators of 52
Administration of
  drugs, safety measures in 151
  oxygen, safety precautions during 154
Adolescence *See* Puberty, changes in
Adolescence, behavioral problems of 182
Adolescent
  problems 175
    classification 175
    developmental disorders 175
  reactions of 139
Adrenal glands, disorders of 396
Age for toilet training 128
Allergic reactions, types of 167
Allergies 167
  management of 168
Altered consciousness, stages of 363
Ambiguous genitalia 397
  management 397
Amebic
  dysentery 279
  liver abscess 298
Anal
  agenesis 292, 292*f*
  stenosis 292, 292*f*
Ancylostomiasis *See* Hook worms
Anemia 318
  causes of 319
  classification of 319
  clinical grading of 319
  complications 320
  management 320
  nursing management 320

Anencephaly 381
Anorectal malformations 291, 292*f*
  classification of 291
  complications 293
  diagnosis 292
  management 293
Anorexia nervosa 184
Antisera 37
Antitoxins *See* Antisera
Anti-tuberculosis antibiotics 479
Aorta, coarctation of 308, 308*f*
Aortic
  regurgitation 314
  stenosis 308
Apgar scoring 66*t*
Aplastic anemia 323
Apparent hepatomegaly 297
Appendicitis 288
  complications 288
  diagnosis 288
  management 288
  pathophysiology 288
Arthritis management 436
Artificial feeding 57
  principles of 57
Ascariasis *See* Round worms
Ascorbic acid deficiency *See* Vitamin C
Asphyxia
  neonatorum *See* Birth asphyxia
  pathophysiology of 77
Astigmatism 409
Atelectasis 265
  complications 265
  diagnosis 265
  management 265
  prognosis 265
Atonic cerebral palsy 375
Atrial septal defect 304, 304*f*
Attention deficit disorders 182

B

Baby friendly hospital initiative 24
Bacillary dysentery 278
Bacterial meningitis *See* Pyogenic meningitis
Bag mask ventilation 80*f*

Balanced diet
  for adolescents 59*t*
  for children 59, 59*t*
Ballard *See* Gestational age assessment
Basic care of baby birth 447
BCG vaccination 38
Bed wetting *See* Enuresis
Behavioral disorders
  causes of 177
  faulty parental attitude 177
  in children 177
    introduction 177
  inadequate family environment 177
  influence of
    mass media 178
    social
      change 178
      relationship 178
  mentally sick and physically sick 178
  of children, nursing responsibilities in
    184
Belt restraints 147*f*
Birth asphyxia 76, 78, 81
  bag 79
  chest compression 80
  definition 77
  endotracheal intubation 81
  initial steps of resuscitation 79
  of perinatal asphyxia 77
  preparation for resuscitation 78
  TABCs of resuscitation 78
Birth injuries 93
Bites and stings 170
Bladder management, exstrophy of 339
Bleeding disorders 332
Blindness 410
Blood
  disorders 191
  examination 342
  specimens, collection of 151
Body
  build
    ectomorph 117
    endomorph 117
    mesomorph 117
    types of 117
  fluids 208
  preparation from birth to adolescence
    117*f*
  surface area burnt by rule of five,
    estimation of 355*f*
Bone
  disorders of 425
  marrow transplantation 326
  tumor 433
    osteosarcoma 433
Bowed leg 76, 428*f*
Bowleg *See* Genu varus

Brain
  concussion of 387
  swelling 387
  tumors 385
    management 386
Brainstem glioma 385
Breast milk
  colostrum, different composition of 52
  expression of 55*f*
Breast, anatomy of 52*f*
Breastfeeding 50
  advantages of 50
  baby who
    does not suckle, problems of 54
    refused on breast, problems of 55
  breast
    abscess, problems of 55
    engorgement, problems of 55
  contraindications of 54
  digestibility, advantages of 51
  family, advantages of 51
  initiation of 51
  inverted nipples, problems of 55
  maternal benefits, advantages of 51
  nutritive value, advantages of 50
  preparation for 51
  problems of 54
  protective value, advantages of 51
  psychological benefits, advantages of 51
  sore nipple, problems of 55
  technique of 53
  working mother, problems of 55
Breath-holding spell 179
Bronchial asthma 267
  classification 268
  complications 269
  diagnosis 269
  etiological factors 267
  management 269
  status asthmaticus 269
Bronchiectasis 262
  complications 264
  diagnosis 264
  management 264
Buckle 430*f*
Burn injury
  depth of 353
  extent of 354
  severity of 354
Burns
  disease 352
  in children 352
    classification of 353
    complications 357
    first aid measures 355
    fluid replacement 356
    management 355
    nutritional support 356

    rehabilitation 357
    wound management 356
  surface area, estimation of 354

C

Calcium 205
  deficiency 205
  prevention 205
  sources 205
Candidiasis 358
Caput succedaneum 93*f*
Carbohydrate malabsorption 279
Cardiomyopathy
  in children 316
    definition 316
    secondary 317
    therapeutic management 317
  types of 316
Cardiopulmonary resuscitation, basic life
    support maneuvers of 459
Central nervous system
  defects 189
  diseases of 362
  introduction, diseases of 362
Cephalhematoma 93*f*
  minor problems of 75
Cerebellar
  astrocytoma 385
  concussion *See* Brain, concussion o*f*
  contusion 387
  involvement *See* Atonic cerebral palsy
  palsy 374
    classification of 374
    etiology 374
    management 375
    prevention of 375
    types 374, 375
Cerebrospinal fluid constituents 456
Chemical buffer system of body 209
Chemoprophylaxis 480
Chemotherapy 277
Chest
  circumference, measurement of 120*f*
  compression 80*f*
Child
  abuse 34
  adoption 443
    procedures 443
  approach to 152
  care, guidance to parent for 134
  development 113
  education 10
  from accidents in hospitals, protection of
    145
  growth 113
  guidance clinic 442

health 10
    care in India 9
    care, trends in 3
    concept of 1
    factors affecting 1
    in India 8
    problems 5, 5f
immunization, nursing responsibilities
        for 44
in coma 362
    immediate management 363
    management 363
    pathology 362
    specific management 364
in disaster 5f
labor 31, 443
marriage, prohibition of 444
mortality rate See Under-five mortality
        rate
neglect 34
of rich family 2f
placement 442
reaction to hospitalization and prolonged
        illness 138
rights of 9
survival components 24
undergoes dialysis
        care of 350
        methods, care of 351
welfare
    agencies 441
    services 441
with anemia, nursing process for 321
with ARI, nursing process of 263
with colostomy, care of 290
with fever, management of 163
with leukemia 331
with nephrotic syndrome 345f
        nursing process of 347
Childhood
    behavioral problems of 179
    blood dyscrasias 318
        introduction 318
    cataract 408
Children
    Act 11
    approach to child, physical examination
            of 143
    general principles, physical examination
            of 143
    in difficult circumstances 444
    in need for support services 4f
    in refugee camp 5f
    preoperative nursing management
            of 159
    undergoing surgery
        physical preparation 160
        protective measures 160

undergoing surgery
    care of 159
    psychological preparation 160
with normal physique, weight in 452
Cholera vaccine 42
Chromosomal abnormalities 191
Chronic
    glomerulonephritis 343
        management 344
    myelocytic leukemia 331
    renal failure 349
        complications 350
        etiology 349
        management 350
    sinusitis 415
    suppurative otitis media 413
Cleft lip 189f, 420, 421
    palate complications 421
    palate complications long-term
            problems 421
    palate complications problems 421
    types of 421
Cleft palate 189f, 420, 421
    causes 421
    complications 421
        long-term problems 421
        problems 421
    types of 421
Club foot 427f
Cold
    boxes 44
    chain 43
        equipment 43
Coma
    causes of 363
    grades of 363
Combined DPT-HB
    HIB vaccines 42
    vaccines 42
Common
    accidental injury in different age
            groups 132
    bacterial infections 232
    behavioral problems in children 178
    brain tumors 385
    neonatal medical problems 472
    ophthalmic problems, categorization
            of 406
    skin diseases in children 358
        acne 360
            management 360
        atopic dermatitis 360
            management 361
        psoriasis 360
        scabies 358
            management 358
    types of fracture in children 430
    viral infections 217

chickenpox 224, 225
    complications 225
    diagnosis 225
    epidemiology 224
    management 225
    pathology 225
    preventive measures 226
    prognosis 226
dengue syndrome 227
    epidemiology 227
hepatitis A 222
    epidemiology 222
    investigations 222
    management 222
    pathology 222
    preventive measures 223
hepatitis B 223
    epidemiology 223
    investigations 223
    management 224
    preventive measures 224
measles 217
    complications 218
    epidemiology 217
    investigations 218
    management 218
    pathological changes 218
    preventive measures 219
    prognosis 219
mumps 226
    complications 226
    diagnosis 227
    epidemiology 226
    management 227
    pathology 226
    preventive measures 227
poliomyelitis 219
    complications 221
    diagnosis 220
    epidemiology 219
    management 220
    pathology 219
    preventive measures 221
    prognosis 221
viral hepatitis 222, 224
Communicable diseases
    in children 217
        introduction 217
    prevention of 29
Communicating hydrocephalus 382
Community
    benefits, advantages of 51
    nutrition programs 207
Complementary feeding 56
    different age 56
        12 to 18 months 57
        6 months 56
        6 to 9 months 57
        9 to 12 months 57
    qualities of 56

Congenital
adrenal hyperplasia 396
management 396
anomalies 185, 188
concepts of 185
definitions, concepts of 185
etiology of 186
genetic factors
chromosomal abnormalities,
etiology of 186
etiology of 186
polygenic, etiology of 187
single gene disorders, etiology
of 186
incidence, concepts of 185
miscellaneous 191
nursing responsibilities towards 192
prevention of 191
preventive measures, prevention of
191
club foot 426
complications 428
diagnostic evaluation 427
etiology 427
incidence 427
management 427
diaphragmatic hernia 295
heart disease 190, 303
classification 303
etiology 303
hemolytic anemia 323
hydrocele 76
hydrocephalus 382
intestinal obstruction 285
nasolacrimal duct obstruction 407
nephrotic syndrome 344
Congestive cardiac failure 310
etiology 310
management 311
prognosis 311
Congestive cardiomyopathy 316
Conjoined twin 190f
Conjunctiva, diseases of 406
Conjunctivitis 408
Constipation 165
causes of 165
nonorganic, causes of 165
organic causes, causes of 165
Constrictive cardiomyopathy 316
Convulsive disorders 370
in children, causes of 370
management of 373
Cooley's anemia 324
Copper 207
Corneal diseases 406
Craniocerebral trauma *See* Head injury
Croup's syndrome 418
acute
epiglottitis 419
laryngotracheobronchitis 418

Cry
assessment, excessive 164
treatment, excessive 165
types of 164
Cryptorchidism *See* Undescended testes
Cryptosporidiosis 253
CSF
circulation 382
pathways 382
Cultural influences 195
Cyanocobalamin 204
Cystic fibrosis 272
complications 272
diagnostic evaluation 272
management 272
nursing management 272
prognosis 272

D

Dacryostenosis *See* Congenital nasolacrimal
duct obstruction
Day carriers 44
Deafness *See* Hearing impairment
Decerebrate posture 363f
Decorticate posture 363f
Deep freezers 43
Dehydration 210
assessment of 210, 275t
management of 211
Delayed eruption of teeth 419
Delayed puberty *See* Delayed sexual
development
Delayed sexual development 399
amenorrhea 401
management 401
dysmenorrhea 400
etiology 399
management 400
menorrhagia 401
premenstrual syndrome 400
Delivery devices 458
Deltoid 153f
Dengue
fever 228
hemorrhagic fever 228
syndrome
complications 228
diagnosis 228
management 228
preventive measures 228
prognosis 228
Dental
caries 419
etiology 419
management 420
fluorosis 420
problems 30, 419
Dermatophytosis 359

Developmental
disorders short stature 174
milestones 124
important developmental milestones
at glance up to 3 years 126
infants 124
preschooler 125
school age 126
toddlers 125
Diabetes
insipidus 392
classification 392
complications 392
management 392
mellitus 402
classification 402
complications 403
etiopathogenesis 403
management 404
diet therapy 404
exercise and physical activity 404
insulin therapy 404
type I 402
type II 402
Diabetic
education 404
ketoacidosis, management of 404
Diagnosis of
convulsive disorders 373
tuberculosis 239
Diagnostic approaches 187
Diarrhea 165
secretory 274
types of 274
Diarrheal diseases 274
Diet therapy 373
Dietary management 277
Different congenital anomalies in still birth
baby 188f
Dilated cardiomyopathy 316
Diphtheria 232
complications 233
diagnosis 233
epidemiology 232
management 233
pathology 232
preventive measures 233
prognosis 233
Discharging criteria 110
Disease patterns in children 6
Disseminated intravascular coagulation 334
causes 334
complications 335
management 335
Distribution of total body water 208t
Dog bites 170
diagnosis 170
management 170
Domiciliary management 198

Double headed monster 189*f*
Down's syndrome 378
   management 379
   types 378
Downe's score interpretation 87*t*
DPT vaccination 39
Drowning
   and near-drowning 271
   management 272
Drug
   dosage, calculation of 151
   therapy 373
Dysentery 278
   complications 279
   epidemiology 278
   management 278
   pathology 278
   prognosis 279
Dysplasia 338
Dysraphism *See* Myelodysplasia

E

Ear problems in children 411
Echinococcosis *See* Hydatid disease
Ectopia vesicae *See* Exstrophy of bladder
Effective handwashing, steps of 148*f*
Electrolyte
   composition of body fluids 209, 209*t*
   daily maintenance requirements of 215*t*
   imbalance 211
      monitoring of 215
Emergency care 30
Emerging challenges in pediatric nursing 16
Emotional
   development 123
   support 404
Emphysema 264
   management 264
Empyema 266
   complications 266
   management 266
   prognosis 267
Encephalitis 368, 369
Encephalocele 381
Encephalopathies 368
   complications 369
   etiology 368
   management 369
Encopresis 180
Endocrinal abnormalities 191
Endocrine disorders in children 390
   introduction 390
Endogenous obesity 401
Enemas 158
ENT problem in children 406
Enteric fever *See* Typhoid fever
Enuresis 180

Environmental factors 187
Ependymoma 385
Epidemic parotitis *See* Common viral
     infections mumps
Epigastric hernia 295
Epilepsy 371
   classification of 371
   management of 373
   neonatal seizures 373
   partial seizures 372
   pathophysiology 371
Epispadias 339
   classification 339
   management 339
Epistaxis 416
Epstein pearl 76
Erb's palsy 95*f*
Erikson's psychosocial stage 123
Eruption of teeth 121*t*
   assessment of 120
Erythema toxicum 75
Esophageal atresia
   types of 482*f*
   with tracheoesophageal fistula 282
     classification 282
     diagnosis 283
     etiology 282
     management 283
     pathophysiology 282
Ewing's tumor 433
Excessive cry 163
   causes of 163
   emotional conditions, causes of 163
   management of 164
   nonpathological conditions,
     causes of 163
   pathological conditions, causes of 163
Exogenous obesity 401
Exomphalos 294
   complications 294
   management 294
Exstrophy of bladder 339
External ear
   dermatitis, problems of 411
   furunculosis, problems of 412
   otitis externa, problems of 411
   problems of 411
Extra-abdominal causes 287
Extradural hematoma 387
Extrahepatic biliary atresia 298
Extrapyramidal cerebral palsy 375
Eye
   diseases of 406
   health 30
   movement and alignment,
     diseases of 407
   problem in children 406
Eyelids, diseases of 406

F

Facial palsy, left 95*f*
Factors influencing
   development of child 114, 115
     genetic factors 114
     postnatal factors 115
     prenatal factors 115
   growth of child 114, 115
     genetic factors 114
     postnatal factors 115
     prenatal factors 115
Familial acholuric jaundice 323
Far sightedness 409
Febrile convulsions 371
   management 371
   type 371
Fecal ostomies, placement of 291*f*
Feeding
   gastrostomy, techniques of 156
   gavage, techniques of 156
   oral, techniques of 155
   problems 58
     dehydration fever 58
     excessive crying 58
     overfeeding 59
     regurgitation 58
     suckling and swallowing
      difficulties 58
     underfeeding 58
     vomiting 58
   resistance to 178
   techniques of 155
Female feticide 33
Femoral hernia 295
Fetal circulation 301
   before birth 302*f*
   birth, changes of 302*f*, 303
Fetal-infant growth chart for
     preterm infants 473
Fever 162
   in children
     causes of 162
     investigations 163
First aid 30
Floppy baby syndrome 424
   causes 424
Fluid
   daily maintenance requirements of 215*t*
   imbalance 210
   monitoring of 215
   requirements of lbw infants 106*f*
Fluorine 206
Folacin deficiency *See* Folic acid
Folates *See* Folic acid
Folic acid 204
   supplementations 326
Foot, abnormal position of 427*f*

Fore milk, different composition of 52
Foreign bodies 172
    in alimentary tract 172
    in external auditory canal 412
    in eyes 173
    in respiratory tract 172
        diagnosis 172
        emergency management 172
Fracture 429
    in children 430
        sites of 429
    of skull 386
Fragilitas ossium *See* Osteogenesis
    imperfecta
Free flow oxygen therapy 80*f*
Freud's psycho-sexual stages 123
Functional nutritional status,
    assessment of 60

G

Gastroesophageal reflux disease 284
    complications 285
    management 284
Gastrointestinal system
    abnormalities 190
    diseases of 273
    related to 287
Gastroschisis 189*f*, 294
Gender bias 32
General body growth 116
Genetic counseling 192
Genital growth 116
Genitourinary system abnormalities of 191
Genu
    valgum 428
    varus 428
Geophagia 181
Gestation age birth, assessment of 67*t*
Gestational age assessment 468
Giardiasis 251
    clinical manifestations 251
    diagnosis 251
    management 251
    pathology 251
    preventive measures 252
Girls, protection for 10
Goiter 394
Gomez classification 196
Great arteries, transposition of 307, 307*f*
Growth
    and development
        brain, systemic changes during 121
        cardiovascular changes, systemic
            changes during 121
        gastrointestinal system, systemic
            changes during 121
        hormonal changes, systemic changes
            during 122

immunity, systemic changes
        during 122
lymphoid tissue, systemic changes
        during 122
of child 113
    characteristics of 114
    definitions of terms 113
    development 113
    growth 113
    maturation 113
    postnatal period, stages of 114
    prenatal period, stages of 114
    stages of 114
respiratory changes, systemic
        changes during 121
sexual development, systemic
        changes during 122
systemic changes during 121
urinary system, systemic changes
        during 121
assessment by baby weighing 28*f*
assessment of 117
body mass index, assessment of 118
chart 28*f*
chest circumference, assessment of 120
curve 119*f*
dentition, assessment of 120
fontanelle closure, assessment of 120
head circumference, assessment of 118
hormone deficiency 391
length, assessment of 118
mid upper arm circumference,
    assessment of 120
of child, importance of learning 113
osseous, assessment of 120
span, assessment of 121
stem stature index, assessment of 121
technique of 117
weight, assessment of 117
Guillain-Barré syndrome 369
    management 370

H

Habit spasm *See* Tics
Haemophilus influenzae vaccines 41
Handicapped children 437
    and child welfare 437
    causes 438
    classification 438
        mentally handicapped children 438
        physically handicapped children 438
        socially handicapped children 438
    concept of disability 437
        impairment 437
    education of 30
    management of 439
    rehabilitation of 439

Handicapped conditions *See* Behavioral
    disorders mentally sick and
    physically sick
    in children, prevention of 438
Handicaps
    distribution of 374
    motor deficit of 374
Hansen's disease *See* Leprosy
Hare lip *See* Cleft lip
Harlequin color change 76
Head
    circumference, measurement of 119*f*
    injuries of 93, 386
    injury
        causes of 386
        complications 388
        emergency management 388
        management 388
        medical management 388
        pathology 386
        prognosis 389
        types of 386
Health
    appraisal 29
    education 30
    problems
        during childhood 162
        of newborn baby 73
    promotion during
        adolescence 136
        infancy 134
        preschool age 135
        school age 135
        toddlerhood 134
    promotion of children 134
Healthful school environment 29
Healthy
    adolescents in play 130*f*
    child 2*f*, 113
        of poor family 2*f*
        needs of 127
    girl children 33*f*
    infants of
        6 months age 2*f*
        7 months 125*f*
    mother 2*f*
    neonates 64*f*
        physical characteristics of 64
        physiological characteristics of 65
    newborn infant 64
    school children 126*f*
    toddler 125*f*
Hearing impairment 413
    causes of 413
    classification of 413
    consequence of 414
    management 414
    types 414
Heart diseases in children 301
    introduction 301

Height and weight of Indian boys and girls from 1 to 18 years 450
Height, assessment of 118
Helminthiasis *See* Worm infestations
Helminthic infestations, other 258
Hemodialysis, complications related to 351
Hemolytic disease of newborn 98
Hemophilia 327
    classification 327
    complications 329
    in children
        probability of 327*t*
        transmission of 327*t*
    management 328
    pathophysiology 327
Hepatitis
    A vaccines 42
    B vaccination 40
Hepatobiliary system, related to 287
Hepatomegaly 297
    causes of 297
    investigations 298
Hereditary spherocytosis 323
Hermaphroditism, types of 397
Hernia 294
    causes 294
    in children 295
Hiatal hernia 295
Hind milk, different composition of 52
Hip
    complications, developmental dysplasia of 426
    developmental dysplasia of 425
    etiology, developmental dysplasia of 425
    management, developmental dysplasia of 426
Hirschsprung's disease 289, 289*f*
    complications 290
    management 290
    nursing management 290
HIV/AIDS in children 229
    clinical staging 230
    complications 230
    epidemiology 229
    major criteria 230
    management 230
    minor criteria 230
    nursing interventions 231
    pathogenesis 229
HIV/AIDS, prevention of 231
Hook worms 255
    management 256
    preventive measures 256
Horse-shoe kidney 338
Hospital acquired infections 244
    causes in children 244
    common 245
    control measures 245
    mode of transmission 244

prevention 245
risk factors 244
Hospitalization
    of sick child 138
    on family of child, effects of 139
Hospitalized children, importance of play for 148
Humpback 428
Hunchback *See* Humpback
Hydatid disease 257
Hydrocephalus 381, 383*f*
    complications 384
    etiology of 382
    management 383
    types 382
Hydronephrosis 338
Hyperalimentation *See* Total parenteral nutrition
Hyperkalemia 213
    management 213
Hypermetropia *See* Far sightedness
Hypernatremia 212
    management 212
    etiology of 212
Hyperopia 409
Hypertrophic
    cardiomyopathy 316
    pyloric stenosis 281, 281*f*
        complications 281
        etiology 281
        management 281
        pathology 281
Hypokalemia 212
    etiology of 212
    management 212
Hyponatremia 211
    etiology of 211
    management 211
Hypoparathyroidism 395
    management 395
Hypospadias 340
    classification 340
    management 340
    problems related to 340
Hypothermia, prevention of 84*f*
Hypothyroidism, causes of 393

I

Ice
    lined refrigerators 44
    packs 44
Icterus *See* Jaundice
Identifying intrauterine growth retardation in newborn 467
Idiopathic nephrotic syndrome 345
Immune thrombocytopenic purpura 333
    classification of 333
    management 334

Immunization 36, 127
    introduction 36
    killed 37
    live attenuated vaccines 37
    of children 38
    of HIV positive children 232
    vaccine 36
        preventable diseases 36
Immunizing agents 36
Immunodeficiency 335
    states, presentations of 336
    types 335
        management 336
        primary immunodeficiency 335
        secondary immunodeficiency 336
Immunoglobulins 37
IMNCI
    case management process 474
    protocol 482
Impacted cerumen, wax 412
Impaired appetite *See* Feeding, resistance to
Impaired digestion 279
Imperforate anal membrane 292, 292*f*
Inactivated vaccines *See* Immunization killed
Inadequate health 195
Incompetence *See* Aortic regurgitation
Incompetence, mitral regurgitation 313
Increased intraocular pressure 407
Indian Academy of Pediatrics, classification by 196
Indian childhood cirrhosis 299
    diagnosis 300
    epidemiology 299
    etiology 299
    management 300
Indications of toddler's readiness for toilet training 128
Infancy, behavioral problems of 178
Infant mortality rate 7
Infantile spasms *See* Myoclonic seizures
Infants of
    diabetic mothers 110
    HIV positive mothers 111
        diagnosis 111
        prevention 111
        treatment 111
Infants, reactions of 139
Infections
    and disease conditions 195
    in neonates 88
Infective endocarditis 315
    complications 315
    management 315
    prevention 316
Infective polyneuritis *See* Guillain-Barré syndrome
Influenza vaccines 42

Ingredients of oral rehydration salts 276*t*
Inguinal hernia 295
Insects stings 171
    management 171
Insulin injection, sites for 153*f*
Integrated child development
    delivery of services 26
    services 25
        for adolescent girls 11 to 18 years 26
        for children
        in age group 3 to 6 years 26
        less than 3 years 26
        for nursing mothers 26
        for pregnant women 26
        objectives 25
        other women of 15 to 45 years age
            group 26
Integrated management of neonatal and
        childhood illness 31
Intestinal
    amebiasis 252
        complications 252
        diagnosis 252
        epidemiology 252
        management 253
        pathology 252
        preventive measures 253
    malabsorption 279
    obstruction 285
        causes of 285
        diagnosis 286
        initial management 286
        management 286
        pathology 286
Intracranial
    hemorrhage 386
    injuries to
        bones 95
        muscles 95
        nerves 94
        skin 95
    injury 93
    prevention of birth injuries 96
    space occupying lesions 385
    visceral injuries 96
Intramuscular injection in children, sites of
    153*f*
Intrarenal causes 346
Intrauterine growth retardation, high risk
    106
Intravenous infusion 157
    calculation of flow rates 157
    equipment and procedure 157
    preparation of parents and child 157
    veins used for intravenous infusion 157
Intussusception 286*f*
Iodine 206
Iron 206
    chelation therapy 325

deficiency anemia 320
    complications 320
    management 322
    prevention 322
IUGR baby at birth of 1800 g, 38 weeks 104*f*

J

Jacket restraints 147*f*
Japanese encephalitis vaccines 43
Jaundice 296
    in children, causes of 297
    investigations 297
    management 297
    pathological 96
    physiological 96
Joints, diseases of 434
Juvenile
    delinquency 183
        prevention 183
    Justice Act
        2000 11
        1986 442
    rheumatoid arthritis 434
        complications 435
        etiology 434
        management 435
        types 434

K

Kala-azar 249
    complications 250
    diagnosis 250
    epidemiology 249
    management 250
    preventive measures 251
    prognosis 250
Kangaroo mother care 107
    baby's clothing, preparation for 109
    benefits of 108
    components of 108
    counseling, preparation for 109
    definition 107
    discontinuation of 110
    duration of 110
    eligibility criteria for 108
    feeding, monitoring during 109
    for baby, eligibility criteria for 108
    for mothers, eligibility criteria for 109
    implementation, requirements for 108
    initiation of 109
    introduction 107
    monitoring during 109
    preparation for 109
    prerequisites of 108
    procedure 109
    time of 109

Kangaroo mother's clothing, preparation for
    109
Kangaroo positioning 109
Kidney
    congenital abnormalities of 337
    disorders of 337
Knock knee *See* Genu valgum
Knocked knee 428*f*
Krammer's rule for cutaneous levels of
        jaundice 98*f*
Kwashiorkor 197
Kyphosis 428

L

Lacrimal system, diseases of 406
Lactation, failure of 55
Language development 123
LBW babies, prevention of 103
Length by infantometer, measurement of
        119*f*
Lens, disease of 407
Leprosy 242
    classification 243
    diagnosis 243
    epidemiology 242
    management 243
    preventive measures 244
    prognosis 244
Leukemia 329
    classification 329
    etiology 329
Limping 424
    causes of 424
Liver
    abscess 298
    diseases of 273
    introduction, diseases of 273
Low birth weight babies terminology 102
Lung
    abscess 267
        management 267
    and disorders in newborn 86*f*
Lymphatic filariasis 248
    diagnosis 249
    epidemiology 248
    management 249
    preventive measures 249
    prognosis 249
Lymphoid growth 116

M

Magnesium 206
Maintenance of adolescent health 176
Major types of accidents 132
Malabsorption syndrome 279
    causes 279
    investigations 279

management 280
nursing management 280
Malaria 245
diagnosis 247
epidemiology 245
management 247
pathology 246
preventive measures 247
prognosis 247
Malnourished child 196*f*
of 2 years 4*f*
of urban slum 4*f*
with multiple worm infestations 253*f*
Malnutrition
definition of 194
ecology of 194
Malocclusion of teeth 419
Management of PEM, nursing
responsibilities for 199
Marasmic kwashiorkor 198
Mask ventilation 79
Mastoiditis 413
Masturbation 182
Maternal and child health 23
Maturational assessment of gestational age 469
Mature milk, different composition of 52
Mean urine output at different ages 452
Measles vaccination 40
Meatal stenosis 339
Medical aseptic technique 147
Medications
administration of 151, 152
history 151
routes of 152
Mediterranean anemia *See* Cooley's anemia
Medulloblastoma 385
Megaloblastic anemia 322
Meningitis 365
complications 366
etiology 365
management 366
nursing management 366
Meningocele 380, 380*f*
Meningococcal vaccine 43
Meningoencephalocele 190*f*
Meningomyelocele 380
Menstrual abnormalities 400
Mental
health 30
retardation 376, 377*f*
classification 376
etiology of 377
management 378
preventive management 378
Metabolic
acidosis 213
etiology of 213
management 214

alkalosis 214
etiology 214
management 215
disorders 191
Metatarsus
valgus 427*f*
varus 427*f*
Milia 75
Minerals
and deficiency disorders 205
daily requirements of 50*t*
Minor developmental peculiarities 75
Mitral
regurgitation 313
stenosis 314
Mixed acid-base disorders 215
Mixed type cerebral palsy 375
Modified Glasgow coma scoring system 457
Mongolian blue spots 75
Mongolism *See* Down's syndrome
Moniliasis *See* Candidiasis
Mother
continue kangaroo mother care during sleep and resting 110
privacy, psychological support to 109
psychological support to 109
Motility diarrhea 275
Motor development 123
Mucoid secretions, minor problems of 75
Multifactorial inheritance, etiology of 187
Multiple
congenital anomalies 190*f*
injury 173
Mummy restraints 147*f*
Mumps vaccine 42
Muscles, disorders of 423
Muscular dystrophies 423
diagnosis 424
management 424
Musculoskeletal
abnormalities 191
disorders in children 423
Myelodysplasia 379
Myelomeningocele 381*f*
Myelomeningocele *See* Meningomyelocele
Myoclonic seizures 372
Myopia 409

N

Nail biting 180
Natal teeth *See* Predeciduous teeth
National
Health Programs for Children in India 34
immunization schedule 37, 38*t*
Nutritional Policy 62
long-term measures 63
short-term measures 63

Plan of Action on Nutrition 63
Policy for Children 11
Programs on Nutrition 63
Rural Health Mission 26
Nearsightedness 409
Necrotizing enterocolitis 91
diagnostic evaluation 92
management 92
prognosis 92
Neonatal
care, grades of 112
conjunctivitis 89
convulsions 101
etiology of 101
investigations 101
management 102
prognosis 102
types of 101
death 5*f*
drug chart 477
hypoglycemia, causes of 100
hypoglycemia 100
management 101
prognosis 101
hypothermia 82, 83
concept of warm chain 84
consequence of 84
definition 83
factors responsible for 83
management of 85
prevention of 84
process of thermoregulation 83
stages of 83
infections 88
factors responsible for 88
prevention of 92
sources of 88
jaundice 96
management of 99
types of 96
mortality rate 7
period 370
follow-up *See* Newborn baby subsequent
resuscitation program 465
guideline-2005 463
seizures 101
sepsis 90
types of 90
Neonates
breath holding spells, minor problems of 74
caput succedaneum, minor problems of 75
common indications for referral, high risk 102
constipation, minor problems of 73
cradle cap, minor problems of 74
daily routine care of 70

dehydration fever, minor problems of 74
diarrhea, minor problems of 73
evening colic, minor problems of 74
excessive crying, minor problems of 73
excessive sleepiness, minor problems of 74
hiccups, minor problems of 74
high risk 102
immediate basic care of 70
in incubator, care of 155
low birth weight babies, high risk 102
mastitis neonatorum, minor problems of 75
minor problems of 73
napkin rash, minor problems of 74
obstructed nasolacrimal duct, minor problems of 74
physiological
    jaundice, minor problems of 75
    phimosis, minor problems of 75
ponderal index, high risk 107
poor prognostic factors 82
preterm infants, high risk 103
reactions of 139
small for dates babies, high risk 106
sneezing, minor problems of 74
superficial infections, minor problems of 75
umbilical granuloma, minor problems of 75
vaginal bleeding, minor problems of 75
vomiting, minor problems of 73
with congenital obstructive jaundice 190f
Nephroblastoma See Wilms' tumor
Nephrotic syndrome 344
complications 345
management 346
secondary 345
types 344
Neural
growth 116
tube defects 379
    etiology 380
    types of 380
Neutral thermal environmental temperatures 462
Nevus simplex See Stork bites
New ballard score See Maturational assessment of gestational age
Newborn baby
assessment of 65
daily observation of neonates 70
examination on discharge 70
initial assessment 66
of gestational age at birth 66
subsequent 67

Newborn
infant 64
    routine examination of 470
    resuscitation algorithm 464
Niacin 203
Noncommunicating hydrocephalus 382
Nonthrombocytopenic purpura 334
Normal
biochemical values 453
blood pressure values various ages 451
hematological values 455
neonate, reflexes of 69t
Nose
block, minor problems of 74
disorders of 415
rhinitis, disorders of 415
sinusitis, disorders of 415
Nosocomial infections See Hospital acquired infections
Nursing
assessment 17
care of
    healthy neonates 70
    sick child, adaptations in 141
diagnosis 17
    list of approved 18
interventions 141, 165, 168, 309
management of
    anemia 322
    child with urologic surgery 341
    childhood eye diseases 411
        assessment 411
        diagnoses 411
        interventions 411
    children with congenital heart diseases 309
    diabetes mellitus 405
    handicapped children 440
planning 17
process 17f
    steps in 16, 17f
responsibilities 184
Nutrition 10
in children 46
    introduction 46
Nutritional
counseling 61, 127
    during infancy 61
    for preschooler 62
    for toddler 61
deficiency disorders 194
    introduction 194
dwarfing 198
guidance 61
    to adolescents 62
    to school age child 62
marasmus 197
problems, assessment of 195

rehabilitation center, management in 198
requirements in children 46
calories 47
carbohydrates 48
fats 48
minerals 49
proteins 47
vitamins 49
water 47
services 30
status
anthropometry, assessment of 60
assessment of 60
biochemical evaluation, assessment of 60
dietary history, assessment of 60
weaning 127

O

Obesity 401
causes of 401
developmental disorders 175
in age of 7 years 402f
management 402
Obstructive lesions of urinary tract 338
Omphalitis See Umbilical sepsis
Omphalocele See Exomphalos
One twin baby without head 190f
Ophthalmia neonatorum See Neonatal conjunctivitis
Optic nerve diseases 407
Oral
cavity, problems of 420
thrush 89
Orbital diseases and disorders 406
Organizing sex education 133
Orodental problem in children 406
Osmotic diarrhea 274
Osteogenesis imperfecta 425, 425f
management 425
types 425
Osteomyelitis 432
complications 433
etiology 432
management 433
types 432
Ostomies 158
Otitis media 412
with effusion 412
Over hydration 211
Oxygen
administration, methods of 154
therapy 154, 458
    by oxygen hood 154f
    complications of 154

need for 154
purpose of 154
Oxytocin reflex 54f
Oxyuriasis See Threadworm

P

Pancreas, related to 287
Pancreatitis 296
  causes 296
  complications 296
  diagnosis 296
  management 296
Paraphimosis 340
Parasitosis in children 245
Parathyroid glands, disorders of 395
Parents
  approach to 152
  need guidance 134
Patent ductus arteriosus 305, 305f
Pediatric
  drug dosages/regimens 478
  illness care delivery, setting of 137
  nurse
    functions of 14
    qualities of 13
    role of 14
  nursing
    concept of 13
    definition 16
    goals of 13
    history 142
    process related to 16
    purposes 16
    trends in 15
  techniques, safety measures during 145
  tuberculosis, treatment of 479
  unit in hospital 138
Peeling skin 75
Pelvi-ureteric junction stenosis 338
PEM
  complications of 199
  early
    diagnosis, preventive management of
      199
    treatment, preventive management of
      199
  health promotion, preventive
    management of 199
  management of 198
    hospital 198
  preventive management of 199
  prognosis of 199
  rehabilitation, preventive management
    of 199
  specific protection, preventive
    management of 199

Perinatal
  HIV disease 111
  mortality rate 7
Personality development 123
Pertussis See Whooping cough
Pes
  valgus 427
  varus 427f
Phimosis 340
Phosphorus 205
Pica See Geophagia
Pinworm 255
  clinical manifestations 255
  diagnosis 255
  management 255
  preventive measures 255
Pituitary glands
  disorders of 391
  etiology 391
  management 392
Plastic deformations 430f
Play
  and play materials 129
  for hospitalized children, types of 149
  importance of 129
  materials, selection and care of 130
  types of 129
Plea of baby birth 447
Pleural effusion 265
  complications 266
  diagnosis 266
  management 266
Pneumococcal vaccine 43
Pneumothorax 267
  management 267
Poisoned children, management of 168
Poisoning 168
  agents 168
  ecology of 168
Polio vaccination 39
Poliomyelitis, types of 219
Polycystic kidneys 338
Ponderal index management 107
Poor maternal health 5f
Poor socioeconomic status 195
Postasphyxia management of neonates 81
Postdischarge follow-up 110
Posterior urethral valve 338
Postnatal
  diagnosis 188
  growth
    curves, types of 117f
    patterns of child 116
Postneonatal mortality rate 7
Postoperative nursing management of
  children 160
Postrenal causes 346
Posturing in unconscious state 363f

Potassium 205
  deficiency 205
  hyperkalemia 206
Precocious puberty 399
Predeciduous teeth 76
Predispose accidental injury in children 131
Prekwashiorkor 198
Prenatal diagnosis 187
Prerenal causes 346
Preschool child, reactions of 139
Press areola behind nipple between finger
  and thumb 55f
Preterm
  babies 105
    34 weeks 104f
  birth, causes of 103
  infants, characteristics of 103
  milk, different composition of 52
Prevention of accidents, nursing
  responsibilities in 133
Preventive pediatrics 22, 25f
  concept of 22
  family health 23
  nursing responsibilities in 35
Primary delayed sexual development 399
Primary nephrotic syndrome 345
Prohibition and Regulation Act, 1986
  See Child labor
Prolactin reflex 54f
Protecting child 157
Protein allowances, recommended 48t
Protein-energy malnutrition 195
  classification of 196
Pseudocryptorchidism See Retractile testis
Pseudohermaphroditism 397
Psychosexual development 123
  stages of 123t
Puberty
  changes in 122
    boys, order of 122
    girls, order of 122
Pupillary tract abnormalities 407
Purpura See Bleeding disorders
Pyoderma 90
Pyoderma See Superficial bacterial
  infections
Pyogenic
  arthritis 435
    management 436
  liver abscess 299
  meningitis 365
Pyridoxine 203

R

Rabies vaccines 41
RCH program, component of 24f

Recommended dietary allowance of
    vitamins 49*t*
Rectal
    agenesis 292
    prolapse 296
Rectoperineal fistula 292
Rectovaginal fistula 292
Rectus femoris 153*f*
Reflexes in baby 54*f*
Refractive errors 407, 409
Rehydration therapy 276
Renal
    agenesis 337
    hypoplasia 338
    mechanisms 210
Repeated blood transfusion 325
Reproductive
    and child health 23
    system, related to 287
Respiratory
    acidosis 214
        management 214
    alkalosis 215
    diseases 259
        introduction 259
    distress in neonates 86
        common causes 86
        diagnostic evaluation 86
        management 86
        prognosis 87
    distress syndrome in preterm neonates,
        prevention of 87
    regulatory mechanism 210
    system abnormalities 191
Restraints 146
    hazards of 147
    types of 146, 147*f*
Restrictive cardiomyopathy 316
Retina, diseases of 407
Retinoblastoma 410
Retinopathy of prematurity 407
Retractile testis 398
Retrolental fibroplasia *See* Retinopathy of
    prematurity
Rheumatic
    fever, prevention of 313
    heart disease 313
Riboflavin 203
Ringworm infections *See* Dermatophytosis
Road to health card 119*f*
Rotavirus vaccine 42
Round worms 254
    diagnosis 254
    management 254
    preventive measures 254
Rubella vaccine 42
Rule of Five of estimation of burns surface
    area 354*f*

S

Sacrococcygeal teratoma 189*f*
Safe disposal of hospital waste 481
Safe motherhood components 24
Salmon patches 76
School
    aged children, reactions of 139
    health
        records 30
        service 29
        aspects of 29
        objectives 29
    phobia 182
    refusal *See* School phobia
Sclera, abnormalities of 407
Scoliosis 429
    etiology 429
    management 429
Second gravida *See* Teenage mother
Seeking genetic counseling, reasons for 192
Sensory development 123
Separation anxiety *See* Stranger anxiety
Septic arthritis *See* Pyogenic arthritis
Severe birth asphyxia, systemic
    manifestations of 81
Sex education 133
    need for 133
Sexual
    development, secondary delayed 399
    problems of adolescents 133
Shigellosis *See* Bacillary dysentery
Short
    sightedness *See* Near sightedness
    stature 390
        causes of 390
        chronic organic diseases 391
        drug induced 391
        endocrine disorders 391
        genetic cause 390
        management 391
        nutritional disorders 391
        psychosomatic 391
Sick child 137
    introduction 137
    nursing care of 141
    proforma for assessment of 475
    therapeutic play 148
Sick neonates, transport of 112
Sickle cell anemia 323
Silverman
    anderson score 87*t*
    score for assessing magnitude of
        respiratory distress 86*f*
Site of infusion 157
Skin disease 352
Sleep disorders 182
Small for dates babies

causes of 107
problems of 107
Snake bites 170
    first aid management 171
    hospital management 171
Sodium 205
    deficiency 205
Spastic cerebral palsy 375
Speech problems 181
    cluttering 181
    delayed 181
    dyslalia 181
    stuttering 181
Spina bifida 380
    occulta 380
Splenectomy 325
Sputum, collection of 151
Squint *See* Strabismus
Stammering *See* Speech problems stuttering
Statistics related to child health 6
Status
    asthmaticus, case of 270
    epilepticus 372
Stool specimens, collection of 150
Stork bites 76
Strabismus 408
    management 409
Stranger anxiety 179
Street
    child 5*f*
    children 32
Subconjunctival hemorrhage 76
Substance abuse 183
    preventive measures 183
Sucking callosities 76
Suitable play material according to age 131
Superficial
    bacterial infections 359
        impetigo 359
    fungal infections 358
Supportive management 326
Swimmer's ear *See* External ear otitis
    externa, problems of
Syndromal classification 196
Syringe for treatment of inverted nipples,
    preparing and using 55*f*

T

Talipes
    calcaneovalgus 427
    equinovalgus 427
    equinovarus 427
Tapeworms 256
    diagnosis 257
    management 257
    preventive measures 257

Tectile stimulation 79*f*
Teenage mother 4*f*
Temper tantrums 179
Temperature in neonates, assessment of 85
Teniasis *See* Tapeworms
Tetanus 235
    clinical manifestations, types of 236
    complications, types of 236
    diagnosis, types of 236
    epidemiology 235
    management, types of 236
    pathology 236
    preventive measures, types of 237
    prognosis, types of 237
    types of 236
Tetralogy of Fallot 306, 306*f*
Thalassemia 324
    classification 324
    complications 325
    intermedia 324
    major 324, 325
    management 325
    minor 324
Therapeutic play, nursing responsibilities for 149
Thiamine 203
Threadworm *See* Pinworm
Three months colic *See* Neonates evening colic, minor problems of
Thrive
    causes, failure to 174
    failure to 173
    management, failure to 174
    nursing management, failure to 174
Throat
    disorders of 416
    pharyngitis, disorders of 416
    swab
        collection of 151
        culture 342
    tonsillitis
        acute, disorders of 417
        adenoidal hypertrophy, disorders of 417
        chronic, disorders of 417
        disorders of 417
Thrombocytopenia 332
    causes 332
    management 333
Thumb sucking 179
Thyroid glands
    disorders of 393
    hyperthyroidism
        disorders of 393, 394
        management, disorders of 393, 394
Thyromegaly *See* Goiter
Tics 181
Tocopherol *See* Vitamin E deficiency 202

Toddlers, reactions of 139
Toilet training 127
    problems of 129
    process of 128
Tongue tie 76
Torus *See* Buckle
Total parenteral nutrition 157
Tracheoesophageal fistula 482*f*
Transient abnormalities in first few days of life 471
Transitional milk, different composition of 52
Transporting neonates, principles for 112
Tricuspid
    atresia 307
    regurgitation 314
Trivandrum developmental screening chart 127*f*
True cryptorchidism 398
True hermaphroditism 397
Tuberculosis 237
    epidemiology 237
    management 239
    pathology 238
    preventive measures 240
    prognosis 240
Tuberculous meningitis 367
    complications 368
    management 367
Typhoid fever 240
    complications 241
    diagnosis 241
    epidemiology 240
    management 241
    pathology 241
    preventive measures 242
    prognosis 242
Typhoid vaccination 41

U

Ulcerative colitis 280
    diagnosis 280
    management 280
Umbilical
    hernia 76, 293
    malformations 293
    sepsis 89
Under-five's clinic, concept of 27
    adequate nutrition 27
    care in illness 27
    family planning 27
    health education 28
    immunization 27
    symbol for 27*f*
Under-five's mortality rate 8
Undescended testes 397
    causes 398
    management 398

Universal children's day 10
    overall goals (1990–2000) 10
Urinary
    introduction 337
    system, related to 287
    tract
        congenital abnormalities of 337
        disorders of 337
        infections 344
            management 344
Urine
    examination 342
    specimens, collection of 150
Urticaria neonatorum *See* Erythema toxicum
Use of restraints 146
Uveal tract abnormalities 407

V

Vaccine carriers 41, 44
Varicella *See* Common viral infections chickenpox
Varicella vaccines 42
Vastus lateralis 153*f*
Ventricular septal defect 303, 304*f*
Ventriculoperitoneal shunt 384*f*
Ventrogluteal 153*f*
Visceral leishmaniasis *See* Kala-azar
Visual
    disorders 407, 410
    impairment 410
        categories of 410*t*
Vitamin
    A deficiencies 200
    and deficiency disorders 200
    B complex deficiencies 202
    B_1 deficiency *See* Thiamine
    B_{12} deficiency *See* Cyanocobalamin
    B_2 deficiency *See* Riboflavin
    B_5 deficiency *See* Niacin
    B_6 deficiency *See* Pyridoxine
    C 204
    D deficiencies 201
        important sources 201
        prevention of 202
        rickets 201
    E deficiency 202
    K deficiency 202
        prevention 202
Vitellointestinal duct, abnormalities related to 293
Vitreous, diseases of 407
Volvulus of sigmoid colon 286*f*
Vomiting 164
    causes of 164
    nonorganic causes, causes of 164
    organic causes, causes of 164

W

Walk in cold rooms 43
Water intoxication 211
Weaning *See* Complementary feeding
Weaning foods
    introduction of 56
    principles of 56
Weighing
    baby in digital machine 118*f*
    infant in baby weighing machine 118*f*
Weight, measurement of 118*f*

Welfare *of*
    children 440
    delinquent children 441
        causes 441
    destitute children 442
    working children 443
WHO grading of anemia 319
Whooping cough 233
    complications 234
    epidemiology 234
    investigations 234
    management 235

    pathology 234
    preventive measures 235
    prognosis 235
Wilms' tumor 340
    management 341
    staging of 341
Women, protection for 10
Worm infestations 253

Z

Zinc 206